Stress Testing

Stress Testing

Principles and Practice

Fifth Edition

MYRVIN H. ELLESTAD, M.D., F.A.C.C.

Director of Research

Memorial Heart Institute

Long Beach Memorial Medical Center

Long Beach, California

With contributions by

RONALD H. STARTT SELVESTER, M.D.

FRED S. MISHKIN, M.D.

FREDERICK W. JAMES, M.D.

OXFORD

UNIVERSITY PRESS

2003

OXFORD
UNIVERSITY PRESS

Oxford New York
Auckland Bangkok Buenos Aires Cape Town Chennai
Dar es Salaam Delhi Hong Kong Istanbul Karachi Kolkata
Kuala Lumpur Madrid Melbourne Mexico City Mumbai
Nairobi São Paulo Shanghai Taipei Tokyo Toronto

Published by Oxford University Press, Inc.
198 Madison Avenue, New York, New York, 10016
http://www.oup-usa.org

Library of Congress Cataloging-in-Publication Data
Stress testing : principles and practice / Myrvin H. Ellestad ; with contributions by
Ronald H. Startt Selvester, Fred S. Mishkin, Frederick W. James. — Ed. 5.
p. ; cm.
Includes bibliographical references and index.
ISBN 978-0-19-515928-8
1. Heart function tests. 2. Exercise tests. 3. Stress (Physiology)
I. Ellestad, Myrvin H., 1921–
[DNLM: 1. Exercise Test — methods. 2. Stress. WG 141.5.F9 S915 2003]
RC683.5.H4 S776 2003
616.1′20754—dc21
2002030793

Printed in the United States of America
on acid-free paper

Dedicated to my lovely and loving wife, Lera.

Preface

The first edition of this book was released in 1975. When the 4th edition was published I planned that it should be the last. As before however, new information on exercise testing has stimulated a desire to revise the previous text and integrate our present state of knowledge with what went before.

It is of some concern that many cardiologists and others doing exercise testing have little interest in the newer information now available on exercise physiology. Fortunately, there is still a significant cadre of investigators asking tough questions and proposing unconventional ideas. There will always be many practitioners who want to know everything they can about a technique that they are using every day. For this group this book will be required reading.

Because of the book's popularity the general format has not been changed but every chapter has been revised to not only include new information but to make it more readable. The chapter on electrocardiographic changes has been completely reorganized to emphasize the importance of unconventional markers of ischemia, which are rarely applied in most exercise laboratories. To emphasize important points, *take home* messages are sprinkled throughout some chapters to help emphasize various concepts. Two new chapters provide information on exercise echocardiography and exercise testing in congestive heart failure. Many of the figures have been redrawn for clarity.

Some of the new concepts proposed recently include the idea that ST depression occurring in premature ventricular contractions (PVCs) can indicate ischemia. It appears that horizontal ST changes during exercise may indicate subendocardial ischemia while Downsloping ST segments represent a more severe process that is probably most commonly seen with multivessel disease and possibly posterior wall subepicardial dysfunction. There are a number of patterns that can localize the area of the myocardium and the culprit stenotic vessel, a capacity that was once the exclusive claim of nuclear scintigraphy. New concepts on the physiology of ischemia are presented as well as the new information on chronotropic incompetence.

As an example of the new format a summary of the patterns that suggest false-positive ST depression include (1) complexes with a short PR interval, (2) complexes with steep PQ slopes, (3) when there are prominent enlarged septal Q waves, (4) when ST depression is confined to the inferior leads, especially if P waves are large and (5) the ST segment is convex or "humped."

It is hoped that students of the physiology of exercise induced ischemia will find this work a valuable reference and will be stimulated by its contents to add new ideas to this important field of cardiology.

An acknowledgement of the support staff at Memorial Heart Institute and especially the diligent labor of my secretary, Carole Sweet, is in order. Without their help this book could not have been completed.

Long Beach, California M.H.E.

Contents

Contributors **xi**

1. History of Stress Testing **1**
2. Cardiovascular and Pulmonary Responses to Exercise **11**
3. Physiology of Cardiac Ischemia **43**
4. Indications **77**
5. Contraindications, Risks, and Safety Precautions **85**
6. Parameters to Be Measured **103**
7. Stress Echocardiography **127**
8. Stress Testing Protocol **135**
9. Memorial Heart Institute Protocol **157**
10. Stress Testing After Myocardial Infarction **169**
11. Stress Testing After Surgical Intervention and Coronary Angioplasty **179**
12. ECG Patterns and Their Significance **189**
13. Rhythm and Conduction Disturbances in Stress Testing **241**
14. Predictive Implications **271**
15. Stress Testing in Women **309**
16. Exercise Testing in Congestive Heart Failure **319**
17. Chest Pain and Normal Coronary Arteries **327**
18. Blood Pressure Measurements During Exercise **335**
19. Silent Myocardial Ischemia **353**
20. Sports Medicine and Rehabilitation **367**
21. Pediatric Exercise Testing **381**
22. Radionuclide Techniques in Stress Testing **413**
23. Metabolic Abnormalities and Drugs **481**
24. Computer Technology and Exercise Testing **513**

Index **535**

Contents

Contributors

Frederick W. James, M.D.
Professor and Chair
Department of Pediatrics
Charles R. Drew University
Los Angeles, California

Fred S. Mishkin, M.D.
Professor of Radiological Sciences
Director, Division of Nuclear Medicine
University of California, Los Angeles
Department of Radiology
Harbor-UCLA Medical Center
Torrence, California

Ronald H. Startt Selvester, M.D.
Professor Emeritus
University of Southern California School of Medicine
Director of Electrocardiography Research
Memorial Heart Institute
Long Beach Memorial Medical Center
Long Beach, California

Stress Testing

1
History of Stress Testing

The cornerstone of modern stress testing is based on the empirical discovery that exercise in patients with coronary disease produces ST-segment depression. This discovery might be credited to Bousfield,[1] who recorded ST-segment depression in the three standard ECG leads during a spontaneous attack of angina in 1918; or, it might be credited to Feil and Siegel,[2] who, in 1928, actually exercised patients with known angina to bring about pain and, concurrently, the ST- and T-wave changes we now recognize as showing evidence of ischemia. These researchers described the changes as being due to a decrease in blood flow to the heart, and they published tracings showing a return to normal after the pain had subsided and also after administration of nitroglycerin. Feil and Siegel conducted their stress tests by having the patients do sit-ups; in selected cases, they held their hands on the patient's chest to increase the resistance and therefore the energy required to perform this maneuver. Einthoven[3] may have actually recognized the changes associated with ischemia. He published a tracing in 1908 showing ST-segment depression after exercise, but did not comment on this finding. Felberbaum and Finesilver[4] probably published the first paper describing a step test in 1927. Using a footstool 12 inches high, they regulated the rate of stepping and monitored the heart rate before and after exercise.

Master, with Oppenheimer,[5] published his first paper on an exercise test in 1929 but did not recognize the value of the ECG in the demonstration of ischemia. He used only pulse and blood pressure to evaluate the patient's cardiac capacity. Master claimed Felberbaum and Finesilver's method was inadequate for a number of reasons. The contribution of Master must be labeled as being related to an exercise protocol rather than to the use of the ECG for the evaluation of ischemia in these early years. Master also popularized the idea of evaluating exercise capacity with some type of a standard test. In 1931, Wood and Wolferth[6] also described ST-segment changes with exercise and indicated the usefulness of exercise in diagnosis, but claimed it was too dangerous to deliberately exercise patients with coronary disease. They claimed that the precordial lead (lead 4) was more useful in revealing ischemic changes than were the standard leads.

In 1932, Goldhmammer and Scherf[7] reported that ST-segment depression was present in 75% of 40 patients with angina and proposed the use of exercise to confirm the diagnosis of coronary ischemia. It is interesting to note that the percentage of their false-negatives is similar to that of some of the data being published at this time.

Katz and Landt[8] confirmed Wood and Wolferth's findings in 1935 in terms of precordial leads but found lead 5 to be better in terms of discrimination than lead 4. They also demonstrated that the number of negative responses in patients with a history of classic angina, could be reduced by using precordial leads. They tried to standardize their exercise test by having the subjects lift dumbbells while lying on a table. Katz and Landt also discussed the mechanism of pain and ischemia and implicated some irritative substance related to catabolism in the myocardium. In addition, they reported on the use of anoxia to bring about characteristic changes in the ST segment. They went on to produce the same changes with intravenous epinephrine.[8]

By 1938, Missal[9] studied normal patients by having them run up from three to six flights of stairs; he may have been the first to use a maximum stress test. For convenience, Missal later elected to use Master's 9-inch steps to exercise his patients. He had his patients exercise to the point of pain and emphasized the necessity of taking the recording as quickly as possible thereafter. He cited a case report in which the stress test contributed to the management of a woman with hypothyroidism and angina who had an earlier onset of angina and ST-segment depression after taking thyroid hormone. Missal also described the use of the Master's test in evaluating increases in exercise tolerance after nitroglycerin.

In 1940, Riseman and colleagues[10] published an excellent review of the use of anoxia in the evaluation of ischemia. They compared exercise with the anoxemia test and suggested that the latter was more specific because fewer negative test results occurred in patients believed to have coronary disease. They also described for the first time the use of continuous monitoring and thus discovered that ST-segment depression usually appeared before the onset of pain and persisted for a time after the pain subsided. Riseman and colleagues demonstrated the protective effects of oxygen breathing and described the presence of mild ST-segment depression (1.0 mm or less) in normal subjects as contrasted with 2.0- to 7.0-mm depression in some of their patients. In spite of all this information, these researchers concluded that the exercise test was of little practical value because of its poor discrimination between normal and abnormal subjects.

In 1941, 12 years after his original paper on an exercise test, Master, in collaboration with Jaffe,[11] proposed for the first time that an ECG could be taken before and after his exercise tolerance test to detect coronary insufficiency. In the same year, Liebow and Feil[12] reported that digitalis caused ST-segment depression and would confuse the diagnosis of ischemia in the exercise ECG. They also suggested the possibility of the drug's reducing coronary flow.

Johnson and associates,[13] working at the Harvard Fatigue Laboratory, developed the Harvard Step Test, which was similar in many ways to the original Master's test. It was used widely in athletic circles to measure fitness, and a form of it (the Pack Test) was used for military purposes. A variation of this called the Schneider was also popular in evaluating military personnel. These tests used pulse counts during recovery and provided an index of physical fitness, a technique that was to be carried forward in the indexes of fitness and aerobic power for a number of years. Brouha and Heath[14] also used this methodology to evaluate the cardiovascular response to various occupations and emphasized the influence of environmental factors such as room temperature. In 1949, Hellerstein and Katz[15] performed their classic studies describing the direction of the vector associated with subendocardial injury in various areas of the right and left ventricle. They also used direct-current electrograms and established that ST depression is primarily a diastolic injury current manifested during the TQ interval.

By 1949, Hecht[16] was reporting his experience with the anoxemia test and claiming 90% sensitivity in coronary disease. He emphasized the important fact that pain is an unreliable end-point and accompanies ischemia in only 50% of the cases. He also pointed out that ST-segment changes associated with anoxemia may not be present if previous myocardial necrosis has occurred. Since then, Castellanet and colleagues[17] have confirmed that infarction tends to mask the ECG expression of ischemia.

In 1950, Wood and associates[18] at the National Heart Hospital in London described their experience with an effort test. They had patients run up 84 steps adjacent to their laboratory and also claimed that it was necessary to push the patients to the maximum level of their capacity. Wood and associates established several points that still have validity:

1. The amount of work performed should not be fixed, but adjusted to the patient's capacity.
2. The more strenuous work (resulting in a heart rate greater than 90 beats per minute) would produce a higher percentage of positive tests in patients with known coronary disease than if the heart rate were not accelerated above this level.
3. The reliability of the test (in effect, a maximum stress test) was 88% overall compared with 39% in the Master's test.

Wood and colleagues, as Hecht before them, definitely recommended the use of the stress test to uncover latent myocardial ischemia, to determine the severity of the disease, and to evaluate therapy.

In 1951, Hellerstein and colleagues[19] used stress testing as a method of evaluating the work capacity of cardiac patients and began to amplify the work pioneered by Brouha. They deserve credit for demonstrating to employers that their cardiac employees might safely return to work. Thus, the continuing interest in the oxygen cost of various activities and in the analysis of ischemia at various workloads planted the seed that flowered into our present cardiac rehabilitation program.

In 1952, Yu and Soffer[20] reported on the use of the Master's stairs with continuous monitoring and cited the following changes in the ECG indicating ischemia:

1. ST-segment depression of 1.0 mm or more
2. Alteration of the T wave from upright to inverted or from inverted to upright
3. Increase in the amplitude of the T wave of 50% or more over the resting deflection
4. Prolongation of the QT/TQ ratio during exercise to more than 2

The last finding may still be a useful element in the evaluation of ischemia, but it has not been fully explored. Yu and Soffer again emphasized the value of continuous monitoring previously described by Riseman and associates[10] and pointed out that the QT interval should be carefully measured.

Yu and coworkers[21] had previously reported a test using a motor-driven treadmill elevated to a 10% or 20% grade with continuous monitoring. They suggested that the lead system be set up as a bipolar lead from the right scapula to the V_5 position, a lead configuration that Bruce used for many years.

In 1953, Feil and Brofman[22] reviewed the bundle branch block patterns. They referred to transient bundle branch block developing with exercise and pointed out that this was first described by Bousfield[1] in 1918. They reported that ST-segment depression, when coexisting with the block pattern, indicates ischemia in both right and left bundle branch block. They also reported false-positive stress tests in two or three patients with Wolff-Parkinson-White syndrome, an observation subsequently confirmed by Sandberg[23] and Gazes.[24]

By 1955, the Master's test had become widely accepted as a standard because of its simplicity. Its failure to apply adequate stress and the fact that information was lost by not observing the pulse response and the ECG patterns during exercise were rarely appreciated, even though these limitations had been pointed out by many of the earlier investigators. Although the Master's test was originally proposed to provide information about the patient's functional classification, it remained for others to begin to combine a fairly satisfactory test of cardiac function with one that would provide information on the presence or absence of ischemic heart disease. Bruce[25] and Hellerstein and Katz[15] were early workers in this area.

An important push in the evolution of treadmill stress testing came from the work classification units. In 1950, Hellerstein's unit in Cleveland,[26] patterned after the original one in Bellevue Hospital in New York established by Goldwater in 1944, set the stage for a proliferation of these clinics in many areas, sponsored by the American Heart Association. My introduction to the treadmill test came when I worked in the Los Angeles Work Classification Unit. Familiarity with testing of postmyocardial infarction patients led to the realization that treadmill testing offered a more comprehensive evaluation than the Master's test.

Modern stress testing might be dated from 1956 when Bruce[27] reported a work test performed on a treadmill and established guidelines that would more or less group patients into the New York Heart Disease Classifications I through IV. Many of the protocols for stress testing now in vogue have been based on an extension of the principles Bruce established at that time. Shortly before this, Åstrand and Rhyming[28] had documented that maximum oxygen uptake or aerobic capacity could be predicted by the heart rate at submaximal exercise. Thus, the groundwork necessary to establish the progressive exercise test as a physiological exercise tolerance test had been laid.

About this time, Taylor and colleagues,[29] based on the work of Hill and Lupton,[30] proposed an index for circulatory performance that emphasized that if the strongest muscle was used, the amount of exercise would usually be limited by the cardiac output rather than by muscle weakness. Therefore, in walking or running, increases in pulse could be correlated with increases in cardiac output, and thus with the aerobic capacity of the individual. In the late 1950s, Balke and Ware,[31] working in the Department of Physiology and Biophysics at Randolph Air Force Base, established the importance of stress testing in evaluating military personnel. They published a formula that is still useful in estimating the oxygen uptake associated with treadmill walking.

In the early 1960s, numerous articles were written attempting to refine the criteria for ischemia ST-segment changes and the appropriate leads for recording.[23] Blackburn's work[32] in 1969 and the work of Blackburn and associates[33] in 1966 demonstrated the incidence of ST-segment depression in various leads. Blackburn's findings that 90% of the ischemic changes could be demonstrated in the CM_5 or V_5 lead made it possible to do stress testing with a relatively simple ECG recording system. This had a considerable impact because it extended the use of progressive testing outside the research laboratory. The CM_5 is still in use today.

As the Air Force and NASA prepared to launch a man into space, Lamb[34] and Fascenelli and colleagues,[35] in a continuation of the work pioneered by Balke and Ware,[31] refined the methods necessary for accurate monitoring of multiple variables during exercise. Shortly after, in 1967, Robb and Marks[36] published follow-up data on 2224 male applicants for life insurance and for the first time gave us statistical verification of the predictive value of the ST-segment depression. They demonstrated that the presence of horizontal or downsloping ST segments after the double Master's test was more reliable in predicting subsequent coronary abnormalities than was the patient's medical history. They also established that deep ST-segment depression carries with it a more serious prognosis than a moderate degree of depression. By 1969, Bruce and associates,[37] Winter,[38] and Sheffield and colleagues[39] had reported on the use of computers to analyze ST segments, and the correlation of these changes with coronary angiographic data was published by Najmi and associates,[40] Martin and McConahay,[41] Lewis and Wilson,[42] and Balcon and associates.[43]

Because ST depression and angina-type chest pain were believed for a long time to be almost synonymous with coronary disease, many subjects underwent angiography and were found to have normal coronary arteries. This provided us with insight into the limitations as well as the benefits of stress testing. We now understand more about the pathophysiology of the coronary system and recognize that many parameters besides the ST segment need to be scrutinized to make maximum use of the procedure.

The late 1970s and early 1980s might be labeled "The Decade of Bayesian Analysis."

Our understanding of probability and its use in large populations has been advanced by many workers, including George Diamond,[44,45] Victor Froelicher,[46,47] Bernard Chaitman,[48] and a number of others.[49–51] We have also recognized that there are a number of changes in physiology that can be better analyzed by combining data such as chronotropic incompetence and heart rate recovery.[52] The predictive value of these methods is now being documented and tested. The ST Over Heart Rate Index by Kligfield and Okin,[53] the Duke Score by Mark,[54] and the Athens Score by Michaelides[55] as well as some other scores may add to our ability to categorize patients better so that we may be able to arrive at rational decisions as to how to proceed with therapy. A recent series of papers by Lauer and Associates[50,51] seems to be confirming our report from 1975 that chronotropic incompetence is going to be very useful.

THE RELIABILITY OF EXERCISE TESTING

Technology has been enriched by the proliferation of imaging techniques, the most important of which are nuclear scintograny[56] and exercise echocardiography.[57] For those patients who cannot and will not exercise, the use of Adenosine or Dipyridamole produce vasodilatation or of Dobutamine to increase myocardial work has vastly expanded the utility of stress testing.[58] We are also probably on the verge of another new methodology—stress magnetic resonance imaging.[59] In only a few years the reliability of these techniques will undoubtedly improve so that the cardiac physiology identified by these new methods will tell us as much or more than the angiogram.

These techniques, when combined with conventional testing, improve the diagnostic certainty and often help to localize the diseased vessels.

We are beginning to realize that there are different types of ischemia, several of which are unrelated to fixed coronary obstruction. We will have to revise our ideas about the character of the coronary lesions[60] that restrict flow as we study patients by new methods using dynamic measurements of flow reserve as well as anatomical analysis of the vessel caliber.[60] We are also understanding more about redistribution of myocardial blood flow.

There is evidence that at times ischemia is caused by a redistribution of flow from subendocardium to the subepicardial tissue, probably mediated by adenosine.[60]

There was a long period when we correlated our noninvasive tests with the perceived degree of narrowing of the coronary arteries. Arbitrarily assigning normal function to lesions under 50% and abnormal function to lesions over 50% hardly passes the straight face test today.[60] No wonder we have always had trouble with "false negatives and false positives." Recently, analysis of flow by intravascular ultrasound (IVUS) and flow reserve has forced us to take another look at what really constitutes exercise-induced ischemia.[61] It will take some time to sort this all out but I predict in the next few years we will reevaluate many of our previous dogmas—and probably find that we can diagnose ischemia with exercise testing better than previously believed.

If I were to select one person who has made the greatest contribution to the technique of stress testing, it would be Robert Bruce of Seattle, whose protocol is the standard in most laboratories in the United States. His meticulous work has given us a body of knowledge that provides a foundation for most other investigators. His large study, the Seattle Heart Watch, was especially important in our understanding of the limitations of exercise testing in asymptomatic persons.[62]

Many other workers not mentioned here have made major contributions to the understanding of stress testing. Their work will be discussed in the appropriate sections in the chapters that follow. As with the brilliant description of angina by Heberden, the understanding of basic physiology displayed by some of the pioneers in stress testing is remarkable. They have given us a tool that has improved and will continue to improve our understanding of cardiac physiology and that continues to play a major role in the detection and evaluation of coronary heart disease.

REFERENCES

1. Bousfield, G: Angina pectoris: Changes in electrocardiogram during paroxysm. Lancet 2:457, 1918.
2. Feil, H and Siegel, M: Electrocardiographic changes during attacks of angina pectoris. Am J Med Sci 175:225, 1928.
3. Einthoven, W: Weiteres uber das Elektrokardiogramm. Arch ges Physiol 172:517, 1908.
4. Felberbaum, D and Finesilver, B: A simplified test for cardiac tolerance. Medical Journal and Record 126(1):36, 1927.
5. Master, AM and Oppenheimer, EJ: A simple exercise tolerance test for circulatory efficiency with standard tables for normal individuals. Am J Med Sci 177:223, 1929.
6. Wood, FC and Wolferth, CC: Angina pectoris: The clinical and electrocardiographic phenomena of the attack and their comparison with the effects of experimental temporary coronary occlusion. Arch Int Med 47:339, 1931.
7. Goldhammer, S and Scherf D: Electrokardiographische untersuchungen bei kranken mit angina pectoris. Z Klin Med 122:134, 1932.
8. Katz, L and Landt, H: Effect of standardized exercise on the four-lead electrocardiogram: Its value in the study of coronary disease. Am J Med Sci 189:346, 1935.

9. Missal, ME: Exercise tests and the electrocardiograph in the study of angina pectoris. Ann Intern Med 11:2018, 1938.
10. Riseman, JEF, Waller, J, and Brown, M: The electrocardiogram during attacks of angina pectoris: Its characteristics and diagnostic significance. Am Heart J 19:683, 1940.
11. Master, AM and Jaffe, HL: The electrocardiographic changes after exercise in angina pectoris. J Mt Sinai Hosp 7:629, 1941.
12. Liebow, IM and Feil, H: Digitalis and the normal work electrocardiogram. Am Heart J 22:683, 1941.
13. Johnson, RE, Brouha, L, and Darling, RC: A practical test of physical fitness for strenuous exertion. Rev Can Biol 1:491, 1942.
14. Brouha, L and Heath, CW: Resting pulse and blood pressure values in relationship to physical fitness in young men. N Engl J Med 228:473, 1943.
15. Hellerstein, HK and Katz, L: The electrical effects of injury at various myocardial locations. Am Heart J 36:184, 1948.
16. Hecht, HH: Concepts of myocardial ischemia. Arch Intern Med 84:711, 1949.
17. Castellanet, MJ, Greenberg, PS, and Ellestad, MH: The predictive value of the treadmill test in determining post-infarction ischemia. Am J Cardiol 42:29, 1978.
18. Wood, P, et al: The effort test in angina pectoris. Br Heart J 12:363, 1950.
19. Hellerstein, HK, et al: Results of an integrative method of occupational evaluation of persons with heart disease. J Lab Clin Med 38:821, 1951.
20. Yu, PNG and Soffer, A: Studies of electrocardiographic changes during exercise (modified double two-step test). Circulation 6:183, 1952.
21. Yu, PNG, et al: Variations in electrocardiographic response during exercise (studies of normal subjects under unusual stresses and of patients with cardiopulmonary disease). Circulation 3:368, 1951.
22. Feil, H and Brofman, BL: The effect of exercise on the electrocardiogram of bundle branch block. Am Heart J 45:665, 1953.
23. Sandberg, L: Studies on electrocardiographic changes during exercise tests. Acta Med Scand 169(Suppl 365):1, 1961.
24. Gazes, PC: False-positive exercise test in the presence of Wolff-Parkinson-White syndrome. Am Heart J 78:13, 1969.
25. Bruce, RA, et al: Observations of cardiorespiratory performance in normal subjects under unusual stress during exercise. Arch Indust Hyg 6:105, 1952.
26. Hellerstein, HK: Cardiac rehabilitation: A retrospective view. Heart Disease and Rehabilitation 509, 1979.
27. Bruce, RA: Evaluation of functional capacity and exercise tolerance of cardiac patients. Mod Concepts Cardiovasc Dis 25:321, 1956.
28. Åstrand, PO and Rhyming, I: Nomogram for calculation of aerobic capacity (physical fitness) from pulse rate during submaximal work. J Appl Physiol 7:218, 1954.
29. Taylor, HL, Buskirk, E, and Henschel, A: Maximal oxygen intake as objective measure of cardiorespiratory performance. J Appl Physiol 8:73, 1955.
30. Hill, AV and Lupton, H: Muscular exercise, lactic acid, and supply and utilization of oxygen. Q J Med 16:135, 1923.
31. Balke, B and Ware, RW: An experimental study of physical fitness of Air Force personnel. US Armed Forces Med J 10:675, 1959.
32. Blackburn, H: The electrocardiogram in cardiovascular epidemiology: Problems in standardized application. In Blackburn, H (ed): Measurement in Exercise Electrocardiography. Charles C Thomas, Springfield, IL, 1969.
33. Blackburn, H, et al. The electrocardiogram during exercise (Findings in bipolar chest leads of 1449 middle-aged men, at moderate work levels). Circulation 34:1034, 1966.
34. Lamb, LE: The influence of manned space flight on cardiovascular functions. Cardiologia 48:118, 1966.
35. Fascenelli, FW, et al: Biomedical monitoring during dynamic stress testing. Aerospace Medicine 9:911, 1966.
36. Robb, GP and Marks, H: Postexercise electrocardiogram in arteriosclerotic heart disease. JAMA 200:110, 1967.
37. Bruce, RA, et al: Electrocardiographic responses to maximal exercise in American and Chinese population samples. In Blackburn, H (ed): Measurement in Exercise Electrocardiography. Charles C Thomas, Springfield, IL, 1969.

38. Winter, DA: Noise measurement and quality control techniques in recording and processing of exercise electrocardiograms. In Blackburn, H (ed): Measurement in Exercise Electrocardiography. Charles C Thomas, Springfield, IL, 1969.
39. Sheffield, LT, et al: Electrocardiographic signal analysis without averaging of complexes. In Blackburn, H (ed): Measurement in Exercise Electrocardiography. Charles C Thomas, Springfield, IL, 1969.
40. Najmi, M, et al: Selective cine coronary arteriography correlated with hemodynamic response to physical stress. Dis Chest 54:33, 1968.
41. Martin, CM and McConahay, D: Maximal treadmill exercise electrocardiography: Correlation with coronary arteriography and cardiac hemodynamics. Circulation 46:956, 1972.
42. Lewis, WJ, III and Wilson, WJ: Correlation of coronary arteriograms with Master's test and treadmill test. Rocky Mt Med J 68:30, 1971.
43. Balcon, R, Maloy, WC, and Sowton, E: Clinical use of atrial pacing test in angina pectoris. Br Med J 3:91, 1968.
44. Diamond, GA: Bayes' theorem: A practical aid to clinical judgment for diagnosis of coronary-artery disease. Practical Cardiology 10(6):47, 1984.
45. Diamond, GA, et al: Application of conditional probability analysis to the clinical diagnosis of coronary artery disease. J Clin Invest 65:1210, 1980.
46. Miranda, C, et al: Comparison of silent and symptomatic myocardial ischemia during exercise testing in men. Ann Intern Med 114:649, 1991.
47. Froelicher, VF, et al: The electrocardiographic exercise test in a population with reduced workup bias: Diagnostic performance, computerized interpretation, and multivariable prediction. Veterans Affairs Cooperative Study in Health Services #016 (QUEXTA) Study Group. Quantitative Exercise Testing and Angiography. Ann Intern Med: 128(12Pt)1:965, 1998.
48. Chaitman, B. Does the angiogram still qualify as the gold standard for the evaluation of noninvasive tests? In Ellestad MH and Amsterdam EA (eds): Exercise Testing: New Concepts for the New Century. Kluwer Academic Publishers, Boston, Dordrecht, London, 2001.
49. Morise, AP. Exercise electrocardiography in women with suspected coronary disease. In Ellestad MH and Amsterdam EA (eds): Exercise Testing: New Concepts for the New Century. Kluwer Academic Publishers, Boston, Dordrecht, London, 2001.
50. Lauer, MS, et al: Impaired heart response to graded exercise: Prognostic implications of chronotropic incompetence in the Framingham Heart Study. Circulation 93:1520, 1996.
51. Lauer, MS, et al: Impaired chronotropic response to exercise stress testing as a predictor of mortality. JAMA 281:524, 1999.
52. Tsuji, H, et al: Reduced heart rate variability and mortality risk in an elderly cohort. The Framingham Heart Study. Circulation 90:878, 1994.
53. Kligfield, P and Okin, PM: Heart rate adjustment of exercise ST segment depression: The ST/HR index. In Ellestad MH and Amsterdam EA (eds): Exercise Testing: New Concepts for the New Century. Kluwer Academic Publishers, Boston, Dordrecht, London, 2001.
54. Mark, D, et al: Prognostic value of a treadmill exercise score in outpatients with suspected coronary artery disease. New Engl J Med 325:849, 1991.
55. Michaelides, AP, et al: New coronary disease index based on exercise induced QRS changes. Am J Heart 120:292, 1990.
56. Shaw, LJ, et al: The economic consequences of available diagnostic and prognostic strategies for the evaluation of stable angina patients: An observational assessment of the value of precatheterization ischemia. J Am Coll Cardiol 33:559, 1999.
57. Armstrong, WF, et al: Effect of prior myocardial infarction and extent and location of coronary disease on accuracy of exercise echocardiography. J Am Coll Cardiol 10:531, 1987.
58. Falcone, RA, et al: Intravenous albunex during dobutamine stress echocardiography: Enhanced localization of left ventricular endocardial borders. Am Heart J 130:254, 1995.
59. Kim, RJ, et al: Relationship of MRI delayed contrast enhancement to irreversible injury, infarct age, and contractile function. Circulation 100:1992, 1999.
60. Gasparodine, A, et al: Bamiphylline improves exercise-induced myocardial ischemia through a novel mechanism of action. Circulation 88:502, 1993.
61. Ellestad, MH: The time as come to reexamine the gold standard when evaluating noninvasive testing. Am J Cardio 87:100, 2001.
62. Bruce, RA, et al: Value of maximal exercise tests in risk assessment of primary coronary heart disease events in healthy men. Am J Cardiol 46:371, 1980.

2
Cardiovascular and Pulmonary Responses to Exercise

Preload and Stroke Volume
Stroke Volume and Training
Contractility
Effect of Muscle Mass
Heart Rate
Effect of Age
Effect of Gender
Heart Rate with Training
Training Methods
- Frequency
- Intensity
- Duration
- Mode

Age and Conditioning
Coronary Blood Flow
Coronary Resistance
Myocardial Oxygen Demand
Tension Time Index
Intramyocardial Tension
Systolic and Diastolic Time Intervals
Oxygen Uptake and Metabolism
- Maximum Oxygen Uptake ($\dot{V}O_2max$)
- Carbon Dioxide, pH, and Bicarbonate

Substrate Use in the Heart
- Carbohydrates
- Noncarbohydrates
- Role of Nucleotides and Phosphorylase

Aerobic Metabolism
Anaerobic Metabolism
Hypoxia and Ischemia
Temperature
- Heat
- Cold

Respiration
- Exercise Hyperpnea
- Rate Versus Depth
- Diffusion

A review of the mechanisms leading to the changes in cardiac output and other circulatory adaptations associated with activity will be helpful in understanding the body's cardiovascular and pulmonary response to exercise. Various factors, including venous tone, body position, blood volume, and depth of respiration, control the input to the heart. The heart responds by pumping into the arterial circulation the volume delivered from the venous side. The amount per beat in milliliters is called the *stroke volume.* The total cardiac output (measured in liters per minute) is the stroke volume (usually 50 to 80 mL of blood) multiplied by the heart rate. For example, if each beat pumped 80 mL out and there were 70 beats per minute, the cardiac output would be 80 × 70 or 5600 mL, or 5.6 L of blood per minute. This is an average value for a 70-kg adult at rest. The output increases with exercise, depending on the efficiency of the system, up to about 30 L/min in a well-conditioned athlete. An individual's ability to increase pumping volume is the most important factor limiting the ability to increase physical work capacity.

When exercise signals the cardiopulmonary system to increase its output, a complex set of events influences the heart to increase pumping. The most important is the heart rate. However, if the stroke volume were to remain constant at 80 mL and the heart rate were to increase to its maximum (approximately 195 beats per minute for a 25-year-old man), the limit of the cardiac output would be 80 × 195 or 15,600 mL, or 15.6 L/min. We know that the peak heart rate for a man at a given age falls within a predictable range. How then is it possible to increase cardiac output to approximately double the above value, or 30 L/min? The only solution is to increase the stroke volume during the early phases of increased work. The increase in stroke volume occurs in different degrees, depending on fitness, age, and sex.[1]

PRELOAD AND STROKE VOLUME

When exercise begins, a complex set of events can be measured, which sets the stage for the events to follow. Probably the first event is the increase in venous tone, which is mediated by autonomic reflexes.[2] This squeezes the blood from the large veins into the right side of the heart, increasing the effective filling pressure. In a normal heart, the right ventricle is very distensible and accepts the increased volume of blood during diastole with very little increase in pressure (the filling pressure of both the right and left sides of the heart is usually from 5 to 10 mm Hg). Cardiac output increases immediately as a result of the increased filling and tachycardia (Fig. 2–1). At this stage an increase in stroke volume cannot always be detected, but there is a wide variation among individuals.[3]

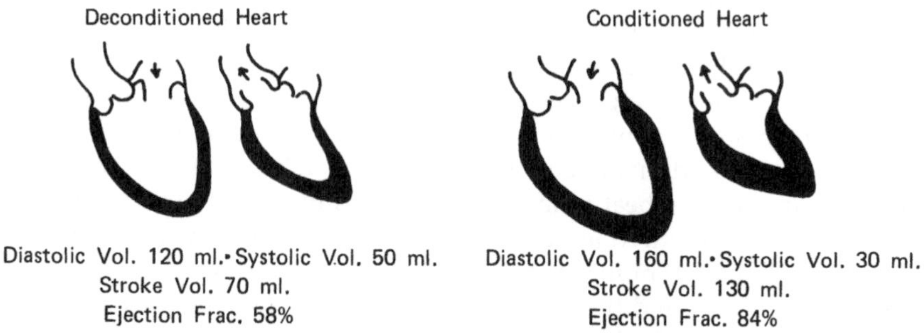

FIGURE 2–1. As training increases, the increase in diastolic volume is accompanied by a simultaneous decrease in systolic volume. This results in an increase in stroke volume and in the percentage of the diastolic volume expelled with each systole (ejection fraction).

Evidence that the baroreceptor reflexes are progressively inhibited as exercise increases is suggested by denervation experiments.[4]

Obviously the heart cannot pump out more blood than it takes in; thus, the increased return is central to the problem of increased output. Besides the constriction in the veins, mediated by the sympathetic nervous system's forcing of more blood into the heart, the pumping action of the muscles, especially those in the legs, propels the blood toward the heart. The increased negative pressure of deep inspiration, termed the *abdominal thoracic pump,* also tends to encourage this process. The tendency for blood to be preferentially shunted from certain organ systems, such as the kidney and splanchnic bed, the liver, and the spleen, also increases the venous return.

When exercise is initiated, the stroke volume tends to increase as the increased venous flow takes place, but levels off somewhat short of the maximal pumping capacity[5] (Fig. 2–2).

Body position has considerable influence on stroke volume at rest. For example, the return to the heart is greater in the supine position, since it is easier for the veins to move blood into the right heart when the gravity effect is removed. Thus, exercise in the supine position, as in swimming,

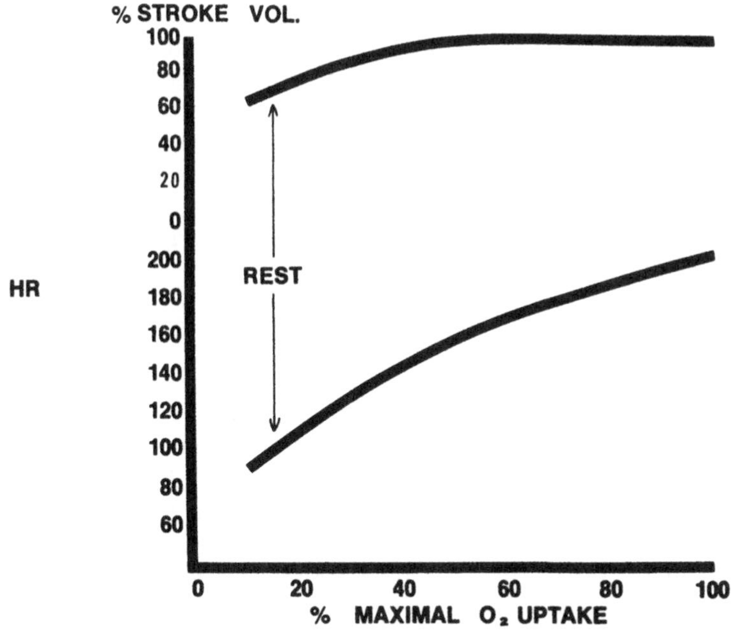

FIGURE 2–2. As the heart rate increases with exercise, there is a moderate increase in stroke volume, which reaches a maximum at approximately midway during the buildup of the exercise capacity.

would be expected to be associated with a larger stroke output and a lower heart rate. At low levels of horizontal exercise, however, the heart rate is the main source of the increase.[6] Chapman and colleagues[7] also have shown that after strenuous physical exercise is under way, the difference in stroke volume related to posture is minimized. The increased stroke volume in trained athletes is aided by a marked decrease in peripheral resistance.[8] The cardiac dimensions are directly related to the diastolic volume and contractility. The heart gets slightly smaller near peak exercise, but the systolic volume decreases even more than the diastolic so that the stroke volume is maintained. As we will later see, the alteration of this normal response by those with some disease states provides a mechanism for evaluating function during exercise.

STROKE VOLUME AND TRAINING

Numerous studies have demonstrated progressive increases in stroke volume after prolonged exercise programs.[9] The stroke volume of endurance athletes has been reported to be 50% to 75% higher than that of sedentary individuals.[10] This enables those who are physically well conditioned to operate at a slower heart rate. An increased volume load has been shown to be the most efficient method of increasing cardiac output in terms of myocardial oxygen consumption. Studies done with nuclear blood pool imaging[11] confirmed previous measurements in normal subjects and suggested that the increased stroke volume and maximal cardiac output seen in normals can to some degree also be achieved by coronary patients who are subjected to training.[12–14] The stroke volume can be correlated with heart volume estimated from a roentgenogram of the patient's chest. The volume averages for various athletes are indications of the changes associated with various types of sports (Fig. 2–3). The isometric type of exercise (weight lifting) produces no significant change in heart volume.

CONTRACTILITY

The mechanical response of the ventricle is based on *Starling's law,* which states that the force of contraction is a function of the degree of stretch during diastole (Fig. 2–4). Thus, as more blood enters the heart during each diastolic interval, the muscle is subjected to more stretch, which increases the force of contraction. During this process not only is more energy expended, but also the increased fiber length results in a larger stroke volume if other factors such as blood pressure are not altered.[15] The force of contraction is related to the inherent strength of the heart muscle as well as to the amount of

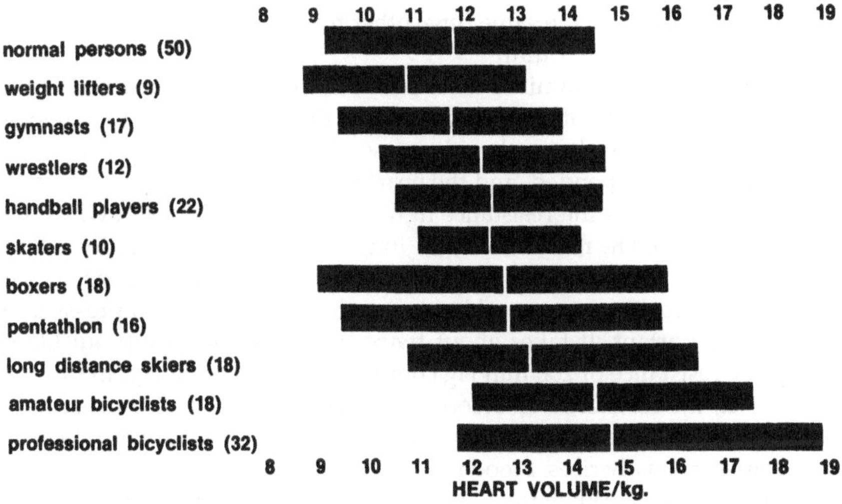

FIGURE 2–3. Heart volume estimated from the roentgenogram of the chest showing correlation with the type of physical activity. (Originally published in *Canadian Medical Association Journal* Vol. 96, March 25, 1967)

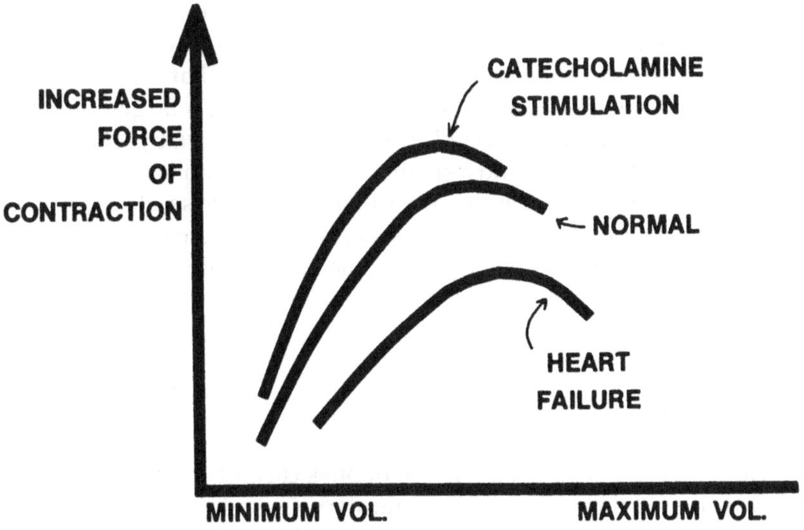

FIGURE 2–4. Starling's curves: the greater force generated by increasing the stretch on the myocardial fibers is influenced by many metabolic and mechanical factors. The effects of catecholamines and the still poorly understood state of heart failure are depicted.

stretch taking place. At the same time, other mechanisms influence the final ability of the ventricle to pump.

Circulating catecholamines exert the most important influence. By stimulating the production of adenyl cyclase and thereby increasing the release of adenosine triphosphate, they increase the force of contractility, the amount of energy expended, and the heart rate.

Another factor is the resistance in the vascular bed through which the heart must pump. The resistance in the lungs is so low in the healthy subject that it plays very little role as a limiting factor in exercise. The resistance in the systemic circuit, as measured by the brachial or aortic blood pressure, is extremely important. It takes about twice the energy to pump out blood against the resistance of 200 mm Hg compared with 100 mm Hg. In the normal subject, the resistance to blood flow decreases as exercise progresses. This may not be obvious to someone measuring blood pressure during exercise because it usually rises. Blood pressure is the product of blood flow multiplied by resistance. When the heart pumps more blood, the cardiac output usually increases more than the resistance drops; therefore, a modest increase in systolic blood pressure occurs during exercise in most patients.

Training has been shown to improve the inotropic properties of the myocardium,[16] probably due to an increase in velocity of enzyme activity.[17]

EFFECT OF MUSCLE MASS

The volume of muscle mass has a major effect on cardiac output, mainly due to the magnitude of the venous return from the working muscles. Studies on arm and leg exercise have demonstrated that arm exercise results in a greater increase in catecholamines and thus a larger increase in heart rate than would be expected from equivalent work by a larger muscle.[18] The higher heart rate and a smaller amount of venous return produce a smaller stroke volume. On the other hand, leg exercise utilizing 40% to 50% of the total body muscle mass causes a larger increase in venous return, relatively less workload, a smaller increase in catecholamines, and a lower heart rate.[19]

HEART RATE

The heart rate is the result of a number of physical and emotional influences that are mediated through the autonomic nervous system. These include excitement, fear, anticipation, temperature alterations, respiratory maneuvers, and physical work. Both the vagal and the sympathetic nerves are constantly stimulating the sinoauricular node so that if the influence of either is increased or decreased, a change in rate will be manifested. A number of complex inhibitory as well as stimulating reflexes in the vascular system affect the heart rate. During exercise, the sympathetic reflex is the most important, since vagal tone is gradually withdrawn as the workload increases.[20] At the onset of exercise, the heart rate has been shown to increase within 0.5 second, probably secondary to an abrupt inhibition of a significant portion of the vagal tone.[21] An interesting sawtooth effect in the heart rate has been described in the first few seconds of exercise, suggesting that the autonomic nervous system is "searching" for the proper balance.[22]

Stimulating the sinus node with a pacemaker accelerates the heart rate, but the filling pressure does not increase; therefore, the stroke volume decreases. The result is a stable rather than an increased cardiac output in spite of the faster heart rate. On the other hand, administering adrenaline or other catecholamines causes both heart rate and venous return to increase, resulting in a net increase in cardiac output. Studies with dogs suggest that about 50% of the cardiac acceleration is due to sympathetic drive, primarily beta stimulation.[20] A study has indicated that the right stellate ganglion is an important pathway in this system.[21]

A curious property of the heart is its apparent age-related ceiling on rate. The anatomy and physiology of cardiac function are so designed that when the body calls for the heart to increase its pumping, it can accelerate only to a predetermined peak and does not further increase its rate of pumping or its output, regardless of the demands of the body. As far as we know, pushing the heart to its maximum in a normal person does no damage. If a person tries to push physical exertion past this maximum pumping capacity, the peripheral tissues become anoxic because of inadequate oxygen delivery. The individual then rapidly builds up lactic acid and other metabolites, which terminate the ability to function in only a few minutes. Lactic acid depresses cardiac function and produces peripheral vascular dilatation, which then decreases blood pressure.

Knowledge of the peak heart rate in various age groups makes it possible for physicians to know when a subject has exercised to maximum pumping capacity. Although some disagreement exists about the range and variation around the mean, and about the mean rates, the data adapted from Robinson[22] have been very useful in my experience. The maximum heart rate varies among individuals about 15% from age-predicted formulas (Fig. 2–5).

Bates[8] has studied cardiac output in relation to its limiting effect on exercise. He has demonstrated that with an oxygen uptake of up to 1500 mL/min (Fig. 2–6), cardiac output, heart rate, and oxygen consumption increase in a linear relationship. However, near peak capacity (above 80% of maximum capacity), both heart rate and cardiac output tend to level off. It was possible at this point, however, to increase the peripheral oxygen consumption by another 300 to 500 mL, which was attributed to a widening

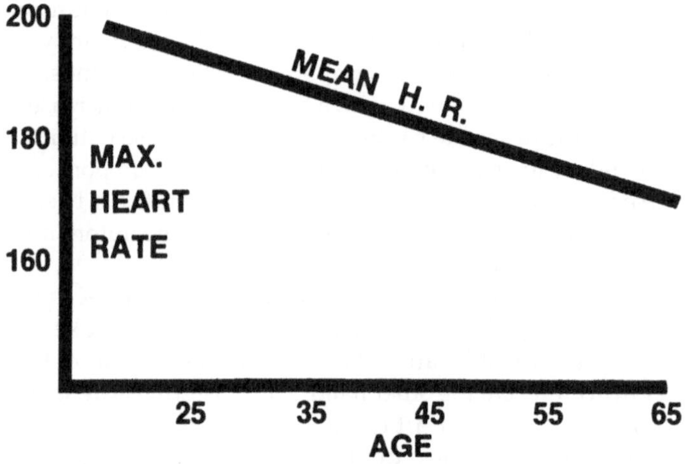

FIGURE 2–5. The maximum predicted heart rate is age-related. When the subject exercises to maximum capacity, the cardiac pumping reaches its maximum possible output at about the same time that the peak rate is attained.

of the arteriovenous oxygen difference. This ability of the peripheral tissues to extract more oxygen, especially when the subject is well conditioned, is a very important element of the circulatory adaptations to exercise. During the period when the oxygen consumption is increasing near peak workload, a very rapid increase in respiratory rate ensues.[23] It is postulated that the increase in oxygen consumption after the heart rate levels off is used for the extra work of breathing and is not available for useful external work.

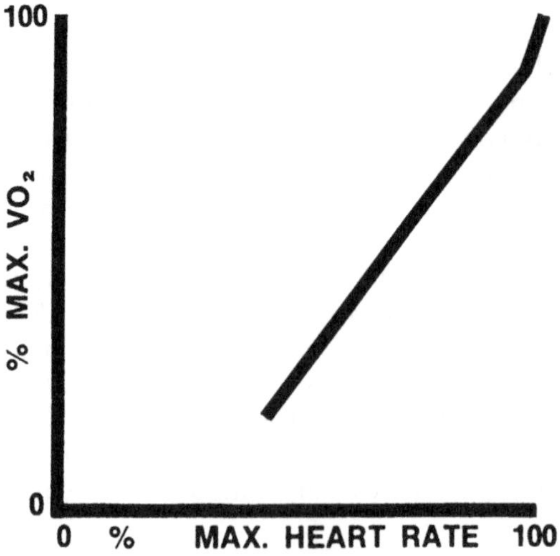

FIGURE 2–6. The relationship between maximum oxygen uptake by the body as a whole and the increase in heart rate tends to be almost linear until about 85% or 90% of maximum capacity is reached. At this point, a slight further increase in oxygen uptake occurs without a significant increase in heart rate.

EFFECT OF AGE

The aging process is associated with a wide range of changes, some of which are due to "natural aging," some due to disuse, and some due to degenerative diseases that accompany the aging process.[24,25]

The peak aerobic capacity decreases 3% to 8% per decade.[26] This is partly due to a reduced heart rate.[27] A radionuclide study has suggested that the change in cardiac output in older versus younger men is due more to a decrement in arteriovenous oxygen (AV-O_2) difference than to a decline in cardiac function.[28] A decline in cardiac receptors, increased myocardial stiffness, and a decrease in velocity of contraction suggest that a considerable increase in stroke volume is necessary to compensate for age.[28,29]

EFFECT OF GENDER

Women have a lower exercise capacity than men when corrected for weight.[27] The AV-O_2 difference has been reported to be lower in women, possibly because of their lower hemoglobin concentrations. As a result, cardiac output is increased for female patients for any given level of work tested.[30] Although the ejection fraction increases in exercising men, Higgenbotham and associates[28] have demonstrated that it remains fixed with increasing exercise in women. On the other hand, women increase their diastolic volume with exercise more than do men, thus achieving equivalent stroke volumes.[28]

HEART RATE WITH TRAINING

The most dramatic and easiest alteration to measure in the physiology of physical conditioning is the heart rate response to a standard workload.[31] Typical responses are depicted in Figure 2–7. At high workloads, the heart rate may be 40 beats per minute higher in an unconditioned subject than in a conditioned one.

As previously mentioned, the heart rate correlates well with the oxygen consumption of the heart, so that the heart of the well-conditioned subject is at least 25% more efficient. The decrease in resting heart rate is usually significant in trained individuals and is proportional to the duration of the period of increased activity. Note that 14,400 total heartbeats are saved daily by a decrease in average heart rate of 10 beats per minute. Glagov and associates[29] actually measured the total number of heartbeats in a 24-hour period by a cumulative counter and found that it varied from 93,615 to 113,988. The factors leading to a heart rate decrease at any give workload are probably multiple. Not only the increase in stroke volume, but also a decrease in circulating catecholamines, an increase in AV-O_2 difference in the working muscles, and an increased vagal tone probably are important. The optimum

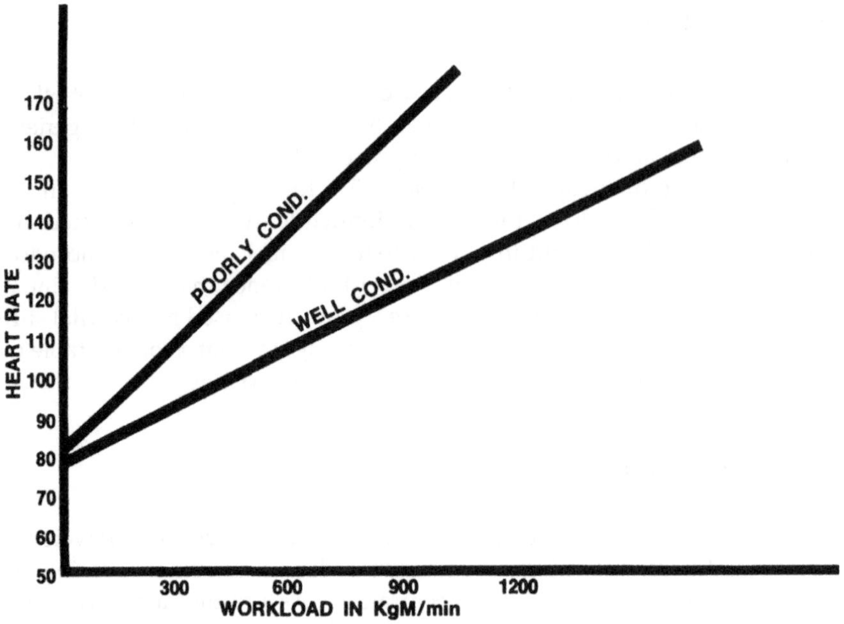

FIGURE 2–7. Heart rate response to exercise: as the workload is increased, the increment of pulse rise is more marked in the poorly conditioned subject.

duration of exercise and repetition rate necessary to obtain the best pulse response from conditioning is still in doubt. However, a discussion by Pollack[30] suggests some guidelines of importance (see the following).

TRAINING METHODS

Frequency

Although fairly strenuous training 2 days each week will result in almost as much training effect as three sessions, exercising a minimum of 3 days allows the subject to get a good training effect with a less strenuous workout.[32] The time demands of training more than 3 days a week are unrealistic for many people. Enthusiasts may train 5 days a week but their injury rate is likely to be much higher.[35] Injuries to the foot, ankle, and knee, which are common in middle-aged adults, can be minimized by limiting the training. The body appears to need rest between workouts.

Intensity

Most studies suggest that a minimal threshold for a satisfactory training response is 60% of the maximum capacity.[33] In younger people, this means training to heart rates of 130 to 150 beats per minute; in older persons, to as low as 110 to 120. Studies comparing very high levels of training with more moderate levels fail to show any significant increase in benefits as far as general health is concerned.[34] Obviously, a higher aerobic capacity can be obtained by pushing the intensity and time of work, but many studies have shown that the dropout rate in very-high-intensity or interval training programs tends to be much higher than in programs of lower intensity work. The problem of intensity is highly related to the subject's ego and his or her initial level of physical fitness.

Duration

Improvement in cardiovascular respiratory fitness is directly related to duration of training.[35] A moderate improvement in fitness can be obtained from 5 or 10 minutes of regular training, but improvement in maximal oxygen uptake probably is optimum when the duration of training is from 30 to 45 minutes. On the other hand, a significant training effect can be shown in 15 minutes if the intensity is increased. Programs using longer periods of training at a slightly slower pace are better tolerated, as reflected by lower dropout and injury rates.[36] I am inclined to urge people to strive for at least 30 minutes of exercise; if they are vigorous, young, and not prone to injuries, they might attempt 45 minutes. Individualization of the exercise prescription to account for age, fitness, and motivation is essential.

Mode

Although some enthusiasts believe that jogging or running is a formula for eternal life, this has yet to be proved. Any type of rhythmic training that burns calories and increases the heart rate, such as running, walking, bicycling, swimming, or jumping rope, is equally effective. Exercise that fails to produce a significant increase in caloric demands, such as bowling, golfing, or moderate calisthenics, does not have much value. Weight lifting has been shown to be useful in a cardiovascular sense only when very light weights are used with multiple repetitions; even in these programs, the improvement in aerobic capacity has been minor. However, weight lifting might be added to an exercise program to gain muscle strength, which is often very important to the individual.

AGE AND CONDITIONING

In the absence of neurological or orthopedic handicaps, conditioning can be achieved at any age.[37] Improvements in aerobic capacity of 10% to 15% have been demonstrated in older subjects when they are able to persist on a regular program for several months.[38] To prevent injuries, increases in work should be gradual.

Seals and colleagues[39] trained a group of men aged 60 to 69 for 1 year. The men increased their aerobic capacity by 12% the first 6 months, and after increasing the intensity for another 6 months, they were able to gain another 18%. A study by Pollack and coworkers[40] of 70-year-old Master runners who had trained for many years found that their aerobic capacity was less than 5% lower than measurements taken 10 years earlier. Lifelong high-level physical activity thus appears to reduce the rate of decline in $\dot{V}O_2max$ and, in the minds of some, the rate of aging.[41,42]

CORONARY BLOOD FLOW

In the peripheral circulation of humans, about 25% to 30% of the oxygen is extracted from the blood as it runs through muscle or other tissues at rest. As the metabolic demands of the tissues rise or the blood flow decreases, a larger percentage of oxygen is extracted.[43] Thus, in a normal human at rest, the arterial saturation can be 95% and the venous 75%, resulting in an AV-O_2 difference of 20%.[44] This pattern is altered in cardiac patients with low outputs, so that the AV-O_2 difference may be as high as 40% due to a drop in venous oxygen to 55% or 60%. The coronary circulatory system does not have the capacity to adapt to this degree, however, because of its relatively high extraction rate of oxygen at normal work levels. Coronary sinus blood returning from the capillary bed of the myocardium is usually from 10% to 25% saturated, resulting in an AV-O_2 difference across the myocardium of 75% or more. This high degree of extraction is near the limits of the ability of hemoglobin to release oxygen, thereby producing an absolute need for more blood whenever the heart requires more nourishment. Thus, in a normal man, there is almost a linear relationship between the increase in work done by the heart and the coronary blood flow[45] (Fig. 2–8). Fourfold increases in coronary blood flow during exercise, from 60 mL/100 g of ventricular myocardium per minute to 240 mL/min, are achieved by a marked reduction in coronary vascular resistance.

CORONARY RESISTANCE

The aortic pressure minus the resistance in the terminal arterioles and capillaries during diastole and the pressure of contraction during systole provide the driving pressure that nourishes the heart.

The resistance to flow has been subdivided into three types. *Viscous resistance* is defined as resistance due to blood viscosity and the surface tension in the arterioles and capillary bed. *Autoregulatory resistance* is mediated through the smooth muscle in the arterioles and precapillary sphincters. This

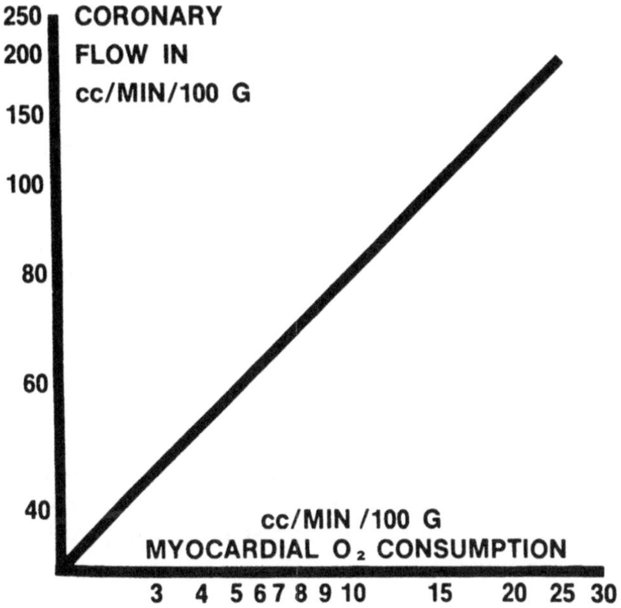

FIGURE 2–8. Because the heart extracts almost all the oxygen possible from the blood at rest, it is necessary for the coronary blood flow to increase linearly as myocardial demands increase.

resistance is controlled by metabolic processes in the heart muscle. *Compressive resistance* is due to the force of myocardial contraction. This compressive effect inhibits the flow during systole and, depending on diastolic compliance, has considerable effect during relaxation.[46]

Studies involving the left anterior descending coronary artery actually demonstrate retrograde blood flow during the isometric phase of systole.[46] Not only is the diastolic blood flow two or three times that of the systolic, but also, during this period, it preferentially goes to the subendocardium, an area relatively starved during systole[47] (see Chapter 3).

Methods of blood flow regulation are still being studied, but certain factors have been established. Anoxia decreases the resistance in the coronary bed, possibly directly because of the action of a low partial pressure of oxygen (PO_2) level or indirectly because of the liberation of metabolites such as adenosine.[45]

These changes would be classified as autoregulatory. Flow is also subject to local pH changes, partial pressure of carbon dioxide (PCO_2), bradykinins, nitric oxide, and very likely other factors still to be discovered.[48] This type of regulatory function controls flow in a patient who becomes hypertensive, so that perfusion is restricted to the exact needs of the muscle in spite of the increase in diastolic driving pressure.

A great deal of interest has recently centered around the effect of adrenergic influences on coronary flow and resistance. The ability to block either alpha or beta receptors has made it possible to study this process in more detail. Intracoronary norepinephrine has been shown to reduce coronary flow in humans[49,50] as does dopamine.[51] Stellate ganglion stimulation and isoproterenol (Isuprel) in dogs reduce the inner/outer layer flow ratio,[52] but propranolol increases this ratio and favors subendocardial perfusion.[53] In spite of these findings, the direct role of adrenergic influences on the coronary circulation in normal and diseased individuals is still under study but may have considerable importance. It has been demonstrated that it has a short-term beneficial effect but in excess a long-term detrimental impact.[54]

MYOCARDIAL OXYGEN DEMAND

The myocardium uses 8 to 10 mL of oxygen per 100 g of muscle per minute when a person is at rest. Even when the heart is not beating, about 30% of this amount is still required.[53] The efficiency of the heart can be estimated by knowing its level of oxygen use both at rest and during work, as illustrated by the following formula[55]:

$$\text{Efficiency of heart} = \frac{\text{Work of heart in kg-m/min}}{\text{Oxygen consumption in mL/min} \times 2.059 \times 0.806}$$

Here, 2.059 is the energy equivalent (kg-m/mL) of oxygen at a respiratory quotient of 0.82, and 0.806 is the fraction of oxygen used in the contractile work of the heart only.

According to these calculations, myocardial efficiency is approximately 37% in the dog and 39% in man.[56] With exercise, the oxygen consumption of the heart may increase 200% or 300%. Contributing factors would include the initial muscle fiber length or diastolic volume, the afterload or blood pressure, the velocity of contraction, and probably other elements not yet completely understood, such as the ability to use anaerobic metabolism in some cases.

Figure 2–8 illustrates that the increase in coronary blood flow correlates well with myocardial oxygen consumption. Also, the heart rate increases with exercise and also correlates well with coronary blood flow (Fig. 2–9). Therefore, observation of the heart rate in an exercising individual allows us to predict how hard the heart is working or how well it is performing. If the peripheral resistance or afterload (blood pressure) increases excessively during work, the myocardial oxygen consumption will have to be increased considerably more per unit of pulse elevation than if it were to remain low. Therefore, it becomes evident that the work of the heart, the cardiac output, the coronary blood flow, and the heart rate all increase in a parallel manner and attain a peak together. This means that when the cardiac output has reached its maximum, so have the coronary blood flow and the heart rate; hence, it is possible to make predictions about one based on another within certain limitations.

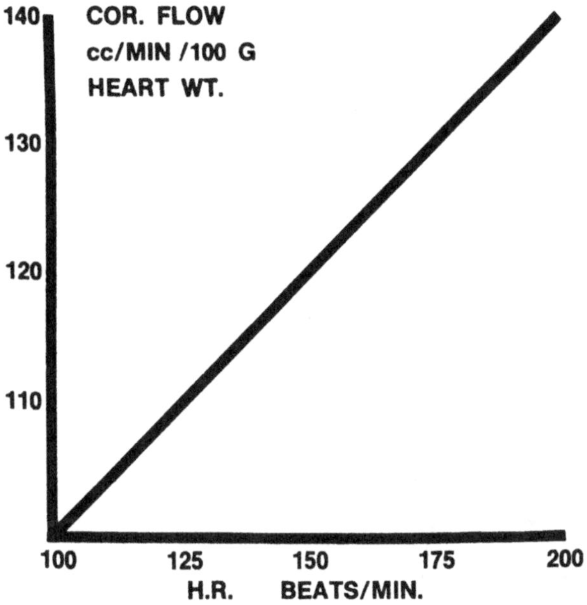

FIGURE 2–9. The coronary blood flow and pulse rate increase in a linear relationship as exercise progresses.

TENSION TIME INDEX

No discussion of coronary blood flow or myocardial oxygen requirements is complete without a discussion of the work on tension time index by Sarnoff and associates.[53] By controlling most of the variables with a heart-lung preparation, it is possible to correlate coronary blood flow and myocardial oxygen needs with a number of parameters. Sarnoff and colleagues found a positive correlation among heart rate, increase in blood pressure, diastolic volume, and myocardial oxygen consumption. The best correlation was with the so-called tension time index, which was determined by multiplying the heart rate by the systolic blood pressure by the time of systolic contraction. Thus, the tension time index per heartbeat is proportional to the area underneath the left ventricular pressure curve as shown in Figure 2–10. Because it is relatively easy to approximate this by noninvasive methods, it constitutes an important landmark in the physiology of exercise.[53] Subsequent studies have demonstrated the importance of other determinants of myocardial needs.[56] These are mentioned later.

Another important finding of the same research, often overlooked, was that the increase in stroke volume against a low systemic resistance has a relatively small extra cost in myocardial oxygen consumption. This may explain why the heart responds to exercise with this type of mechanism in a well-conditioned subject.

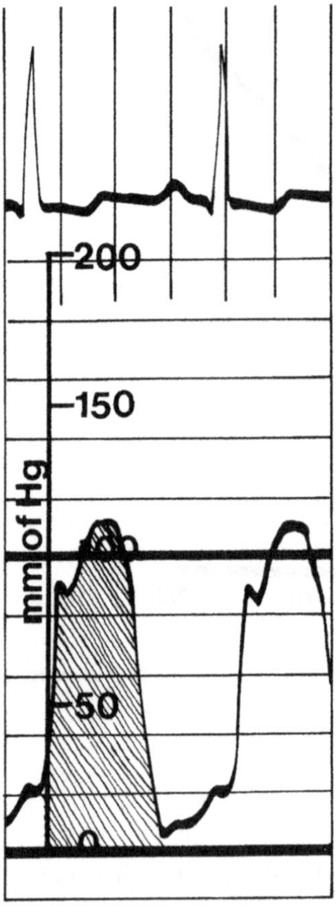

FIGURE 2–10. The area under the pressure curve *(shaded area)* tends to correlate with the myocardial oxygen uptake per beat. If the systolic pressure increases or the length of systole is prolonged, the oxygen requirements of the myocardium rise rapidly.

INTRAMYOCARDIAL TENSION

The tension or pressure developed by the ventricular wall has a very important influence in myocardial oxygen needs. It is not only related to the pressure of the blood in the ventricular cavity but also to the thickness of the wall and the radius of the ventricle.[56] Therefore, at a fixed pressure and wall thickness, an increase in ventricular volume will increase the tension and thus the oxygen consumption. The work performed by contractile elements in stretching the elastic components of the myocardium has been termed the *internal contractile element work*.[56]

The discovery that wall tension is such an important determinant of myocardial oxygen consumption casts doubt on the validity of the tension time index as a reliable indicator of heart muscle demands. The double product (systolic blood pressure times heart rate) is considered more reliable than the triple product (systolic blood pressure times heart rate times systolic ejection time).[57] This is because the systolic ejection time becomes shortened with increasing exercise and tends to decrease the total index with relationship to heart rate and blood pressure. When the time is excluded, the wall tension factor, which would increase oxygen uptake with increasing exercise and catecholamine load, approximately equals the negative influence left out of the equation when the ejection time is excluded.

No discussion of wall tension is complete without a comment on the relationship of ventricular diameter to the magnitude of tension. Laplace's law states that the wall tension is equal to the pressure within a cylinder times the radius of the curvature of the wall. Thus, the greater the ventricular volume, the less the curvature and the greater the radius, which in turn will increase the tension. This is probably why dilatation is almost invariably associated with hypertrophy, so that the increased tension can be contained by the larger muscle fibers. It follows that that larger fibers also increase the oxygen demand as well as protect the heart against the increased tension. A schematic diagram summarizing the factors involved in the myocardial supply/demand equation is depicted in Figure 2–11.

SYSTOLIC AND DIASTOLIC TIME INTERVALS

During rest, the systolic interval time is about one third of the total cardiac cycle. As previously mentioned, most of the coronary blood flow at rest takes place during diastole, which is allotted two thirds of the cycle when the heart rate is between 60 and 70. The time relationships become very significant in our understanding of the physiology of the coronary flow. As the heart rate

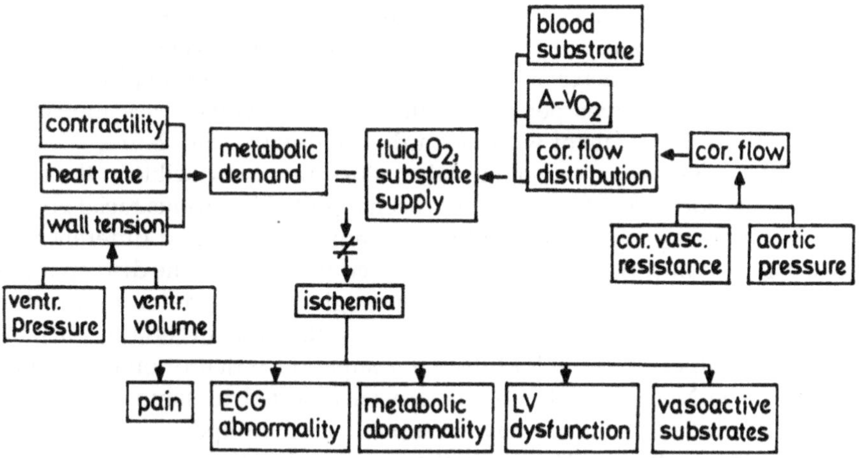

FIGURE 2–11. The oxygen supply/demand relationships are illustrated in subjects with ischemic heart disease. It can be seen that the supply and delivery are influenced by multiple factors. When contractility, wall tension, heart rate, or other parameters in the left side of the diagram are increased, there must be a corresponding increase in delivery. If not, ischemia may result.

accelerates, systole shortens, but not nearly as much as diastole. As a result, the heart is forced to do more and more work, but is given less and less time to obtain nourishment. This shortening of the diastolic interval was believed to be the most important factor limiting heart rate. As the heart rate increases and diastole shortens, it was thought that not enough blood flow was available in the time allowed to supply the demands of the heart.[58] It is now known that this effect is compensated for to some degree at high heart rates by an increase in coronary flow during systole. Increasing diastolic stiffness as aging progresses might slow myocardial blood flow and also be a factor in the progressive decrease in maximum heart rate with age. The tendency of patients with severe coronary disease and decreased myocardial compliance to have low peak heart rates, and thereby a longer diastolic time, tend to support this concept.

OXYGEN UPTAKE AND METABOLISM

Maximum Oxygen Uptake ($\dot{V}O_2max$)

Although $\dot{V}O_2max$ pertains to the oxygen consumption of the total body during a maximal response to exercise, a brief discussion is warranted in this section.

Many years ago, the oxygen uptake at maximum exercise, termed $\dot{V}O_2max$, was found to correlate well with the degree of physical conditioning, and it has been accepted as an index of total body fitness by researchers in this field.[59] The capacity to take in oxygen is related not only to the effectiveness of the lungs but also to the ability of the heart and circulatory system to transport the oxygen and to the ability of the body tissues to metabolize it. The $\dot{V}O_2max$ is a reproducible value, especially when corrected for body weight, which increases and decreases with the degree of physical conditioning.[60] In any given person, the intake of oxygen increases almost linearly with the heart rate or with the cardiac output (see Fig. 2–6).

Although maximal oxygen uptake values are reproducible in the same subject, considerable differences have been reported in various racial groups and in different geographic locations. Cummings[61] reported differences in data collected in various areas and suggested that some of the discrepancies seen between Europeans and Americans might be less pronounced if they were corrected for lean body mass (Table 2–1). Even so, in certain areas, the fitness of both children and adults is far superior to that of other societies studied. The Norwegian Lapps have been reported to stand out among adults as being more fit than any other population group.[45]

$\dot{V}O_2max$ is influenced by the method used to elicit the exercise. For a time there was considerable controversy as to the limiting factor or factors affecting the capacity of the organism to take up oxygen. The data now suggest that the heart and cardiovascular capacity are the major determinants, but

Table 2–1. **Mean Values for Maximal Oxygen Uptake (mL/kg/min)**

CHILDREN					
Age	**Stockholm**	**Philadelphia**	**Indianapolis**	**Lapland**	**Winnipeg**
6	48	—	—	—	52
8	55	—	—	—	49
10	52	29	—	51	40
12	50	30	28	48	42
14	46	34	—	44	38
16	47	23	—	42	39
18	47	19	—	42	44

MEN									
						Norway		*Winnipeg*	
Age	**Boston**	**Stockholm**	**Dallas**	**Lapland**	**Lumber**	**Industry**	**Office**	**Industry**	**Office**
20–29	53	52	45	54	45	44	44	44	44
30–39	41	40	39	54	46	44	42	38	38
40–49	40	39	35	—	44	38	39	38	33
50–59	37	33	32	44	39	34	36	36	31
60	30	31	—	—	—	—	—	—	—

the capacity of the muscle groups exercised is also critical. The oxygen demand of the working muscles is directly related to their mass and metabolic efficiency; therefore, exercise involving a larger mass of muscle is likely to be associated with a higher oxygen uptake. Indeed, running has been shown to result in a greater uptake than bicycling,[23] and working both the arms and legs results in a greater $\dot{V}O_2$max than running.[62]

Carbon Dixoide, pH, and Bicarbonate

Alterations in carbon dixoide content affect coronary resistance, as discussed more fully in Chapter 22. The remarkable increase in coronary resistance produced by hypocapnia, with its resultant drop in myocardial oxygen extraction and coronary sinus oxygen content, was demonstrated by Case[63] (Fig. 2–12). He showed that a reduction in arterial PCO_2 of less than 20 mm Hg will almost double the coronary vascular resistance and that a severe reduction in coronary flow, possibly to the point of ischemia, can be produced by hypocapnia. This effect appears to be somewhat independent of the pH changes.[64] Also, an increase in PO_2 in the coronary blood has been demonstrated to decrease coronary flow, and a decrease will cause a marked increase in perfusion.[65] The fact that carbon dioxide has such a potent effect on flow questions the previously held view that the oxygen content of the myocardium is the primary regulator of coronary vascular resistance.

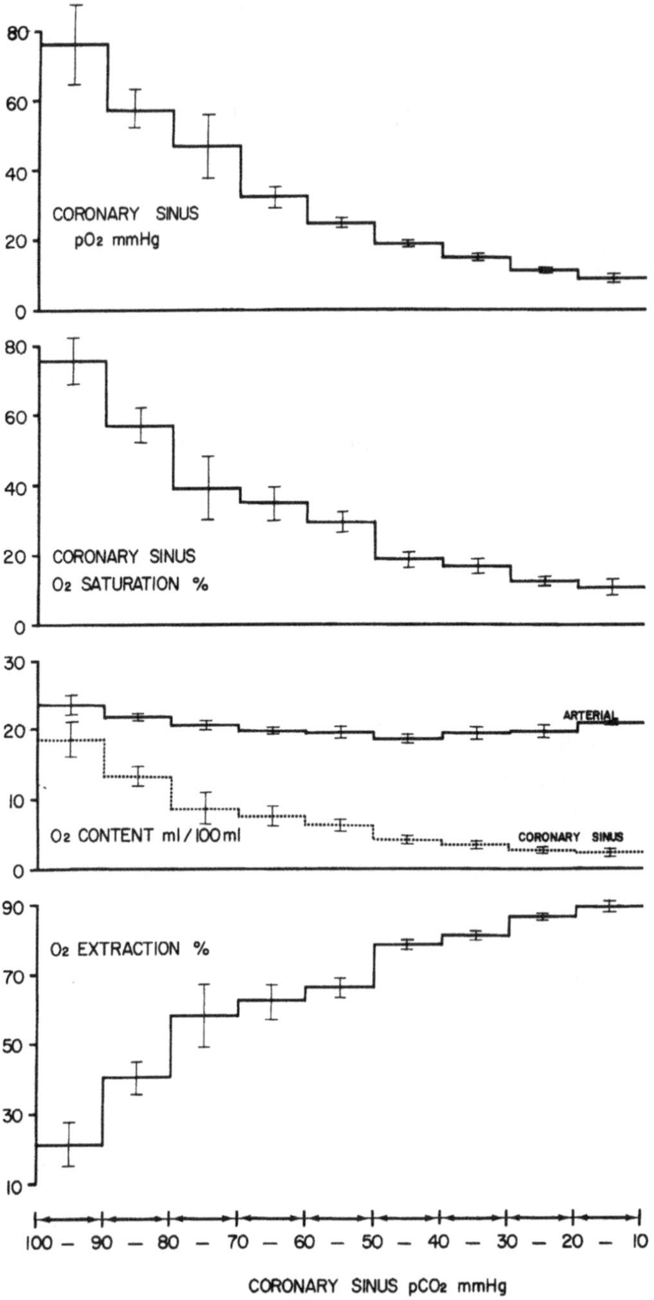

FIGURE 2–12. When the P_{CO_2} in the coronary arterial blood is varied in dogs, an inverse effect is registered on the coronary sinus oxygen content and P_{O_2}. As the coronary sinus P_{CO_2} is decreased, the extraction of oxygen from the arterial blood increases as flow decreases.

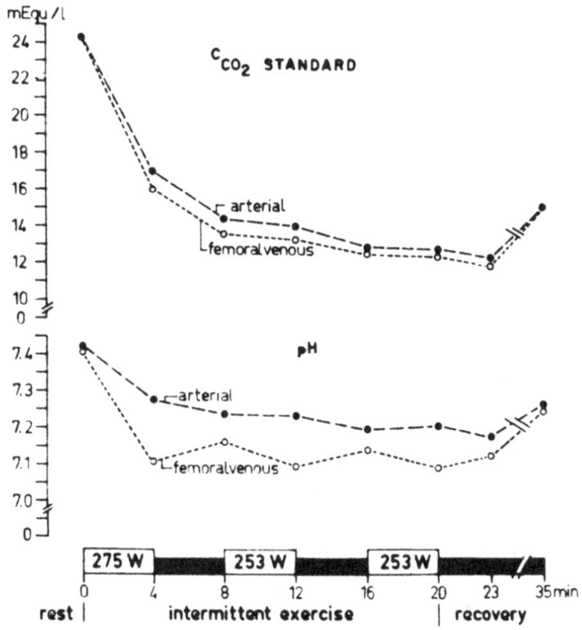

FIGURE 2–13. The pH and standard sodium bicarbonate buffer in arterial and venous blood both decrease during intermittent exercise.

As exercise progresses, there is a consistent decrease in pH and sodium bicarbonate that correlates with a rise in blood lactate. The response to intermittent exercise, as reported by Keul and Doll[66] is presented in Figure 2–13. Note that the lactic acid in the working muscle is only partly liberated into the blood, thus decreasing the tendency toward acidosis, which would have a deleterious effect on the organism and its response to exercise if the pH fell much below 7.1.[67]

SUBSTRATE USE IN THE HEART

Carbohydrates

It is becoming increasingly clear that the cardiac metabolism varies considerably when comparing normal subjects with those with hypoxic or ischemic conditions.[68] *Hypoxia* is used here to indicate adequate coronary flow with reduced oxygen content, as distinct from a reduced or interrupted flow of blood with normal oxygen tension, constituting *ischemia*.

The metabolism of glucose, pyruvate, and lactate by the heart is determined by their levels of concentration in the arterial blood. Glucose and lactate are used at normal levels of concentration in about equal proportions in the blood, but the pyruvate level is so low that it plays a limited role.[69]

The total aerobic metabolism of carbohydrates accounts for about 35% of the total oxygen consumption. Some evidence exists that the arterial insulin level is important in the regulation of glucose use by the heart.[57] Under normal conditions, the human heart uses about 11 g of glucose and 10 g of lactate per day. Thus, the concentration levels in the coronary sinus of both lactate and glucose are lower than in the arterial blood.

Acidosis has not only been demonstrated to increase coronary blood flow but also, to some degree, to increase glucose and lactate uptake. Alkalosis, on the other hand, decreases coronary blood flow and the uptake of both glucose and lactate.[70] The heart is unable to use fructose.

Noncarbohydrates

Bing[57] and Detry[60] have demonstrated that the human heart has a predilection for fatty acids as fuel. About 67% of the oxygen extracted by the heart goes toward the metabolic use of fatty acids. Ketones, triglycerides, cholesterol, lipoprotein, and the various free fatty acids make up this fraction, depending on their level of concentration and on certain hormone and enzyme influences. For instance, diabetes decreases the relative use of oleic acid, at least in animals.[18]

It is often said that when the heart has access to carbohydrates and lipids together, it will preferentially use the lipid,[71] although some investigators[72] have questioned this. It has been clearly shown that an isolated, perfused heart can maintain contractility for a long time by oxidizing endogenous lipids.[73] A buildup of long-chain acylcoenzyme A (acyl-CoA) ester will inhibit adenine nucleotide translocase, which causes early loss of functional integrity of the mitochondrial membrane.[66] Giving carnitine can inhibit this loss and may restore the membrane's ability to mobilize calcium.[74] A nicotinic acid analog that reduces plasma free fatty acids has been reported to minimize the ST changes generated by ischemia in humans during exercise testing.[75]

Role of Nucleotides and Phosphorylase

The activity of nucleotides and phosphorylase is intimately related to coronary flow. Ischemia leads to a significant diminution of creatinine phosphate and an increase in inorganic phosphate. This results in a decrease in adenosine triphosphate (ATP) and an increase in adenosine diphosphate (ADP). The latter may be a major reason for coronary dilatation in myocardial anoxia.

AEROBIC METABOLISM

The accepted figure for oxygen consumption of the normally beating left ventricle is about 8 to 10 mL of oxygen per 100 g per minute. When the output increases sixfold to eightfold in champion athletes, the oxygen consumption must increase to at least 35 to 40 mL per 100 g per minute, and the ATP production must rise to 15 to 20 mmol of ATP per 100 g per minute. This very high energy demand can be met because of the high concentration of mitochondria in the well-conditioned heart.[76] Under low metabolic rates, the oxidation rate is determined by the availability of the free fatty acids and the rate of acyl-CoA oxidation of the citric acid cycle and, at high metabolic rates, by the rate of acyl translocation across the intermitochondrial membrane.

ANAEROBIC METABOLISM

Although the ATP concentration in the heart is about the same as in the skeletal muscle, the glycogen content is about 5 g/kg, one third of the content in the skeletal muscle.[77] The heart begins to deteriorate about 8 to 12 beats after oxygen delivery ceases, but not because of depletion of high-energy phosphates.[78] This must mean that the ATP available to the contractile protein compartment is limited or that the rapid buildup of metabolic end-products in some way inhibits contraction. In the experimental perfused heart, oxygen can be given without any other substrate, and the myocardium will function for at least 40 minutes before glycogen is depleted, indicating that the experiment has washed out an inhibitor that is normally present.[79]

HYPOXIA AND ISCHEMIA

From the previous discussion, it is evident that the metabolic effects of hypoxia (reduced oxygen content) and ischemia (reduced flow) are different. Biopsy material from ischemic hearts shows that contraction stops when ATP is only 20% depleted, but when the flow is maintained and ATP is reduced 40%, contraction continues to be almost normal.[71] Studies in the working rat heart clearly show the difference between hypoxia and ischemia. When coronary flow is maintained, but oxygen is replaced with nitrogen, a threefold increase in glucose use occurs within 5 minutes, which is maintained for 30 minutes.[80] Glycogen stores drop by 70% in 4 minutes when these same animals are made ischemic by reduction in coronary flow of 50% or more. Glucose use drops immediately and decreases to 50% of that of the control within 12 minutes.[81] After 30 minutes of anoxia with normal coronary flow, intercellular lactate doubles, but after 30 minutes of ischemia with low coronary flow, the lactate increases 10-fold.

The accumulation of lactate appears to be a significant factor; the low pH reduces the rate of energy production by interfering with subcellular calcium transport. The above data are important because even a moderate reduction in blood flow (50%) triggers biochemical changes and decreases myocardial function. Cardiologists have tended to assign some arbitrary number (a percentage of luminal coronary narrowing, usually 70% to 80%) to the degree of stenosis necessary to produce ischemia. It can be seen, however, that a host of factors, especially those related to pH in the muscle, will alter substrate use and therefore cardiac function. The factors leading to the ischemic changes reflected in the ECG and the associated decrease in contractility are further discussed in Chapter 3.

TEMPERATURE

External environment has a profound effect on the organism and its ability to adapt to exercise, primarily because of the need to dissipate the heat generated by the contraction of the muscles.

Heat

Not only does the heart rate increase with a higher body temperature, but its total efficiency also seems to decrease[18] (Fig. 2–14). Burch[82] and Brouha[83] have shown that the heart works less efficiently as the temperature rises, and that a hot, humid environment results in a marked increase in cardiac work for any given level of external work. Also, recovery from work is much

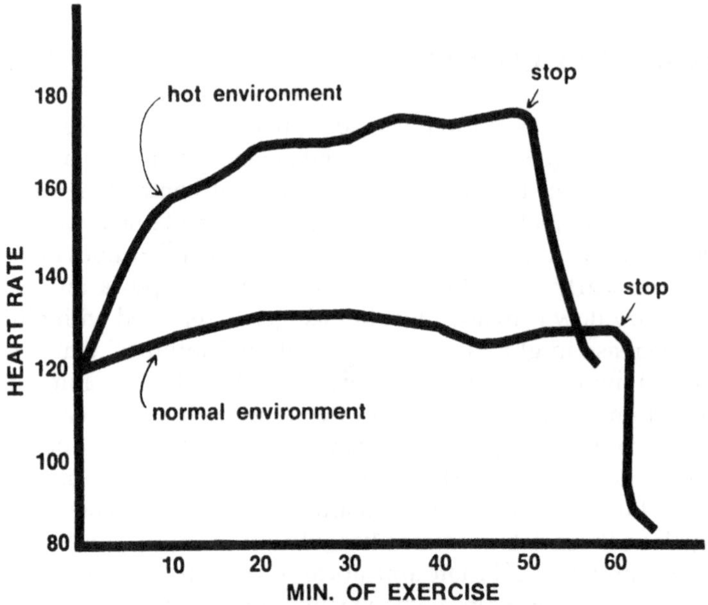

FIGURE 2–14. As illustrated by these findings from a well-conditioned college oarsman, the increase in heart rate associated with a hot environment during exercise demonstrates the need for an increased cardiac output as the body temperature rises. This increased demand may be excessive if heart disease is present and the increased cardiac output cannot be generated.

slower, apparently because of the body's failure to dissipate the heat generated. As temperature and humidity rise, the heart rate is increased for any given workload as well as at rest. If the body temperature rises much over 107°F (41.6°C), heat stroke can result from central nervous system changes followed by a complete loss of vascular tone.

It is well known that the skin blood flow is reduced in subjects who have a cardiac output lower than their metabolic needs at any particular level of exercise.[84] A gray skin color is easily recognized as clinical evidence of this condition; the body not only is signaling its failure to provide adequate total blood flow but also is now unable to dissipate heat generated by muscle contraction. The resultant rising core temperature then further inhibits cardiac output, thus initiating a vicious cycle.

In subjects with a normal cardiovascular system, repeated exposure to high temperatures alters the ability to cope with this problem by inhibiting sodium loss and thus reducing the expected decrease in central blood volume. With a larger blood volume and therefore a better stroke volume, cardiac output will be greater and more blood will be available to augment skin blood flow, improving heat loss and cardiovascular function in general. Robinson[22] reported that after conditioning, the effect of heat on performance is considerably reduced, confirming the adaptive mechanism described above.

Cold

The oxygen uptake at rest in a cool environment (50°F [10°C]) has been demonstrated to be considerably higher than when a subject is exposed to moderate temperatures (60°F to 70°F [15.5°C to 21.1°C]). After exercise is under way, the oxygen consumption in a cool environment is about the same as in a warm one.

Even though no measurable increase in oxygen uptake per unit of work has been documented, the general efficiency of the organism is less than optimum at a low temperature. Athletic endurance records are never established in extreme cold.

Patients with coronary insufficiency have an earlier onset of angina in the cold because of a rise in peripheral resistance with exercise, perhaps due to vasoconstriction in the skin and other superficial vascular beds.

Physical fitness improves cold tolerance. This has been demonstrated by Hart,[85] of Ottawa, who also reports that training and the resultant changes in $\dot{V}O_2$max are not altered by cold.

RESPIRATION

A detailed description of pulmonary function in respiration is not included here, but a few remarks about the respiratory adaptation to exercise are appropriate. The heart has long been recognized as the limiting factor in the oxygen delivery system during exercise in the healthy individual. However, the respiratory apparatus is obviously involved and its basic function should be appreciated.

Exercise Hyperpnea

The ventilatory response to the onset of exercise is characterized by a rapid, almost instantaneous, increase in ventilation. It has been argued that because this increase occurs before any metabolite from the exercising limbs could reach an appropriate sensor, it must be due to a neurogenic stimulus. If this were totally true, one would expect to find a concomitant early drop in PCO_2, which is usually not present. Casaburi and colleagues[86] have shown that cardiac output increases abruptly at the onset of exercise, with delivery of an increased carbon dioxide load to the lungs, so that the ventilatory response is appropriately adequate to maintain the PCO_2 in the normal range. Later, the respiration gradually increases in accordance with the metabolic needs, a process believed to be under hormonal control. The exact pathways regulating volume of ventilation during exercise are still not completely established. The hypoxic component seems to be large, varying from 13% to 54%.[87] There is a smaller nonhypoxic component, probably mostly carbon dioxide, so that the sensitivity of subjects to oxygen drive increases with exercise, but not to carbon dioxide. The endurance athlete seems to have less of a hypoxic drive than a sedentary counterpart, which allows the athlete to function at a slightly lower level of PO_2.

Rate Versus Depth

The rate and volume or depth of respiration are the obvious major mechanisms to be altered in increasing oxygen uptake. The respiratory muscles must overcome two types of resistance; the elastic resistance of the chest wall, the muscles, and the lungs themselves, and the airway resistance caused by the friction of air movement in the trachea, bronchi, and alveoli. The anatomical dead space between the alveoli and the mouth must be considered when the determination of optimal tidal volume and respiratory rate for any given increase in ventilation is appraised.

In normal subjects, the increased ventilation at low levels of power is achieved by an increase in tidal volume up to a maximum of about 60% of the subject's vital capacity. Increasing the rate may merely move the air in the dead space in and out without increasing alveolar ventilation significantly. Therefore, as the demand for a greater total volume of air ensues, there must be an associated increase in tidal volume over and above that needed to fill the dead space. Increases in tidal volume are, however, more costly in terms of muscle work, especially if the airway or elastic resistance is greater than normal. The tidal volume at rest is usually about 500 mL (about 150 mL being dead space), with a respiratory rate of about 12 to 15 per minute. This produces a minute volume of about 6 L/min, but an effective alveolar ventilation of only about 4.2 L/min. Strenuous exercise may result in a minute volume of 140 L/min or more, produced by respiratory rates of 60 to 70 and tidal volumes around 2 L. When the respiratory rate and depth are increased, the extra oxygen expended on respiration reaches a point at which it becomes a major metabolic burden.

The oxygen cost of breathing assumes considerable importance. Conditions that increase airway resistance, such as emphysema or bronchospasm, or that increase the elastic resistance, such as pulmonary fibrosis or lung edema, markedly increase the work of breathing and thus reduce the efficiency of the lungs. Bouhys[88] believes that the ability to function at higher tidal volumes decreases rapidly with age, making age one of the limiting factors in oxygen transport as well as in cardiac output.

Diffusion

The rate at which gas passes through the alveolar wall into the capillaries is often decreased by lung disease. There has been some question as to whether the rate of diffusion is a significant limiting factor in ventilation at high levels of performance. Measurements of diffusing capacity during exercise are markedly increased over the resting values, but it is not known whether this is merely a function of increased pulmonary capillary blood flow or an actual physiological alteration in the characteristics of the barriers to the passage of oxygen and carbon dioxide. The steady-state diffusing capacity measured during exercise has been found to correlate with the vital capacity, which in turn correlates with the degree of physical conditioning and the $\dot{V}O_2$max.[89]

SUMMARY

This chapter has reviewed the current concepts believed to best describe how the cardiovascular system responds to exercise. Our knowledge of these complex changes has increased dramatically. One must marvel at the capacity of the intricately interrelated systems to adjust to the wide range of stresses, such as a sevenfold increase in cardiac pumping capacity, the elimination of heat in a variety of climatic extremes, and the provision of the broad range of metabolic requirements of the various tissues of the body. When we consider that the mitochondria, the metabolic machines making it possible to increase our aerobic capacity to such extremes, may well be the product of what was once the symbiotic association between one-celled organisms, it is even more amazing to realize how well the complex metabolic, chemical, mechanical, and neurogenic mechanisms fit together.

As we continue to learn about the intricate steps necessary to integrate the whole organism, our ability to deal with its dysfunctions will certainly be enhanced. For a more detailed discussion of the coronary circulation, the reader should consult the monograph on the physiology of exercise by Pollock and Willmore[90] and the excellent short summary by Higgenbotham.[91]

REFERENCES

1. Gorlin, R, et al: Effect of supine exercise on left ventricular volume and oxygen consumption in man. Circulation 32:361–371, 1963.
2. Clausen, LP: Circulatory adjustments of dynamic exercise and effects of physical training in normal subjects and in patients with coronary artery disease. Prog Cardiovasc Dis 18:459–495, 1976.
3. Brutsaert, DL and Sonnenblick, EH: Cardiac muscle mechanics in the evaluation of myocardial contractility. Prog Cardiovasc Dis 16:337–361, 1973.
4. McRitchie, RJ, et al: Roles of arterial baroreceptors in mediating cardiovascular response to exercise. Am J Physiol 230:85, 1976.
5. Sheffield, LT, Holt, JH, and Reeves, TJ: Exercise graded by heart rate in electrocardiographic testing for angina pectoris. Circulation 32:622, 1965.
6. Horwitz, DL, Atkins, MJ, and Leshin, SJ: Role of the Frank-Starling mechanism in exercise. Circ Res 31:868–875, 1972.
7. Chapman, CB, Fisher, NJ, and Sproule, BJ: Behavior of stroke volume at rest and during exercise in human beings. J Clin Invest 30:1208, 1960.
8. Bates, DV: Commentary on cardiorespiratory determinants of cardiovascular fitness. Can Med Assoc J 96:704, 1967.
9. Sarnoff, HJ and Mitchel, JS: The regulation of the performance of the heart. Am J Med 30:747–771, 1961.
10. Braunwald, E, et al: An analysis of the cardiac response to exercise. Circ Res 20–21 (suppl):44–58, 1967.
11. Sheps, DS, et al: Effect of a physical conditioning program upon left ventricular ejection fractions determined serially by a noninvasive technique. Cardiology 64:256, 1979.
12. Hindman, MC and Wallace, AG: Radionuclide exercise studies. In Cohen, LS, Mock, MB, and Ringqvist SI (eds): Physical Conditioning and Cardiovascular Rehabilitation. John Wiley & Sons, New York, 1981, p 33.
13. Wallace, AG, et al: Effects of exercise training on ventricular function in coronary disease [abstract]. Circulation II. 1970.
14. Roskamm, H: Optimum patterns of exercise for healthy adults. Can Med Assoc J 96:895, 1967.
15. Harrison, DC, et al. Studies on cardiac dimensions in an intact, unanesthetized man. Effects of exercise. Circ Res 13:460–467, 1967.
16. Penpargkul, S and Scherer, J: The effects of physiological training upon the mechanical and metabolic performance of the rat heart. J Clin Invest 49:1959, 1970.
17. Scherer, J: Physical training and intrinsic cardiac adaptations. Circulation 47:677, 1973.
18. Finkelstein, LJ, Spitzer, JJ, and Scott, JC: Society for the study of atherosclerosis: Myocardial uptake of free fatty acids in dogs. Circulation 22:679, 1960.
19. Petro, JK, Hollander, AP, and Bouman, LM: Instantaneous cardiac acceleration in man induced by a voluntary muscle contraction. J Appl Physiol 29:794, 1970.
20. Fagraeus, L and Linnarsson, D: Autonomic origin of heart rate fluctuations at the onset of muscular exercise. J Appl Physiol 40:679, 1976.
21. Schwartz, PJ and Stone, HL: Effects of unilateral stellectomy upon cardiac performance during exercise in dogs. Circ Res 44:637, 1979.
22. Robinson, S: Experimental studies of physical fitness. Arbeits-physiologic. 10:251, 1930.

23. Borst, C, Hollander, AP, and Bouman, LM: Cardiac acceleration elicited by voluntary muscle contractions of minimal duration. J Appl Physiol 32:70, 1972.
24. Manyari, DE, et al: Left ventricular diastolic function in a population of healthy elderly adults. J Am Geriatr Soc 33:758–763, 1985.
25. Hossack, KF and Bruce, RA: Maximal cardiac function in sedentary normal men and women: Comparison of age related changes. J Appl Physiol 53:799–804, 1982.
26. Rodeheffer, RJ, et al: Exercise cardiac output is maintained with advancing age in healthy human subjects: Cardiac dilatation and increased stroke volume compensate for a diminished heart rate. Circulation 69:203–213, 1984.
27. Åstrand, I: Aerobic work capacity in men and women with special reference to age. Acta Physiol Scand 169(suppl): 1–92, 1960.
28. Higgenbotham, MB, et al: Sex-related differences in the normal cardiac response to upright exercises. Circulation 70:357–366, 1984.
29. Glagov, S, et al: Heart rates during 24 hours of unusual activity. J Appl Physiol 29:799, 1970.
30. Pollock, ML: How much exercise is enough? Phys Sportsmed 6:4, 1978.
31. Hill, JS: The effects of frequency of exercise on cardiorespiratory fitness of adult men. Master's Thesis. London, University of Western Ontario. 1969.
32. Pollock, ML, et al: Effects of frequency and duration of training on attrition and incidence of injury. Med Sci Sports 9:31–36, 1977.
33. Katch, FI and McArdle, WD: Nutrition, Weight Control and Exercise, ed. 3. Lea & Febiger, Philadelphia, 1988.
34. Coyle, EF, et al: Time course of loss of adaptation after stopping prolonged intense endurance training. J Appl Physiol 57:1857–1864, 1984.
35. Wenger, NA and Bell, GJ: The interactions of intensity, frequency and duration of exercise training in altering cardiorespiratory fitness. Sports Med 3:346–356, 1986.
36. Sharkey, BJ: Intensity and duration of training and the development of cardiorespiratory fitness. Med Sci Sports Exerc 2:197–202, 1970.
37. DeVries, HA: Physiological effects of an exercise training regimen upon men age 52 to 88. J Gerontol 24:325–336, 1970.
38. Thomas, SG, et al: Determinants of the training response in elderly men. Med Sci Sports Exerc 17:667–672, 1985.
39. Seals, DR, et al: Endurance training in older men and women. J Appl Physiol 57:1024–1029, 1984.
40. Pollock, ML, et al: Effect of age and training on aerobic capacity and body composition in master athletes. J Appl Physiol 62:725–731, 1987.
41. Robinson, S, et al: Training and physiological aging in man. Fed Proc 32:1628–1634, 1973.
42. Grimby, G and Saltin, B: Physiological analysis of physically well trained middle-aged and old athletes. Acta Med Scand 179:513–526, 1986.
43. Klocke, FJ: Coronary blood flow in man. Prog Cardiovasc Dis 19:117, 1976.
44. Scott, JC: Physical activity and the coronary circulation. Can Med Assoc J 96:853, 1967.
45. Andersen, KL and Hermansen, L: Aerobic work capacity in middle aged Norwegian men. J Appl Physiol 20:432, 1965.
46. Greenfield, JC, et al: Studies of blood flow in aorta to coronary venous bypass grafts in man. J Clin Invest 51:27–34, 1972.
47. Ross, G: Adrenergic responses of the coronary vessels. Circ Res 39:463, 1976.
48. Egashira, K, et al: Effects of endothelian-dependent vasodilatation of resistance coronary vessels by acetycholine. Circulation 88:77, 1993.
49. Midal, G and Bing, RJL: Myocardial efficiency. Ann NY Acad Sci 72:555, 1959.
50. Becker, LC, et al: Effect of ischemia and antianginal drugs on the distribution of radioactive microspheres in the canine left ventricle. Circ R28:263, 1971.
51. Dole, VF: The relations between non-esterified fatty acids in plasma and the metabolism of glucose. J Clin Invest 35:150, 1956.
52. Uchida, Y and Ueda, H: Nonuniform blood flow through the ischemic myocardium induced by stellate ganglion stimulation. Jpn Circ J 36:673, 1972.
53. Sarnoff, SJ, et al: Hemodynamic determinants of oxygen consumption of the heart with special reference to the tension-time index. In Rosenbaum, FF (ed): Work and the Heart. Paul B. Hoeber, Harper & Bros., New York, 1959.
54. Feliciano, L and Henning, RJ: Coronary artery blood flow: Physiologic and pathophysiologic regulation. Clin Cardiol 22:775, 1999.
55. Gobel, FL, et al: The rate-pressure product as an index of myocardial oxygen consumption during exercise in patients with angina pectoris. Circulation 57:549, 1978.

56. Sonnenblick, EH, et al: Oxygen consumption of the heart. Newer concepts of its multifactorial determination. Am J Cardiol 22:328, 1968.
57. Bing, RJ: Cardiac metabolism. Physiol Rev 45:2, 1965.
58. Najmi, M, et al: Selective cine coronary arteriography correlated with the hemodynamic response to physical stress. Dis Chest 54:33, 1968.
59. Taylor, HL, et al: Maximal oxygen intake as objective measure of cardiorespiratory performance. J Appl Physiol 8:73, 1955.
60. Detry, JR: Exercise Testing and Training in Coronary Heart Disease. Williams & Wilkins, Baltimore, 1973.
61. Cummings, GR: Current levels of fitness. Can Med Assoc J 96:868, 1967.
62. Hermansen, L: Oxygen transport during exercise in human subjects. Acta Physiol Scand (suppl)39:91, 1973.
63. Case, RB: The response of canine coronary vascular resistance to local alterations in coronary arterial Pco_2. Circ Res 39:558, 1976.
64. Kittle, CF, et al: The role of pH and CO_2 in the distribution of blood flow. Surgery 57:139, 1965.
65. Case, RB, et al: Changes in coronary resistance and ventricular function resulting from acutely induced anemia and the effect thereon of coronary stenosis. Am J Med 18:397, 1955.
66. Keul, J and Doll, E: Intermittent exercise, metabolites, Po_2 and acid base equilibrium in the blood. J Appl Physiol 34:220, 1973.
67. Simson, E: Physiology of Work Capacity and Fatigue. Charles C Thomas, Springfield, IL, 1971.
68. Jennings, RB: Early phases of myocardial ischemia injury and infarctions. Am J Cardiol 24:753, 1969.
69. Braun-Menendez E, et al: Usage of pyruvic acid by the dog's heart. Q J Exp Physiol 29:91, 1939.
70. Goodyear, AVN, et al: The effect of acidosis and alkalosis on coronary blood flow and myocardial metabolism in the intact dog. Am J Physiol 200:628, 1961.
71. Gudbjarnason, S, et al: Functional compartmentalization of ATP and creatine phosphate in heart muscle. J Mol Cell Cardiol 1:25, 1973.
72. Opie, LH: Metabolism of the heart in health and disease, II. Am Heart J 77:100, 1969.
73. Olson, RE and Hoeschen, RJ: Utilization of endogenous lipids by the isolated perfused rat heart. Biochem J 103:796, 1967.
74. Skrogo, E, et al: Control of energy production in myocardial ischemia. Circ Res 38 (suppl 1): 75, 1976.
75. Luxton, MR, et al: Antilipolytic therapy in angina pectoris, reduction in exercise-induced ST depression. Br Heart J 38:1200,1976.
76. Gibbs, CL: Cardiac energetics. Physiol Rev 58:174, 1978.
77. Fisher, RB and Williamson, JR: The oxygen uptake of the perfused rat heart. J Physiol (Lond) 158:86, 1961.
78. Kubler, W and Spiekermann, PG: Regulations of glycolysis in the ischemic and anoxic myocardium. J Mol Cell Cardiol 1:351, 1970.
79. Thorn, WG, et al: Function, substrate supply and metabolic content of rabbit heart perfused in situ. Am J Physiol 214:139, 1968.
80. Neely, JR, et al: Effects of ischemia on function and metabolism of the isolated working rat heart. Am J Physiol 225:651, 1973.
81. Opie, LH: Effects of regional ischemia in metabolism of glucose and fatty acids. Circ Res (suppl 1)38:152, 1976.
82. Burch, GE: Influence of hot and humid environment upon the work of the heart. In Rosenbaum, FF (ed): Work and the Heart. Paul B. Hoeber, Harper & Bros., New York, 1959.
83. Brouha, LA: Effect of work on the heart. In Rosenbaum, FF (ed): Work and the Heart. Paul B. Hoeber, Harper & Bros., New York, 1959.
84. Andersen, KL: The effect of physical training with and without cold exposure upon physiological indices of fitness for work. Can Med Assoc J 96:801, 1967.
85. Hart, JS: Commentaries on the effect of physical training with and without cold exposure upon physiological indices of fitness for work. Can Med Assoc J 96:803, 1967.
86. Casaburi, R, et al: Ventilating central characteristics of the exercise hyperpnea as discerned from dynamic forcing techniques. Chest (suppl 20th Aspen Lung Conference) 73:2280, 1978.

87. Martin, B, et al: Chemical drives to breathe as determinants of exercise ventilation. Chest (suppl 20th Aspen Lung Conference) 73:2283, 1978.
88. Bouhys, A: Commentary to cardiorespiratory determinants of cardiovascular fitness. Can Med Assoc J 96:704, 1967.
89. Holmgren, A: Cardiorespiratory determinants of cardiovascular fitness. Can Med Assoc J 96:697, 1967.
90. Pollock, MI and Willmore, HE: Exercise in Health and Disease, 2nd ed. WB Saunders, Philadelphia, 1990.
91. Higgenbotham, MB: Cardiac performance during submaximal and maximal exercise in healthy persons. Heart Failure 4:68, 1988.

3
Physiology of Cardiac Ischemia

Supply Versus Demand
Coronary Arteries
Vasomotion
Collaterals
Stimulus to Coronary Collateral Formation
Exercise Stimulus to Collateral Formation
Coronary Size Related to Workload
Trigger Mechanisms for Ischemia
Intramyocardial Perfusion
Physiology of Bloodflow Regulation
Nitric Oxide
Adenosine
Transmural Flow Distribution
Vasodilator Reserve
Pressure Relationships of Left Ventricle and Coronary Arteries
Time Intervals
Relationship of Left Ventricle to Pulmonary Artery Pressures
Posture and Filling Pressures
Systemic Blood Pressure
Contractility and Wall Motion
Abnormal Relaxation
The Pericardial Hypothesis
Left-Ventricular Stroke Volume
Stroke Work
Pain
Endorphins
Comment
Biochemical Changes in the Ischemic Myocardium
Lactate
Free Fatty Acids
Prostaglandins
Mechanism of ST-Segment Depression
Direction of ST Vector
ST-Segment Elevation

In this chapter, I review current concepts that help to explain the pathophysiology of myocardial ischemia. Although our understanding of these mechanisms is constantly changing, a review is important because it provides a framework on which to organize clinical observations.

SUPPLY VERSUS DEMAND

Ischemia results from an imbalance between the oxygen supply and the myocardial demand. In simple terms, supply is primarily a function of coronary artery luminal diameter times the driving pressure minus the noncoronary resistance to flow, modified by hemoglobin content and blood viscosity. Myocardial demand is primarily influenced by heart rate, wall tension, and contractile state. An imbalance in the supply/demand ratio may be either global or, more often, localized in certain areas of the heart muscle. This imbalance may be silent clinically or manifested by chest pain, arm or jaw pain, dyspnea, sudden weakness, or arrhythmias.

CORONARY ARTERIES

Vasomotion

For many years, we viewed the coronary epicardial arteries as passive conduits, with the main regulatory process being located in the arterioles. Evidence presented by Maseri and colleagues[1–3] and others,[4,5] has clearly demonstrated that spasm in the large epicardial coronary arteries often reduces blood flow enough to result in clinically important ischemia. This may occur in what appears to be a normal artery, but it usually occurs in a section of the arterial wall already altered by an atheromatous plaque. Thus, the dynamic aspect of the coronary tree becomes important in our understanding of the pathophysiology of the coronary artery.

A number of maneuvers can precipitate arterial spasm. These include intravenous ergonovine, methacholine, histamine, cold pressor maneuvers, anxiety, fear, hostility, exercise, hyperventilation, and probably many other stimuli. The reduction in flow can be reversed by nitroglycerin, pentolamine, calcium blockers, nitric acid, and, in some cases, acetylcholine. Pentolamine is an alpha-adrenergic agent that may affect epicardial coronary vessels or, more likely, the coronary arterioles.

A coronary dilator that acts on the precapillary sphincter would only send more blood through normal regions, so that if nitroglycerin acts in the heart, it must do so mainly by redistributing blood toward areas of reduced perfusion. A good deal has been written about the degree of coronary narrowing necessary to produce clinical signs of ischemia. It is well established that function in a dog's heart begins to deteriorate when perfusion pressure drops to around 55 mm Hg, and as the reduction in flow increases, the loss of contractility progresses rapidly.[6] It has also been demonstrated that the drop in perfusion pressure is related to the velocity of the blood as well as to the magnitude of the obstruction. The work of Young and associates,[6] who demonstrated the relationship of velocity to magnitude of obstruction and its effect on pressure drop, is illustrated in Figure 3–1. It can be seen that even restrictions of 50% to 60% can produce important pressure drops at high velocity. This suggests that previous statements claiming that 70% narrowing or more is required to compromise function must be viewed with some skepticism.[7] The resistance to flow secondary to muscle pressure during systole, left-ventricular filling pressure during diastole, and the lack of available filling time in a patient with tachycardia, are discussed on pages 84 to 87. It is now established that nitric acid, elaborated by the cells lining coronary arteries, is an important moderator of vasodilatation.[8] Its absence or a deficit in production may result in severe vasoconstriction, especially with exercise.[9]

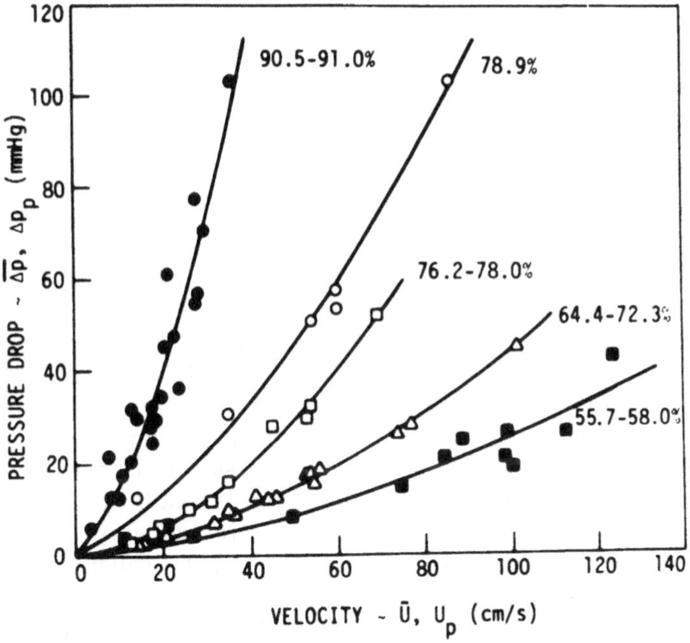

FIGURE 3–1. The pressure drop induced by various degrees of coronary narrowing as related to velocity of blood flow. The drop in pressure with high-grade stenosis is manifested at low velocities, while a high velocity is necessary to cause a significant drop when the obstructions approach 50%. (From Young, et al,[6] with permission.)

Now that we realize that endogenous agents may further restrict flow in the region of a relatively small stenotic plaque, our faith in a coronary angiogram must be reconsidered. A patient who has typical angina or ischemic ST changes, especially at rest, with an angiogram demonstrating as little as 30% narrowing of a major coronary trunk, must be suspected of having temporary decreases in the stenotic orifice due to coronary spasm or due to constriction of the microcirculation.[10]

Collaterals

Intracoronary collaterals, connecting an ischemic arterial network to another coronary arterial bed, have definite functional benefit in providing improved perfusion to the starved myocardium. However, it appears that at best, these vessels replace up to about 40% of normal coronary flow. Thus, the flow is never enough during increased oxygen demand.[11,12] That is, the improved perfusion may provide protection against myocardial infarction during low levels of metabolic activity, but when metabolic demands on the heart muscle increase, ischemia almost invariably occurs. Thus, cardiac function is reduced to some degree, especially when significant increases in cardiac work are required, even in the face of well-developed collaterals. Also, we now know that collaterals that are visible during coronary angiography constitute a variable and often small portion of the actual intracoronary flow.

Stimulus to Coronary Collateral Formation

In animals, especially dogs, epicardial collateral vessels connecting to vascular beds seem to develop very rapidly, sometimes within a few minutes after a myocardial infarction.[8] If narrowing in the affected artery is slow enough, the rapidly developing collaterals protect the heart from infarction altogether.[12] This is probably not always the case in humans, although a well-formed collateral system certainly reduces the likelihood of myocardial necrosis, or reduces the size of the ultimate scar. In humans, coronary narrowing of greater than 75% is probably necessary to stimulate collateral circulation[13]; however, the efficiency of this process, which may be inherited, differs greatly among individuals. It also appears that the more rapidly the occlusion occurs, the less likely adequate collaterals will form, and that complete obstruction of an artery is the best stimulus for collateralization.[14–16] When patients are compared, those with good collateralization to ischemic areas invariably have better function, especially when the muscle is stressed either by exercise or atrial pacing.

Exercise Stimulus to Collateral Formation

In 1967, Ekstein[17] performed a classic and often-quoted study. He exercised dogs with partly occluded coronary arteries and found marked improvement in coronary flow compared with dogs that were kept at rest. Coronary collaterals are very sensitive to extravascular compressive forces; Ekstein's failure to account for this, the errors inherent in using retrograde flow as a measure of collateral flow, and the fact that he frequently used vascular beds where only 80% or 90% antegrade obstruction was present probably led to erroneous conclusions. More recent work by Schaper and colleagues,[18] in a rigidly controlled dog model, found that exercise in dogs, at least, had no effect on collateral flow.

Heaton and colleagues[19] have studied myocardial blood flow to the epicardium compared with that to the subendocardial areas in dogs. They found that in ischemic areas caused by previous coronary constriction, prolonged exercise improved the subendocardial flow when compared with controls, as estimated by radioactive microspheres. Scheel and colleagues,[20] Burt and Jackson,[21] and Kaplinsky and associates,[22] like Schaper and associates,[23] were unable to find that exercise was a stimulus to collateral growth in dogs. The epicardial collaterals in dogs and men are not exercise-induced, but intramyocardial collaterals as seen in pigs can be stimulated by exercise.

In an extensive review of the stimulus to collateral flow, Sasayama and Fujita[24] provide interesting insights into this still unsettled question. They report that exercise in combination with heparin definitely increases collateral flow in humans exercised daily on a treadmill. They found not only angiographic evidence of increased coronary flow but also improved exercise tolerance and double product achieved. They believe ischemic myocytes stimulate DNA replication and growth of endothelial and smooth muscle cells. Many patients in coronary rehabilitation programs exercise religiously because of the belief that it will stimulate coronary collaterals. We now know that exercise stimulates the release of nitric oxide from the endothelium thus improving coronary flow.[25]

MacAlpin and colleagues[26] have stated that 50% of patients who improved their exercise capacity during a coronary rehabilitation program also showed an improved collateral pattern on angiography, which supports this concept. The one point on which everyone seems to agree is that the best stimulus to collateral formation is ischemia. We have seen collaterals associated with high-grade coronary disease disappear within a few minutes after the ischemia is relieved by percutaneous transluminal angioplasty. Thus, the collaterals visible on angiography, at least, respond very quickly to changes in myocardial demand.

Coronary Size Related to Workload

There is no doubt that increased myocardial work increases the size of epicardial coronary arteries. Linzbach[27] has shown in autopsies and MacAlpin and colleagues[26] have shown in coronary arteriograms that the coronary size increases appropriately for the increased myocardial work. We tend to confuse the process of collateral proliferation associated with atheromatous disease with the increased blood flow to heart muscle that has been overworked either by exercise or by valvular abnormalities. These two processes probably have little to do with each other. MacAlpin and associates[26] have shown significant alterations in cross sections of coronary arteries of patients who have abnormalities that place excessive demands on their heart, such as aortic stenosis and mitral insufficiency.

Studies in rats, ducks, and cats by Stevenson[28] have been consistent in showing an increase in the absolute volume of coronary vasculature and an increase in the ratio of blood vessels to heart size with exercise. He found that forcing rats to exercise 2 days a week produced a greater increase in coronary size than exercising them 5 days a week. One hour per day of exercise produced the same increase in blood vessel volume as did 5 hours a day. A possible conclusion is that moderate exercise is as good for the coronary circulation as strenuous exercise if collaterals act in the same way. The animal experiments cited and the angiographic studies by MacAlpin and associates[26] are in accord with the large coronary arteries reported in Clarence Demarr (Mr. Marathon) after his death from cancer. It is very tempting to correlate the increase in size found in Demarr's arteries with his long history of marathon running. It is also possible that he was an outstanding marathon runner *because* he was congenitally endowed with unusual coronary flow.

TRIGGER MECHANISMS FOR ISCHEMIA

Ischemia, with or without anginal pain, comes on at unexpected times. Several mechanisms may trigger this reduction in flow. One theory is that when blood flows across a stenotic area, a passive collapse may occur, especially if the velocity of flow is increased. Coronary spasm in patients with Raynaud's syndrome and migraine headaches suggests that altered autonomic tone may be a factor in some cases. The long-held belief that vagal tone, and thus the release of acetylcholine, is always terminated with the onset of exercise has recently been discredited by the work of Marraccini and colleagues,[29] who have demonstrated an improvement in the double product at the time of onset of ischemia followed by atropine. Another mechanism is thought to be platelet aggregation on the surface of the plaques. Prostacyclin, and nitric oxide elaborated in the vascular endothelium, are important regulators of the interaction between platelets and the vessel wall.[30] Activation of the prostaglandin mechanism in platelets results in an increased synthesis of thromboxane A_2, which is both a vasoconstrictor and a promoter of platelet aggregation. The relative balance between this agent released from the platelets and prostacyclin, a vasodilator and an inhibitor of platelet adhesiveness manufactured in the endothelium, is probably crucial. Factors known to shift this balance in the direction of thromboxane, thus favoring spasm and thrombosis formation, are aspirin in large doses, coronary atherosclerosis, age, increased low-density lipoproteins, diabetes, mental stress, catecholamines, and vascular trauma.[30–32] There is no doubt that plaque rupture, which exposes an ulcerated area and thus attracts platelets, is a trigger for ischemia. Hyperventilation has been demonstrated to increase coronary resistance and decrease oxygen release from red blood cells to the point where myocardial ischemia develops.[33] Other complex chemical mechanisms in the coronary endothelium and arterial wall probably alter this process, but as yet are incompletely understood. New information about the dynamic process that regulates changes in coronary blood flow is summarized below.

INTRAMYOCARDIAL PERFUSION

Even though considerable narrowing may occur in epicardial coronary arteries, the flow may not be significantly reduced because the resistance in the precapillary sphincters is greater than in the areas of the plaque in the proximal large artery. Figure 3–2 illustrates that resistance to flow can come from any of a number of anatomical sites or from several in combination.

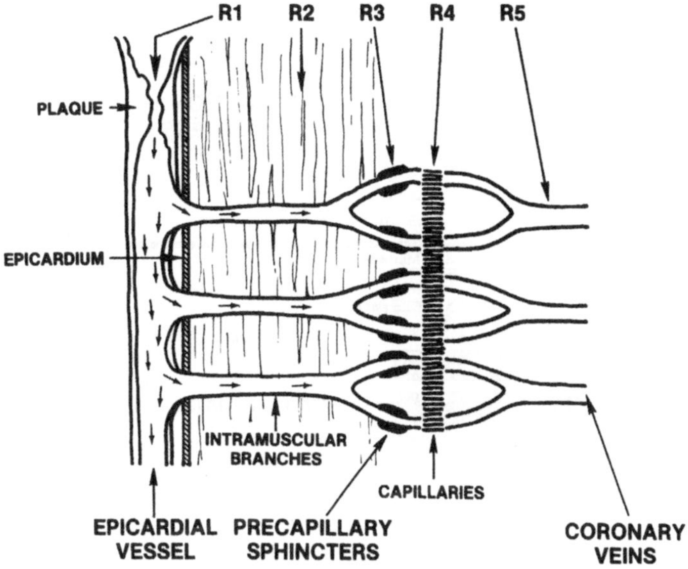

FIGURE 3–2. The diagram depicts the various resistances that influence blood flow, from a plaque at R1 to the effect of coronary venous pressure at R5. When the heart is at basal state, the precapillary sphincters at R3 probably play the most important role.

A patient whose heart is well perfused at rest may become ischemic when exposed to maximum metabolic demands shortly after the metabolic chemoreceptors in the myocardium dilate the precapillary sphincters and increase coronary flow to the point where the upstream narrowing becomes manifest.

The function of shunt pathways to aid in these compensating adjustments is illustrated in Figure 3–3. Maximal dilatation of these pathways can sometimes compensate for a complete obstruction of a large coronary epicardial artery, especially if the patient rarely places increased metabolic demands on the system. When the heart is pushed to a point where this system fails, the subendocardium becomes ischemic (Fig. 3–3). When this recurs over time, it may result in propagation of more ischemia, as proposed by Guyton and associates,[30] who demonstrated an increased resistance downstream from a critical narrowing. This could result in the death of myocardial cells or in a reduction in function termed *myocardial stunning*.

Physiology of Blood Flow Regulation

An excellent review of our understanding of the mechanisms operative in the control of myocardial blood flow in ischemia was published by Feliciano and Henning and should be reviewed by the serious student.[25] A simplified

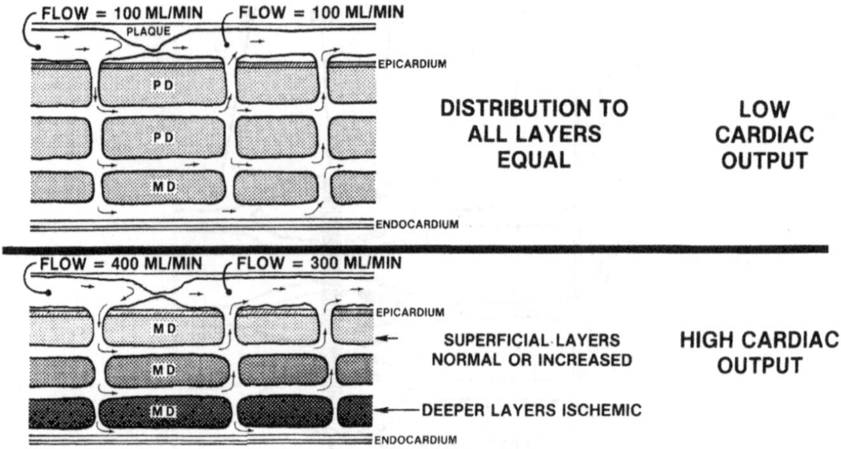

FIGURE 3–3. *(Top)* The capacity of the collateral shunt pathways to compensate for severe epicardial narrowing when the patient is at rest. *(Bottom)* The same heart when the patient is exercising, requiring a greater cardiac output. The shunt pathways, maximally dilated with a low output, cannot increase flow to compensate for the greater metabolic demands, resulting in subendocardial ischemia. (MD = maximally dilated; PD = partially dilated.)

summary is as follows. A large number of vasoactive substances have been extensively studied in the last few years. These include acetylcholine, bradykinin, adenosine triphosphate (ATP), prostacyclin, serotonin, substance P, histamine, ADP (adenosine diphosphate), nitric oxide, as well as norepinephrine, endothelian, vasopressin, aldosterone, and many others.

Nitric Oxide

Probably the most important of these is nitric oxide, which is elaborated by the coronary endothelium and plays an important role in not only vasodilitation but also inhibiting platelet adhesion. This material is elaborated by NO synthase from L'Arginine and becomes deficient when atherosclerosis destroys significant amounts of the endothelial lining of the coronary circulation. Most of the modulators of coronary flow have some effect on the release of nitric oxide. When acetylcholine is administered to a subject with normal endothelial function the coronaries dilate but when destruction of the endothelium by atherosclerosis has occurred, vasoconstriction occurs.[25]

Adenosine

Another very important endogenous vasoactive substance that modulates coronary flow is adenosine, which comes into play when myocardial hypoxia occurs. The small coronary arteries with diameters less than 100 microns, providing for at least 50% of the total coronary resistance, are the sight of action.

As we learn more about how these work in patients with coronary disease it may well be that pharmacological manipulation may become an important part of therapy. As yet however, their role during exercise-induced ischemia is not completely understood.

Transmural Flow Distribution

Transmural bloodflow in mammals of widely varying body sizes are so consistent that there is no reason to predict that it will be different in humans. Flow increases from the epicardium to the endocardium owing to the increase in metabolic demands probably related to the increased wall stress on the inner layers. This increase of about 20% to 50% is maintained with increasing heart rates under normal conditions but is profoundly altered in pathological states, as seen in Figure 3–3. Flow is also altered by the definite reduction in driving pressure as the vessel penetrates the myocardium. The aortic pressure or epicardial coronary pressure is far higher than that found in the inner third of the myocardium (see Chapter 2). Also, the tissue pressure is not determined only by the force of contraction, but by a combination of chemical and other neuroendocrine influences difficult to quantify. Increased vagal tone increases flow by 40%, whereas stimulation of the stellate ganglion reduces flow initially and later stimulates flow by coronary vasodilatation.[33] Epinephrine and dopamine reduce coronary resistance and increase flow, and angiotensin causes a profound vasoconstriction. Of course, adenosine, glucagon, histamine, serotonin, the kinins, and other substances produced in the myocardium and vascular epithelium also play an important role.

Recently, transmural flow has been studied by positron emission tomography (PET), which allows evaluations in patients with coronary artery disease. A surprise finding revealed that flow to areas where the coronary arteries appeared normal on angiography, in patients with "single vessel disease" was reduced when myocardial oxygen consumption was augmented by atrial pacing.[33] Flow in these areas could however be returned to normal by Dipyridamol. This report suggests that endothelial damage in arteries appearing normal may limit the required increase in perfusion that would occur with exercise. Equally important was the finding that those who had lost their ability to dilate their "normal" coronary arteries were the ones that had ST depression with pacing. This may help explain the reason why exercise testing has been unable to localize the culprit vessel in most cases. When endothelial function is destroyed by atheroma, even if they are not obvious on an angiogram, the ability for the heart to meet the metabolic demands during exercise may be compromised.[34]

Microvascular flow responds not only to the above vasoactive agents but patients with ischemia seem to have a paradoxical response to increased heart rate and myocardial work.[34] Until recently it was believed that capillary flow was maximal downstream to a stenotic lesion within the coronary artery.[34] New information now suggests that coronary resistance paradoxically increases downstream to a stenotic lesion. This concept has also been supported by studies using contrast echocardiography.[35–37]

Vasodilator Reserve

Studies by Wright and associates[38] in the operating room with Doppler flowmeters have documented that the ability of an area of the myocardium to increase flow is subject to a number of factors, some of which are still poorly understood. When they compressed the coronary artery for about 20 seconds, they found that reactive hyperemia increased the flow about eightfold in normals. While stenosis in the coronary circulation progressed, this reserve capacity was reduced and became abolished when the stenosis was near 90%. On the other hand, the researchers could not predict this response when coronary lesions, sized angiographically, were less than 90%. Some subjects with apparent obstructions of as little as 30% would have a severely compromised flow reserve, whereas others with stenosis of 70% to 80% would have a near-normal reserve. Thus, angiographically measured coronary stenosis of less than 90% may have different dynamic implications for ischemia from patient to patient (Fig. 3–4). It is now easy to understand why the reliability of ischemic ST depression in predicting coronary anatomy as estimated from angiography is limited. Patients with left-ventricular hypertrophy and so-called syndrome X (ischemia with normal coronary arteries)

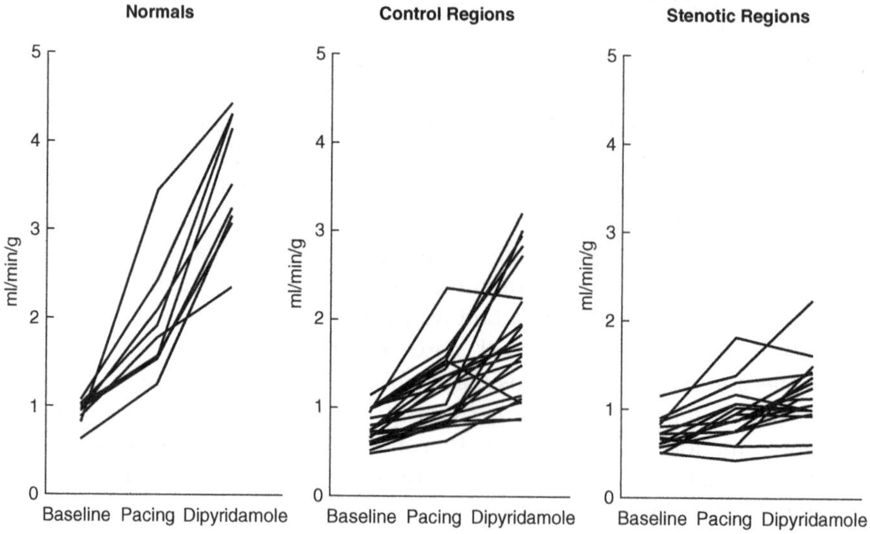

FIGURE 3–4. After administration, notice that the flow in angiographically normal arteries in patients with significant coronary artery disease is only slightly better than arteries with critical narrowing. With permission of publisher.[34]

have been found to have a reduced ability to increase flow even when the coronary vessels appear normal on angiography.[39] The reasons for this are more easy to understand in view of the recent reports on the function of endogenous agents such as nitrous oxide, adenosine, prostaglandin, and others.[34,40]

PRESSURE RELATIONSHIPS OF LEFT VENTRICLE AND CORONARY ARTERIES

If we recall the concepts reviewed previously and examine the myocardial circulation in relation to the anatomical pathways and pressure gradients in dogs (Figs. 3–5 and 3–6), it can be seen that the flow gradient during diastole favors adequate perfusion in the normal heart (Fig. 3–6). In the ischemic heart, however, the previously mentioned factors, which foster a decrease in ventricular compliance and promote the rise of end-diastolic pressure, result in a decrease in the driving pressure gradient across the myocardium, which then inhibits total myocardial perfusion.[41,42] This process is a vicious cycle because, as the stiffness of the ventricle increases, the decrease in total coronary flow is more profound. This would be even more marked if plaques in the proximal coronary arteries decrease the driving pressure gradient from epicardium to endocardium, as illustrated in Figure 3–7. As progressive ischemia develops, the endocardium and subendocardial tissue are selectively starved.

This series of events explains why the end-point of exercise and ST-segment depression is so reproducible in the patient with angina.[43,44] Nuclear perfusion studies confirmed the marked decrease in myocardial perfusion with exercise-induced angina.[45] The chain of events finally results in a global restriction of the necessary increased myocardial flow at a time when metabolic demands are increasing, so that power failure in the ischemic segment eventually ensues.

TIME INTERVALS

Along with the variables related to pressure, we should understand the relative duration of systole and diastole. As the heart rate increases, relative diastolic time shortens. This may well be one of the major factors in limiting the increase in heart rate associated with exercise. Buckberg and coworkers[46] have produced dramatic decreases in subendocardial flow with a shortening of the diastolic time as well as with a diastolic pressure increase in dogs (Fig. 3–8). They proposed using a diastolic pressure time index to estimate the relative decrease in blood flow to the subendocardial layers of the myocardium

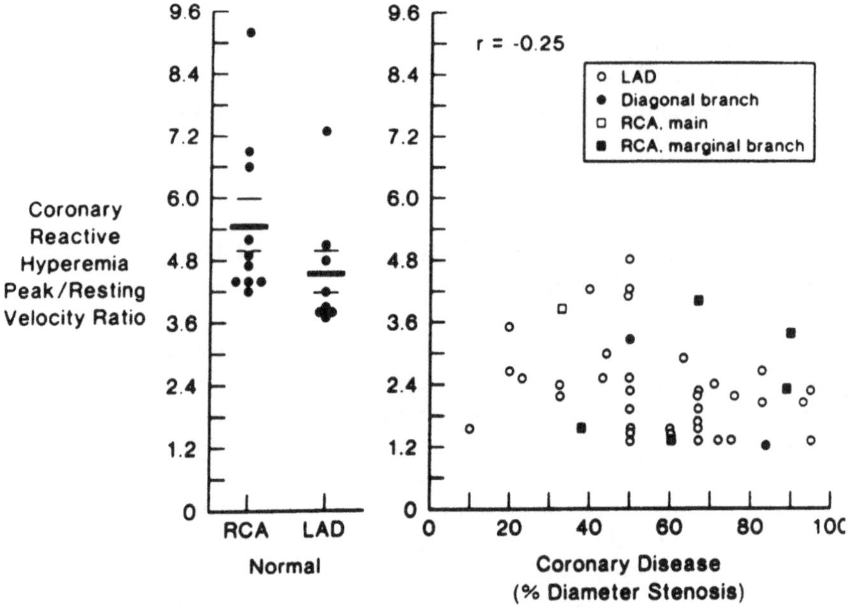

FIGURE 3–5. The response of the coronary flow measured in the operating room after mechanical occlusion for 20 seconds. *(Left Panel)* Note that normal coronary arteries will increase flow approximately five times during reactive hyperemia but that this increase shows almost no correlation with the magnitude of coronary narrowing as determined by angiography. Some with LAD artery obstructions of 85% can increase flow almost threefold while some with only 20% are in the same range. (LAD = left anterior descending; RCA = right coronary artery.) (From White, CW, et al: Does visual interpretation of coronary angiogram predict the physiological importance of a coronary stenosis? N Engl J Med 310: 819–824, 1984, with permission.)

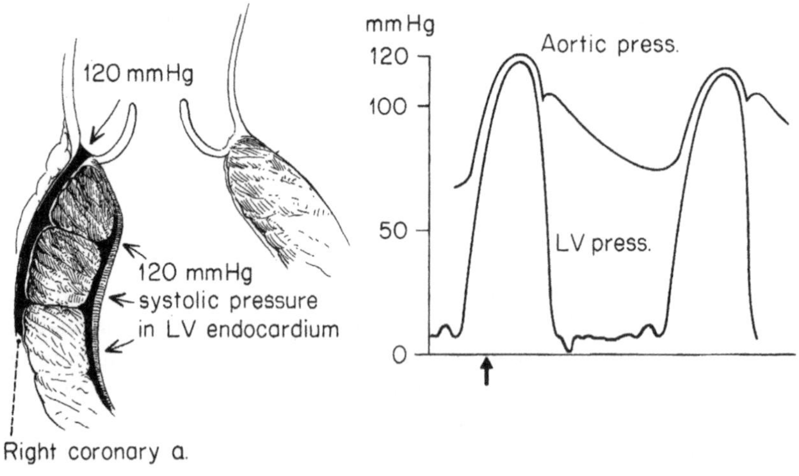

FIGURE 3–6. During systole in the normal heart, intraventricular pressure is the same as coronary artery pressure. Therefore, very little coronary flow occurs.

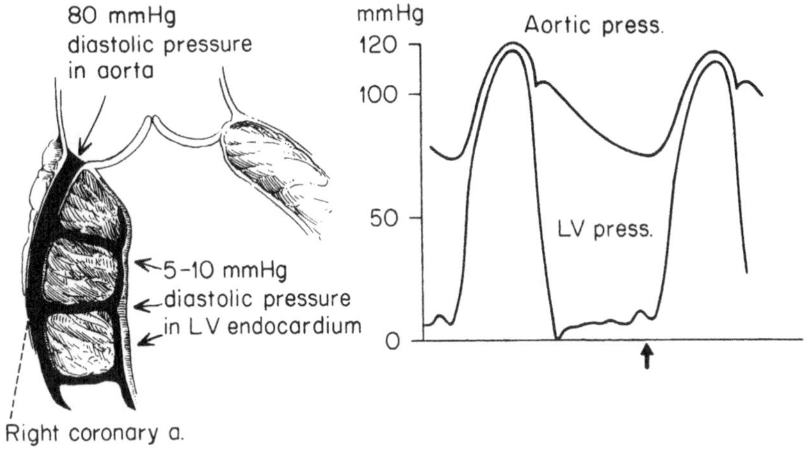

FIGURE 3–7. Normal diastole results in a fall in intraventricular pressure, allowing for a flow gradient to develop, thus perfusing the myocardium.

and have shown with radioactive microspheres that this flow may decrease even as the total coronary flow increases. Barnard and associates[47] have shown ST-segment depression in apparently normal men who were exercising very vigorously without a warm-up. They demonstrated that the subjects had inordinate shortening of diastolic filling time, thus postulating a decrease in endocardial perfusion very similar to that which occurred in Buck-

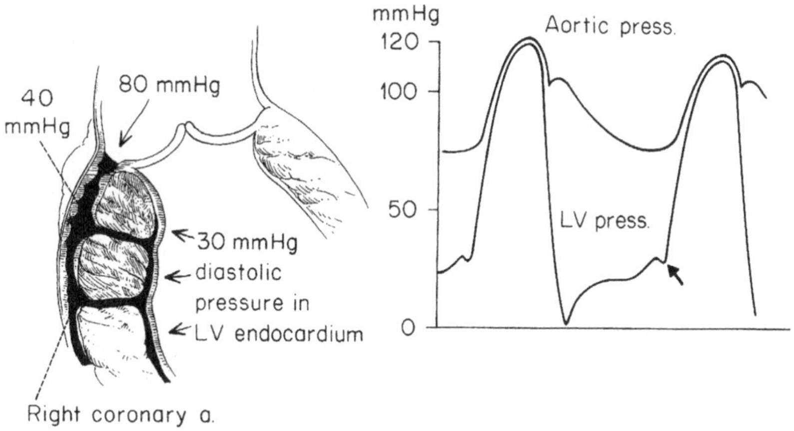

FIGURE 3–8. A large coronary plaque decreases the pressure in the coronary artery during diastole and at the same time the intraventricular pressure rises. The result is a very low flow gradient (40 − 30 = 10); consequently, there is very little myocardial perfusion.

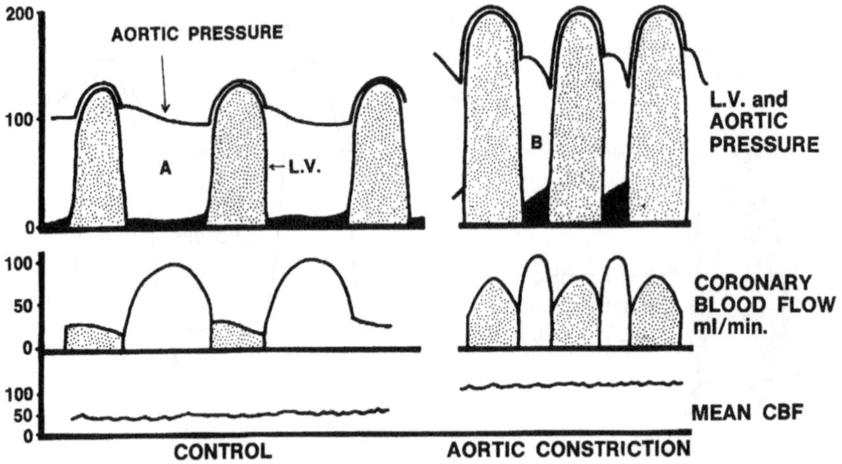

FIGURE 3–9. *(A)* The area under the aortic diastolic pressure becomes much smaller after aortic constriction and *(B)* with an increase in heart rate when related to the systolic area *(Shaded)*. This results in a decrease in diastolic (endocardial) coronary blood flow as compared with the total flow, most of which must go to the more superficial layers of the myocardium.

berg's dogs.[46] Although these data are appealing, Gregg[48] has shown that in instrumented greyhounds, exercise causes a rapid increase in coronary flow well into systole. During strenuous exercise, the short diastolic period appears to leave insufficient time for myocardial perfusion and, at least in dogs, systolic flow can exceed diastolic flow (Fig. 3–9). Prodigious athletic performance with cardiac outputs of 25 L or more per minute suggests that this happens also in humans.[49]

Although concepts just discussed help us to conceptualize the mechanisms of flow in a working ventricle, efforts to predict thresholds by the ratio of the systolic to the diastolic pressure time interval (SPTI/DPTI) are based on some invalid assumptions.[50] The influence of inertial factors, coronary capacitance, and blood velocity may also be considerable. Also, the original assumption that the stop flow pressure (see Figs. 3–5 and 3–6) is the same as diastolic pressure has been demonstrated to be in error; it is nonuniform across the left-ventricular wall. Thus, diastolic pressure time ratios help understand physiology but do not provide accurate thresholds.[51]

RELATIONSHIP OF LEFT VENTRICLE TO PULMONARY ARTERY PRESSURES

Because left-ventricular ischemia has been associated with a high filling pressure, we sometimes fail to remember that this is a function not only of myocardial compliance but also of the volume and velocity of filling, which depend on the right side of the heart. An example is illustrated by a patient

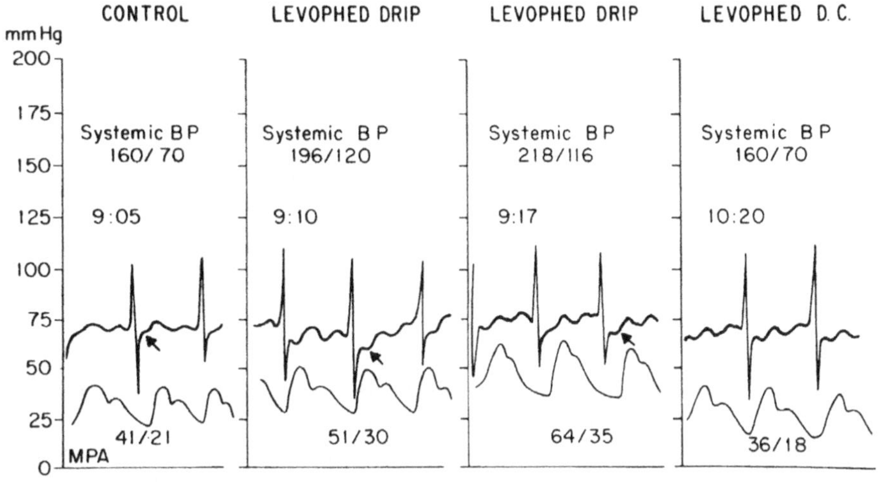

FIGURE 3–10. Two days after this patient obtained relief from his symptoms through the use of a vasodilator, he was subjected to measurements of his pulmonary artery diastolic pressure at rest and after a rapid Levophed drip. As the systemic pressure was increased by the alpha stimulator, the increasing left-ventricular diastolic pressure, as reflected by the rising pulmonary diastolic pressure, resulted in transient ST-segment depression in the V_5 precordial lead.

treated in our hospital for pulmonary edema (Fig. 3–10). The pulmonary artery diastolic pressure has been demonstrated to be a fairly reliable indicator of the left-ventricular diastolic pressure.[49] The increase in systemic resistance and arterial blood pressure that followed resulted in a return of chest pain and shortness of breath and an increase in pulmonary artery pressure reflecting the rise in left-ventricular diastolic pressure and a depression of the ST segment. This rapidly abated when the peripheral resistance was allowed to return toward normal.

POSTURE AND FILLING PRESSURES

Occasionally ST-segment depression associated with treadmill exercise can be accentuated by placing the patient in a supine position.[52] When a person assumes the horizontal position, the central circulation is increased by 200 to 300 mL, increasing the filling pressure of the left ventricle.[53] If there is ischemia and an increased stiffness of the ventricle, the end-diastolic pressure increases, accentuating the ST-segment depression. This process was further investigated by placing polyethylene catheters in the pulmonary arteries of 10 patients with known ischemic heart disease in an attempt to correlate the pulmonary diastolic pressure (and thus, indirectly, the left-ventricular filling pressure) with ST-segment depression. It was found that when using the pulse as a guide to the amount of stress applied, the end-diastolic pressure

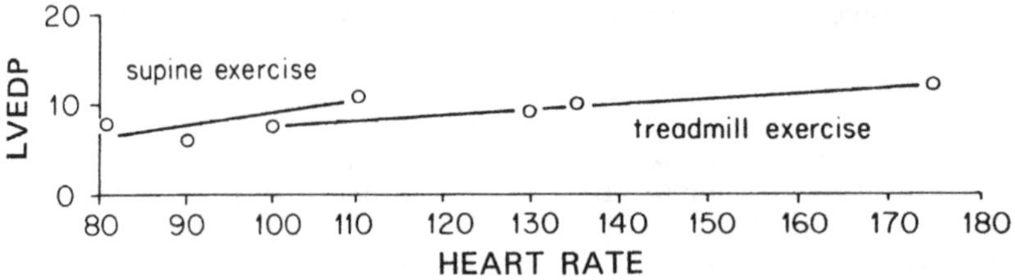

FIGURE 3–11. Pulmonary diastolic pressure responses of normal subject to supine and treadmill exercise.

increased much faster in the horizontal position, and with it came an earlier onset of ST-segment depression (Figs. 3–11 and 3–12).

Case and coworkers[54] have eloquently demonstrated the relationship of ST-segment depression to the left-ventricular end-diastolic pressure (LVEDP) elevation and also have correlated this with metabolic changes. These data have dramatized the importance of taking into consideration the metabolic and mechanical events associated with ischemia (Fig. 3–13).

A patient's heart may have normal compliance, as evidenced by a normal left-ventricular diastolic pressure, at one time, and then a few minutes later, when subjected to exercise or anoxia, may suddenly become stiff, only to return to normal when the workload allows the muscle to equilibrate with its oxygen supply.[55] Echocardiographic studies of posterior wall motion by Fogelman and coworkers[56] reveal the rate of relaxation to be markedly reduced during or immediately after an angina attack. This change also has been demonstrated by Barry and associates[57] with left-ventricular angiograms done at the time of atrial pacing, measuring pressure volume relationships, and by a number of other workers.[57–59]

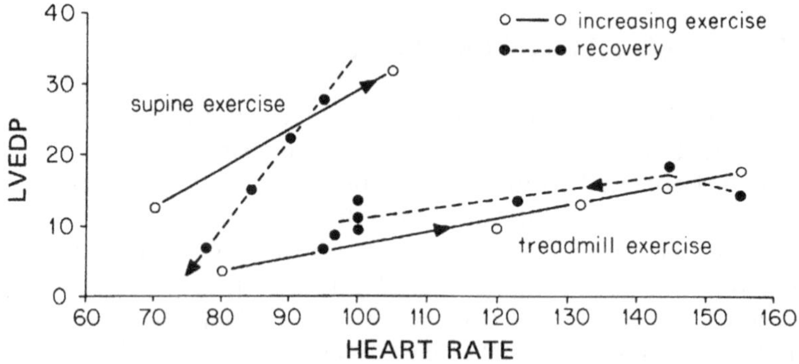

FIGURE 3–12. Pulmonary artery diastolic pressure (reflecting LVEDP) in patient with coronary disease in the supine position and on the treadmill.

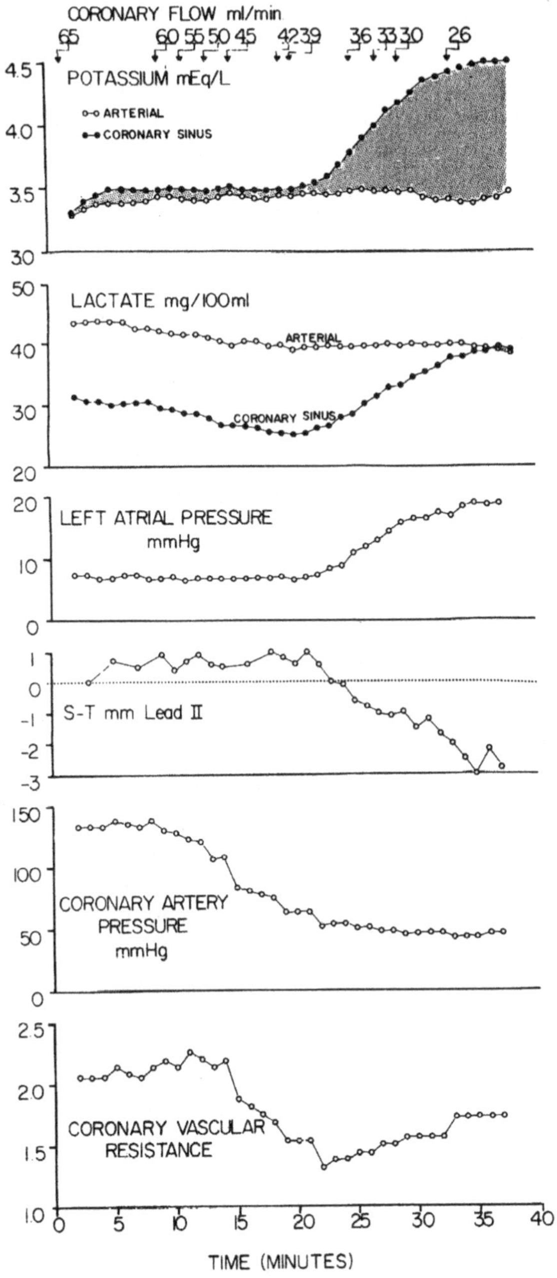

FIGURE 3–13. Data adapted from the work of Case and colleagues[54] demonstrates that the pressure, metabolic, and electrical changes occur at about the same degree of coronary ischemia.

SYSTEMIC BLOOD PRESSURE

Systemic blood pressure usually increases normally with exercise in coronary patients, but evidence suggests that the peripheral resistance often increases inappropriately with the onset of myocardial ischemia. This has two effects: (1) the driving pressure in the coronary circulation is increased in diastole, thus favoring better coronary perfusion; and (2) the work necessary to eject blood is increased, and the myocardial wall tension is increased, which requires an increase in myocardial oxygen use, the magnitude of which is often difficult to discern. The extra work is more of a burden than can be compensated for by the increased coronary perfusion as a function of the increase in diastolic pressure. Blood pressure in relationship to stress testing is reviewed in Chapter 18.

CONTRACTILITY AND WALL MOTION

Although patients with decreased coronary flow and near-normal left-ventricular function may have fair contractility as evidenced by observing an angiogram, it is definitely less than that of normal subjects. This can be measured in a number of ways in the catheterization laboratory with the use of Vmax,* $\Delta P/\Delta T$,† and circumferential fiber shortening. They all show a decrease when carefully measured, and as might be expected, the amount of decrease is related to the severity of the ischemia (Fig. 3–14).[60]

Often the contractility is augmented by an excess of catecholamines, but the ability of the muscle to respond to these agents is somewhat depressed. Note that the systolic ejection rate index (which equals the velocity of ejection over stroke input) is reduced so that under the stress of exercise, the time during systole (corrected for the heart rate) is actually longer. This can be measured from the aortic pressure with a catheter or from external recordings of the carotid artery or other peripheral arteries.

The contractility is often reduced in a localized segment so that a reduction in wall motion, or even a paradoxical bulge, becomes manifested during an ischemic episode.[61] This phenomenon occurs early in ischemia, even before the adenosine triphosphate (ATP) in the involved muscle is depleted.[62] One can see how effective such a mechanism can be in preventing infarctions. As the ATP in muscle begins to deplete, some metabolic trigger mechanism suspends contraction, which then promotes increased blood flow to the ischemic segment by eliminating the resistance inherent in the systolic squeeze. Methods for detecting these local wall motion abnormalities are now serving to identify ischemia when initiated by an exercise test.[62,63]

---

*Vmax is the maximum velocity of pressure rise extrapolated to 0 pressure.
†Delta pressure over delta time characterizes the velocity of ventricular contractions.

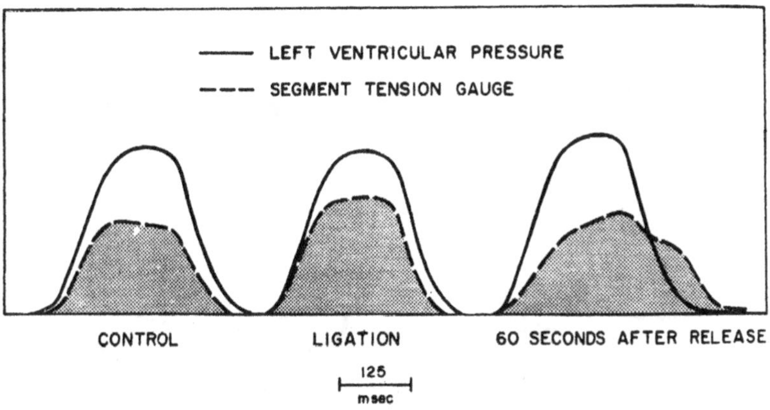

FIGURE 3–14. Isometric tension gauge tracings are superimposed on left-ventricular pressure recordings of an open-chested dog during a control period, 3 minutes after coronary artery ligation and 60 seconds after release. Note the prolongation of tension—thus incomplete relaxation is demonstrated. (From Bing, OH, et al,[65] by copyright permission of the American Society of Clinical Investigation.)

Abnormal Relaxation

What is the metabolic process that alters compliance and slows relaxation? Calcium ions that leave the sarcoplasmic reticulum and unlock the actin-myosin gate to initiate contractions must be returned by a calcium pump to bring about the muscle relaxation.[64] Langer[65] estimates that 15% or more of total myocardial energy costs may be expended to bring about this process, which involves moving about 50 mmol of calcium ions per kilogram of heart muscle back to the sarcotubular system. Hypoxia was thought to deplete the supply of ATP, which mediates this transfer, resulting in a cell with an excess of calcium ions and incomplete muscle relaxation.[64] Support for this concept comes from the work of Bing and associates,[65] who have shown that myocardial tension development extends into diastole. This is particularly true immediately after the hypoxia is relieved by adequate reoxygenation (Fig. 3–15).

There is evidence that a trigger mechanism halts contraction before the ATP or other substrates are depleted.[66] This may be due to a drop in myocardial pH, since it has been shown that the reversal of acidosis in ischemic muscle improves the suppressed contraction.[67] The possibility has also been proposed that some cells maintain their ATP and in others it is rapidly depleted, causing contracture in enough cells to decrease compliance markedly.[68] As this sequence of events takes place, lactate release, probably the reason for the increase in hydrogen ion concentration, occurs prior to the recording of ST-segment shifts sampled at the epicardium.[69] At the same time, the increase in stiffness is associated with little total increase in diastolic volume except in the underperfused segment, together with some decrease in systolic contraction.[70]

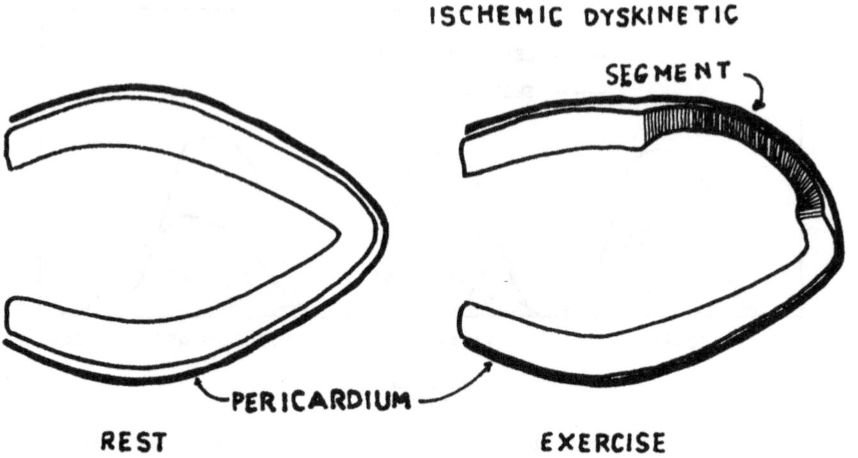

FIGURE 3–15. Pericardial constraint. As the dyskinetic myocardium bulges during exercise, it uses up the maximum pericardial distensibility so that the normal diastolic expansion cannot occur, thus resulting in a restrictive process that causes an increase in LVEDP.

The Pericardial Hypothesis

Although there is still some conflicting evidence, the idea that pericardial constraint may play an important role in the increase in LVEDP with ischemia has been gathering supporters. Tyberg and Smith,[71] in an extensive review, point out that the pericardial restrictive force is equivalent to the LVEDP. They show that increases in right-ventricular or right-atrial volume, as might occur with a volume load, translate linearly to left-ventricular diastolic volume in intact animals, because of the limited distensibility of the pericardium. Thus, an ischemic segment of the ventricular wall may bulge outward, resulting in a more distended pericardium, which then limits normal left-ventricular diastolic expansion. This mechanism has been supported by Kass and associates[72] in patients studied during angioplasty and by Janicki[73] in patients with heart failure (Fig. 3–15.)

We have seen constrictive pericarditis apparently causing ST depression with exercise in the absence of coronary disease.[74] Also, remember that the increased resistance to filling results in an increase in left atrial pressure and size, which affects left atrial conduction time.[75] Figure 3–16 illustrates ST depression in a patient with normal coronary arteries and constrictive pericarditis.

LEFT-VENTRICULAR STROKE VOLUME

The normal tendency to increase stroke volume with exercise is not altered much in patients with coronary narrowing if the left ventricle is

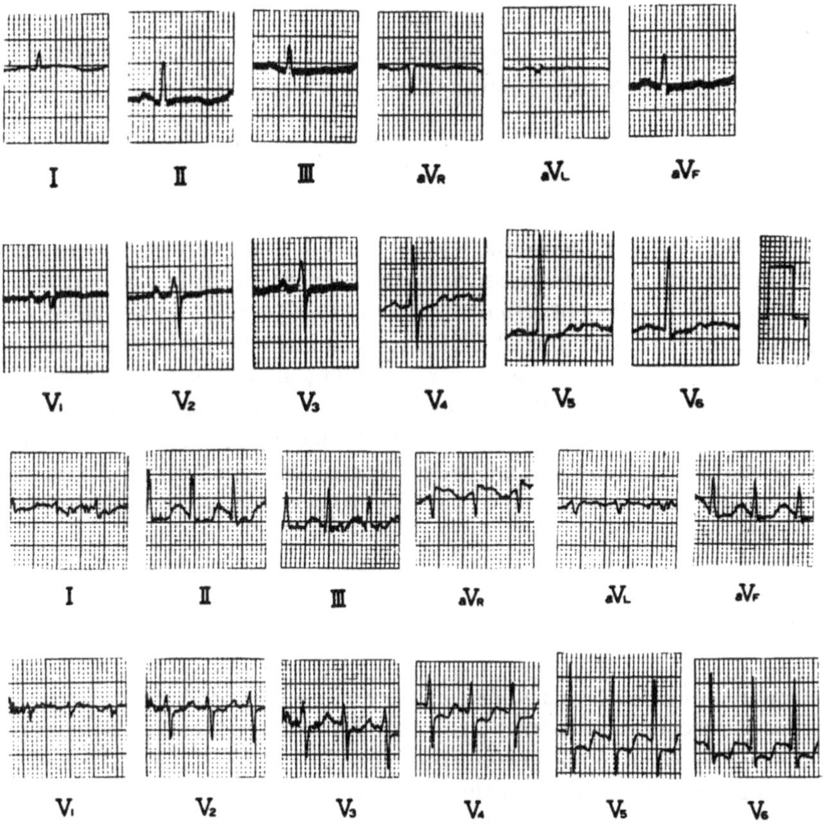

FIGURE 3–16. Percarditis. *(A)* The resting tracing of a patient with constrictive pericarditis. *(B)* ST depression occurring with exercise, where the restriction in diastolic expansion produces an increase in LVEDP and thus inner-layer ischemia.

relatively normal and if the magnitude of coronary narrowing is not too severe. Lichtlen[60] actually found it to be slightly, but not significantly, greater in a group of patients with angina when compared with normal subjects.

When there is left main disease or severe three-vessel disease, the normal stroke volume cannot be maintained with increasing myocardial demand in the face of inadequate delivery of oxygen. When this imbalance becomes manifest, the diastolic and the systolic volume both increase, resulting in a net drop in stroke volume and ejection fraction.[62] As this trend progresses, the cardiac output and systolic blood pressure begin to drop, resulting in the termination of exercise. It is obvious also that as the left ventricle is replaced by increasing amounts of scar tissue, the stroke volume decreases, especially during exercise.

A compensatory increase in contractility of the normally perfused muscle has been recognized by echocardiographers. The cardiac output required in patients with coronary disease after a training program may be less for a given workload than before, because of the increased oxygen extraction and the decrease in vascular resistance in peripheral tissues.[76]

STROKE WORK

The inefficiency of the ischemic left ventricle is characterized by the stroke work index (left ventricle pressure minus LVEDP multiplied by stroke volume index). The left-ventricular function curves correlating left-ventricular work and cardiac index and LVEDP clearly indicate that when patients with coronary disease are performing normally, they are doing so at an increased metabolic cost. It is also rather obvious that the heart usually performs much better before a myocardial infarction takes place than after, even though the patient may be free from angina pain as a result of the infarction. Thus, those involved in patient care should work toward preventing the infarction or at least reducing its size.

PAIN

The anginal pain in coronary insufficiency, considered to be the hallmark of myocardial ischemia, is poorly understood. Although a classic anginal pattern is a fairly reliable marker for coronary disease, the exact metabolic and physiological pathways responsible for its genesis are an enigma. As early as 1935, Katz and Landt[77] postulated that the pain might be due to the release of metabolites by the anoxic myocardium. They also suggested that the pain and the ischemic ECG changes may be due to separate but coexisting processes. The work done on myocardial ischemia since that time has provided little improvement in our understanding. When a patient with coronary insufficiency is stressed, as shown in Figure 3–17, the elevation in LVEDP consistently precedes the onset of pain, but in our experience, anginal pain rarely develops in the absence of the rise in diastolic pressure.

The patient whose ECG is depicted in Figure 3–17 had pain at the time of the deep ST-segment depression and high LVEDP, but it was relieved shortly after the diastolic pressure began to fall and several minutes before the ST-segment depression had improved. This sequence of events is predictable. Subendocardial ischemia could be assumed to be closely correlated with pain, as it is with the ST-segment changes, but it often occurs without pain.

The absence of pain is of no value in predicting the absence of coronary disease. A good deal has been written about the incidence of silent myocardial infarction, but the incidence of silent coronary disease is much harder to determine. We studied 1000 subjects referred for stress testing in 1968 and found that only 37% of those with ischemic changes had chest pain during

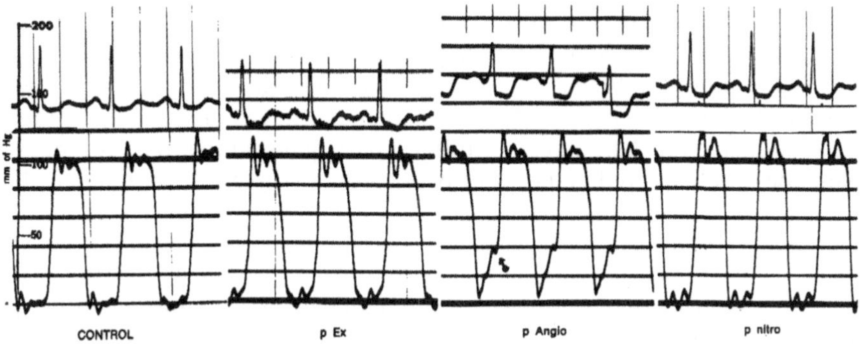

FIGURE 3–17. Left-ventricular pressures and ECG recorded during exercise in a catheterization laboratory. Immediately after the angiogram, the patient developed angina that was associated with a very high LVEDP and deep ST-segment depression. Administration of nitroglycerin resulted in relief from the angina pain and a drop in LVEDP, but there was a delay in the resolution of the ST-segment depression.

the test. A group of executives believed to be normal were found to have ischemic changes at or near their peak exercise capacity; yet pain was uniformly absent.[52]

Endorphins

There has been increasing interest in endorphins, the natural opiumlike compounds manufactured by the body.[78,79] When these substances are released by the brain, they are thought to reduce pain. Therefore, we postulated that patients with ischemia who are not experiencing pain may have higher levels of endorphins.[79] To test this concept, we exercised 10 subjects who had severe coronary narrowing to the point of ST-segment depression and injected naloxone, expecting to neutralize their endorphins and initiate pain.[80] Naloxone is known to neutralize endorphins as well as other opiumlike drugs. None of our subjects had pain, nor could we detect any other effect attributable to the agent. Some have measured endorphins in the blood and find that when they are very high, anginal pain is usually absent. Thus, we appear to be not much closer than before to understanding the absence of anginal pain in ischemic patients. Others have suggested that bradykinins and prostaglandin may be implicated in anginal pain.[80,81] Droste and Roskamm[82] studied the pain threshold in asymptomatic coronary patients and found it to be higher than in the patient with classic angina. Convincing evidence to implicate any mechanism in the final expression of coronary pain is still lacking.

Some patients also discover that their angina returns if they stop their exercise regimen but will again disappear if conditioning is resumed. For many years, therapeutic decisions have been made on the basis of pain patterns, yet it is now well known how fallacious this can be. Our experience is that moderate angina is usually unpredictable, but as the degree of disability increases, the threshold at which pain occurs becomes more constant.

Thus, although there is a good deal of knowledge about the physiology of ischemic heart disease, we do not understand the factors limiting or initiating anginal pain. A number of studies have suggested that the presence of pain does not help predict the severity of coronary disease.[82] See Chapter 19.

Comment

In some ways, the circulatory pattern and high metabolic requirements of the heart seem to be poorly designed, leaving it extremely susceptible to injury. On the other hand, we often see patients with 90% narrowing of all main coronary arteries who still have not only good left-ventricular function at rest, but also surprisingly good exercise tolerance. The trigger mechanism, as yet poorly understood, that decreases or halts contraction in an ischemic segment prior to the depletion of ATP is an effective safeguard. It allows the most ischemic part of the myocardium to stop contraction prior to permanent injury, whereas the segments of the heart muscle with normal perfusion pick up the load to maintain pumping capacity.

The decrease in heart rate response of any given workload seen in some ischemic patients is also an effective way to improve myocardial circulation.[83] The relatively longer diastole seen with a slow heart rate is very effective in providing more perfusion when the rate of flow through a coronary artery is reduced by a high-grade obstruction.

Finally, considering the remarkable performance required for a patient with coronary narrowing to complete a 26-mile marathon, the redistribution of flow from normal to ischemic areas, still incompletely understood, must be extremely effective in some patients.

BIOCHEMICAL CHANGES IN THE ISCHEMIC MYOCARDIUM

For a time, the loss of contraction in the ischemic area, which occurs soon after the onset of inadequate perfusion, was assumed to be due to a loss of high-energy phosphates (ATP). However, biopsies in experimental preparations demonstrated normal ATP for a time after contraction had ceased.[84] It is likely that the increase in intracellular hydrogen ion following anaerobic metabolism interferes with the interaction of calcium in the contractile proteins and also restricts the release of calcium from the sarcoplasmic reticulum.[66] The increased lactate may also inhibit phosphorylase kinase, which suppresses use of glycogen. The mechanism that switches off contraction is really protective because when the flow of adequate oxygenated blood is reestablished so that abnormal metabolites can be washed out, adequate ATP is still present to resume contraction, thus preventing permanent damage during temporary supply/demand imbalance. The metabolic changes during ischemia and especially during the early stages of recovery from ischemia impair ventricular relaxation so that the left-ventricular filling pressure, with its attendant reduction in subendocardial flow, is increased. The ability to metabolize free fatty acids (FFA) also profoundly influences the effect of ischemia. It reduces the activity of carnitine palmitoyl coenzyme A, a key enzyme responsible for the oxidation of fatty acids, the usual substrate for myocardial metabolism when adequate oxygen is available.

Lactate

In normal subjects, increasing lactate levels in the blood are associated with increased lactate metabolism in the heart when adequate myocardial oxygenation is available. Both cardiac and skeletal muscle produce excess lactate when using anaerobic pathways, liberating hydrogen ions and reducing pH. Not only does acidosis reduce the ability to metabolize lactate and fats and thus rapidly deplete myocardial glycogen, but the increasing level of FFA causes further deterioration of myocardial contactility.[85] The mechanisms for this are incompletely understood, but they probably include inhibition of cellular enzyme systems and membrane transport functions. Studies in swine indicate a reduction in activity of adenine nucleotide transferase and a reduction in cytosolic free carnitine. The coronary sinus lactate rise has been shown to be more profound with greater ischemia, initiating a rapid deterioration in cardiac output, which further reduces myocardial perfusion. A number of reports implicating adenosine in this process are appearing. Much remains to be discovered.

Free Fatty Acids

During ischemia the heart preferentially switches from fatty acid to glucose metabolism. Because high FFA and low carnitine levels decrease myocardial contractility, carnitine has been used in both animals[86] and humans[87] to improve cardiac function at times of ischemia. Whether this will become a practical clinical tool is yet to be determined. Other agents that favor conversion to glucose metabolism during ischemia include Renolazine, Dichloracetate, and Troglitazone.[88] Oliver and associates[89] have used a nicotinic acid analog to reduce FFA during myocardial infarction and found that it suppresses arrhythmias. How the level of FFA correlates with exercise-induced arrhythmias in ischemic patients is yet to be studied thoroughly but is of considerable interest.

Prostaglandins

Berger and colleagues[28] have reported the release of prostaglandin F in the coronary sinus of ischemic patients after atrial pacing. The hemodynamic effects are yet unknown, but the material may have some type of protective effect, possibly by stabilization of lysosomes in the ischemic area. Many other vasoactive substances probably play some role in cardiac function during exercise. Staszewski-Barczaks and colleagues[81] believe prostaglandin and bradykinin are the mediators of anginal pain, but evidence for this is still fragmentary.

MECHANISM OF ST-SEGMENT DEPRESSION

The normal ST segment, registered as a positive voltage, is due to a differential between the depolarization from the epicardium versus the endocardium. Endocardial depolarization activation starts early and ends early, and thus repolarization of the endocardium does the same. This results in a residual voltage differential late in repolarization and thus a positive ST and T wave. Because ischemia is usually more severe in the endocardium, delaying impulse propagation, this process reverses, resulting in inversion of ST or T waves or both.

Extensive animal studies and data in humans have given information about the factors leading up to and responsible for the ST-segment changes that have long been empirically correlated with myocardial ischemia. Ischemia should be distinguished from hypoxia and anoxia. Ischemia is oxygen deprivation due to reduced perfusion, whereas hypoxia is decreased oxygen supply despite adequate perfusion. Anoxia is the absence of oxygen in association with adequate perfusion. When the delivery of blood becomes inadequate, the subendocardial area is the first to suffer, whether the inadequacy is due to a temporary reduction in flow (as might be caused by a coronary spasm), a sudden drop in cardiac output (as with an intense vagal episode), or an increase in myocardial demand in association with a significant coronary stenosis.

The onset of ischemia is associated with a rapid loss of intracellular potassium, resulting in a diastolic current of injury, outward toward the epicardium (Fig. 3–18). The figure depicts the outward diastolic current caused by the potassium leak with its resultant effect on the ECG baseline or the TQ segment. The P and QRS are then inscribed on this elevated baseline. When ventricular depolarization occurs, inscribing the QRS, all the myocardial cells, including those injured, are depolarized. There is *no* current flow. At this point, the time of the onset of the ST segment, the galvanometer deflection relates to the original 0 or null point, which is located below the previously elevated diastolic baseline. The result is ST-segment depression, which, when systole is completed, is followed by the elevated diastolic baseline due to the current of injury.

These changes have been associated with a shortening of the refractory period and a prolongation of the QT interval.[90] The transmembrane potential undergoes a reduction in amplitude and some prolongation, as depicted in Figure 3–19.[91]

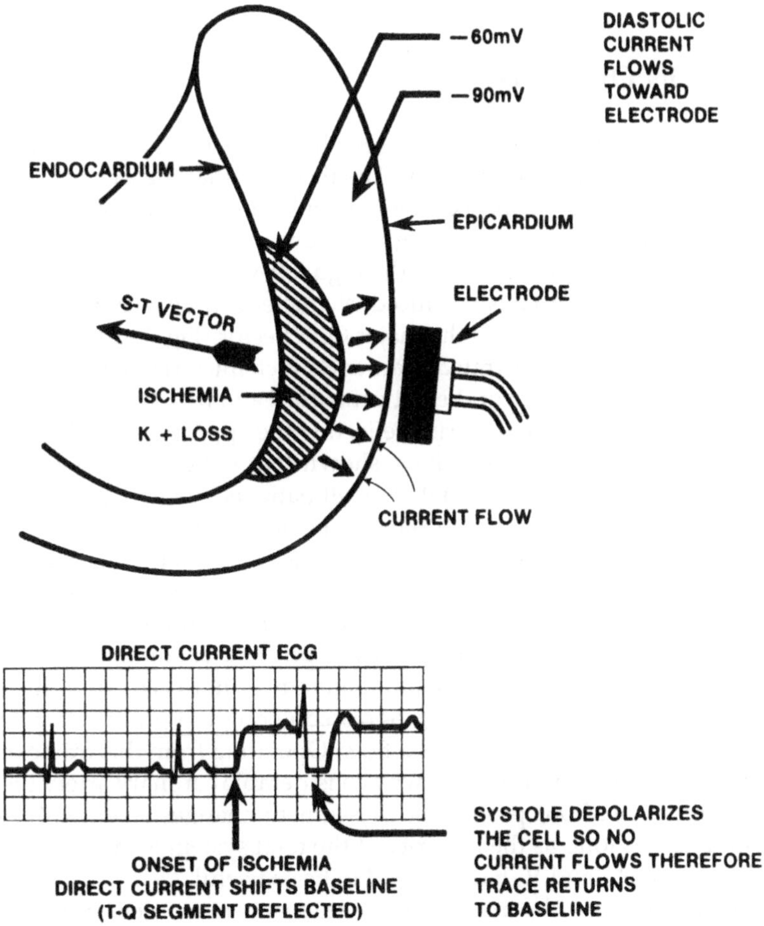

FIGURE 3–18. Mechanism of ST-segment depression. As the subendocardium becomes ischemic, potassium is lost from the cells, resulting in a diastolic current flow toward the epicardium and the monitoring electrode. This would deflect the baseline inward but is not recognized in our standard ECG because of the balancing current, until depolarization terminates the other potentials, resulting in the inscribed ST-segment depression.

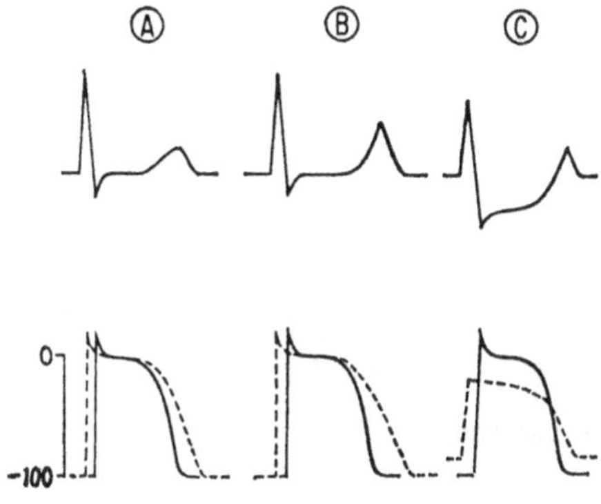

FIGURE 3–19. As ischemia is increased *(A to C)* the transmembrane potential alterations (dotted line of lower row) reveal a prolongation of electrical systole as the ECG in the top row reflects ST-segment depression. (From Sodari-Pollares, et al,[91] with permission.)

DIRECTION OF ST VECTOR

As subendocardial ischemia progresses, the vector of a depressed ST segment is fairly consistent in direction. The theory is that the ischemic zone of endocardium appears to be relatively evenly distributed throughout the whole ventricular cavity, even though only one area of the heart may have a severe perfusion defect. Because of the high left-ventricular filling pressure, a diastolic injury potential is produced, characterized by a consistent vector force, opposite in direction to the major QRS vector (Fig. 3–20). The subendocardial ischemia demonstrated years ago[92] is characterized by ST-segment elevation within the cavity of the left ventricle[93] and by ST-segment depression on the precordium in the leads reflecting the appropriate area of injury.

Blackburn and associates[93] have shown that ischemic ST-segment depression is best demonstrated in 90% of all patients by using a bipolar lead system with the negative electrode near V_5 position. Kaplan and colleagues[94] have shown that no matter what area of heart wall is ischemic (as determined by coronary angiography), the incidence of ST-segment depression in the CM_5 configuration is very similar and the amount or number of collaterals detected by angiography does not alter this process. Therefore, it would appear that ST-segment depression and angina may not occur until the ischemia of the subendocardium has progressed enough to produce a generalized change in subendocardial blood flow. Operating from this frame of reference, it is possible to understand why considerable coronary artery disease may be present without producing ST-segment changes, even with maximum exercise, as long as the integrity of the total system is maintained,[94–96] and also why CM_5 and V_5 have proved to be so useful.

Statements about the inadequacy of lead systems to demonstrate local ischemia imply that even the most minute areas of ischemia would be re-

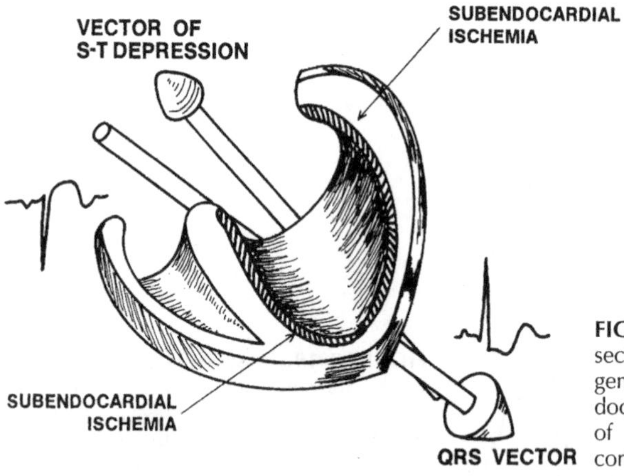

FIGURE 3–20. Schematic cross-section of the heart demonstrating generalized left-ventricular subendocardial ischemia and the vector of ST-segment depression most commonly recorded.

vealed by ST-segment depression if we used sufficient electrodes. There is no doubt that multiple leads identify more diseased patients than a single lead.[97] Selvester and associates,[98] using a computer model of the ECG, have generated data suggesting that subtle changes might always be identifiable, but clinical confirmation has yet to be published. Selvester's recent work in our laboratory suggests that careful analysis of at least 32 leads will identify ischemia now often overlooked. More data on multiple lead systems can be found in Chapter 8. In most cases, the decrease in total myocardial blood flow with its generalized subendocardial changes produces a consistent ECG pattern when the heart is disabled enough to cause a decrease in ventricular compliance and a rise in the diastolic pressure.

ST-SEGMENT ELEVATION

For a long time, ST elevation in leads with Q waves was believed to indicate a scar and an aneurysm.[99,100] Recent work suggests it is more likely that there is a good deal of viable muscle in the area represented.[101] This may even turn out to be a way of detecting "stunned myocardium." It may be that ST elevation reflects transmural ischemia, whereas ST depression is mainly a marker for subendocardial ischemia. This is suggested by the transient ST changes seen in the catheterization laboratory with coronary spasm or during angioplasty when the balloon causes complete closure of the artery being dilated. When no permanent cell death is present and flow is reintroduced, the ECG changes resolve within 1 or 2 minutes, suggesting that transmural or subepicardial ischemia is the usual source of these changes.

In patients with very high-grade proximal left-anterior descending stenosis, ST elevation occurs with exercise in leads with R waves, probably representing a very severe degree of ischemia.[102]

SUMMARY

More than one sequence of events can lead to ST-segment depression. The most common is probably an increase in myocardial oxygen demand in a patient who has a "significant" atheromatous plaque. The magnitude of obstruction by the plaque, combined with obstruction by endothelin-mediated constriction, or failure to adequately dilate during increased demand, results in inadequate perfusion to some or most all segments of the myocardium. This initiates a process in the myocardial cells that inhibits contraction and in some cases the myocardial segment will bulge outward into the pericardial space. The bulge is inhibited by an inelastic pericardium, restricting the diastolic expansion necessary to accommodate the increase in venous inflow.

The diastolic restriction results in a high filling pressure, causing an area of global subendocardial ischemia. This pressure not only starves the subendocardium, but also inhibits antegrade flow, increasing the total coronary resistance. The subendocardial ischemia causes potassium ion to leak out of the cells and produce a current flow toward the endocardium, usually opposite to the mean QRS vector (ST-segment depression).

The same process can be produced by a reduction of coronary flow due to spasm in the endocardial coronary arteries or in the microvasculature. It can also be caused by diastolic restriction due to left-ventricular hypertrophy or constrictive pericarditis. More work needs to be done to establish some of these scenarios, but they seem to fit our current knowledge.

This chapter deals with myocardial ischemia as it pertains to exercise stress testing. For a complete work on the coronary circulation, I recommend the excellent text by Melvin Marcus.[37]

REFERENCES

1. Maseri, A, et al: Coronary artery spasm as a cause of acute myocardial ischemia in man. Chest 68:625, 1975.
2. Maseri, A, et al: "Variant" angina: One aspect of a continuous spectrum of vasospastic myocardial ischemia. Am J Cardiol 42:1019, 1978.
3. Maseri, A, et al: Pathogenic mechanisms of angina pectoris: Expanding view. Br Heart J 43:648, 1980.
4. Schang, SJ, Jr and Pepine, CJ: Transient asymptomatic ST segment depression during daily activity. Am J Cardiol 39:396, 1977.
5. Severi, S, et al: Long-term prognosis of "variant" angina with medical treatment. Am J Cardiol 46:226, 1980.
6. Young, DF, et al: Hemodynamics of arterial stenosis at elevated flow rates. Circ Res 41:99, 1977.
7. Humphries, JO, et al: Natural history of ischemic heart disease in relationship to arteriographic findings. Circulation 49:489, 1974.
8. Zeiher, AM, et al: Modulation of coronary vasomotor tone in humans. Circulation 83:391, 1991.
9. Gordon, JB, et al: Atherosclerosis influences the vasomotor response of epicardial coronary arteries to exercise. J Clin Invest 83:1946, 1989.
10. De Bruyne, B, et al: Abnormal epicardial coronary resistance in patients with diffuse atherosclerosis but « normal » coronary angiography. Circulation 104:2401, 2001.
11. Berne, RM and Rubio, R: Acute coronary occlusion: Early changes that induce coronary dilatation and the development of collateral circulation. Am J Cardiol 24:776, 1969.
12. Schwartz, F, et al: Effect of coronary collaterals on left ventricular function at rest and during stress. Am Heart J 95(5): 570, 1978.
13. Wilson, J, et al: Regional coronary anatomy in rest angina: Comparison of patients with rest and exertional angina using quantitative coronary angiography. Chest 82(4):416, 1982.
14. Elliot, E, et al: Day to day changes in coronary hemodynamics secondary to constriction of circumflex branch of left coronary artery in conscious dogs. Circ Res 22:237, 1968.
15. Schaper, W: The Collateral Circulation of the Heart. American Elsevier Company, New York, 1971.
16. Elliot, E, et al: Direct measurement of coronary collateral blood flow in conscious dogs by an electromagnetic flowmeter. Circ Res 34:374, 1974.
17. Ekstein, R: Effect of exercise and coronary artery narrowing in collateral circulation. Circ Res 5:230, 1967.
18. Schaper, W, et al: Der Einfluss korperlichen Training auf den kollateralkreislauf des herzens. Vereh Dtsch Ges Kreislaufforsch 37:112, 1971.

19. Heaton, W, et al: Beneficial effect of physical training on blood flow to myocardium perfused by chronic collaterals in the exercising dog. Circulation 57:575, 1978.
20. Scheel, K, et al: Effects of exercise on the coronary and collateral vasculature of beagles with and without coronary occlusion. Circ Res 48(4):523, 1981.
21. Burt, J and Jackson, R: The effects of physical exercise on the coronary collateral circulation of dogs. J Sport Med Phys Fit 5:203, 1965.
22. Kaplinsky, E, et al: Effects of physical training in dogs with coronary artery ligation. Circulation 37:556, 1968.
23. Schaper, W, et al: Quantification of collateral resistance in acute and chronic experimental coronary occlusion in the dog. Circ Res 39:371, 1976.
24. Sasayama, S and Fujita, M: Recent insights into coronary collateral circulation. Circulation 85:1197, 1992.
25. Feliciano, L and Henning, RJ. Coronary artery blood flow: Physiologic and pathophysiologic regulation. Clin Cardiol 22(12):775, 1999.
26. MacAlpin, R, et al: Human coronary artery size during life. A cinearteriographic study. Radiology 108:567, 1973.
27. Linzbach, AJ: Heart failure from the point of view of quantitative anatomy. Am J Cardiol 5:370, 1960.
28. Stevenson, JA: Exercise, food intake and health in experimental animals. Can Med Assoc J 96:862, 1967.
29. Marraccini, P, et al: Effects of parasympathetic blockade on ischemic threshold in patients with exercise-induced myocardial ischemia. Am J Cardiol 68:539,1991.
30. Berger, H, et al: Cardiac prostaglandin release during myocardial ischemia induced by atrial pacing in patients with coronary artery disease. Am J Cardiol 39(4):481, 1977.
31. Pitt, B, et al: Prostaglandins and prostaglandin inhibitors in ischemic heart disease. Ann Intern Med 99:83, 1983.
32. Guyton, R, et al: Evolution of regional ischemia distal to a proximal coronary stenosis. Am J Cardiol 40:381, 1977.
33. Uren, NG, et al: Relation between myocardial blood flow and the severity of coronary artery stenosis. New Engl J Med 330(25):1782, 1994.
34. Sambuceti, G, et al: Paradoxical increase in microvascular resistance during tachycardia downstream from a severe stenosis in patients with coronary artery disease. Circulation 103:2352, 2001.
35. Wei, K, et al: Noninvasive quantification of coronary blood flow reserve in humans using myocardial contrast echocardiography. Circulation 103:2560, 2001.
36. Neill, WA and Hattenhauer, M: Impairment of myocardial oxygen supply due to hyperventilation. Circulation 52:854, 1975.
37. Marcus, ML: The Coronary Circulation in Health and Disease. McGraw-Hill, New York, 1983.
38. Wright, C, et al: A method for assessing the physiologic significance of coronary obstructions in man at cardiac surgery. Circulation 62:111, 1980.
39. Opherk, D, et al: Reduction of coronary reserve: A mechanism for angina pectoris in patients with arterial hypertension and normal coronary arteries. Circulation 69(1):1, 1984.
40. Cohen, RA and Shepherd, JT: The inhibitory role of the endothelium in the response of isolated coronary arteries to platelets. Science 221:273, 1983.
41. Sonnenblick, E, et al: Oxygen consumption of the heart: Newer concepts of its multifactorial determination. Am J Cardiol 22:328, 1968.
42. Mann, T, et al: Factors contributing to altered V diastolic properties during angina pectoris. Circulation 59:14, 1979.
43. Castellanet, M, et al: The predictive value of the treadmill stress test in determining postinfarction ischemia. Am J Cardiol 42:24, 1978.
44. Grossman, W and McLaurin, SP: Diastolic properties of the left ventricle. Ann Intern Med 84:316, 1976.
45. Zaret, B, et al: Noninvasive assessment of regional myocardial perfusion with potassium 43 at rest, exercise and during angina pectoris [abstract}. Circulation 46(suppl 11):18, 1972.
46. Buckberg, GD, et al: Some sources of error in measuring regional blood flow with radioactive microspheres. J Appl Physiol 31:598, 1971.
47. Barnard, JR, et al: Ischemic response to sudden strenuous exercise in healthy men. Circulation 48:936, 1973.
48. Gregg, DE: Physiology of the coronary circulation. Circulation 27:1128, 1962.

49. Saltin, B and Astrand, O: Maximal oxygen uptake in athletes. J Applied Physiol 23:353, 1967.
50. Bouchard, R, et al: Evaluation of pulmonary arterial end diastolic pressure as an estimate of left ventricular end diastolic pressure in patients with normal and abnormal left ventricular performance. Circulation 44:1072, 1971.
51. Myers, B, et al: Correlation of electrocardiographic and pathologic findings in ringlike subendocardial infarction of the left ventricle. Am J Med Sci 222:417, 1951.
52. Ellestad, MH, et al: Maximal treadmill stress testing for cardiovascular evaluation. One year follow-up of physically active and inactive men. Circulation 39:517, 1969.
53. Wang, TG, et al: Central blood volume during upright exercise in normal subjects [abstract]. Fed Proc 21:124, 1962.
54. Case, R, et al: Biochemical aspects of early myocardial ischemia. Am J Cardiol 24:766, 1969.
55. Epstein, SE, et al: Angina pectoris: Pathophysiology, evaluation, and treatment. Ann Intern Med 75:263, 1971.
56. Fogelman, AM, et al: Echocardiographic study of the abnormal motion of the posterior left ventricular wall during angina pectoris. Circulation 46:905, 1972.
57. Barry, WH, et al: Analysis of ventricular compliance curves following pacing induced angina. Circulation 46(suppl 11):483, 1972.
58. Cohn, PF: Maximal rate of pressure fall (peak negative Dp/Dt) during ventricular relaxation. Cardiovasc Res 6:263, 1972.
59. Mathey, D, et al: Left ventricular relaxation and diastolic stiffness in experimental myocardial infarction. Cardiovasc Res 8:583, 1974.
60. Lichten, P: The hemodynamics of clinical ischemic heart disease. Ann Clin Res 3:333, 1971.
61. Langer, GA: Ionic Movements and the Control of Contraction: The Mammalian Myocardium. John Wiley & Sons, New York, 1974.
62. Rerych, SK, et al: Cardiac function at rest and during exercise in normals and in patients with coronary artery disease. Ann Surg 187:449, 1978.
63. Sharma, B and Taylor, SH: Localization of left ventricular ischemia in angina pectoris by cineangiography during exercise. Br Heart J 37:963, 1975.
64. Katz, AM and Tada, M: The "stone heart": A challenge to the biochemist. Am J Cardiol 29:578, 1972.
65. Bing, OH, et al: Tension prolongation during recovery from myocardial hypoxia. J Clin Invest 50:660, 1971.
66. Hillis, LD and Braunwald, E: Myocardial ischemia. N Engl J Med 296:971, 1977.
67. Regan, TJ, et al: Myocardial ischemia and cell acidosis: Modification by alkali and the effects on ventricular function and cation composition. Am J Cardiol 37:501, 1976.
68. Hearse, DJ, et al: Ischemic contracture of the myocardium: Mechanisms and prevention. Am J Cardiol 39:986, 1977.
69. Waters, DD, et al: Early changes in regional and global left ventricular function induced by graded reductions in regional coronary perfusion. Am J Cardiol 39:537, 1977.
70. Braunwald, E, et al: Studies on Starling's law of the heart. Circ Res 8:1254, 1960.
71. Tyberg, JV and Smith, ER: Ventricular diastole and the role of the pericardium. Herz 15(6):354, 1990.
72. Kass, DA, et al: Influence of coronary occlusion during PTCA on end systolic and end diastolic pressure-volume relations in humans. Circulation 81:447, 1990.
73. Janicki, JA: Influence of the pericardium and ventricular interdependence on left ventricular diastolic and systolic function in patients with heart failure. Circulation 81(suppl 3):3-16, 1990.
74. Masumi, K, et al: False positive exercise test due to constrictive pericarditis. Am J Noninvas Cardiol 8:47-50, 1994.
75. Myrianthiefs, M, et al: Significance of signal averaged P-wave changes during exercise in patients with coronary artery disease. Am J Cardiol 68:1619, 1991.
76. Clausen, JP, et al: Physical training in the management of coronary artery disease. Circulation 40:143, 1969.
77. Katz, L and Landt, H: The effect of standardized exercise on the four-lead electrocardiogram. Its value in study of coronary disease. Am J Med Sci 189:346, 1935.
78. Buchsbaum, MS, et al: Opiate pharmacology and individual differences. I. Psychophysical pain measurements. Pain 10:357, 1981.
79. Buchsbaum, MS, et al: Opiate pharmacology and individual differences. II Somatosensory evoked potentials. Pain 10:367, 1981.

80. Ellestad, MH and Kuan, P. Naloxone and asymptomatic ischemia. Failure to induce angina during exercise testing. Am J Cardiol 54:982, 1984.
81. Staszewski-Barczaks, J, et al: An excitatory nociceptive cardiac reflex elicited by bradykinin and potentiated by prostaglandins and myocardial ischemia. Cardiovasc Res 10:314, 1976.
82. Droste, C and Roskamm, H: Experimental pain measurement in patients with asymptomatic myocardial ischemia. J. Am Coll Cardiol 1:940, 1983.
83. Cohn, PF: Silent myocardial ischemia in patients with defective anginal warning system. Am J Cardiol 45:697, 1980.
84. Covell, JW, et al: Effects of acutely induced ischemic heart failure on myocardial high energy phosphate stores. Proc Soc Exp Biol Med 124:131, 1967.
85. Bourassa, MG, et al: Myocardial lactate metabolism at rest and during exercise in ischemic heart disease. Am J Cardiol 23:771, 1969.
86. Liedtke, AJ and Nellis, SH: Effects of carnitine in ischemic and fatty acid supplemented swine hearts. J Clin Invest 64:440, 1979.
87. Thomsen, JH, et al: Improved pacing tolerance of the ischemic human myocardium after administration of carnitine. Am J Cardiol 43:300, 1979.
88. Taegtmeyer, H: Metabolism—The lost child of cardiology: J Am Coll Cardiol 36(4):1386, 2000.
89. Oliver, MF, et al: Effect of reducing circulating free fatty acids on ventricular arrhythmias during myocardial infarction and on S-T segment depression during exercise-induced ischemia. Circulation 53(3;suppl 1):210, 1976.
90. Harumi, K, et al: Ventricular recovery time changes during and after temporary coronary occlusion [abstract]. Am J Cardiol 25:26, 1970.
91. Sodi-Pallares, E, et al: Polyparametric electrocardiography concerning new information obtained from clinical electrocardiogram. Prog Cardiovasc Dis 13:97, 1970.
92. Hellerstein, HK and Katz, L: The electrical effects of injury at various myocardial locations. Am Heart J 36:184, 1948.
93. Blackburn, H, et al: The exercise electrocardiogram during exercise: Findings in bipolar chest leads of 1449 middle aged men at moderate work levels. Circulation 34:1034, 1966.
94. Kaplan, MA, et al: Inability of the submaximal stress test to predict the location of coronary disease. Circulation 47:250, 1973.
95. Blomqvist, CG: Use of exercise testing for diagnostic and functional evaluation of patients with arteriosclerotic heart disease. Circulation 44:1120, 1971.
96. Tucker, SC, et al: Multiple lead ECG submaximal treadmill exercise tests. Angiology 27:149, 1976.
97. Kornreich, F, et al: Discriminant analysis of the standard 12 lead ECG for diagnosing non-Q wave infarction. J Electrocardiography 24(suppl), 1991.
98. Selvester, RH, et al: Find grid computer simulation of QRST-T and criteria for the quantitation of regional ischemia. J Electrocardiology (suppl Oct) 1–8, 1987.
99. Manvi, KN, et al: Elevated S-T segments with exercise in ventricular aneurysm. J Electrocardiol 5:317, 1972.
100. Simonson, E: Electrocardiographic stress tolerance tests. Prog Cardiovasc Dis 13:269, 1970.
101. Morgonato, A and Capelletti, A: Exercise induced ST elevation on infarct related leads: A marker of residual viability. Circulation (suppl 1):86:1, 1992.
102. Chaitman, BR, et al: Improved efficiency of treadmill exercise testing using a multiple lead system and basic hemodynamic response. Circulation 57:71, 1978.

4
Indications

Evaluation of Patients with Chest Pain
Prognosis and Severity of Disease
Evaluation of Therapy
Screening for Latent Coronary Disease
Early Detection of Labile Hypertension
Evaluation of Patients with Congestive Heart Failure
Evaluation of Arrhythmias
Evaluation of Functional Capacity
Congenital Heart Disease and Valvular Dysfunction
Stimulus to Motivate Change in Lifestyle
Sports Medicine

During the heyday of the Master's test, stress testing was primarily used to identify or confirm the presence of ischemic heart disease. Prior to World War II, it was mainly a research tool applied to problems related to exercise in athletes. More recently, as the method again evolved into a measure of functional capacity as well as a means of diagnosing coronary disease, the applications have been extended to a number of areas previously excluded, such as the prognosis in coronary artery disease and the evaluation of treatment in congestive heart failure, stable angina, and certain arrhythmias.

In spite of the occasional editorials and articles criticizing the usefulness of exercise testing, there has been an enormous increase in its use as cardiologists and other physicians have discovered how helpful stress testing can be in patient management.[1,2] This chapter lists some of the indications for stress testing and attempts to add perspective to the present controversy.

Coronary artery disease has reached epidemic proportions. Not only does the death rate average about 600,000 a year in the United States, but it also exceeds all other causes of death. Death or a myocardial infarction is the first symptom in 55% of patients with coronary heart disease. An enormous amount of energy is being expended in a search for the cause and a way to control this malignant process. Although it would be desirable to be able to map and quantitate the evolution of plaques in the coronary tree, an acceptable noninvasive means of doing this is not yet available. Recent reports on imaging calcium in the coronary tree suggest that this may be one method,[3] and magnetic resonance imaging also holds some promise. Although the stress test is far from perfect, it has emerged as the most practical means of uncovering latent disease, and even though the coronary obstructive lesions may have to reach 50% or more in one vessel to reduce flow significantly, most such lesions are probably still asymptomatic as far as the patient is concerned.[4] The study in dogs by Wegria and associates[5] suggests that blood flow must be reduced 75% before changes are routinely seen in the ECG.

Kaplan and associates[6] reported on the correlation of stress tests and coronary angiograms in 200 subjects. They found that 19 (9.5%) had positive tests, but a few had no more than 25% narrowing in a single artery. It must be concluded that some of these stenotic lesions were underestimated, but it points to the usefulness of the test in some patients with mild degrees of stenosis. Work by Marcus[7] illustrates the difficulty in predicting the metabolic significance from the coronary angiogram, suggesting the importance of a dynamic measure of function. Although an abnormal exercise test has definite predictive value, many plaques that are not "flow limiting" may rupture and produce unstable coronary syndromes or even sudden death.[8] Eventually, some noninvasive method to detect these "time bombs" will become available.

There are many forms of stress testing, such as the well-known polygraph or lie detector, the anoxia test, and the use of an isometric handgrip. Several of these will be reviewed, but this chapter will concentrate on the common indications for exercise testing, which include:

- Evaluation of the patient with chest pain or with other findings suggestive of, but not diagnostic of, coronary disease
- Determination of prognosis and severity of disease
- Evaluation of the effects of medical and surgical therapy
- Screening for latent coronary disease
- Early detection of labile hypertension
- Evaluation of congestive heart failure
- Evaluation of arrhythmias
- Evaluation of functional capacity and formulation of an exercise prescription
- Evaluation of congenital heart disease
- Stimulus to a change in lifestyle

EVALUATION OF PATIENTS WITH CHEST PAIN

If the pain pattern is suspicious, but not classic for angina, the presence or absence of disease can often be established by a maximum stress test. Although there is a significant percentage of false-negatives when compared with coronary angiography (depending on what is considered significant disease), the reliability depends on the magnitude and time of onset of the ST changes, on the heart rate and blood pressure response, and very importantly, on the prevalence of disease in the population under study. The influence of prevalence on the reliability of the ST-segment change is discussed in more detail in "Bayesian Analysis," Chapter 14. Suffice it to say that in patients with chest discomfort selected because they are clinically apt to have coronary disease, exercise testing remains one of the more practical approaches to diagnosis, especially when using a number of parameters in combination with ST changes.

PROGNOSIS AND SEVERITY OF DISEASE

Numerous studies have confirmed that severity of disease, which is a major factor in prognosis, can be estimated with considerable accuracy with exercise testing.[9,10] The details are presented in Chapter 14; however, it must again be emphasized that a clinical approach, considering multiple variables along with the presence of the ST changes, will provide insight into the future course of the patient's disease process. In the past few years, evidence points to the fact that the heart rate response during exercise[11] and during recovery,[12] maximum exercise time,[13] and frequency of ventricular ectopy are also predictors of coronary events.[14]

EVALUATION OF THERAPY

An objective method of evaluating therapy in coronary disease is essential. The sham operation for internal mammary ligation established dramatically how difficult it is to evaluate coronary disease by depending on the patient's reported symptoms. A good stress testing protocol should measure the patient's relative myocardial blood flow, onset of ST depression in terms of the work applied, and aerobic capacity before and after treatment. Knowledge of this type can give us much more useful information than just asking patients how they feel. Because it is known that a myocardial infarction will terminate angina, it certainly follows that the presence or absence of pain is often a rather crude and misleading indicator of coronary disease.

One of the logical applications is the evaluation of coronary patients before and after surgery and angioplasty. Stuart and Ellestad[15] and others[16,17] report that stress testing has considerable value in predicting postoperative graft patency, but a certain amount of caution is indicated. When various medical regimens rather than invasive approaches have been instituted, the test will also be helpful. Cardiotoxic agents such as doxorubicin (Adriamycin) are being used more frequently, and stress testing provides an evaluation of these effects.

SCREENING FOR LATENT CORONARY DISEASE

It was once believed that significant coronary disease usually produces angina and that a good historian can typically elicit evidence of this process during a complete medical workup by questioning the patient about chest pain. As noted in Chapter 3, however, our data indicate that only about 30% of those with ischemia have concurrent chest pain.[18] When symptoms of typical angina are described by the patient, coronary disease can be predicted with considerable reliability, but when no history of pain is present, there is still a strong possibility of significant narrowing in the coronary tree in patients with appropriate risk factors.

The exact reliability of the positive stress test in predicting coronary disease is discussed in detail in Chapter 14, but using ST-segment changes alone, it is at least twice as useful as a high cholesterol level or any of the other risk factors usually mentioned. It could in some cases be one of the clues to the presence of unsuspected coronary narrowing, even though the false-positive rate in most asymptomatic groups is high.

Figure 4–1 illustrates the relative capacity of the stress test to predict coronary events among the various risk factors used in the Framingham study,[19] compared with the stress test.[20,21] Chapter 14 discusses how the reliability of the test in asymptomatic persons is reduced because of the lower prevalence of the disease. In spite of the inherent limitations, the stress test remains a useful, cost-effective approach in evaluating asymptomatic individuals believed to be at risk. Once an abnormal test has been discovered, appropriate follow-up studies can be instituted to confirm the results and identify appropriate therapy.

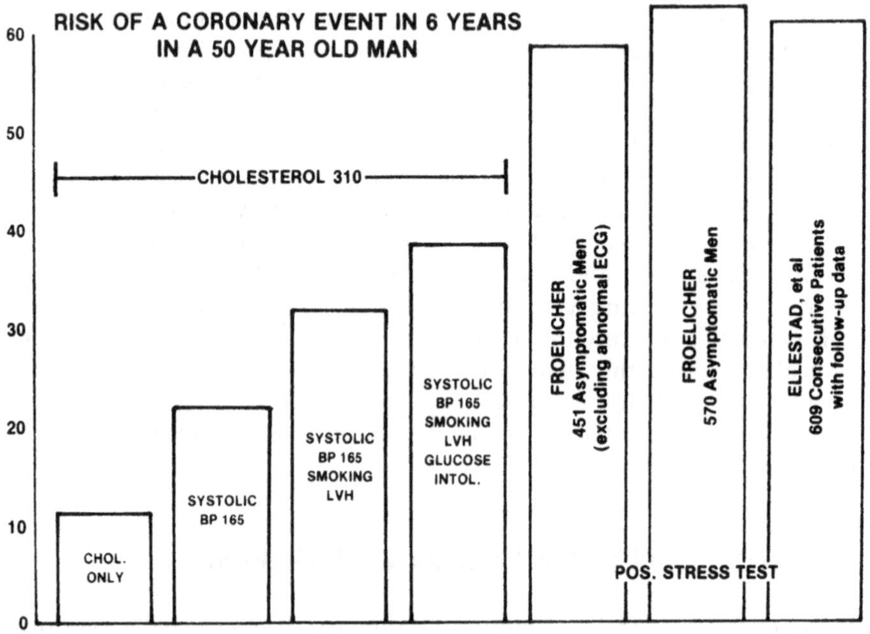

FIGURE 4–1. Graph of the relative capacity to predict coronary events among the various risk factors used in the Framingham study as compared with the stress test.

EARLY DETECTION OF LABILE HYPERTENSION

The normal response to exercise is an increase in blood pressure. Experience has taught us the range of responses seen in a normal population (see Appendix). Several studies have demonstrated that an unusually high pressure in persons who are normotensive at rest suggests that they may become hypertensive in the future.[22] This finding may be predictive even in teenagers.[23]

EVALUATION OF PATIENTS WITH CONGESTIVE HEART FAILURE

Until recently, congestive heart failure was considered an absolute contraindication to exercise testing. A number of workers have used this approach to try to understand functional changes, to establish mechanisms, and to measure response to therapy.[24,25] At this time, exercise testing is being used more and more to evacuate severity and determine benefit from the new therapeutic interventions being developed.

EVALUATION OF ARRHYTHMIAS

Many rhythm disturbances are initiated by exercise, and it is very important to document them. It is also important to establish that some abnormalities in rhythm are terminated by exercise. When we treat an arrhythmia that is influenced by exercise, we are deluding ourselves if we believe that the efficacy of the therapy can be determined by observing the patient only at rest. The significance of exercise-induced arrhythmias on the ability to predict future events in coronary patients has been determined and is reviewed in Chapter 13. The presence of exercise-induced arrhythmias also becomes an important public health issue when the arrhythmias develop in subjects engaged in hazardous activities or occupations in which coordination and alert performance affect the lives of others. Young and colleagues[26] have used the symptom-limited exercise test routinely to evaluate malignant arrhythmias referred to their group.

EVALUATION OF FUNCTIONAL CAPACITY

One of the most important decisions a physician must make in the case of a patient who has angina or who has had a myocardial infarction is how much exercise the patient can tolerate. Testing 2 to 3 weeks after a myocardial infarction has been established as a safe and useful adjunct to patient management. If the patient has a strenuous job, this is especially critical. All too often, the patient's physician is inclined to be conservative and insists on

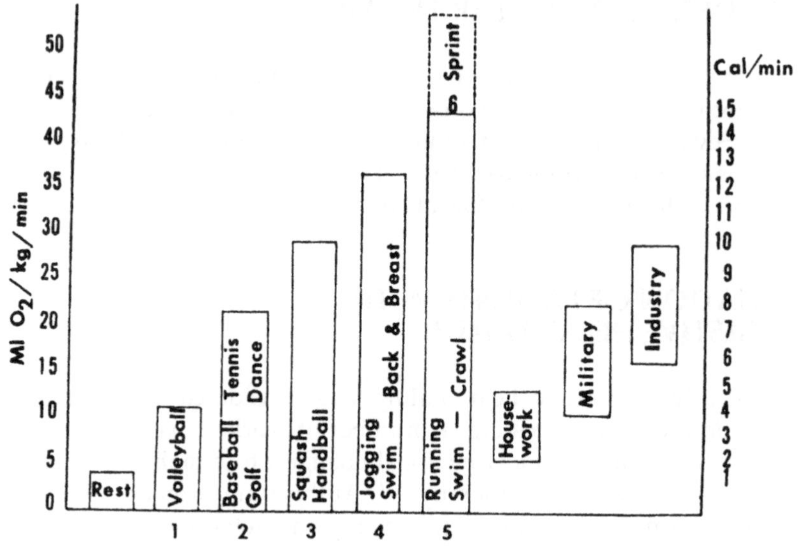

FIGURE 4–2. Various types of exercise presented in relation to oxygen uptake in milliliters per kilogram of body weight and calories expended per minute. (Adapted from classification schema of Wells, Balke, and Van Fossan by Falls, HB. In J SC Med Assoc [suppl], December 1969.)

restrictions based on an unsubstantiated guess rather than on hard data. There is no substitute for watching the patient exercise. The next best thing is to have a detailed report from someone knowledgeable in exercise physiology who has watched the subject exercise.

It is also important to be able to advise patients with coronary insufficiency, either latent or manifest, about how much exercise they can do during their leisure time or in some anticipated new endeavor requiring a higher degree of stress. Good data are available as guides to the metabolic demands for various occupations and sports.[27] From a properly designed stress test, the response can be translated into a proper exercise prescription (Fig. 4–2).

The ability to predict a patient's aerobic capacity is now well established, and this knowledge can be useful in noncardiac conditions as well as in those with valvular and other forms of noncoronary cardiac disability.[21]

The cardiac rehabilitation unit was formulated on the concept that a safe exercise prescription can be predicated on the results of the stress test. This is being expanded to patients who have had coronary bypass surgery and angioplasty as well as angina and a previous myocardial infarction.

CONGENITAL HEART DISEASE AND VALVULAR DYSFUNCTION

The management of children with congenital heart disease is being determined after function as well as anatomy has been considered. Stress testing has been especially useful in congenital aortic stenosis[28] and in studying postoperative patients with tetralogy and other complex defects[29,30] (see Chapter 21).

One of the most difficult decisions in cardiology is deciding when to replace damaged valves. Exercise testing provides invaluable guidelines. This is especially true in aortic and mitral insufficiency when it is used in conjunction with nuclear blood pool imaging.

STIMULUS TO MOTIVATE CHANGE IN LIFESTYLE

One of the most serious problems in our sedentary population or in those with coronary disease is the need to motivate patients to stop smoking, to follow a diet, to exercise regularly, and to make other necessary changes in their lifestyles. Because the results associated with such changes in their habit patterns are not readily apparent to them, a stimulus of some sort is often needed. The patient's performance on a stress test often serves just such a function. In our cardiac rehabilitation program, the stress test response is explained to the patient, and its meaning in regard to progress often motivates cooperation not otherwise forthcoming. This has been the experience of cardiac rehabilitation units across the country.

SPORTS MEDICINE

Over the years, there has been more and more research in exercise physiology in sports medicine.[31–33] In a large number of these reports, exercise testing plays an indispensable role. A significant segment of the new information in exercise testing is now coming from this sector. As fitness becomes more and more of an obsession in our culture, the stress test emerges as a useful method for measuring this parameter. This is often desirable prior to sports training, so that a baseline may be established in order to judge the efficacy of a certain program.

SUMMARY

Albert Kattus who wrote the Foreword to the first edition of this book, stated "we have progressed beyond the take it easy mentality and realize the importance of evaluating cardiovascular function during exercise as well as rest." The indications discussed here will undoubtedly be expanded in future years including its use in the field of pediatric cardiology and congestive heart failure. The work by Marcus[7] and others emphasizes that even the coronary angiogram needs to be correlated with functional testing to provide the information needed to make sound clinical decisions.

REFERENCES

1. Borer, JS, et al: Limitations of the electrocardiographic to exercise in predicting coronary artery disease. N Engl J Med 293:367, 1975.
2. Redwood, DR, et al: Whither the ST segment during exercise. Circulation 54:703, 1976.
3. Janowitz, WR, et al: Comparison of serial quantitative evaluation of calcified coronary artery plaque by ultrafast computed tomography in persons with and without obstructive coronary artery disease. Am J Cardiol 68:1, 1991.
4. Astrand, I: Exercise electrocardiograms recorded twice with an 8-year interval in a group of 204 women and men 48–63 years old. Acta Med Scand 118:27, 1965.
5. Wegria, R, et al: Relationship between reduction in coronary flow and appearance of electrocardiographic changes. Am Heart J 38:90, 1949.
6. Kaplan, MA, et al: Inability of the submaximal treadmill stress test to predict the location of coronary disease. Circulation 47:250, 1973.
7. Marcus, ML: The Coronary Circulation in Health and Disease. McGraw-Hill, New York, 1983.
8. Taubes, G: Does inflammation cut to the heart of the matter. Science April:242, 2002.
9. Dagenais, GR, et al: Survival of patients with a strongly positive exercise electrocardiogram. Circulation 65(3):452, 1982.
10. Goldschlager, N, et al: Treadmill stress tests as indicators of presence and severity of coronary artery disease. Ann Intern Med 85:277, 1976.
11. Lauer, MS, et al. Impaired heart rate response to graded exercise: prognostic implications of chronotropic incompetence in the Framingham Heart Study. Circulation 93:1520, 1996.
12. Cole, CR, et al. Heart rate recovery following submaximal exercise testing as a predictor of mortality in a healthy cohort. Ann Internal Med 132:552, 2000.
13. Myers, J, et al: Exercise capacity and mortality among men preferred for exercise testing. New Engl J of Med 346 (11):793, 2002.
14. Jouven, X, et al: Long-term outcome in asymptomatic men with exercise-induced premature ventricular depolarizations. N Engl J Med 343:826, 2000
15. Stuart, RJ and Ellestad, MH: Postoperative stress testing. Angiology 30:416, 1979.
16. Assad-Morell, JL, et al: Aorta-coronary artery saphenous vein bypass surgery: Clinical and angiographic results. Mayo Clin Proc 50:379, 1975.
17. Frick, MH, et al: Persistent improvement after coronary bypass surgery: Ergometric and angiographic correlations at 5 years. Circulation 67(3):491, 1983.
18. Kemp, GL and Ellestad, MH: The incidence of -silent+ coronary heart disease. Calif Med 109:363, 1968.
19. Kannel, WB (ed): Framingham Study: An Epidemiological Investigation of Cardiovascular Disease. Pub National Heart, Lung and Blood Institute. 1948 to present.
20. Ellestad, MH and Wan, MCK: Predictive implication of stress testing. Circulation 51:363, 1975.
21. Froelicher, VF, et al: The correlation of coronary angiography and the electrocardiographic response to maximal treadmill testing in asymptomatic persons. Circulation 48:597, 1973.
22. Olin, RA, et al: Follow-up of normotensive men with exaggerated blood pressure response to exercise. Am Heart J 106(2):31, 1983.
23. Kannel, WB, et al: Labile hypertension. A faulty concept. Circulation 61:1183, 1980.
24. Franciosa, JA: Exercise testing in chronic congestive heart failure. Am J Cardiol 53:1447, 1984.
25. Kramer, BL, et al: Controlled trial of captopril in chronic heart failure: A rest and exercise hemodynamic study. Circulation 67:807, 1983.
26. Young, DZ, et al: Safety of maximal exercise testing in patients at high risk for ventricular arrhythmia. Circulation 70:184, 1984.
27. Thompson, PD. Exercise and Sports Cardiology. McGraw-Hill, 2001.
28. Bruce, RA, et al: Maximal oxygen intake and nomographic assessment of functional aerobic impairment in cardiovascular disease. Am Heart J 85:546, 1973.
29. James, FW and Koplan, S: Exercise testing in children. Prim Cardiol 3:34, 1977.
30. Strieder, DJ, et al: Exercise tolerance after repair of tetralogy of Fallot. Am Thorac Surg 19:397, 1975.
31. Corquiglini, S (ed): Biomechanics III. Medicine and Sport, Vol. 8. Karger, Basel, 1971.
32. Keul, et al. (eds): Energy metabolism of human muscle. Medicine and Sport, Vol. 7. Karger, Basel, 1972.
33. Wilson, PK (ed): Adult Fitness and Cardiac Rehabilitation. University Park Press, Baltimore, 1976.

5

Contraindications, Risks, and Safety Precautions

When Not to Stress (Absolute Contraindications)
Relative Contraindications
Aortic Stenosis
Suspected Left Main Equivalent
Severe Hypertension
Idiopathic Hypertrophic Subaortic Stenosis and Asymmetrical Septal Hypertrophy
Severe ST-Segment Depression at Rest
Congestive Heart Failure
When to Terminate the Exercise Test
Indications for Test Termination: Comments
Submaximal Target Heart Rates
ST-Segment Elevation
Equipment and Supplies Necessary to Test Safely
Drugs
Defibrillator
Management During the Postexercise Period
Case Histories of Patients Who Died
Discussion
Risks Reported in the Literature
Legal Implications

A good deal of controversy has occurred over the safety of exercise in various population groups. Because Americans have gone on a health binge, with millions jogging and entering in organized runs, some understanding of the risks involved warrant discussion. Some of these same issues pertain to the prescribing of exercise and exercise testing. Shephard,[1] of the University of Toronto, has taken the position that a certain level of risk is involved in initiating an exercise program for a sedentary asymptomatic middle-aged man. He advises against an exercise test because of the evidence that a high percentage of abnormal electrocardiographic (ECG) stress tests are false-positives in this population, and he believes the information may lead to other unnecessary tests, such as angiography.

The American Heart Committee on Exercise,[2] however, recommends stress testing prior to the initiation of exercise programs in normals older than 40 years of age or in others with risk factors for coronary artery disease. Fletcher and colleagues[3] and others[4–7] concur in this decision. Data from the Seattle Heart Watch study[8] clearly indicate that in asymptomatic persons with two or more risk factors, stress testing can identify a cohort with a risk of a coronary event at least 15 times greater than the negative responders. Such a group warrants careful scrutiny to determine the presence of a life-threatening process. If exercise testing is used in these subjects, or in cardiac patients in general, safety is an important aspect of the procedure.

The most important safety factor in stress testing is a knowledgeable and experienced physician in charge. Knowing when to stop and when not to start a stress test requires considerable knowledge and experience with exercise physiology, cardiology, and ECG. This experience and knowledge are essential for the physician undertaking the risk of exercising cardiac patients. On the other hand, even maximum testing is safe if the physician follows available guidelines after receiving some degree of training and experience.[9,10] Verbal but unpublished reports of deaths occurring with enthusiastic untrained novices come to us frequently.

A reasonable knowledge of the patient's medical history and present problems is essential. A fairly good idea of the patient's capacity to exercise can be obtained when this information is combined with auscultation of the heart and inspection of the resting ECG. Then, careful observation of the patient's response to the early stages of the exercise protocol can alert the physician to potential dangers so that steps can be taken to avoid harm.

WHEN NOT TO STRESS (ABSOLUTE CONTRAINDICATIONS)

It is generally agreed that stress testing should not be done on the following patients:

1. Patients with an acute myocardial infarction.
2. Patients suffering from acute myocarditis or pericarditis.
3. Patients exhibiting signs of unstable progressive angina. This includes the patient who has long periods of angina of fairly recent onset while at rest. (Note commentary following.)
4. Patients with rapid ventricular or atrial arrhythmias at the time of the test.
5. Patients with second- or third-degree heart block and patients with known severe left main disease.
6. Acutely ill patients, such as those with infections, hyperthyroidism, or severe anemia.
7. Patients with locomotion problems.
8. Severe symptomatic aortic stenosis.

Over the years, exercise was believed to be dangerous in certain conditions, which led to the above list of absolute contraindications to exercise testing. Some contraindications may be justified by common sense; others, such as unstable angina, by experience. But every so often one of the absolutes is moved to the list of relative contraindications. This has happened to both aortic stenosis and congestive heart failure, and may happen to left main coronary disease and various types of heart block before long. Thus, the preceding list outlines the current consensus but may change as new knowledge is accumulated.

Some evidence suggests that unstable angina may be relegated to the list of relative contraindications, but this will require complete agreement on the definition of this entity. There has been a trend toward exercising patients who come to the emergency room with chest pain syndromes, many of whom are classified as having unstable angina. For example, if these patients have no enzyme or ECG evidence of a myocardial infarction, an exercise test is used to decide whether it is safe to send them home. Keep in mind that if there is resting evidence of ischemia, great caution should be used.

Concepts regarding the risks of stress testing are evolving, and I recommend that such testing be done only in a hospital where much stress testing is carried out.

RELATIVE CONTRAINDICATIONS

Aortic Stenosis

Early reports of cardiac arrest from stress testing in patients with aortic stenosis resulted in a cautious approach in patients with this valvular lesion. The following guidelines should be applied. If the auscultatory findings, clinical symptoms, and laboratory data suggest very high grade stenosis in adults, stress testing should be avoided. This is particularly true if there is a history of synchope. In adults with moderate valvular disease, it can be a very useful procedure with an acceptable risk when used cautiously. (We have never had a serious problem with a patient with aortic stenosis.) In children, stress testing has been found to be useful and safe (see Chapter 21).

Suspected Left Main Equivalent

Because we frequently fail to identify this lesion before the stress test and discover later what we have done, considerable experience is necessary. Most patients tolerate the test safely but have a limited exercise capacity. Our practice is to withhold stress testing if we have knowledge that the left main lesion is greater than 70% or if there is left main equivalent (very high grade proximal obstruction in all branches of the left coronary artery). One of our deaths was in a patient with left main disease.

Severe Hypertension

If the patient has severe resting hypertension (240/130) requiring multiple medications, the test should be withheld or used with extreme caution. The clinical status, such as history of stroke, carotid bruits, age, and heart size must be taken into consideration. If hypertension can be brought under control with medication, the exercise testing may be done with safety.

Idiopathic Hypertrophic Subaortic Stenosis and Asymmetrical Septal Hypertrophy

In conditions in which outflow obstruction may be severe, caution is important. Sudden death after exercise occasionally occurs even in young patients, regardless of the degree of obstruction.[11]

Severe ST-Segment Depression at Rest

In a patient with a history of angina who is not on digitalis, ST-segment depression at rest should be viewed with caution because it may indicate severe subendocardial ischemia. Such a patient failed to tolerate a stress test in our laboratory, and I have reviewed other case reports (see "Case 3"). If these patients with ST-segment depression at rest are tested, it should be done with extreme caution.

Congestive Heart Failure

Patients with basal rales and leg edema who are being evaluated for ischemia as a rule should not be tested until they are compensated; however, the evaluation of patients with compensated heart failure is often helpful in regulating their exercise schedule. Recent studies on patients with congestive heart failure have been accomplished without complications.[12] (See Chapter 16.)

WHEN TO TERMINATE THE EXERCISE TEST

In a patient with known or suspected heart disease, the physician or trained technician administering the exercise test must continually observe the patient and the monitor and have the ability to record the ECG on paper for further analysis. The ECG printout is often more informative than the image on the oscilloscope and must be available for immediate inspection. The proper application of electrodes and the capacity to filter the signal are also very important. In addition, some filtering designed to minimize baseline wandering may eliminate the ST-segment depression. Details on electrical filtering and standards for ECG equipment are discussed in Chapter 8.

It is generally agreed by most workers in the field that the test should be terminated when:

1. Premature ventricular contractions (PVCs) develop in pairs or with increasing frequency as exercise increases, or when ventricular tachycardia develops (runs of four or more PVCs).
2. Atrial tachycardia, atrial fibrillation, or atrial flutter supervenes.

3. There is onset of heart block, either second or third degree.
4. Anginal pain is progressive (grade 3 pain if grade 4 is the most severe in patient's experience).
5. ST-segment depression has become severe. Some would terminate with 3 mm or more, but if the patient looks good and feels good and has no history of severe angina, it has been safe in our experience to proceed with changes of greater magnitude. On the other hand, the Joint Committee of the American Heart Association and the American College of Cardiology in their recommended standards, published in 1997, suggest termination if the ST-segment depression is greater than 2 mm. We have found that when the magnitude of the ST depression is increasing rapidly at low workloads, it is safer to terminate when ST depression begins to exceed 2 mm.
6. ST depression is present at rest and there is a progressive increase in ischemia with modest exercise.
7. ST elevation is 2 mm or more in precordial or inferior leads that do not have a resting Q wave.
8. The heart rate or systolic blood pressure drops progressively in the face of continuing exercise.
9. The patient is unable to continue because of dyspnea, fatigue, or feeling of faintness.
10. Musculoskeletal pain becomes severe, such as might occur with arthritis or claudication.
11. The patient looks vasoconstricted—pale and clammy.
12. Extreme elevations occur in systolic and diastolic blood pressures associated with a headache or blurred vision.
13. The patient has reached or exceeded the predicted maximum pulse rate. In this case, one can be satisfied that the patient has performed satisfactorily. However, if the subject is able and willing to continue, it is safe to proceed in the absence of other indications for termination.
14. Equipment problems exist, such as loss of ECG on monitor.

Patients should understand that they can stop voluntarily but are encouraged to try to reach or exceed maximum predicted heart rate.

INDICATIONS FOR TEST TERMINATION: COMMENTS

Submaximal Target Heart Rates

Many investigators in this field discontinue the exercise test at some arbitrary heart rate less than maximum capacity.[13,14] Some use the heart rate of 150 beats per minute for all patients.[15] Some use 75%, 80%, or 90% of maximum predicted heart rate.[16] Any arbitrary cutoff, when not adjusted for age, must be recognized as being unphysiological just as is any predetermined load, such as 150 or 200 watts on the bicycle. Stopping short of maximum heart rate is safer, and the available support for this is presented. In our laboratory, the predicted rate seems to be a safe target but is often exceeded in fit patients. If a predetermined heart rate is used, the ability to estimate aerobic capacity is lost.

ST-Segment Elevation

After exercise is under way, some patients develop ST-segment elevation. In the absence of a previous infarction, this pattern in the anterior precordial leads usually indicates ischemia involving the total thickness of the myocardium rather than just a subendocardial problem.[17] When seen, it is almost always associated with a high-grade obstruction in the proximal left anterior descending coronary artery. If exercise persists, infarction may be imminent, and it would be wise to terminate the test. Sheffield and associates[14] describe a patient with a history suggesting variant angina who had resting ST-segment elevation reverting to normal on exercise. Shortly after the test, the patient sustained an anterior wall infarction. They believe that ST-segment elevation should be treated with extreme caution.

ST-segment elevation in leads reflecting a previous infarction need not generate too much concern but usually reflects dyskinesia and some myocardial scarring. It also reflects ischemia in the myocardium adjacent to the scar and may be a way of identifying a hibernating myocardium.[18] ST-segment elevation on the anterior/posterior lead, either V1 or V2 or the orthogonal Z, may reflect subendocardial changes in the septum and should be considered equivalent to ST-segment depression in other leads.[3] Over the years cardiac arrest in the stress lab comes with ST elevation more often than with any other EKG abnormality. The concepts presented here are in accord with the recommendations of the exercise testing guidelines.[19]

EQUIPMENT AND SUPPLIES NECESSARY TO TEST SAFELY

Although it is generally stated that the Master's test, which requires only a modest workload, is associated with no significant risk, two of the three patients who died in our laboratory exhibited problems at a workload commensurate with the double Master's test. Therefore, it is strongly urged that all stress testing be done in a setting where emergencies can be treated efficiently and expeditiously. Monitoring should be continuous. If, for some reason, interference caused by muscle artifact, lead dislodgement, or the battery effect of the electrode-skin interface produces an uninterpretable tracing, the test should be terminated. Blood pressure monitoring should be done before, during, and after the test. The standard cuff method is still preferred, although a number of automated devices are on the market. As far as I know, no method now in use can accurately record blood pressure in all patients during running, short of intra-arterial catheterization. Fortunately, only those subjects in good condition spend much of the test time jogging at more than 4 miles per hour on most protocols. Those able to reach this level of activity are usually less likely to have sudden changes in blood pressure; therefore, the failure to record accurately the pressure at high workloads is not as serious as it would be for one in poorer physical condition. Fortunately, the pressure immediately after the test is similar to the one just before termination of the test and is much more accurately measured. An early rise may often occur about 1 minute after termination of the test and is usually a sign that the subject has exceeded the anaerobic threshold and has performed at near-maximum capacity.

Drugs

An emergency kit of appropriate drugs should be adjacent to the testing area, along with syringes, intravenous equipment, and an Ambu bag. The medicines to be included will vary with the experience of the physician and the methods and concepts of treatment in the area. Those kept in our unit are listed in Table 5–1.

Defibrillator

It is generally agreed that a DC defibrillator should be on hand and frequently tested to ensure that it is functioning properly. However, it will be used very rarely if the proper care is exercised in testing. The rapid conversion of ventricular tachycardia or ventricular fibrillation will be lifesaving. Those in attendance should be fully trained in the use of a defibrillator, as in other matters of resuscitation.

We have used the defibrillator on three patients with ventricular fibrillation. One, who was converted immediately, did not have an infarction. Another, who also converted immediately, did prove to have an infarction, but recovered. The third patient sustained an infarction and failed to survive.

MANAGEMENT DURING THE POSTEXERCISE PERIOD

If angina or significant ST depression persists more than 2 or 3 minutes into the recovery period, nitroglycerin should be administered. The changes in the ST segment following nitroglycerin administration are helpful in diagnosis, but, more important, eliminating ischemia (ST-segment depression) is good for the patient. It is generally believed that monitoring should not be terminated until all exercise ECG changes have returned to normal. In a few cases in which the ECG does not normalize within 15 to 30 minutes, we have insisted on immediate admission to the hospital.

Table 5–1. **Emergency Kit of Drugs**

MEDICATION STRENGTH AND SIZE	
Albumin, normal serum 5% 50 mL	Hydrocortisone, 250 mg/2 mL vial
Aminophylline IV 500 mg 20 mL vial	Insulin regular, 100 U/mL 10 mL vial
Atropine, 1 mg 10 mL syringe	Isoproterenol, 1 mg/5 mL ampule
Atropine, 1 mg/mL vial	Isoproterenol, 1:5000 5 mL syringe
Bretylium 50 mg/mL 10 mL vial	Isoproterenol, 1:50,000 10 mL syringe
Calcium chloride, 1 g/10 mL syringe	Lidocaine, 100 mg 5 mL syringe
Calcium gluconate, 1 g/10 mL vial	Lidocaine, 2 g/50 mL vial
Dexamethasone, 20 mg/5 mL vial	Metaraminol, 10 mg/mL 10 mL vial
Dextrose, 2.5 g/10 mL vial (25%)	Methylprednisolone, 1 g vial
Dextrose, 25 g/50 mL (50%) syringe	Naloxone, 0.4 mg/1 mL ampule
Diazepam, 10 mg/2 mL syringe	Naloxone, 0.02 mg/mL 2 mL ampule
Digoxin, 0.5 mg/2 mL ampule	Nitroprusside sodium, 50 mg
Digoxin (Peds) 0.1 mg 1 mL ampule	Norepinephrine, 1 mg/mL 4 mL ampule
Diphenhydramine 50 mg 1 mL syringe	Phenobarbital, 65 mg/1 mL
Dopamine, 400 mg vial	Phenylephrine, 10 mg/mL ampule
Dopamine, 800 mg vial	Phenytoin, 100 mg/2 mL
Epinephrine, 1:1000 30 mL vial	Potassium chloride, 40 mEq/20 mL vial
Epinephrine, IC 1:10,000 10 mL 20 g syringe	Procainamide, 100 mg/mL 10 mL vial
Epinephrine, IV 1:10,000 10 mL syringe	Propranolol, 1 mg/1 mL ampule
Furosemide, 100 mg/10 mL ampule	Sodium bicarbonate, 10 mEq/10 mL (8.4%)
Furosemide, 20 mg/2 mL ampule	Sodium bicarbonate, 50 mEq 50 mL syringe
Heparin sodium, 1000 U 10 mL vial	Verapamil, 5 mg/2 mL ampule
CPR	
IV Solutions/sets	IVS regular pump set
IV D5W 250 mL	IVS regular pump volumetric
IV D5W 500 mL	Dopamine, 400 mg/250 mL
IV D51/4NS 500 mL	Dopamine, 200 mg/250 mL
IV D5NS 500 mL	Lidocaine, 0.4% 500 mL
IVS Nonvented pump set	

CASE HISTORIES OF PATIENTS WHO DIED

There has been one death in our exercise lab in the last 20 years. This type of tragedy should always be analyzed carefully. Examples of problem cases to illustrate various concepts are presented.

Case 1

H.G. was a 53-year-old male machine operator with a history of angina subsequent to a myocardial infarction sustained 4 years before. Progression of his angina had recently accelerated to the point where prolonged pain at rest had been common. Examination disclosed a sustained apical heave suggestive of a myocardial aneurysm and a loud fourth sound. The resting ECG revealed an old inferior and an anterior septal infarction. A coronary angiogram and catheterization disclosed a large calcified apical aneurysm and severe three-vessel coronary disease. The left-ventricular end-diastolic pressure was 24 mm Hg at rest and increased to 36 mm Hg with 3 minutes of straight leg-raising.

When the treadmill test was performed, H.G. walked 5 minutes without pain, reaching a pulse of 164 and stopping because of dyspnea. The physician noted several PVCs just before the patient stopped the exercise; ST-segment elevation was also recorded during stress. Two minutes after termination of the test, H.G. suddenly developed ventricular fibrillation, and although he reverted to sinus rhythm several times with cardioversion, ventricular fibrillation repeatedly returned, and he eventually expired. The autopsy revealed a fresh infarction (Fig. 5–1).

Case 2

A.S. was a 53-year-old man with a 2-year history of progressive angina limiting his walking to half a block on level ground. Physical examination was negative except for a loud fourth sound and a double apical impulse. The resting ECG did not show an infarction but did disclose ST-segment depression of 1.0 mm in V_4, V_5, and V_6.

A.S. walked for 2 ½ minutes, reaching a heart rate of 138 beats per minute and stopping because of fatigue, dyspnea, and a slight pressure sensation in his chest. ST-segment depression increased from 2.0 mm at rest on the CM_5 lead to 3.0 mm at peak exercise. Two minutes after the test was terminated, he developed severe dyspnea, a drop in systolic blood pressure to 80, and cold, sweaty skin. No arrhythmia or evidence of infarction was manifested on three monitoring leads. Intermittent closed chest massage failed to improve his condition, and for 2 hours various attempts to improve his status, including massage, ionotropic agents, and oxygen, failed. All during this time, his ECG remained stable (Fig. 5–2). After 2 hours, A.S. succumbed to fibrillation and expired. Autopsy disclosed an acute myocardial infarction of the inferior and lateral walls.

Discussion

What can we learn from these cases? We avoid stressing those patients who have experienced recent rapid acceleration of their angina. If resting ST-segment depression of 2.0 mm or more is present in an anterior precordial lead, we do not subject the patient to a stress test unless we know the condition of the coronary anatomy and can be sure there is good left ventricular function as well as adequate myocardial perfusion.

Cases 3 and 4 were reported from another institution.

Case 3

A 45-year-old man, who jogged 5 miles a day until he developed a sore knee 2 months before, reported to the doctor with chest pain occurring at night but

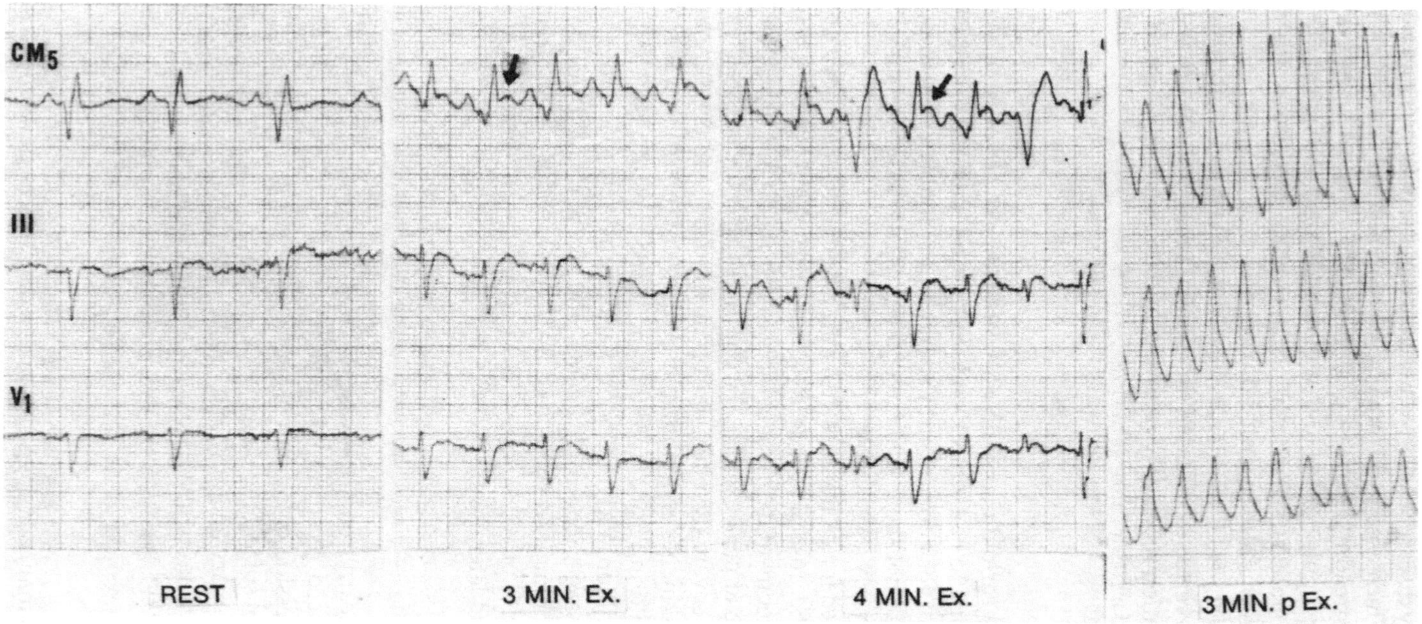

FIGURE 5–1. The ECG shows resting Q waves in CM_5 and ST-segment elevation with exercise as well as an increasing incidence of premature ventricular contractions. Two minutes after exercise, ventricular fibrillation supervened.

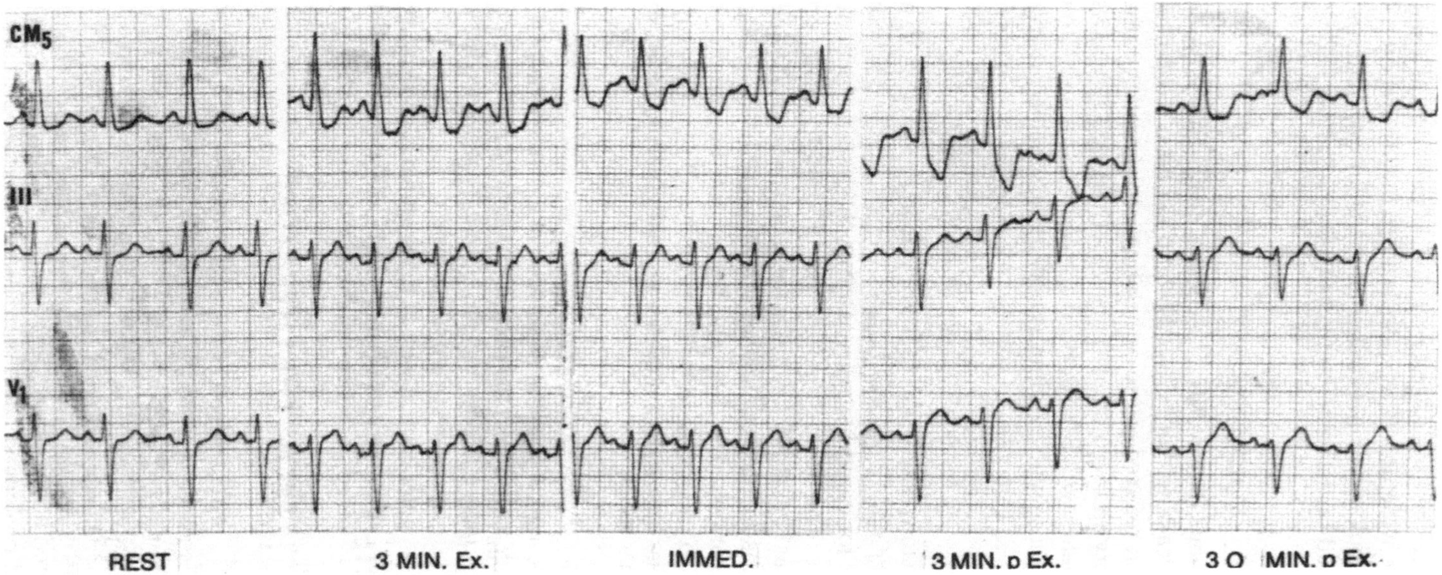

FIGURE 5–2. A 53-year-old man developed a low cardiac output after a stress test without a significant arrhythmia or ECG signs of an acute myocardial infarction. Note stable sinus rhythm after 30 minutes of closed-chest massage, which was associated with almost no significant cardiac output.

not with exercise. The exercise test revealed ST elevation in leads without Q waves and some widening of the QRS but produced no chest pain. He was referred to a cardiologist who recommended thallium scintigraphy, and during the test he had cardiac arrest and died. (Fig. 5–3).

Discussion

This case represents the severity of ischemia that is always associated with ST elevation in leads without Q waves. If it had been recognized, the man would have been referred to the catheterization laboratory rather than the nuclear laboratory and would have survived. Detry and associates[20] have reported that patients with ST elevation are much more prone to serious arrhythmias than those with ST depression. I agree wholeheartedly.

Case 4

A 76-year-old man was worked up for carotid surgery. He gave a history of modest stable angina. An echocardiogram exercise test was scheduled to determine the risk for carotid surgery. During the test, the man developed a drop in pressure. The doctor reported he could not hear the pressure but could palpate it at 90 systolic. Exercise was not terminated, but the resistance on the bicycle was reduced somewhat. Although he had no pain, the man's blood pressure continued to drop and the echocardiogram revealed a dramatic increase in his left-ventricular volume. Prolonged support with dopamine, cardiac resuscitation, and eventually pacing failed to save him (Fig. 5–4).

Discussion

In this case, it was not recognized how serious a significant drop in blood pressure can be, and exercise was not terminated appropriately.

RISKS REPORTED IN THE LITERATURE

Rochimis and Blackburn[9] surveyed 73 medical centers in 1971 to evaluate their procedures with reference to methods and complications present in stress testing. Their data summarized approximately 170,000 tests. Sixty percent of the centers used the treadmill, with Master's test being the next most popular. In 66% of the centers questioned, subjects were stressed to 75% or more of their maximum heart rate. Twenty-five centers, or 34%, used the maximum work capacity of each patient as their end-point. Sixteen deaths were reported, resulting in a mortality rate of about 1/10,000 (0.01%). Four per 10,000 required hospitalization within 1 day of the test for events such as arrhythmias and prolonged chest pain. Brock[16] surveyed 17,000 cases from

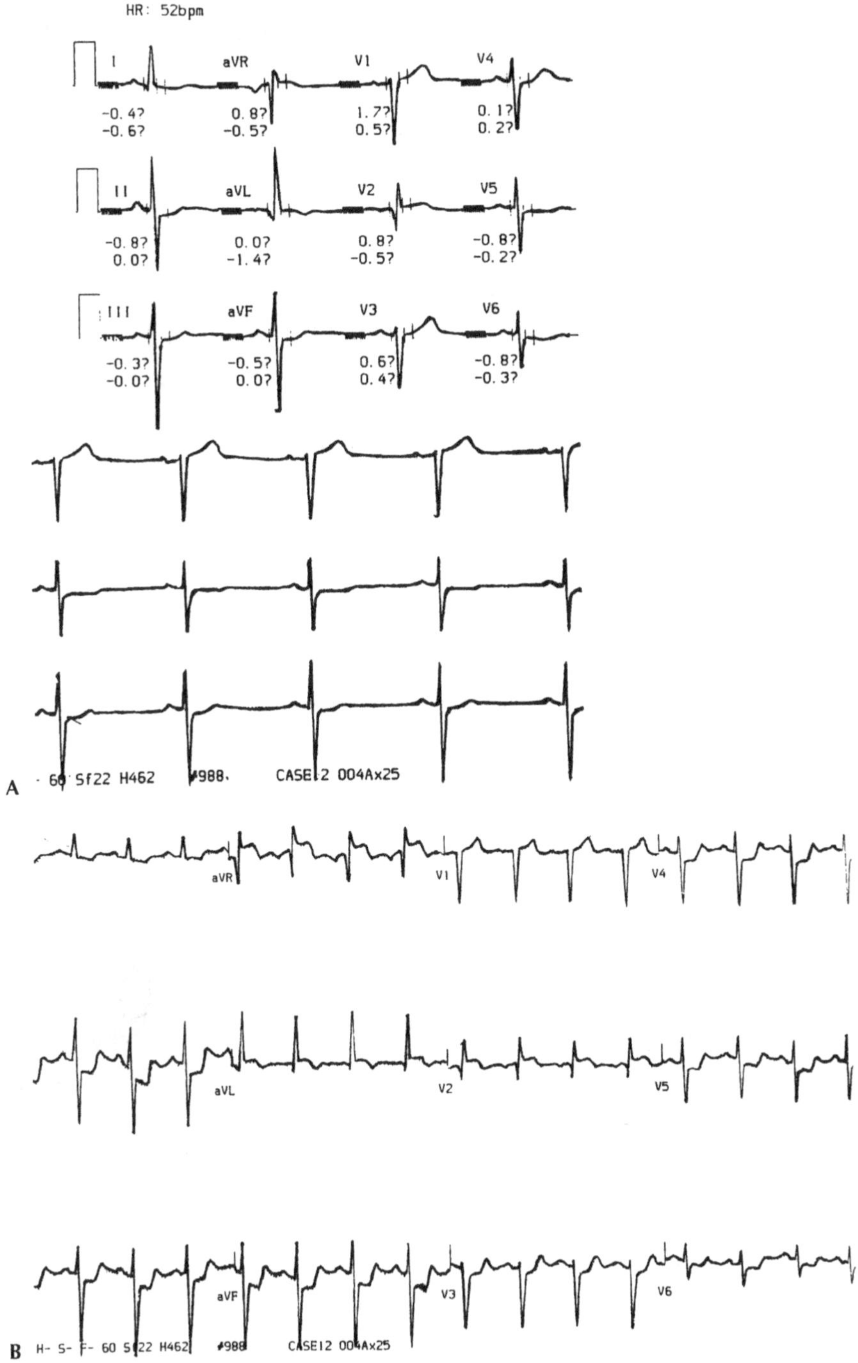

FIGURE 5–3. ECG of a 45-year-old male jogger who started having chest pain a few days prior to the test. The treadmill revealed ST-segment elevation in V_2 and widening of the QRS. (*A*) Resting tracing. (*B*) Exercise tracing.

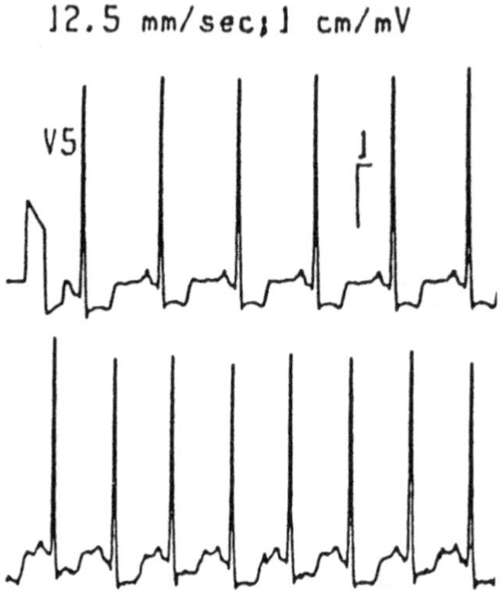

A

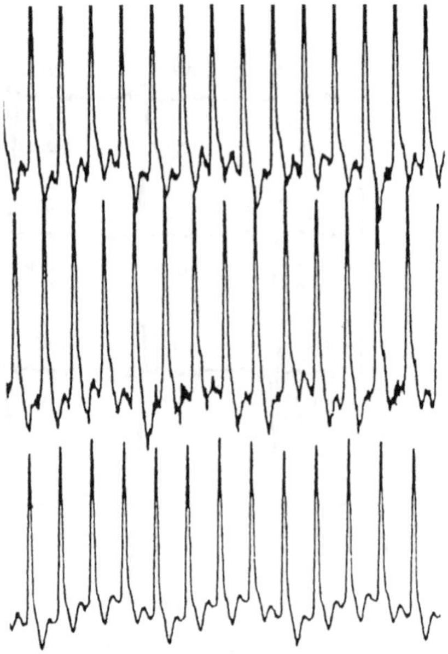

B

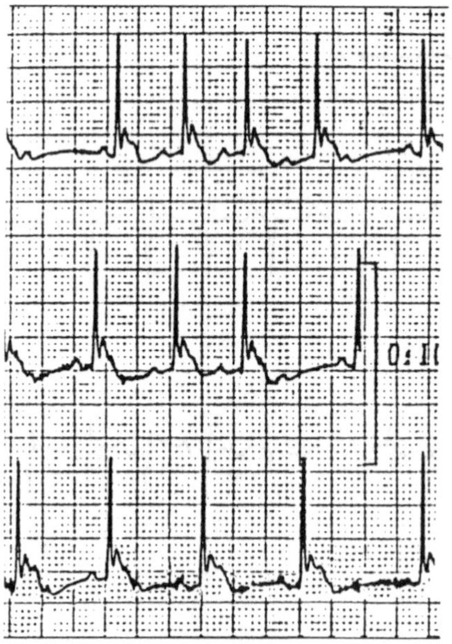

C

FIGURE 5–4. A 67-year-old man who was scheduled for carotid surgery had an exercise echocardiogram done as a screening test. He had no pain but developed widening of the QRS complexes and a drop in blood pressure. The echocardiogram revealed global left-ventricular enlargement. Prolonged treatment with vasopressors had no effect, and after an hour of resuscitation he died. (*A*) Resting—note ST depression. (*B*) Four minutes of exercise—note wide complex tachycardia occurring when blood pressure dropped. (*C*) After exercise terminated, the QRS narrowed but the patient developed ST-segment elevation.

work evaluation units and found 1.7 deaths per 10,000. No information on how many deaths or other complications occurred in the various types of tests was available.

In 1977, we surveyed 1375 centers who reported on 444,396 treadmill tests, 44,460 bicycle stress tests, and 25,592 Master's tests from the previous year's experience.[10] Complications reported were 3.5 infarctions, 48 serious arrhythmias, and 0.5 deaths per 10,000. Scherer and Kaltenbach[21] reported on 1,065,923 tests, mostly bicycle ergometry, done in German-speaking regions of Europe. Stress testing on 353,638 sportspersons had no mortality or morbidity, whereas in 712,285 coronary patients, there were 17 deaths and 96 life-threatening complications, mostly ventricular fibrillation. Thus, bicycle ergometry in a disease population resulted in about 2 deaths in 100,000 in their experience. They found that the recumbent ergometer test resulted in pulmonary edema seven times more frequently than did the upright test, and the mortality increased from 0.6 to 1.2 per 10,000.

Sheffield and associates[22] analyzed the results of the Lipid Research Clinics prevalence study on 9464 patients. They had no mortality with near-maximal testing in this group and attributed the safety to careful patient selection and appropriate termination of the test.

It appears from these data that even in the face of an enormous increase in volume, the mortality rate from stress testing has decreased at least 50% and possibly more. The risks of serious complications in stress testing seem reasonable, and with use of established techniques and continuous monitoring, they can be greatly minimized. Because most deaths on the treadmill are not reported to anyone it may be that problems are more common than previously believed, however.

LEGAL IMPLICATIONS

Although lawsuits against physicians doing stress tests are fairly common, few, if any, have been appealed, so that precedence is not yet established. Sagall[23] has written extensively, however, on the necessity of informed consent and exercising reasonable care. Testing according to published standards seems to be the best protection. When complications arise, the physician should document that he or she was familiar with and able to deal with problems in a manner commensurate with the standards in the community. Having a procedure manual available to show adequate preparation is beneficial. Lawsuits have also been filed for misdiagnosis of the test in patients who later had an infarct, for not informing patients and family of the severity of the test findings, and for not directing the patients to immediate follow-up care when test results suggested very severe ischemia. All those engaged in this procedure need to be up-to-date on the current literature and methodology and to be able to demonstrate this when necessary.

SUMMARY

As in the previous chapter on indications for stress testing, the contraindications are also in a state of flux. Although aortic stenosis used to be an absolute contraindication to stress testing, it is now safe to test if the degree of stenosis is not severe and the patient is watched meticulously. This approach has been successfully practiced in pediatric cardiology for some time. When ST elevation occurs, immediate termination of exercise is mandatory. Patients presenting to the emergency department with chest pain can be tested if they have a normal ECG and cardiac enzymes and have a low probability of CHD.[24]

REFERENCES

1. Shephard, RJ: Do risks of exercise justify costly caution? Physician Sportsmed February: 58–65, 1977.
2. Ellestad, MH (Chairman), Blomqvist, CC, and Naughton, JP: Standards for adult exercise testing laboratories. American Heart Association Subcommittee on Rehabilitation. Circulation 59:421A–443A, 1979.
3. Fletcher, GF, et al: Exercise in the Practice of Medicine. Futura Publishing, Mount Kisco, NY, 1982.
4. McHenry, PL: Exercise in the practice of medicine. J Contin Ed Cardiol 7:17, 1984.
5. Haskell, WI: Design of a cardaic conditioning program. In Wenger, NK (ed): Exercise and the Heart. Cardiovascular Clinics, Vol 15, No. 2, FA Davis, Philadelphia, 1979.
6. Wilson, PK: Cardiac Rehabilitation, Adult Fitness, and Exercise Testing. Lea & Febiger, Philadelphia, 1981.
7. Froelicher, VF and Marion, D: Exercise testing and ancillary techniques to screen for coronary heart disease. Prog Cardiovasc Dis 24:261, 1984.
8. Bruce, RA, Derouen, TA, and Houssack, KF: Value of maximal exercise tests in risk assessment of primary coronary heart disease events in healthy men: Five years experience of the Seattle Heart Watch study. Am J Cardiol 46:371–378, 1980.
9. Rochimis, P and Blackburn, H: Exercise test: A survey of procedures, safety and litigation experience in approximately 170,000 tests. JAMA 217:1061, 1971.
10. Stuart, RJ and Ellestad, NH: National survey of exercise stress testing facilities. Chest 77:94, 1980.
11. Frank, S and Braunwald, E: Idiopathic hypertrophic subaortic stenosis. Circulation 37:159, 1968.
12. Franciosa, JA: Exercise testing in chronic congestive heart failure. Am J Cardiol 53:1447–1450, 1984.
13. Fox, SM, Naughton, JP, and Haskell, WL: Physical activity and the prevention of coronary heart disease. Ann Clin Res 3:404, 1971.
14. Sheffield, LT, et al: Electrocardiographic signal analysis without averaging of complexes. In Blackburn, H (ed); Measurement in Exercise Electrocardiography. Charles C Thomas, Springfield, IL 1967.
15. Borer, JS, et al: Limitations of electrocardiographic response to exercise in predicting coronary artery disease. N Engl J Med 293:367, 1975.
16. Brock, LL: Stress testing incidents in work evaluation units in WEU subcommittee newsletter. American Heart Association, New York, 1967.
17. Takahashi, N: How to evaluate the ST segment elevation during or after exercise. Am Heart J 79:579, 1970.
18. Margonato, A, et al: ST segment elevation at site of recent transmural myocardial infarction during exercise stress testing: A marker for residual tissue viability [abstract]. Circulation 84(suppl 4):1802, 1991.

19. Gibbons, RJ, et al: ACC/AHA guidelines for exercise testing: A report of the American College of Cardiology/American Heart Association task force on practice guidelines (committee on exercise testing). ACC/AHA, 1997.
20. Detry, JMR, et al: Maximal exercise testing in patients with spontaneous angina pectoris associated with transient ST segment elevation. Br Heart J 37:897, 1975.
21. Scherer, D and Kaltenbach, N: Frequency of life-threatening complications associated with stress testing. Dtsch Med Wochenschr 104:1161, 1979.
22. Sheffield, LT, et al: Safety of exercise testing volunteer subjects: The lipid research clinics+ prevalence study experience. J Cardiac Rehab 2(5):395, 1982.
23. Sagall, EL: Malpractice aspects of medically prescribed exercise. Leg Med Ann 30:275, 1975.
24. Amsterdam, EA, et al: Immediate exercise testing for assessment of clinical risk in patients presenting to the emergency department with chest pain: results in over 1,000 patients. Circulation. 98:I-774, 1998.

6
Parameters to Be Measured

Electrocardiographic Specifications
Lead Systems
- Bipolar Leads
- Conventional 12 Leads
- XYZ Orthogonal Leads
- Precordial Maps
- Mixed-Lead Systems

R Waves
P Waves
ST/HR Slope
Blood Pressure
Pressure Pulse Product
Heart Rate Response to Exercise
Delta Heart Rate
Oxygen Consumption
Respiratory Data Other Than Oxygen Uptake During Stress Testing
Respiratory Gas Exchange and Anaerobic Threshold
Walk-Through Phenomenon
Heart Sounds and Other Auscultatory Findings
- First and Second Heart Sounds
- Third Heart Sounds
- Fourth Heart Sounds
- Aortic Murmur
- Mitral Murmur

Palpitation
Pulsus Alternans

As we learn more about the physiology of exercise and the perturbations in the normal process brought on by disease states, it stands to reason that our ability to separate disease from normal function would improve, and indeed it has. One of the most important revelations is the acceptance that ischemia is often due to a reduction in delivery of blood flow to the myocardium rather than just an increase in the demand. Maseri[1] must be credited for this turn-around in our thinking, which also has led to the concept of a reduced coronary vasodilator reserve.

This concept implies that the increased flow required by increasing myocardial action demands is inadequate, probably because of some problem in vasomotion of the myocardial arterioles. For instance, Marcus[2] has shown that reactive hyperemia, caused by mechanical obstruction of a coronary artery for 20 seconds, normally results in a five- to eightfold increase in perfusion. Some patients with normal epicardial coronary arteries can only increase flow to double the resting level, however. Marcus has also demonstrated that reductions in flow associated with coronary plaques vary a great deal when the obstruction is estimated by angiography; thus, the old idea that a 70% obstruction implies reduced perfusion and a 40% obstruction does not is untenable. Some subjects with angiographic narrowing of 30% to 40% show a very poor increase in flow with increased metabolic demand, whereas others with obstruction of 60% to 80% respond almost normally.

The implications of these findings are far-reaching. One reason for the difference is that the degree of vasomotion likely to occur varies from patient to patient due to the effect of the potent vasoactive agent, endothelin.[3] As yet we have no way of predicting how much of a role this plays in each individual. We now know that nitric acid secreted by the endothelium opposes the vasoconstrictive effect of endothelian and its production may be even more important than other functions of these interesting cells.[4]

Many so-called false-positives and false-negatives may be true-positives and true-negatives when one is considering myocardial perfusion rather than coronary anatomy. We should also recognize the need to analyze as many different facets of the exercise response as possible rather than concentrate too heavily on the ST segment. When searching for parameters that are useful in identifying disease, *powerful predictors are infrequent*, and *frequent predictors are rarely powerful.*[5]

Some of the methods described in this chapter, such as the Master's test, are presented primarily for historical interest, either because they have not been used enough to warrant general acceptance or because they are no longer in use for various reasons. Some other methods presented in the previous edition have been deleted.

ELECTROCARDIOGRAPHIC SPECIFICATIONS

The wide recognition of the importance of faithful recording at the lower end of the ECG frequency range has been a significant development in the instrumentation necessary for accurate stress testing.[6,7] The standards recommended by the Committee on Electrocardiography of the American Heart Association in 1967 require errors of less than 0.5 mm (0.05 mV) in the early part of the ST-T segment (0.05 Hz cutoff with a 0 decibel per octave rolloff).[8] Technical aspects of the ECG recording during muscular activity are clearly interdependent. Poor frequency response at the lower end of the spectrum in the older ECG units would smooth the record, giving apparently better records, but obscuring the most important information, the low-frequency ST-segment changes. As impedance at the skin source is reduced by better electrodes and as the skin preparation techniques are improved, the fidelity of the recorder can be improved and still give clean, readable records. Faris and colleagues[9] claim that 10% of the ischemic ST changes appear only during exercise, so good quality is essential. Special systems for noise reduction are considered in Chapter 24.

LEAD SYSTEMS

As early as 1931, Wood and Wolferth[10] noted that the precordial leads gave a greater sensitivity in detecting the ST-segment depression of ischemia than did Einthoven's standard leads. Various types of unipolar and bipolar precordial systems have been in use for a number of years and have produced satisfactory results.

Bipolar Leads

CM_5. This system locates the negative electrode on the upper sternum and the positive one in the V_5 position. The CM_5 was probably the most popular single lead for exercise monitoring for many years and has been demonstrated to have the highest incidence of positive changes in patients with known ischemia.[11]

CC_5. The negative electrode is on the right lateral part of the chest in the axilla, and the positive electrode is in the V_5 position.[12] The CC_5 lead has been credited with showing less contamination by the TA wave (see Chapter 12).

CA Lead. The negative electrode is on the medial scapular ridge on the right side, and the positive electrode is in the V_5 position.

CB Lead. The negative electrode is on the inferior scapular angle on the right, and the positive electrode is in the V_5 position (Fig. 6–1).

CS_5. The negative electrode is just below the right clavicle, and the positive electrode is in the V_5 position.

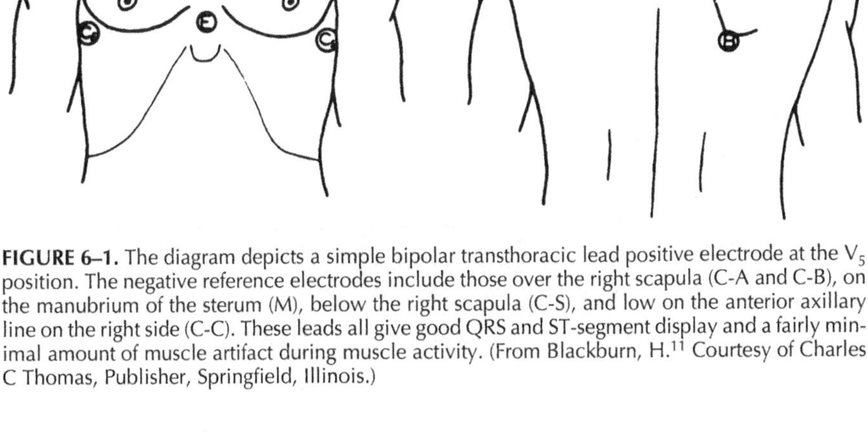

FIGURE 6–1. The diagram depicts a simple bipolar transthoracic lead positive electrode at the V_5 position. The negative reference electrodes include those over the right scapula (C-A and C-B), on the manubrium of the sterum (M), below the right scapula (C-S), and low on the anterior axillary line on the right side (C-C). These leads all give good QRS and ST-segment display and a fairly minimal amount of muscle artifact during muscle activity. (From Blackburn, H.[11] Courtesy of Charles C Thomas, Publisher, Springfield, Illinois.)

When testing patients with ischemic ST-segment depression, the vector of the maximum ST-segment depression is usually 180° opposite the maximum R-wave amplitude. Blackburn and associates[11] studied this phenomenon in 25 men and plotted the R wave as shown in Figure 6–2. It can be seen that by using the various lead systems discussed previously, the CM_5 and CS_5 fall near the regression line of 45°. In the same study, the other parameters of the ECG complexes were tabulated (Table 6–1). Examination of this table reveals that bipolar leads with the exploring electrode at V_5 generally resemble a true V_5 of the Wilson systems except that these have a higher QRS voltage and are more sensitive to ST-segment depression.[13] The bipolar systems that combine the highest R-wave amplitude and the greatest display of ST depression are CM_5 and CS_5. They have been reported to identify 89% of all ST-segment depression found by multiple-lead systems. These leads might be termed *optimally distorted.*

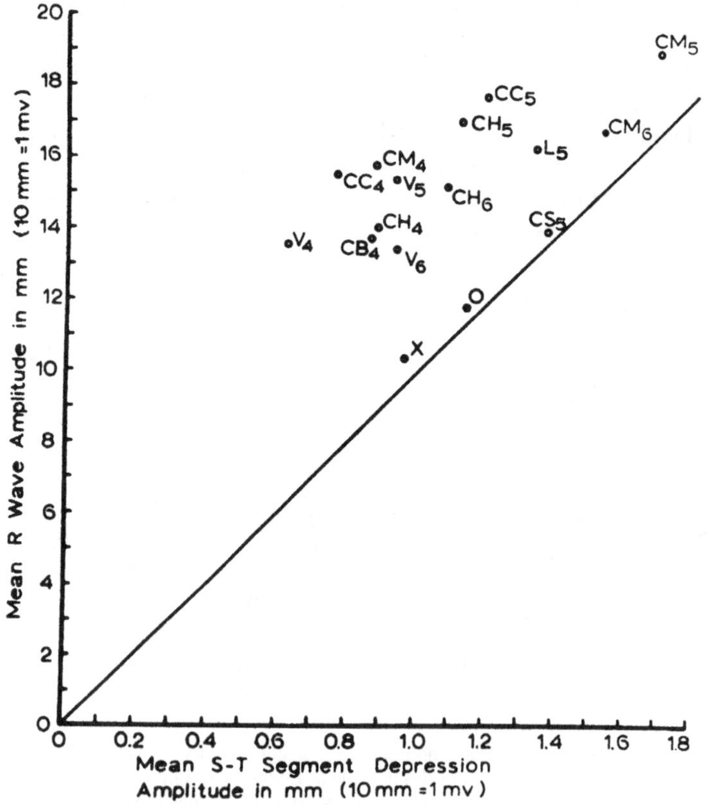

FIGURE 6–2. The ST-segment amplitudes are plotted against the R-wave amplitude in men exhibiting positive ischemic responses. There tends to be a regression line correlating the R-wave amplitude and the amount of ST-segment depression. However, it is not linear. (From Blackburn, H.[13] Courtesy of Charles C Thomas, Publisher, Springfield, Illinois.)

Table 6–1. **Four Simultaneously Recorded Bipolar Monitoring ECG Leads Immediately Postexercise Among a Mixed Group of Normal Subjects and Patients***

		CB N = 25	CA N = 25	CS N = 25	CM N = 25
Q-wave amplitude	M	0.5	0.8	0.9	1.4
	SD	0.7	1.0	0.9	2.0
R-wave amplitude	M	16.0	19.0	17.9	19.9
	SD	7.3	9.1	9.2	9.8
S-wave amplitude	M	4.5	5.8	4.8	3.4
	SD	2.5	3.7	2.2	2.6
T-wave amplitude	M	2.3	2.7	2.7	2.5
	SD	2.1	1.9	2.0	2.2
ST junction maximum	M	−2.5	−2.6	−2.3	−2.4
amplitude	SD	1.6	1.8	1.9	1.9
ST midpoint amplitude	M	1.8	1.8	1.8	1.9
	SD	0.4	0.3	0.3	0.4
ST-segment maximum amplitude when depressed	M	−3.8	−6.0	−5.0	−4.9
% Total Depressed		48	36	36	44

Reference Electrode		*Exploring Electrode*
CB	inferior scapular angle, right	Common to all in position C_5
CA	medial scapular ridge, right	
CS	subclavicle, right lateral	
CM	manubrium sternum	

*Amplitude in mm (10 mm = 1 mV); M = mean; SD = standard deviation. The amplitude of the waves varies somewhat with the different lead systems plotted. The tallest R-wave amplitude is with the CM lead. The highest percentage of positive test results of the four leads was with the CB lead, although it is very similar to that of the CM. (From Blackburn.[13] Courtesy of Charles C Thomas, Publisher, Springfield, Illinois.)

Hakki and associates[14] have demonstrated that a lead with a low R-wave amplitude is likely to exhibit no ST depression even when ischemia is present.

McHenry and Morris[15] locate the bipolar system by examination of the resting precordial leads. They then place the positive monitoring lead at the position of the maximum R-wave amplitude.

Conventional 12 Leads

The use of all 12 leads of the conventional systems has the advantage of wide familiarity, but has the disadvantage of redundancy and some decrease in relative sensitivity to the display of ST-segment depression. Virtually all the ST-segment information in common usage at present is found in leads II, III, aVR, aVF, V_3, V_4, V_5, and V_6. When patients were studied by Blackburn[13] with a 3-minute step test, recording 12 standard leads, a fairly high incidence of 0.5-mm ST-segment depression in one lead or another was recorded. Isolated changes in lead III were 1%; in aVF, 3%; and in both III and aVF, another 3%. The use of multiple leads is much more practical with the newer recorders and has become the standard. The option of adding CC_5 and CM_5 probably provides the optimal approach.

XYZ Orthogonal Leads

Computer programs are available that can synthesize the standard 12 leads from the orthogonal leads, and some excellent studies have been done in normal subjects for standardization.[16] However, with exercising patients, the noise level of muscle activity is considerable, making digital filtering and noise reduction essential when using this approach. Information as to the sensitivity and specificity of the XYZ leads has been published by Simoons,[16] suggesting that with computer measurements the results are excellent. In a limited study, Blackburn[13] reported the XYZ leads to be less sensitive, but Hornsten and Bruce[17] found them to be equal in sensitivity to the bipolar system.

Camp and colleagues[18] compared the orthogonal lead with CM_5 in 93 patients who had stress testing and coronary angiography. They reported the true-positive tests to be 57% in the Y lead, 66% in CM_5, and 69% in the X lead. They found the total sensitivity of the X, Y, and Z leads to be 84%, compared with 71% for CM_5. In 1966, Isaacs and colleagues[19] claimed that the analysis of the vector loop in the Frank system produced better sensitivity than scalar tracing. They found the loop positive in 80%, whereas the scalar ST segments were positive in only 60%. This method has never become popular and has not been confirmed by others using angiograms as a check.

Most of the work on vectorcardiographic analysis of exercise tracings has been done with the Frank system. There seems to be general agreement that the X lead, which is equivalent to a bipolar lead from right to left axilla, provides the most useful information on the ST segment.[20] The other leads are of lesser value. Blomqvist[21] described the greater magnitude of ST-segment depression recorded simultaneously in the CH_4 and CH_6 bipolar leads than in the orthogonal leads. He has also provided excellent data on variations seen during exercise in normal subjects.[21] However, unless one has a computer available to analyze the data and is very conversant with vector loops, use of the orthogonal leads is not practical.

Precordial Maps

Fox and colleagues[22,23] have reported a number of studies using a 16-lead precordial map or grid and report a sensitivity when compared with coronary angiography of about 87%, similar to that obtained by Chaitman and coworkers[24] with their 14 leads. In a more recent report, Chaitman has reported a sensitivity of up to 95%, with a specificity of approximately 78%.[25] It is important to realize that these percentages come from a caseload with a very high proportion of coronary disease and might well be less reliable if the percentage of disease is as low as 50% or less. Chaitman did find that ST elevation had a sensitivity of 100%, although only 4% had this finding. Fox and colleagues[23] reported that they have had enough experience to recommend that the precordial map be used clinically on a daily basis. They also reported that it can be used to localize the coronary artery involved when single-vessel disease is present. Fox and colleagues found a sensitivity of 74% with their map compared with 42% when a standard 12-lead system was used (Fig. 6–3).

An editorial by Spach and Barr[26] from Duke University presents some theoretical insights into the practical application of the precordial map. They suggest that a good deal of work remains to be done before we can accurately identify localized epicardial electrical events on the surface of the torso. Interest in this approach seems to wax and wane, and I cannot predict whether maps will find a broader clinical application. I am convinced, however, that in the future we will abandon the standard 12 leads.

Mixed-Lead Systems

Studies will continue to be published claiming that various lead combination are superior. Chaitman and associates[24] evaluated a number of systems and reported that a 14-lead system including CM_5, CC_5, CL, and the standard 12 leads with the exception of aVR was superior to the others, with a sensitivity of 88% and a specificity of 82%. They reported the two most sensitive single leads in this system to be CM_5 and CC_5. Froelicher and coworkers[12] reported CC_5 and V_5 to be superior to CM_5. However, they excluded the

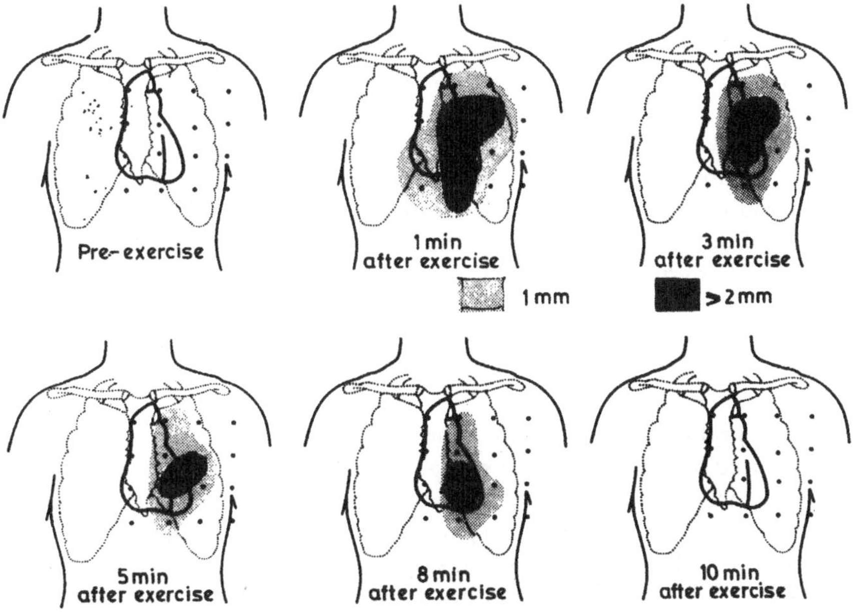

FIGURE 6–3. Example of sequence of contour maps showing areas of ST-segment depression after exercise. Shaded = 1 mm; black = 2 mm. (From Fox et al,[23] with permission.)

upsloping patterns in their abnormal group (see Chapter 11). We evaluated CM_5 and CC_5 simultaneously in our laboratory for 1 year and found more false-positives in CM_5, and more false-negatives in CC_5.

Although the final chapter has not been written on the best lead system, there are important differences among many of the systems. By far the most sensitive exploring electrode position is at the V_5 chest location. The CH (forehead to chest), CC, or C_5R to C_5 (a transthoracic lead) and the CC lead (right back to apex) all provide very good data. The right ear, the ensiform cartilage, and the C_7 position also stand out in this regard. In spite of these reports the standard 12 leads using a Mason-Likar distribution is now the most common configuration in most testing facilities.[27] Even though recent claims for increased sensitivity using 14 or 15 leads have been published.[28]

R WAVES

Although normals usually have a decrease in precordial R waves with exercise, an increase is present in a relatively small number of patients with ischemia. A recent study in our laboratory indicated that this finding is less sensitive than we originally believed, but the R wave still should be measured and considered along with other variables, a discussion of which follows[29] (see Chapter 12).

P WAVES

Myrianthefs and colleagues,[30–32] working in our laboratory, demonstrated that P-wave duration prolongs with ischemia. This is because the elevated left-ventricular end-diastolic pressure (LVEDP) and atrial pressure distend the left atrium and thus slow conduction through the atrial wall. Although this measurement is difficult, both because of the low P-wave voltage and the overlap of the T wave, it is useful in identifying exercise-induced ischemia (see "ECG Patterns," Chapter 12).

ST/HR SLOPE

Although preliminary calculations correcting the ST depression for the heart rate reported by Simoons[16] set the stage, considerable interest was generated by the reports from the group at Leeds, England, claiming that their application of this concept resulted in a perfect identification of patients with coronary disease.[33] They found that the slope not only separated subjects without significant narrowing from those with it, but also could separate single-vessel from double-vessel, and double-vessel from triple-vessel disease.

Although Elamin and associates[33] were convinced of the accuracy of their methods, others have been unable to reproduce their findings.[34] The variation in degrees of myocardial ischemia, related to the number of vessels diseased, negates the kind of results they have reported. Also, a few patients with severe coronary artery disease (CAD) and normal ST segments (a fairly common finding), together with the usual type of false-positive we see all the time, would make these results impossible. Even so, the work has stimulated others to correct ST segments for heart rate in various ways, and some improvement in discrimination have resulted. The most avid proponents of this method are Kligfield and coworkers[35] from New York; although their work has been challenged by other investigators,[36] enough work has been done to warrant serious consideration of its application on a regular basis, and we use their index as part of our routine evaluation.

BLOOD PRESSURE

Observation of the blood pressure response is important both to ensure the safety of the patient and to provide information on the strength of the cardiac contraction and the state of the peripheral resistance. It may also be of value in predicting hypertension in the future.[37] Blood pressure should be recorded before and with exercise at each work level as well as in recovery (see Chapter 18).

PRESSURE PULSE PRODUCT

The systolic blood pressure is multiplied by the heart rate to provide the double product or modified tension time index. As described in Chapter 2, this value gives an index of myocardial oxygen consumption and provides a parameter for comparison of tests before and after some type of intervention. Figure 6–4 illustrates the relative use of myocardial oxygen before and after treatment with propranolol, as reflected in the pressure pulse product or double product. During the second test, the exercise end-point is at about the same pressure pulse value even though it took 2 minutes longer to reach it. Figure 6–5 shows the effect on the pressure pulse product of obstructed coronary blood flow.

Because the double product depends on both blood pressure and heart rate, the finding that they appear to be related variables is of some interest. Thulein and Werner[38] studied the heart rate response in hypertensive persons during stress testing and Holter monitoring compared with normal persons. Those with blood pressure higher than average on casual findings have consistently higher heart rates for a given workload as well as higher systolic and diastolic blood pressures. It would seem that they are hyperreactors, so that as a group they would have a much higher double product

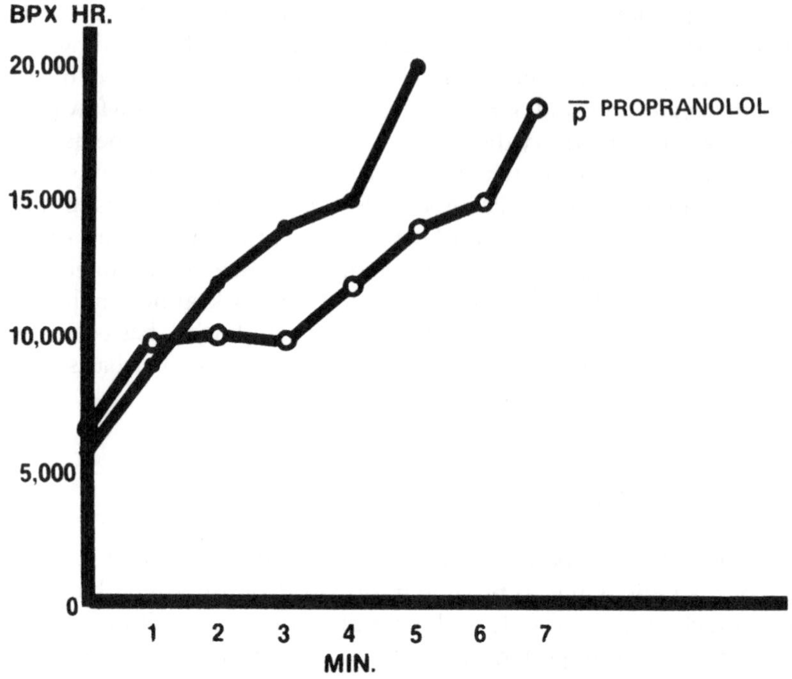

FIGURE 6–4. The double product (systolic blood pressure × pulse) plotted for each minute of exercise until maximum capacity was reached. The patient went longer after treatment with propranolol, but his myocardial oxygen consumption as estimated by the double product was about the same during both tests.

and, accordingly, a higher myocardial oxygen consumption than normal persons.

HEART RATE RESPONSE TO EXERCISE

The heart rate response is the best indicator of the magnitude of exertion. A good estimate of the maximum heart rate obtainable is 220 to 230 minus age. The person doing the test must know the approximate predicted maximum heart rate and be familiar with the average response to the protocol selected for each of the various age groups.

Although it has been long been known that the heart rate gives a reasonably reliable measure of the cardiac output, the tendency to a lower heart rate under a standard exercise load has been frequently considered to be a matter of better conditioning. Indeed, the observable decrease in resting and exercise heart rate after physical fitness programs is regarded as a most desirable result and is carefully recorded.

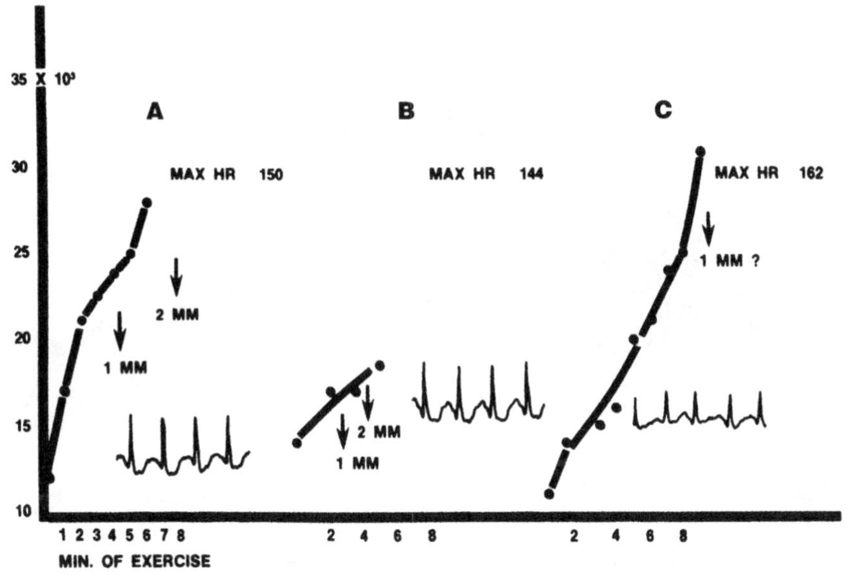

FIGURE 6–5. The double product plotted against time on the treadmill in a 44-year-old man. "A" illustrates the stress test when the patient was first seen. The lower pressure pulse product seen on "B" illustrates the decreasing coronary blood flow approximately 4 months after a saphenous vein bypass graft had become obstructed by a clot. The test labeled "C" illustrates the improvement after reoperation, which established good flow to the left anterior descending coronary artery. Severe anginal pain and a characteristic ischemic ST-segment change were present when the graft was obstructed but not after reoperation.

The work of Jose and Taylor[39] suggests that as myocardial contractility decreases, the so-called intrinsic heart rate becomes slower. After constructing nomograms characterizing the heart rate response to our standard protocol, we began to see patients who had a peculiar lack of chronotropic response to exercise, even though they were severely deconditioned. One of these subjects, who had previously complained of a vague chest pain at night, suddenly died of a myocardial infarction, even though his ST segments during the stress tests appeared perfectly normal. Subsequent study of this phenomenon has led us to believe that "chronotropic incompetence," as we call it, is a fairly reliable sign of poor myocardial function.

Figure 6–6 illustrates the heart rate response to our protocol of a 53-year-old man who had progressive myocardial disease, including one myocardial infarction and progressive angina between the two tests. The change in the slope compared with the predicted normal pulse for his age and sex is easily apparent because the slower heart rate for the same workload was associated with decreasing ventricular function.

Figure 6–7 depicts the heart rate response of another man, aged 51, with severe three-vessel CAD before and after a successful saphenous vein graft operation. His chronotropic response to exercise became normal, and the

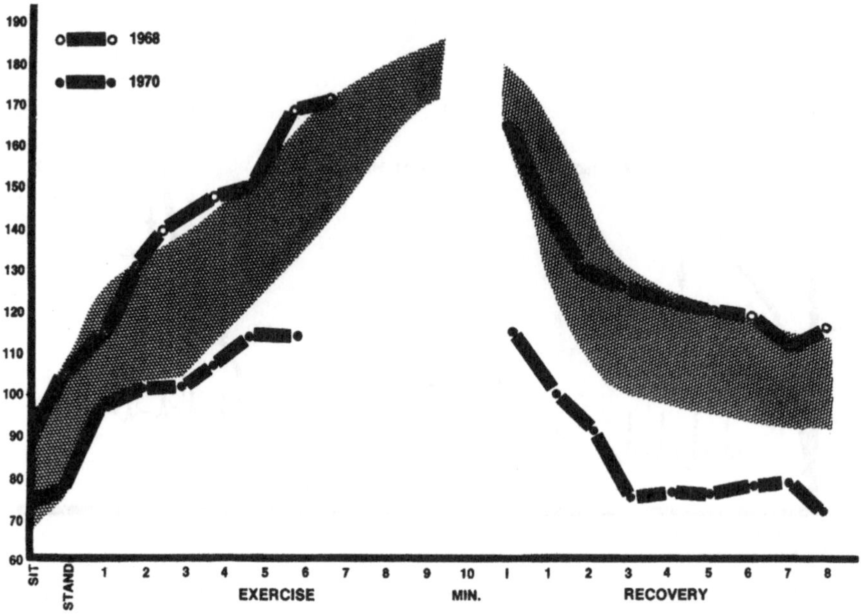

FIGURE 6–6. Chronotropic incompetence. The shaded area illustrates the 95% confidence limits for the average heart rate response at our protocol. The subject was tested twice. In his initial test (*Top Line*), his heart rate response fell along the upper margin of the normal range. Two years later, after a myocardial infarction and continuing angina, the patient's ability to accelerate his heart rate had diminished, and at this time his pulse was far below the normal range.

deep ST-segment depression recorded on his preoperative test disappeared. Hinkle and associates[40] reported this type of response and documented its correlation with CAD and an increased incidence of coronary death. They called it "sustained relative bradycardia." They believed it was due to ischemia of the sinus node and described a 46% mortality rate over a 7-year period (N = 34) compared with a 12% mortality rate in subjects with normal heart rate response (N = 301). Grimby and Saltin[41] found that the peak heart rate capacity in athletes correlated well with the resting rate ($r = 0.81$). We have not found a similar correlation in our patients, most of whom are in poor physical condition.

When we analyzed the 8-year follow-up data on subjects with chronotropic incompetence, the high incidence of CAD was apparent not only in those with ischemic ST segments, but also in those with no electrocardiographic evidence of CAD (see Chapter 14). A subsequent study during catheterization revealed that they have more severe CAD than comparable patients with a normal heart rate response.[42]

Wiens[43] has confirmed our original work and found that a slow heart rate response on the treadmill is a reliable predictor of CAD. To recognize this process, one can construct standard heart rate response graphs for what-

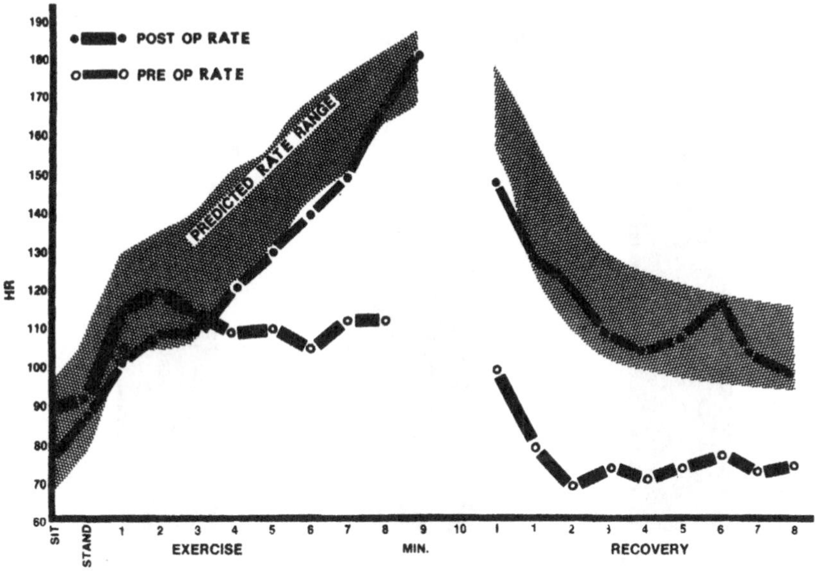

FIGURE 6–7. The pulse response of a 51-year-old man with a severe three-vessel coronary disease shows a very definite plateau with an inability to increase appropriately. Following successful bypass surgery, which completely relieved his pain, his pulse response to the same protocol returned to the normal range.

ever protocol one elects. The information used in our protocol is listed in Appendix 4. Lauer has constructed a chronotrophic index to detect this phenomon and has confirmed in a series of papers that it is predictive of a poor prognosis.[44,45,46]

DELTA HEART RATE

Sandvik et al[47] from Oslo has followed up 2014 normal men and found that the difference between resting and maximum heart rate on a maximum exercise test 20 years ago is predictive of cardiac mortality. The lower the delta heart rate, the higher the mortality rate (Fig. 6–8). Although this finding has yet to be confirmed by other investigators, its correctness seems reasonable. However, we don't know whether this will also be found in patients with established CAD.

OXYGEN CONSUMPTION

Over the years, there has been a great deal of interest in measuring the oxygen consumption of subjects undergoing stress testing.[48] This measurement

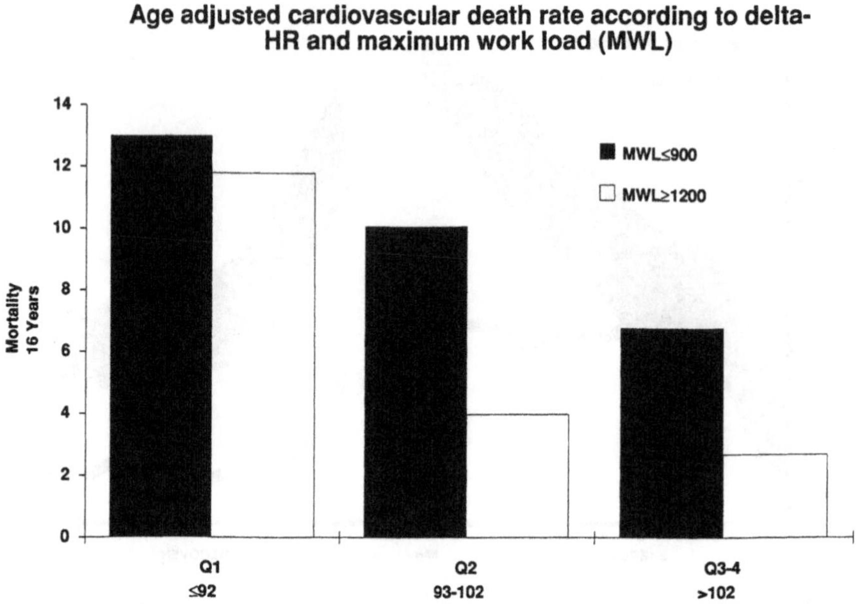

FIGURE 6–8. The difference between the resting and the maximum heart rates (shown as quartiles across the bottom of the graph) has been shown to be predictive of later cardiac mortality. (Adapted from Sandvik's data.[47])

has been accomplished in various centers by collecting expired air in Douglas bags or balloons at measured intervals. This is usually done at rest, during exercise, and at peak stress. Because the amount of work expended by the individual depends a great deal on the type of stress applied, the metabolic cost of walking up stairs is different from the cost of walking on a treadmill, from the cost of running on a treadmill, and from the cost of riding a bicycle. Comparative studies have been published that allow us roughly to estimate one or the other.

The actual measurement of oxygen intake for each patient is expensive, time consuming, and probably not indicated in a routine stress test. Unless patients are familiar with the proceedings, they do not adjust to the mouthpiece, and use of the nose clip is necessary to obtain accurate data. Use of the mouthpiece is especially difficult for cardiac patients, who may be anxious and have chest pain as well as muscular fatigue. Ford and Hellerstein[49] have published data on the energy cost of the Master's test. Balke and Ware[50] published a formula applicable to a treadmill program, which gives a rough estimate of the oxygen requirements of any speed and grade. However, the efficiency of walking and the strength of the subject considerably affect the capacity to walk or run uphill, so that the variation around a mean must be large.

$$\dot{V}O_2 = v \times w \times (0.073 + OC/100) \times 1.8$$

where:

$\dot{V}O_2$	=	oxygen consumption in mL/min (Standard temperature and pressure dry [STPD])
v	=	treadmill speed in m/min
w	=	body weight in kg
OC	=	treadmill angle in percent
1.8	=	factor constituting the oxygen requirement in mL/min for 1 m/kg of work

Mastropaolo and colleagues[51] checked this method of estimating $\dot{V}O_2$ against measured uptake and found it to be satisfactory.

Bruce and associates[52] describe uptake values measured in milligrams per kilogram per minute (Fig. 6–9). This is a simplified approach to the problem for practical application in daily testing. Givoni and Goldman[53] have also published a formula that we have found very reliable at lower workloads. A number of on-line systems have been devised that can measure continuous oxygen uptake (Fig. 6–10).

In daily testing of CAD patients, oxygen measurements probably add little to the understanding of the disease process and are unnecessary.[54] The estimates from the various formulas are satisfactory for clinical purposes.

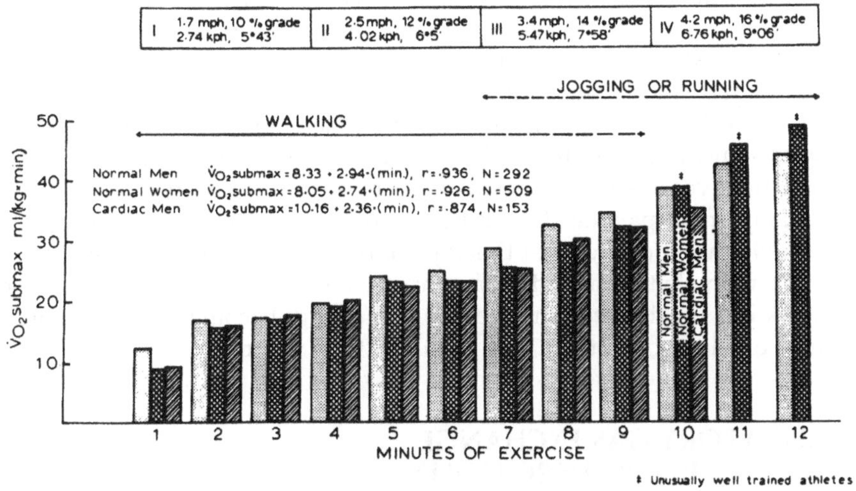

FIGURE 6–9. Aerobic requirements of healthy adult men and women and cardiac men walking without support on a multistage treadmill protocol. The ability to predict the oxygen consumption for each level of work is reliable. (From Bruce et al,[52] with permission.)

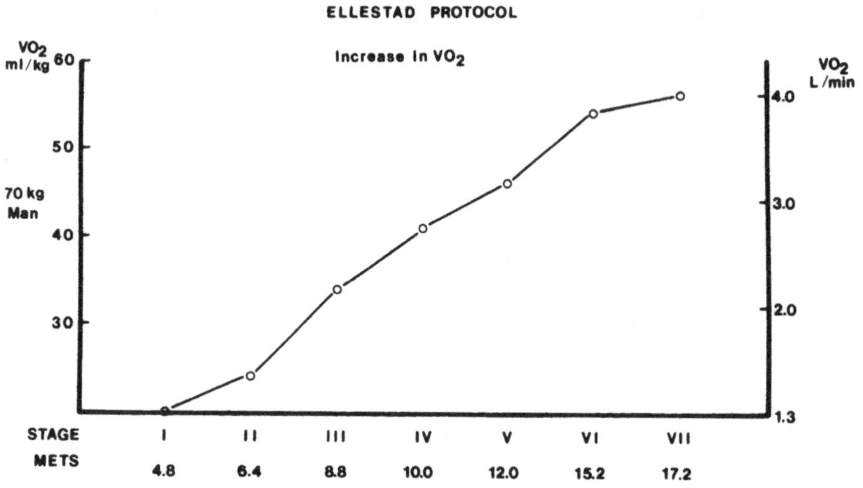

FIGURE 6–10. Oxygen consumption in a 70-kg man according to treadmill stage.

RESPIRATORY DATA OTHER THAN OXYGEN UPTAKE DURING STRESS TESTING

Up to this time, little attention has been paid to respiratory rates or volumes in conjunction with stress testing. In normal subjects, ventilation increases in a linear relationship to oxygen intake and carbon dioxide output, up to power outputs of 50% to 60% of maximal capacity. Beyond this level this, ventilation is more closely related to carbon dioxide output, which increases to a greater extent than oxygen intake. At about this time, the tidal volume increases at a slower rate as the respiratory rate increases more rapidly to compensate[54] (Fig. 6–11). The final tidal volume is a primary function of airway resistance and compliance. The lower the compliance, the more efficient a small tidal volume with its resultant increase in respiratory rate.

Many of our patients discontinue exercise because of extreme dyspnea. Some evidence indicates that this type of dyspnea in patients with CAD is due to a rising left atrial and pulmonary venous pressure. It may be important to know the tidal volume because as the lungs become less compliant, it is more efficient to ventilate with a smaller tidal volume.

RESPIRATORY GAS EXCHANGE AND ANAEROBIC THRESHOLD

In 1964, Wasserman and McElroy[55] proposed a noninvasive method of detecting the onset of anaerobic metabolism during exercise. This occurs earlier than the peak work capacity of the patient and signals the point at which the

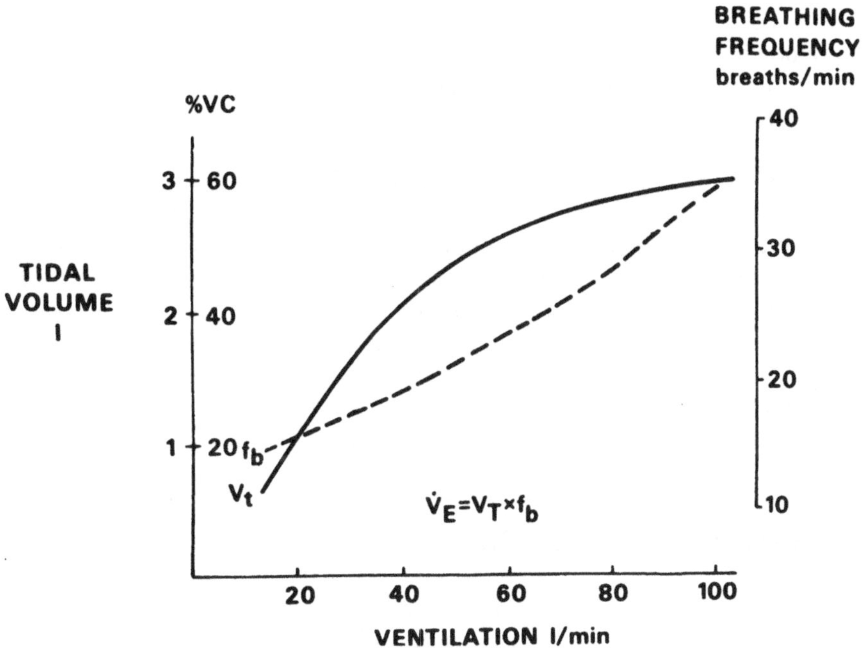

FIGURE 6–11. The *solid line* depicts the rapid change in tidal volume as ventilation increases until about 60% of total capacity and then begins to level off. The frequency of breathing (*dotted line*) increases in a more linear manner but increases excessively after about 80% of maximal capacity is reached.

patient is being deprived of adequate aerobic energy substrates. Although this point during exercise can be detected by an increase in lactic acid concentration in the blood or a decrease in arterial blood bicarbonate or pH, they proposed determination by an increase in the respiratory gas exchange ratio (R) on a breath-by-breath basis. They calculated R from the end-tidal gas concentrations monitored continuously during exercise using the formula:

$$R = \frac{F_ACO_2}{1.26\ F_AN_2 - 1 + F_AN_2}$$

where:

F_ACO_2 = end-tidal carbon dioxide concentration
F_AN_2 = end-tidal nitrogen concentration

R was then determined by a nomogram. Wasserman and McElroy were able to show that the increase in R was related principally to a decrease in end-tidal nitrogen concentration. In a typical subject, they found that the anaerobic threshold was between 60% and 70% of the maximum oxygen capacity when R suddenly changed from 87% to 96%. Experience has shown that R can usually be predicted from a change in the slope of the ventilatory equivalent, as well as the RQ.

Since the original work, Wasserman and Whipp[56] have studied the phenomenon intensely, and the level of anaerobic threshold has been used to estimate $\dot{V}O_2$ max and has been shown to increase with training. Its usefulness in evaluating exercise physiology in patients with CAD has yet to be determined.

This method requires careful monitoring of expired gases and the attendant discomfort to the patient. Unfortunately, many cardiac patients do not tolerate this type of instrumentation well. However, as techniques improve, it may be a worthwhile adjunct to the study of patients with CAD. Some data suggest the possibility that the anaerobic threshold might be detected by integrating electromyographic potentials as exercise progresses.[57] When the slow-twitch fibers become anoxic, the fast-twitch fibers are recruited and increase the potential voltage of the electromyogram. If this method is validated, it may be a useful noninvasive parameter.

WALK-THROUGH PHENOMENON

In 1966, MacAlpin and Kattus[58] reported that when subjects who were having pain while walking on the treadmill could be continued at a set rate, the angina would eventually disappear, even though there was no apparent decrease in their metabolic workload. At the same time, the ischemic ST segments returned to normal. This adaptive capacity can also be demonstrated by repeating the test after the patient has recovered from the first one. The capacity to improve after a warm-up probably reflects a similar process. The investigators reported that the pain usually remains constant at a set workload for about 5 minutes and then begins to decrease. It usually takes approximately 7 to 10 minutes to completely disappear and another 5 to 7 minutes for the ST segments to become isoelectric. Many patients report a similar type of response during their efforts to exercise in their work or recreation. We have not studied this process, but would guess that the adaptive process is less likely to be related to the heart than to peripheral effects. The lowering of peripheral resistance known to accompany exercise might well reduce the myocardial oxygen demands and thus allow the heart to function more efficiently in relationship to the total organism.

HEART SOUNDS AND OTHER AUSCULTATORY FINDINGS

First and Second Heart Sounds

Prior to every stress test, the physician should listen to the patient's heart to note the character of the heart sounds. The fact that the amplitude of the first sound correlates well with the $\Delta P/\Delta T$* of the left ventricle is well established.

Thus it is possible to predict to some degree how well the left ventricle will respond to stress. Paradoxical splitting of the second sound, usually associated with left bundle branch block, also indicates decreased function.

Third Heart Sounds

Third heart sounds are usually associated with very poor left-ventricular function and should cause the physician to seriously reconsider a decision to proceed with the stress test. In most cases, it should be considered a major contraindication to testing. On the other hand, if a third heart sound is heard after the test, it constitutes clear-cut evidence of serious ventricular dysfunction.

Fourth Heart Sounds

A fourth heart sound is a very common finding in ischemic heart disease. If this is fairly loud, the compliance of the left ventricle may be reduced, resulting in an elevation of the LVEDP. If this appears after exercise, it is a useful diagnostic sign. If it gets louder with exercise, it is more significant.[59] However, the fourth heart sound can also occur with primary myocardial disease.

Aortic Murmur

An ejection murmur of aortic stenosis should signal the possibility of an increased risk in testing the patient. Before the stress test is done, a good deal of information regarding the patient's status should be at hand. This is particularly true if the patient is over aged 40. Aortic insufficiency murmurs, however, do not preclude testing, but should be noted and correlated with the patient's blood pressure.

Mitral Murmur

The most commonly heard mitral murmur is associated with papillary muscle insufficiency or a prolapsed mitral leaflet. Short, late systolic murmurs associated with a click should alert one to the possibility that the ST-segment depression recorded may not be due to CAD. Holosystolic murmurs may indicate a more serious degree of mitral insufficiency. These usually do not constitute a significant contraindication to testing, however. The papillary muscle insufficiency murmur usually gets much louder near the peak of exercise. The diastolic murmur of mitral stenosis should tell the examiner that atrial fibrillation may be initiated by the stress. If tight mitral stenosis is present, a very modest increase in cardiac output is all that can be expected.

Figure 6–12 depicts the blood pressure, heart rate, and time of auscultation of a murmur of mitral insufficiency in a man without angina who had severe three-vessel disease.

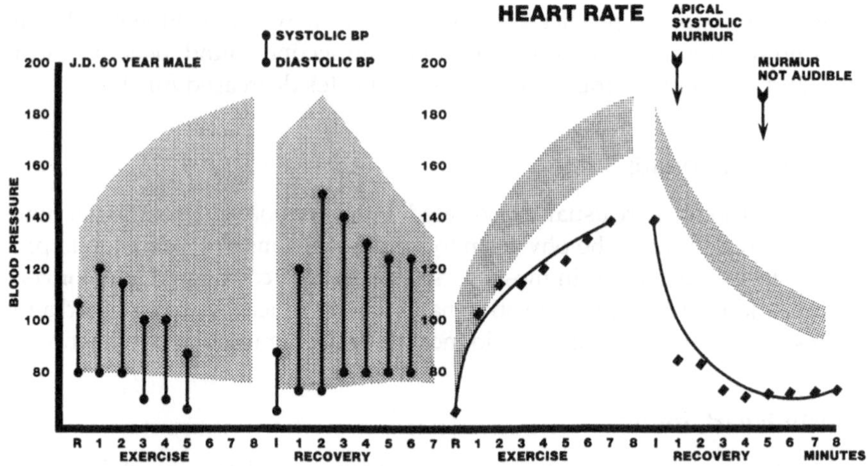

FIGURE 6–12. Blood pressure, heart rate, and time of auscultation of mitral insufficiency in a 60-year-old man without angina who had severe three-vessel disease.

PALPITATION

A double impulse may be felt when a fourth heart sound is heard, confirming the presence of alterations in left-ventricular compliance. Occasionally, a prominent left-ventricular heave is indicative of either a very dilated heart or a large apical ventricular aneurysm. Such a finding should be noted, since it may have a definite bearing on the presence or absence of the characteristic ST-segment changes seen with ischemia (see Chapter 14). An abnormal apical impulse is also common in patients with aortic or mitral valve disease. The typical thrill or vibration palpable on the chest wall, associated with various valvular lesions, is something to be particularly watchful for because it indicates that the physiological abnormality associated with the accompanying murmur is producing an increased workload on the heart.

PULSUS ALTERNANS

Banks and Shugoll[5] described pulsus alternans occurring in 4 of 12 patients during attacks of spontaneous angina. We have not searched for this routinely, but it has been observed occasionally in those with severe angina and poor left-ventricular function. One should be especially alert for pulsus alternans if alternating ST-segment depression or QRS amplitude is observed on the monitor during the stress test (see Chapter 6).

SUMMARY

It is hoped that this chapter has provided enough information to convince the reader that there is more to stress testing than ST-segment depression. An article in the *New England Journal of Medicine* was widely quoted emphasizing that exercise-induced ST depression added little to the diagnosis in patients with classic angina.[73] The authors, however, ignored many of the important parameters demonstrated to be useful in patient evaluation. These will be reviewed again in Chapters 12 and 14. The term *positive* or *negative stress tests,* although still in use, is mostly to help understand some of the concepts relating to prevalence and the Bayes' theorem of probability. It should be abandoned in the clinical setting when based on ST segments only, because it denotes an all-or-none phenomenon that completely distorts our thinking about the use of stress testing. Because so many hemodynamic and other clinical findings are useful in evaluating the stress test, one should never fail to consider all the data available.

REFERENCES

1. Maseri, A: Pathogenic mechanisms of angina pectoris: Expanding views. Br Heart J 43:648, 1980.
2. Marcus, ML: The Coronary Circulation in Health and Disease. McGraw-Hill, New York, 1983.
3. Zeiher, AM, et al: Modulation of coronary vasomotor tone in humans. Circulation 83:391, 1991.
4. Canty, JM and Smith, TP, Jr.: Modulation of coronary autoregulatory responses by endothelium-derived nitric oxide. Int J Cardiology 50;207, 1995.
5. Staneloff, H, et al: The powerful predictor pitfall in prognostication. Circulation 68(111):136, 1983.
6. Banks, T and Shugoll, GI: Confirmatory physical findings in angina pectoris. JAMA 200:107, 1967.
7. Berson, AS and Pipberger, HV: The low frequency response of electrocardiographs: A frequent source of recording errors. Am Heart J 71:779, 1966.
8. Report of Committee on Electrocardiography, American Heart Association: Recommendations for standardizations of leads and of specifications for instruments in electrocardiography and vector cardiography. Circulation 35:583, 1967.
9. Faris, JV, et al: Concepts and applications of treadmill exercise testing and exercise ECG. Am Heart J 95:102, 1978.
10. Wood, FC and Wolferth, CC: Angina pectoris: The clinical and electrocardiographic phenomena of the attack and their comparison with the effects with experimental temporary coronary occlusion. Arch Intern Med 47:339, 1939.
11. Blackburn, H, et al: The standardization of the exercise ECG: A systematic comparison of chest lead configurations employed for monitoring during exercise. In Simonson E (ed): Physical Activity and the Heart. Charles C. Thomas, Springfield, IL, 1967.
12. Froelicher, VF, et al: A comparison of two bipolar exercise ECG leads to lead V5. Chest 70:611, 1976.
13. Blackburn, H. The exercise electrocardiogram: Technological, procedural and conceptual developments. In Blackburn, H (ed): Measurement in Exercise Electrocardiography. Charles C. Thomas, Springfield, IL, 1967.
14. Hakki, AH, et al: R wave amplitude: A new determinant of failure of patients with coronary heart disease t manifest ST segment depression during exercise. JACC 3(5):1155, 1984.

15. McHenry, PL and Morris SN: Exercise electrocardiography: Current state of the art. In Schlant, RC and Hurst, JW (eds): Advances in Electrocardiography. Grune & Stratton, New York, 1976.
16. Simoons, M: Optimal measurements for detection of coronary artery disease by exercise ECG. Comput Biomed Res 10:483, 1977.
17. Hornsten, RR and Bruce, RA: Computed S-T forces of frank and bipolar exercise electrocardiograms. Am Heart J 78:346, 1969.
18. Camp, J, et al: Diagnostic sensitivity of multiple leads in maximal exercise testing. Circulation 44:1120, 1971.
19. Isaacs, JH, et al: Vector electrocardiographic exercise test in ischemic heart disease. JAMA 198:139, 1966.
20. Blomquist, CG: The frank lead exercise electrocaridogram. Acta Med Scand 440(suppl):9, 1965.
21. Blomquist, CG: Heart disease and dynamic exercise testing. In Willerson, JT and Sanders, CA (eds): Clinical Cardiology. Grune & Stratton, New York, 1977.
22. Fox, KM, et al: Projection of ST segment changes on the front of the chest. Br Heart J 48:555, 1982.
23. Fox, KM, et al: Precordial exercise mapping: Improved diagnosis of coronary artery disease. Br Heart J 11:1596, 1978.
24. Chaitman, BR, et al: Improved efficiency of treadmill exercise testing using a multiple lead system. Circulation 57:71, 1978.
25. Chaitman, BR: Unpublished report.
26. Spach, MS and Barr, MC: Localizing cardiac electrical events from body surface maps. Int J Cardiol 3(4):459, 1983.
27. Mason, RE and Likar, I: A new lead system of multiple-lead exercise electrocardiography. Am Heart J 71:196, 1966.
28. Michaelides, A.P., et al: Improved detection of coronary artery disease by exercise electrocardiography with the use of right precordial leads. New Engl J Med 340(5):340, 1999.
29. Saetre, HA, et al: 16 lead ECG changes with coronary angioplasty. J Electrocardiol 24(suppl):152, 1991.
30. Ellestad, MH and Lerman, S: The limitations of the diagnostic power of exercise testing. Am J Noninvas Cardiol 3:139, 1989.
31. Myrianthefs, M, et al: Significance of signal averaged P waves changes during exercise in patients with coronary disease. Am J Cardiol 68:1619, 1991.
32. Myrianthefs, M, et al: Analysis of the signal averaged P wave duration in patients with PTCA. Am J Cardiol 70:728, 1992.
33. Elamin, MS, et al: Accurate detection of coronary heart disease by new exercise test. Br Heart J 48:311, 1982.
34. Quyyumi, AA, et al: Inability of the St segment/heart rate slope to predict accurately the severity of coronary artery disease. Br Heart J 51:395, 1984.
35. Kligfield, P, et al: HR adjustment of ST depression for improved detection of coronary artery disease. Circulation 79:245, 1989.
36. Lachterman, B, et al: Comparison of the ST HR index to standard ST criteria for analysis of the electrocardiogram. Circulation 82:44, 1990.
37. Miller-Crig, M, et al: Use of graded exercise testing in assessing the hypertensive patient. Clin Cardiol 3:236, 1980.
38. Thulein, T and Werner, O: Exercise test and 24-our HR recording in men with high and low casual blood pressure levels. Br Heart J 40:534, 1978.
39. Jose, AD and Taylor, RR: Autonomic blockade by propranolol and atropine to study the intrinsic muscle function in man. J Clin Invest 48:2019, 1969.
40. Hinkle, LE, et al: Slow heart rates and increased risk of cardiac death in middle-aged men. Arch Intern Med 129:732, 1972.
41. Grimby, G and Saltin, B: Physiological analysis of physically well-trained middle-aged and old athletes. Acta Med Scand 179:513, 1966.
42. Chin, CF, et al: Chronotropic incompetence: An analysis of hemodynamic and anatomical findings. Clin Cardiol 2:12, 1979.
43. Wiens, RD, et al: Chronotropic incompetence in clinical exercise testing. Am J Cardiol 54: 74, 1984.
44. J Lauer, MS, et al: Impaired heart rate response to graded exercise: Prognostic implications of chronotropic incompetence in the Framingham Heart Study. Circulation 93:1520,1996.

45. Lauer, MS, et al: Impaired chronotropic response to exercise stress testing as a predictor of mortality. JAMA 1999:524,1999.
46. Goldstein, RE, et al: Impairment of autonomically mediated heart rate control of patients with cardiac dysfunction. Circ Res 36:571, 1975.
47. Sandvik, L, et al: Heart rate increase and maximal heart rate during exercise as predictors of cardiovascular mortality: A 16-year follow-up study of 1960 healthy men. Cor Art Dis 6:667, 1996.
48. Fox, SM, et al: Physical activity and the prevention of coronary heart disease. Ann Clin Res 3:404, 1971.
49. Ford, AB and Hellerstein, HK : Energy cost of the Master's two-step test. JAMA 164:1868, 1957.
50. Balke, B and Ware, RW: An experimental study of physical fitness of Air Force personnel. US Armed Forces Med J 10:675, 1959.
51. Mastropaolo, JA, et al: Physical activity of work, physical fitness and coronary heart disease in middle-aged men. In Karvonen, MD and Barry, AJ (eds): Physical Activity and the Heart. Charles C Thomas, Springfield, IL, 1967, p. 77.
52. Bruce, RA, et al: Maximal oxygen intake and nomographic assessment of functional aerobic impairment in cardiovascular disease. Am Heart J 85:546, 1973.
53. Givoni, B and Goldman, R: Predicting metabolic energy costs. J Appl Physiol30 (3):429, 1971.
54. Jones, HL: Clinical Exercising Testing. WB Saunders, Philadelphia, 1975.
55. Wasserman, K and McElroy, MB: Detecting the threshold of anaerobic metabolism in cardiac patients during exercise. Am J Cardiol 14:844, 1964.
56. Wasserman, K and Whipp, BJ: Exercise physiology in health and disease. Am Rev Respir Dis 112:219, 1979.
57. Moritani, T and Devries, HA: Reexamination of the relationship between the surface EMG and force of isometric contraction. Am J Phys Med 57:263, 1978.
58. MacAlpin, RH and Kattus, AA: Adaptation to exercise in angina pectoris: The electrocardiograms during treadmill walking and coronary angiographic findings. Circulation 33:183, 1966.
59. Gooch, AS and Evans, JM: Extended applications of exercise stress testing. Med Ann Dist Col 38:80, 1969.

7
Stress Echocardiography

Introduction
Treadmill Echocardiography
Indications for Including Echo Imaging
Methodology
Treadmill Echocardiography
Evaluation of Images
Pharmacological Stress
Accuracy of Stress Echocardiography
Accuracy of Various Modes of Stress
Stress Echocardiography in Prognosis
Stress Echo as Compared to Nuclear Studies
Stress Echo to Identify Viable Myocardium

INTRODUCTION

Although it was recognized by Berberich, Zager,[1] and others,[2] as early as 1981, that observing the M-Mode Echocardiogram before and after exercise had diagnostic potential, it was only widely accepted after digitalized 2-dimensional images came into common usage. Development of a system that could digitize a single cardiac cycle at rest and display the rest and exercise images side by side simultaneously immediately after exercise resulted in the general acceptance of this technology.

Recent technical advances in imaging have improved the accuracy of stress echocardiography. Among the most significant of these is the development of tissue harmonic imaging.[3,4] Tissue harmonic imaging is an echocardiographic image technique where the ultrasound beam is sent out at one frequency and received back at twice the initial frequency, resulting in a reduction of noise, thus allowing us to use the power or amplitude signal from the myocardial Doppler.[5] Image segmentation techniques now being generated off line may soon add to the ability to better understand myocardial function such as diastolic stiffness.[6] These techniques allow for increased endocardial border section and thereby provide better visualization of wall motion of the various segments of the heart. Another advancement is the develolpment of intravenous echocardiographic contrast agents, which also allow for improved deliniation of the endocardial border, thus allowing better assessment of wall motion during two dimensional echocardiography, especially during stress echocardiography.[7] Abraham has described a method of measuring time to regional relaxation in various myocardial segments by strain rate imaging.[8] When TR prolongs >20% this indicates ischemia with a sensitivity of 92% and a specificity of 75%. It remains to be confirmed however, before it can be recommended.

The wall motion abnormalities induced by exercise often occur early in the ischemic cascade, often before the electrocardiographic changes and before the onset of chest pain or after pharmacological or pacing induced stress (Fig. 7–1).[9]

Exercise is usually applied with a treadmill or with a supine or upright bicycle. Stress can also be achieved by adrenergic stimulation with Dobutamine, Isopril or Arbutamine.[10] Vasodilatation has also been used with Dipyridamole and Adenosine. At times stress is achieved with pacing, using an esophageal lead or using invasive procedures during a heart cath, such as atrial or ventricular pacing. We have also used atrial pacing in patients who have a permanent pacer by programming their pacer to more rapid rates incrementally.

Each of these methods has their strengths and weaknesses, however exercise clearly provides the best evaluation in our experience.

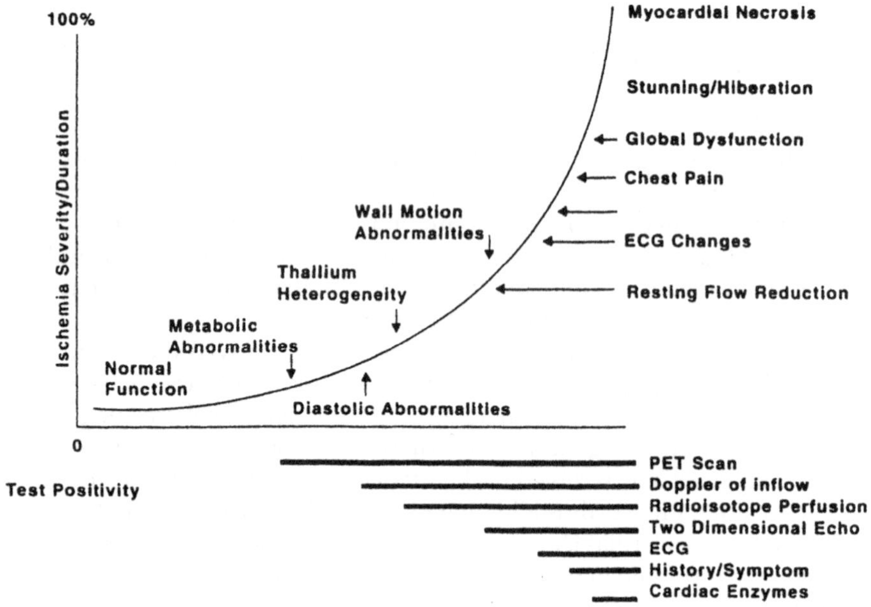

FIGURE 7–1. Representation of the ischemic cascade. After reduction in myocardial blood flow sufficient to result in physiologic abnormalities, a predictable sequence of events occurs, beginning with subclinical diastolic dysfunction and progressing to electrocardiographic abnormalities and the clinical syndrome of anginal chest pain. Of note, wall motion abnormalities as detected by stress echocardiography precede the development of diagnostic electrocardiographic changes and angina. The time points in the ischemic cascade at which different diagnostic tests are presumed to become positive are noted by the bars below the graph.

TREADMILL ECHOCARDIOGRAPHY

The strength of this method is due to the ability to evaluate wall motion changes and at the same time observe the clinical and hemodynamic response as well as the electrocardiogram.

INDICATIONS FOR INCLUDING ECHO IMAGING

Patients with resting electrocardiograms that make the ischemic response difficult to interpret—

1. Digitalis or conduction problems that result in an abnormal resting tracing such as left bundle branch block or left ventricular hypertrophy,
2. Wolf-Parkinson-White Syndrome
3. Very low voltage, as is common in patients who have had an anterior wall infarct
4. Prior bypass surgery
5. Patients whose angiographic images suggest a stenosis of equivocal significance and it is believed a decrease in wall motion during exercise may establish or confirm the presence of ischemia.
6. Patients where an angioplasty might be at high risk in more than one vessel and exercise induced ischemia will often determine which vessel should be the most important to treat.

METHODOLOGY

Treadmill Echocardiography

Patients are exercised according to a standard protocol after a supine Echo is recorded in the left lateral cubitus. The patient is exercised to his maximum capacity and is terminated because of fatigue, chest pain, severe ST depression, arrhythmias, blood pressure drop, etc. As soon as exercise is terminated the patient assumes the same position used prior to the test and images are recorded with as much breath holding as possible (Fig. 7–2).

The images are displayed in standard views as recommended by the American Society for Echocardiography. In our experience the standard 4-chamber view provides the most information.

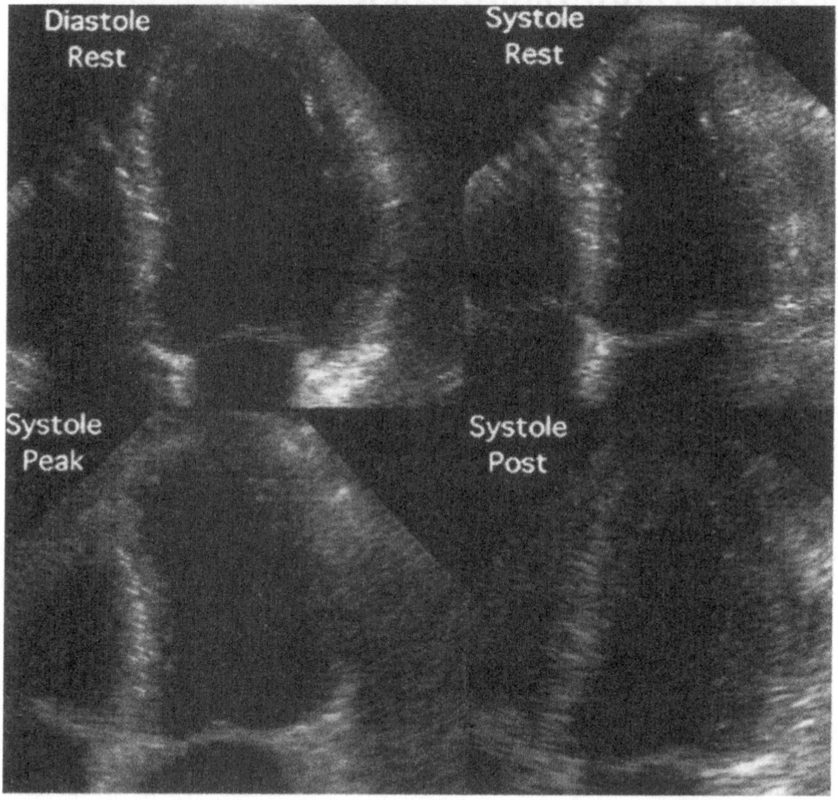

FIGURE 7–2. Images during rest (*Top*) and exercise (*Bottom*) displayed for evaluation of wall motion changes. (From Hecht H, DeBord L, and Sotomayer, N: Supine bicycle stress echocardiography. Cardiology, November: 55, 1993, with permission.)

Evaluation of Images

A normal test is when the myocardial segments visualized have normal contraction at rest and become hyperdynamic with exercise. An abnormal test is characterized by a cardiac segment that changes from normal to hypokinetic, from hyperkinetic to akinetic, or from akinetic to dyskinetic. These changes occur with inducible ischemia and have been reported to have a higher sensitivity and specificity than when the diagnosis is based on EKG changes alone. It is important to realize however, that there have been no studies where electrocardiographic changes other than the standard ST depression is compared, so that when one evaluates multiple electrocardiographic changes, now known to be associated with ischemia, there may be some difference in the comparison of accuracy.

Pharmacological Stress

A significant number of patients are unable to exercise on a treadmill or bicycle. In this population Dobutamine has become the standard agent used to generate an increased metabolic demand.[11] This drug has a strong ionotropic and a modest chronotropic effect. If the heart rate does not accelerate one milligram of IV Atropine can be added,[12] which will usually bring about a significant increase. A new sympathomametic agent, Arbutamine,[10] is under study and seems quite satisfactory as it produces a greater chronotropic response than Dobutamine. Reductions in contractility produced by Dobutamine, that can be detected by Echo, are believed to be similar to that induced by exercise.

Accuracy of Stress Echocardiography

There are a number of reports that are correlating this technology with angiography, some of which are presented in Table 7–1. It is apparent that the reliability is very good. It is reported however, that when exercise blood pressure becomes quite high (over 200) hypokinesis in the apex is common, even in patients without coronary disease.[12a]

Accuracy of Various Modes of Stress

As more and more studies of various types of stress are reported it appears that exercise, Dobutamine, Adenosine and Dipyridamole all have similar sensitivities and specificities.[13,14] The methodology also is quite accurate in patients with LVH and with reduced ejection fraction and in those who are pacemaker dependent (Table 7–1).[15]

Table 7–1. **Studies Using Stress Echocardiography for the Detection of CAD**

Author, Year	Type of Test	No. Patients	Sensitivity (%)	Specificity (%)	Note
Ryan, 1993[26]	Bicycle Exercise	309	91	78	
Hecht, 1993[27]	Bicycle	180	93	86	
Reis, 1995[26]	DSE	30	95	86	ESRD
Marwick, 1995[29]	Exercise	161	80	81	Women
Marwick, 1995[30]	Exercise	79	71	87	Without LVH
		68	71	95	With LVH
Takeuchi, 1996[20]	DSE	70	75	92	Women
Senior, 1996[31]	DSE	43	93	100	With HTN
Kisacik, 1996[32]	DSE	69	94	86	

DSE, dobutamine stress echo; ESRD, end stage renal disease; LVH, left ventricular hypertrophy.

Stress Echocardiography in Prognosis

Prognosis over at least 4 years has been studied and can be estimated with stress echo.[16] Colon reported that event free survival occurred in 97% of those with normal Echoes as compared to 74% in those with wall motion abnormalities in 660 patients.[17] Lin studied patients with unstable angina and found an 81% survival in patients who were positive as compared to 95% in the negatives.[18] It has also been used in diabetics, transplant patients and prior to general surgery.

Stress Echo as Compared to Nuclear Studies

When using coronary angiography as a gold standard, which has its shortcomings, the sensitivity and specificity of stress echocardiography and stress nuclear scintigraphy appears to be similar.[19] In women however, stress echocardiograms appear to be more accurate than nuclear, probably because of the attenuation of tracer caused by breast tissue in women.[20] Olmos compared exercised Echo and exercise Thallium and found them to have almost equal predictive value.[21] This is probably true for both exercise and pharmacological echocardiograms.[22]

Stress Echo to Identify Viable Myocardium

After an infarction revascularization can significantly improve contraction of the myocardial segments that are still viable.[23] Many times they do not contract when visualized on a resting Echo and the question arises, should revascularization be attempted or is the noncontractile segment scar tissue only or is it hibernating and possibly capable of resuming normal function? Low dose Dobutamine Echocardiography has been demonstrated to be of value in making this distinction.[24] If a noncontractile segment of the heart begins to contract with an infusion of 5 micrograms per kilogram but becomes noncontractile or has a reduced function as the concentration is increased it is probably viable and will resume at least some function when revascularization has been achieved. This approach has been compared to Thallium scintigraphy and PET scanning and they all seem to be quite comparable, although in the past PET (positron emission tomography) has been believed to be the most reliable.[25]

SUMMARY

In the last few years stress Echocardiography has taken its place as a clinically useful imaging technique for the diagnosis of cardiac ischemia, for the prediction of future cardiac events and for the determination of viability of noncontractile segments of the heart. It is widely available, reasonable in cost and probably as accurate as the other imaging modalities.

REFERENCES

1. Berberich, SN and Zager, Jr: Hybrid exercise echocardiography. Angiology 32:1, 1981.
2. Mason, DL, et al: Exercise echocardiography: Detection of wall motion abnormality during ischemia. Circulation 59:50, 1979.
3. Skolnick, DG, et al: Enhanced endocardial visualization with noncontrast harmonic imaging during stress echocardiography. J Am Soc Echocardiogr 12:559, 1999.
4. Zaglavara, T, et al: Dobutamine stress echocardiography: Improved endocardial border definition and wall motion analysis with tissue harmonic imaging. J Am Soc Echocardiogr 12:706, 1999.
5. Spencer, KT, et al: Use of harmonic imaging without echocardiographic contrast to improve two-dimensional image quality. Am J Cardiol 82:794, 1998.
6. Chakraborty, A, et al: Deformable boundary finding in medical images by integrating gradient and regional information. IEEE Trans Med Imaging 15:859, 1996.
7. Falcone, RA, et al: Intravenous albunex during dobutamine stress echocardiography: Enhanced localization of left ventricular endocardial borders. Am Heart J 130:254, 1995.
8. Abraham, TP, et al: Time to onset of regional relaxation: Feasibility, variability and utility of a novel index of regional myocardial function by strain rate imaging. JACC 39(9):1531, 2002.
9. Kolias, TJ and Armstrong, WF: Stress echocardiography. Exercise Testing: New Concepts for the New Century. Kluwer Academic Publishers, 2002.
10. Kiat, H, et al: Arbutomine stress using a closed loop delivery system. JACC 26:1159, 1995.
11. Mathias, W, Jr., et al: Safety of dobutamine-atropine stress echocardiography: A prospective experience of 4,033 consecutive studies. J Am Soc Echocardiogr 12:785, 1999.
12. Lewandowski, TJ, et al: Reduced test time by early identification of patients requiring atropine during dobutamine stress echocardiography. J Am Soc Echocardiogr 11:236, 1998.

12a. Ha, JW, et al: Hypertensive response to exercise: A potential cause of new wall motion abnormality in the absence of coronary artery disease. J Am Coll Cardiol 39:323, 2002.

13. Sawada, SG, et al: Upright bicycle exercise echocardiography after coronary artery bypass grafting. Am J Cardiol 64:1123, 1989.
14. Segar, DS, et al: Dobutamine stress echocardiography: correlation with coronary lesion severity as determined by quantitative angiography. J Am Coll Cardiol 19:1197, 1992.
15. Oral, H, et al: Preserved diagnostic utility of dobutamine stress echocardiography in pacemaker-dependent patients with absolute chronotropic incompetence. Am Heart J 138:364, 1999.
16. Marwick, TH, et al: Use of exercise echocardiography for prognostic evaluation of patients with known or suspected coronary artery disease. J Am Coll Cardiol 30:83, 1997.
17. Colon, PJ, III, et al: Prognostic value of stress echocardiography in the evaluation of atypical chest pain patients without known coronary artery disease. Am J Cardiol 81:545, 1998.
18. Lin, SS, et al: Risk stratification of patients with medically treated unstable angina using exercise echocardiography. Am J Cardiol 82:720, 1998.
19. Quinones, MA, et al: Exercise echocardiography versus 201T1 single-photon emission computed tomography in evaluation of coronary artery disease. Analysis of 292 patients [see comments]. Circulation 85:1026, 1992.
20. Takeuchi, M, et al: Comparative diagnostic value of dobutamine stress echocardiography and stress thallium-201 single-photon-emission computed tomography for detecting coronary artery disease in women. Coron Artery Dis 7:831, 1996.
21. Olmos, LI, et al: Long-term prognostic value of exercise echocardiography compared with exercise 201T1, ECG, and clinical variables in patients evaluated for coronary artery disease. Circulation 98:2679, 1998.
22. Previtali, M, et al: Prognostic value of myocardial viability and ischemia detected by dobutamine stress echocardiography early after acute myocardial infarction treated with thrombolysis. J Am Coll Cardiol 32:380, 1998.
23. Afridi, I, et al: Myocardial viability during dobutamine echocardiography predicts survival in patients with coronary artery disease and severe left ventricular systolic dysfunction. J Am Coll Cardiol 32:921, 1998.
24. Bax, JJ, et al: Accuracy of currently available techniques for prediction of functional recovery after revascularization in patients with left ventricular dysfunction due to chronic coronary artery disease: comparison of pooled data. J Am Coll Cardiol 39:1451, 1997.

25. Poldermans, D, et al: Sustained prognostic value of dobutamine stress echocardiography for late cardiac events after major noncardiac vascular surgery [see comments]. Circulation 95:53, 1997.
26. Ryan, T, et al: Exercise echocardiography: detection of coronary artery disease in patients with normal left ventricular wall motion at rest. J Am Coll Cardiol 11:993, 1988.
27. Hecht, HS, et al: Digital supine bicycle stress echocardiography: a new technique for evaluating coronary artery disease. J Am Coll Cardiol 21:950, 1993.
28. Reis, G, et al: Usefulness of dobutamine stress echocardiography in detecting coronary artery disease in end-stage renal disease. Am J Cardiol 75:707, 1995.
29. Marwick, TH, et al: Influence of left ventricular hypertrophy on detection of coronary artery disease using exercise echocardiography. J Am Coll Cardiol 26:1180, 1995.
30. Marwick, TH, et al: Exercise echocardiography is an accurate and cost-efficient technique for detection of coronary artery disease in women. J Am Coll Cardiol 26:335, 1995.
31. Senior, R, et al: Diagnostic accuracy of dobutamine stress echocardiography for detection of coronary heart disease in hypertensive patients. Eur Heart J 17:289, 1996.
32. Kisacik, HL, et al: Comparison of exercise stress testing with simultaneous dobutamine stress echocardiography and technetium-99m isonitrile single-photon emission computerized tomography for diagnosis of coronary artery disease. Eur Heart J 17:113, 1996.

8
Stress Testing Protocol

Requirements
Threshold of Myocardial Ischemia
Preparation for the Test
Single-Load Tests
Master's Test
Intermittent Tests
Continuous Tests
Heart-Rate–Targeted Testing
Bicycle Test
Supine Versus Upright Bicycle Test
Treadmill Test
Bruce Protocol
Comparison of Various Protocols
Cornell Protocol
Ramp Protocol
Estimation of Oxygen Consumption
Exercise Intensity
Maximum Heart Rate
Protocol for Early Stress Testing (After MI)
Isometric Test
Isometric Combined with Isotonic Exercise
Emotional Stress Test
Circadian Influence

Many of the protocols described in the previous edition of this book are of historical interest only and have been deleted. These include Kaltenbach's Climbing Step Test; the hypoxemia test; the Harvard Step Test; the catecholamine, ergonovine, and histamine tests; and the test of left-ventricular wall function using the kymocardiograph.

REQUIREMENTS

The protocol for stress testing should be structured to include the following:

1. Continuous ECG monitoring.
2. Hard copy ECG recording when desired, preferably several simultaneous leads before, during, and after exercise and at 1-minute intervals during exercise. A minimal recording of muscle potential is essential to an artifact-free recording with averaged beats at 1-minute intervals.
3. A type of activity that can be performed by the sedentary, poorly developed, and underconditioned subject as well as by the trained athlete.

4. A workload that can be varied according to the capacity of the individual but is standardized enough to deliver reproducible results and allow comparison with other patients tested.
5. Repeated frequent blood pressure measurements before, during, and after exercise.
6. A way of estimating the aerobic requirements of individuals tested.
7. Maximum safety and minimum discomfort for each individual tested.
8. The highest possible specificity and sensitivity in the discrimination between health and disease.
9. A sufficient body of information available so that the response of normal and cardiac patients can be identified.
10. A first stage long enough for a warm-up to occur.
11. A procedure short enough to be practical.

THRESHOLD OF MYOCARDIAL ISCHEMIA

It has long been believed that patients with coronary artery disease (CAD) will develop angina or ST depression at a fixed threshold, characterized by a constant double product. However, the work of Garber and associates[1] and Carleton and associates[2] at Brown University challenges this concept. These investigators tested a group of patients with known CAD on a standard maximum protocol and repeated the test several days later with a protocol that limited the workload to 70% of the peak heart rate and continued exercise for at least 20 minutes. More patients developed angina on the maximum test; 85% developed ST depression on the submaximum test compared with 100% on the maximum test. Oxygen consumption and the double product at onset of angina or ST depression was lower during the submaximum protocol. Thus, when using exercise testing to establish a threshold, as one might do to evaluate therapy, the exercise protocol must be the same for each test.

PREPARATION FOR THE TEST

In most cases, patients have been advised to come in for their exercise test in the morning before eating, because it has been reported that food causes an increase in cardiac output, oxygen consumption, minute ventilation, and total peripheral vascular resistance and thus would be expected to bring on angina and ST depression at a lower threshold.[3] This dictum was recently challenged by researchers who tested eight patients after a 500-calorie meal and after fasting and reported that the ischemic threshold was the same.[4] This study involved too small a cohort to dismiss the previous work, but it does point out the possibility that a light meal may have little effect on the results. Our policy is not to restrict meals before testing unless we are specifically attempting to compare workloads after some intervention. When doing a diagnostic test, the exact level of the ischemic threshold is not critical to the diagnosis.

SINGLE-LOAD TESTS

Master's Test

The protocol for the Master's test, at one time the most commonly used exercise test, was constructed originally as an exercise tolerance test rather than a screening test for CAD. The subject walked up and over a device two steps high with three steps, two of which were 9 inches above the floor and a top step 18 inches high.[5] Even though Master used three steps in each ascent, two up and one down, it was called a two-step test. After going up and over, the patient then turned and walked over the steps again for a prescribed number of ascents. Blood pressure and pulse were then recorded; by knowing the patient's weight and the time required to complete the test, the work per minute could be derived. It was suggested that the prescribed number of ascents be completed in 1½ minutes. The tables for the number of ascents for men and women are reproduced in Appendix 5.

Many years later, Master added the ECG and suggested that it be recorded before and after the step test. He largely abandoned the original criteria that had been proposed to evaluate exercise tolerance. This test was accepted as the standard until the 1970s and for years was the most widely used in spite of its clinical limitations.

A survey completed in 1978 suggested that the Master's test was decreasing in popularity[6]; now there are only a few of us who have ever seen a set of Master's steps. Because heart rate and blood pressure are not recorded during the test, no measurements are available to evaluate the percentage of maximum work. Master recommended that 0.5 mm of ST depression be accepted as abnormal, which in conjunction with the reduced workload resulted in about 60% false-negative results. Master reported in 1935 that 100 patients with CAD were tested and none developed anginal pain on the test—ample evidence that the workload was too low to induce ischemia in many patients.

INTERMITTENT TESTS

The concept of an intermittent test is basically sound because progressive workloads can be interspersed with short rest periods, thus giving the subject time to recover somewhat before starting the next period of exercise. This time also allows the examiner to take ECGs and make blood pressure determinations without the motion artifact attendant on walking or running. Experience has shown that muscle strength can be restored when frequent rest periods are allowed; therefore, a greater total stress can be applied. Intermittent tests of this sort are often associated with continuous monitoring, and the aerobic capacity can be estimated.

Examples of intermittent tests include Hellerstein and Hornsten's[7] version of the work capacity test (PWC 150) and the widely used Swedish bicycle test[8] and a number of its modifications proposed by Mitchell and associates.[9] Hellerstein, one of the pioneers in stress testing, stated that the intermittent test is more physiological and that he preferred it to a continuous protocol. Although bicycle tests are commonly used for intermittent tests, a treadmill is equally applicable. The chief disadvantage of intermittent tests is the time required for the rest periods between exercise. They have largely been abandoned in the United States.

CONTINUOUS TESTS

Continuous tests are similar to intermittent tests in basic design, but vary in that they may consist of a treadmill, a bicycle, or some type of stepping device. They also vary in the amount of work applied and the duration of effort required. By not allowing the patient to rest between work periods and by progressively increasing the work, the patient's peak capacity or endpoint is reached earlier. The ability to predict aerobic capacity, observe the chronotropic response to stress, measure blood pressure, and continuously record the ECG is similar to that of the intermittent tests.[10]

Heart-Rate–Targeted Testing

Increasing the exercise workload is usually accomplished by selecting some arbitrary increase in bicycle resistance or treadmill speed or grade. Another approach to increasing work is to set a target heart rate for each workload and then increase the work until this rate is reached. This can be done on a bicycle or a treadmill. Because heart rate is a major determinant of myocardial oxygen consumption, the work corresponding to a prescribed heart rate is then a way of estimating the patient's aerobic capacity. Using this method, it might also be possible to evaluate subjects at predetermined percentages of their predicted maximum aerobic capacity. The patient's physiological response theoretically adjusts the heart rate according to individual physical fitness.[11,12] Because individual variation in heart rate at a given workload is very common, if exercise is terminated at a target heart rate, it is not possible to judge the patient's maximum capacity.[13]

Bicycle Test

The use of the bicycle in testing has several advantages. The patient's thorax and arms are relatively stable, allowing ECGs to be recorded with less muscle artifact and making it easier to record blood pressure accurately. The patient's body weight does not influence exercise capacity appreciably, and sitting on a bicycle often produces less anxiety than walking on a mechanically driven treadmill. In addition, the bicycle requires less space in the laboratory and is usually less expensive than a treadmill. It is my feeling, however, that the treadmill applies a more physiological workload. This view seems to be shared by most stress testing laboratory personnel in the United States, and a number of studies have shown that subjects are much more likely to reach their aerobic capacity or their peak predicted heart rate on the treadmill, especially if they are not naturally athletic. The muscles necessary for bicycling are generally not well developed in the American population. We have also found that when patients are somewhat reluctant to push on because of fatigue, it is easier to obtain their cooperation on a treadmill because it is difficult for them to stop voluntarily when the treadmill is still moving.

Bicycle test protocols may be intermittent or continuous but usually involve a progressively increasing workload. The bicycle may be mechanically or electrically braked, and the workload is easily calibrated in watts or kilogram meters and tends to be less dependent on the patient's weight and physical efficiency. A small person may be spending a much larger portion of maximum oxygen intake at a given workload than a large person, but the work applied takes a much less complex set of muscles and therefore is more predictable from one time to another. Nomograms have been constructed, and Table 8–1 lists the aerobic capacity of individuals exercised on a bicycle ergometer. As the subject's weight increases, the oxygen consumption per minute decreases per kilogram of body weight. In one study of both treadmill and bicycle exercise performed in 52 patients, the treadmill was reported to provide a higher oxygen uptake and an increased efficiency in identifying ischemia.[14]

Koyal and colleagues[15] have reported that the small muscle mass used during bicycle tests causes more metabolic acidosis, which cannot be compensated for by increased ventilation. Therefore, the respiratory rate for equivalent workloads was higher.

Supine Versus Upright Bicycle Test

Most bicycle tests are performed sitting upright, but supine bicycle tests have become more popular, especially since exercise echocardiography has come into vogue. Supine bicycling is more likely to result in ischemia than upright pedaling. It may cause more ischemia when used in nuclear tests and thus might be a factor that increases the sensitivity of these tests. Because of increased diastolic filling of the left ventricle in the horizontal posture, left-ventricular diastolic dysfunction resulting in ST depression is more commonly seen in the supine than in the upright position.[16,17] Vellinga and associates[18] have also reported that the increased ST depression is associated with a larger area of myocardial ischemia, as judged by SPECT imaging of the thallium scintigram.

Table 8–1. **Oxygen Requirements of Bicycle Ergometric Workloads***

Workload											
watts		25	50	75	100	125	150	175	200	250	300
kg-m/min		150	300	450	600	750	900	1050	1200	1500	1800
Total oxygen used		600	900	1200	1500	1800	2100	2400	2700	3300	3900
kcal/min		3.0	4.5	6.0	7.5	9.0	10.5	12.0	13.5	16.5	19.5
Body Weight											
(lb)	**(kg)**	***Oxygen Used (mL/min per kilogram of body weight)***									
88	40	15.0	22.5	30.0	37.5	45.0	52.5	60.0	67.5	82.5	97.5
110	50	12.0	18.0	24.0	30.0	36.0	42.0	48.0	54.0	66.0	78.0
132	60	10.0	15.0	20.0	25.0	30.0	35.0	40.0	45.0	55.0	65.0
154	70	8.5	13.0	17.0	21.5	25.5	30.0	34.5	38.5	47.0	55.5
176	80	7.5	11.0	15.0	19.0	22.5	26.0	30.0	34.0	41.0	49.0
198	90	6.7	10.0	13.3	16.7	20.0	23.3	26.7	30.0	36.7	43.3
220	100	6.0	9.0	12.0	15.0	18.0	21.0	24.0	27.0	33.0	39.0
242	110	5.5	8.0	11.0	13.5	16.5	19.0	22.0	24.5	30.0	35.5
264	120	5.0	7.5	10.0	12.5	15.0	17.5	20.0	22.5	27.5	32.5

*Based on data of Fox et al.[13]

Treadmill Test

The use of a treadmill presents a number of advantages because it is possible to adjust the speed and grade of walking to the agility of the subject. For example, Taylor and associates[19] found that groups of young men being studied always contained a few individuals who could not run more than 7 mph, and most middle-aged men find 6 mph to be their peak capacity. The starting speed of 1.7 mph at a 10% grade recommended by Bruce and associates,[20] resulting in an oxygen consumption of about 4 metabolic equivalents (MET) has been very satisfactory. There are also reports of success with higher or lower speeds and inclines.[21,22] In some old or debilitated subjects, 1.7 mph is clearly faster than they can walk, and if stress testing is to be used in this group, a lower speed is useful. We also start with a lower speed when testing patients 2 or 3 weeks after myocardial infarction (MI).

Balke and Ware,[23] Fox and associates,[13] and Naughton and coworkers[22] at one time believed that the treadmill speed should be kept constant and the grade gradually increased. This is because running is difficult for many people, especially the old, sick, and obese. There has been a good deal of disagreement as to how steep the grade of the treadmill should be. We have kept the grade constant at 10% throughout the first four stages of our tests, mainly because walking or running up steep grades often causes pain in the calf muscles, especially in those who are poorly conditioned. Astrand[24] has emphasized that running at the same speed and grade requires more oxygen than walking (Fig. 8–1). A belt speed of more than 4 mph requires all but the very tall to start running.

Bruce Protocol

Bruce,[25] one of the most prolific investigators and an important pioneer in the field, found an increase in both speed and grade to be very satisfactory. He reported that his protocol, by far the most commonly used, produced

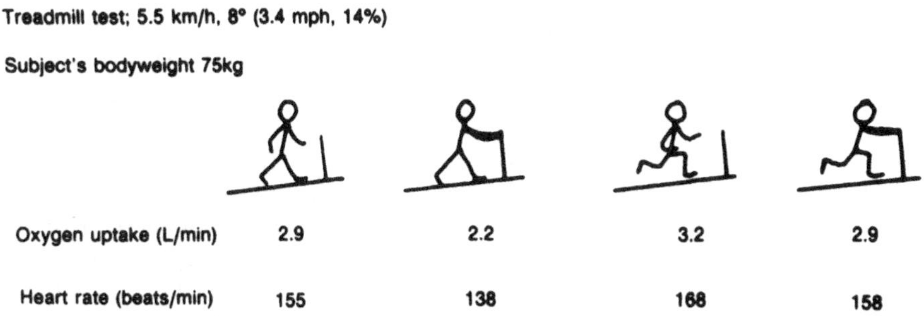

FIGURE 8–1. Figures depict the increased oxygen cost of walking without holding on to the handrail and of running as opposed to walking at the same speed and grade. (From Astrand,[24] with permission.)

STAGE	SPEED	GRADE	TIME	CUMULATIVE TIME
5	5.0	18%	3+	15+
4	4.2	16	3	12
3	3.4	14	3	9
2	2.5	12	3	6
1	1.7	10	3	3

FIGURE 8–2. The incline and speed are both increased every 3 minutes with the Bruce protocol.

nine times as many positive responders as the Master's test. His subjects start out at 1.7 mph on a 10% grade and progress to their maximum capacity at 3-minute intervals (Fig. 8–2). (See Fig. 6–9 for oxygen consumption at each workload.)

COMPARISON OF VARIOUS PROTOCOLS

A number of excellent treadmill protocols have been used by various investigators and are highly satisfactory. An older, well-established protocol is that of Balke and Ware,[23] who keep the speed constant and increase the grade gradually. Astrand and Rudahl,[26,27] also pioneers in exercise physiology, designed their test to start at 3.5 mph at a 2.5% grade with a 5-minute warm-up, followed by a continuous multistage run to exhaustion. This test is probably better suited to testing athletes than CAD patients. Other useful protocols have been published[28–31] (Fig. 8–3). Pollock[32] published an excellent analysis of four popular protocols to determine the relative heart rate response and oxygen cost (Figs. 8–4 and 8–5). From examination of Figures 8–4 and 8–5 it is evident that, although there is some variation in the rate at which the workload increases, the results of most protocols are about the same. Notice the leveling off near maximum workload of heart rate, but not of oxygen consumption. This suggests that the heart rate reaches a plateau prior to reaching the $\dot{V}O_2$max. Redwood,[33] at the National Institutes of Health, demonstrated the importance of warm-up at a reasonably low workload when using the exercise test to quantitate ischemia or to compare various interventions such as medication or surgery. If the initial exercise load was at or greater than the anginal threshold, a higher pulse pressure product or

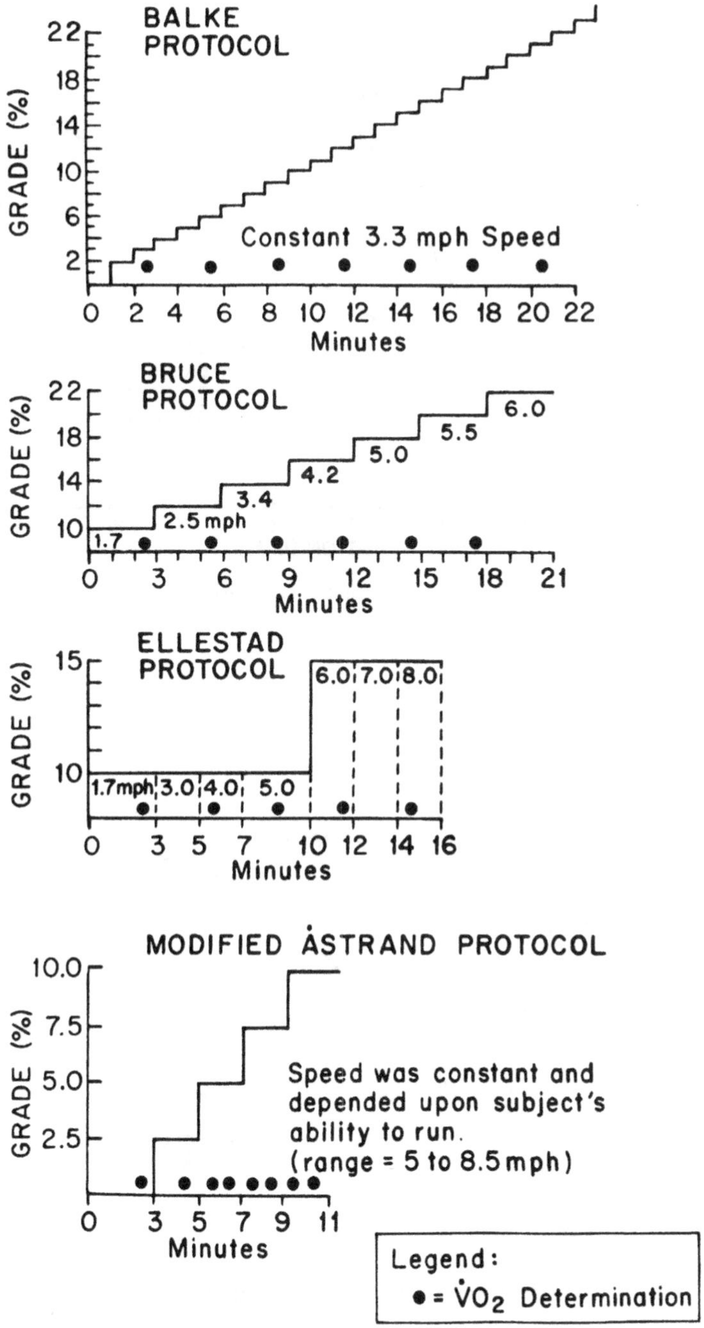

FIGURE 8–3. Diagrams of workloads used on a number of popular protocols. (From Pollock,[32] with permission.) The workload in the ninth minute of the Ellestad protocol has changed (see Figure 9–4).

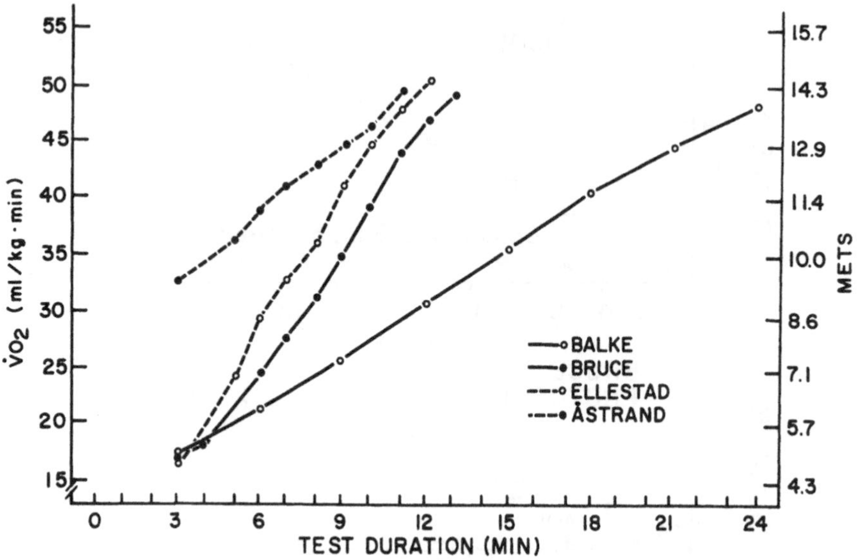

FIGURE 8–4. Mean $\dot{V}O_2$ measured according to time of exercise on four different protocols. (From Pollock,[32] with permission.)

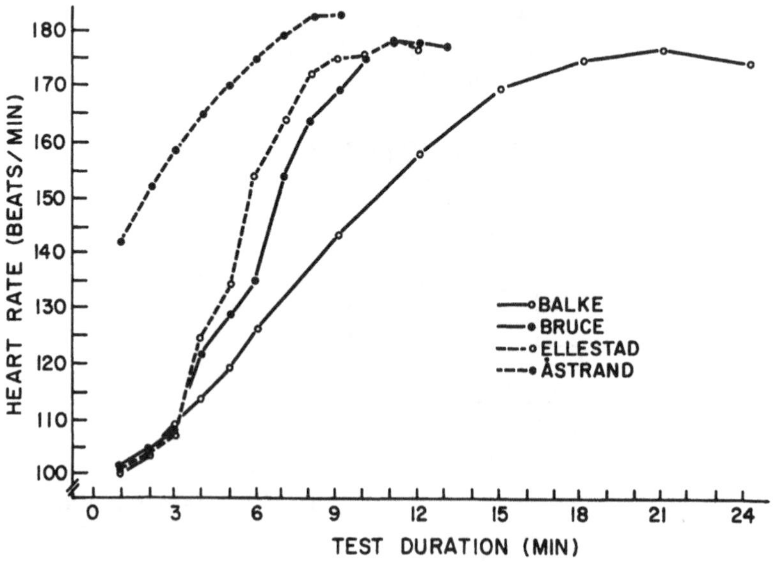

FIGURE 8–5. Mean heart rate response according to time on different protocols. Note in this and the previous figure that starting and stopping points are similar for most protocols. The major difference is how fast you get there. (From Pollock,[32] with permission.)

exercise workload could be achieved than if a warm-up workload were used. When the high initial workload was used, the end-points were also found to have low reproductibility.

Cornell Protocol

Okin and colleagues,[34] who have done the most work on the ST/HR slope, have reported that a gradual increase in exercise gives better diagnostic discrimination than a more rapid progression of work such as the Bruce protocol. They increase the speed and grade slowly to obtain heart rate increments of about 10 beats for each stage (Table 8–2).

Ramp Protocol

Froelicher and colleagues[35] estimate from the history how much total work the patient can tolerate in METS and then set the treadmill to gradually and smoothly accelerate the speed and grade so that patients will reach their peak in 8 to 10 minutes. This group has worked out nomograms that predict maximum oxygen uptake and METS from age and heart rate. They propose that the maximum work achieved be reported in METS rather than in time, to allow for a more standard terminology in describing total work (Fig. 8–6).

ESTIMATION OF OXYGEN CONSUMPTION

Blackburn and associates[36] studied the oxygen consumption and heart rate of 10 men stressed by different protocols using steps, bicycle, and treadmill.

Table 8–2. **Treadmill Speed and Grade for the Cornell Exercise Protocol, Compared with Standard Bruce Stages**

Modified Stage	Elapsed Time (min)	Speed mph	Grade %	Bruce Stage	Elapsed Time (min)
0	2	1.7	0		
0.5	4	1.7	5		
1.0	6	1.7	10	1	3
1.5	8	2.1	11		
2.0	10	2.5	12	2	6
2.5	12	3.0	13		
3.0	14	3.4	14	3	9
3.5	16	3.8	15		
4.0	18	4.2	16	4	12
4.5	20	4.6	17		
5.0	22	5.0	18	5	15

Note the slow progression of the workload.

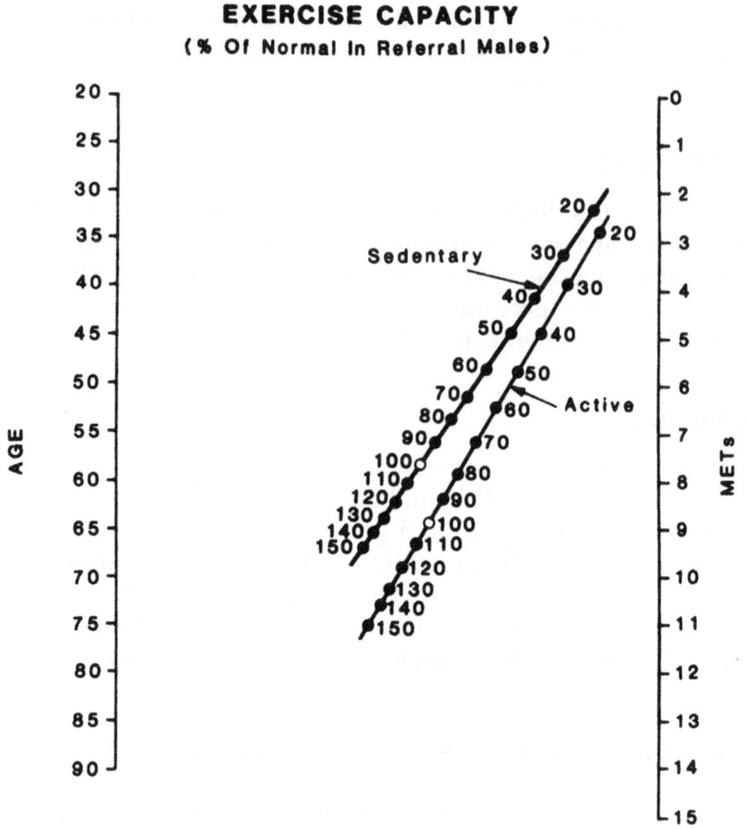

FIGURE 8–6. Nomogram of percentage normal exercise capacity in sedentary and active men. (From Froelicher,[35] with permission.)

As might be expected, the variability of oxygen consumption expressed as liters per minute on the bicycle tests was least because of the constant external load and very small variability of efficiency among subjects. However, since bicycle testing is independent of body weight, a marked variability in oxygen consumption expressed as milliliters per kilogram per minute was found. The treadmill, with its weight-dependent workload, shows a small variation in oxygen reported as milliliters per kilogram per minute and a larger variation when reported as liters per minute. There is no significant difference in the variability of the heart-rate response. Bruce and associates[37] have published oxygen data describing the milliliter per kilogram per minute for subjects using the Bruce protocol, which is excellent. When adjustment was made for the sex and physical activity of the subject, the $\dot{V}O_2max$ was estimated with what appears to be acceptable accuracy[37] (see Fig. 7–10).

Table 8–3. **$\dot{V}O_2$ STPD Estimate Compared with Direct Measurement**

	Ellestad Protocol					
Stage	**Treadmill Speed and Grade**	**Watts**	**Givoni and Goldman (L/M)**	**mL/kg for 70-kg man**	**METS**	**Direct Measurement MMC (L/M)**
I (3 min)	1.7 mph @ 10%	50	1.40	20	4.8	1.28
II (2 min)	3.0 mph @ 10%	100	1.68	24	6.4	1.67
III	4.0 mph @ 10%	150	2.4	34	8.8	2.07
IV	5.0 mph @ 10%	200	2.92	41.7	10.0	2.74
V	5.0 mph @ 15%	250	3.22	46	12.0	3.17
VI	6.0 mph @ 15%	300	4.15	59.3	15.2	3.8
VII	7.0 mph @ 15%	350	4.8	68.5	17.2	3.96

MMC = metabolic cart
$\dot{V}O_2$ = n(W + L) (2.3 + 0.32 [V – 2.5] 1.65 + G[0.2 + 0.07(V – 2.5)])
M = Metabolic rate, kcal/h
n = Terrain factor, defined as 1 for treadmill walking
W = Body weight (kg)
L = External load (kg)
V = Walking speed, km/h
G = Slope (grade) %

Froelicher and coworkers,[38] on the other hand, studied the time on the protocol proposed by Bruce as an estimate of oxygen consumption and found it to be unreliable.

We have used the formula published by Balke and Ware[23] and also by Givoni and Goldman[39] to estimate $\dot{V}O_2$max. Table 8–3 illustrates data from the latter formula and has been fairly accurate at lower workloads (less than about 12 METS).

EXERCISE INTENSITY

Some physicians tend to be reluctant to apply maximum stress to the general population because of fear of producing injury, either cardiac or musculoskeletal. Lester and associates[40] have reported that ventricular and supraventricular tachycardias are most apt to occur at 90% to 100% of maximum heart rate, and they suggest that 90% of maximum predicted pulse be the point of termination. The Scandinavian Committee on Electrocardiogram Classification[41] recommended target heart rates of approximately 85% of the maximum. Sheffield and associates[28] found the maximum predicted heart rate to be 198 (0.14 × age) for conditioned men and 205 (0.41 × age) for nonconditioned men (Table 8–4).

The problem with heart-rate–related end-points is the variability in the maximum heart rate, even when adjusted for age. If a test of 85% of maximum heart rate is used to terminate exercise, it may be much less or more than

Table 8–4. **Maximum Heart Rate Predicted by Age and Conditioning**

Age	20	25	30	35	40	45	50	55	60	65	70	75	80	85	90
Unconditioned	197	195	193	191	189	187	184	182	180	178	176	174	172	170	168
90%	177	175	173	172	170	168	166	164	162	160	158	157	155	153	151
75%	148	146	144	143	142	140	138	137	135	134	132	131	129	128	126
60%	118	117	115	114	113	112	110	109	108	107	106	104	103	102	101
Conditioned	190	188	186	184	182	180	177	175	173	171	169	167	165	163	161
90%	171	169	167	166	164	162	159	158	156	154	152	150	149	147	145
75%	143	141	140	138	137	135	133	131	130	128	127	125	124	122	121
60%	114	113	112	110	109	108	106	105	104	103	101	100	99	98	97

(From Sheffield et al,[28] with permission.)

85% of the individual patient's capacity, depending on the patient's actual—and unknown—maximum heart rate. In using these end-points, one also has to forgo the estimation of aerobic capacity, a useful calculation made from the patient's symptom-limited exercise duration. Although we have long used a symptom-limited maximum test with an age-corrected maximum heart rate as a guide, advocates of submaximum testing claim that the ST changes occurring at heart rates higher than this level have less significance.

Gibbons and colleagues[42] reported a 20-month follow-up of 550 patients with abnormal exercise ECGs. They found that in subjects with known CAD, ST depression occurring at heart rates less than 85% of maximum were six times more predictive of a new event than changes occurring at heart rates greater than 85%. In those with no known disease, ST depression occurring higher and lower than the 85% cutoff had about the same predictive power.

Maximum Heart Rate

The controversy over what constitutes maximum heart rate deserves a few words. The disagreement probably stems from the analysis of different population groups. Our studies are taken from a relatively sedentary population, whereas others have analyzed athletes and other selected groups. The variation higher than and lower than the mean is at least 10 beats, and occasionally subjects are seen with this variance, though rarely. Cooper and colleagues[43] have published data showing the variations associated with fitness (Fig. 8–7). Thus, note that tables are only guidelines and do not require strict adherence.

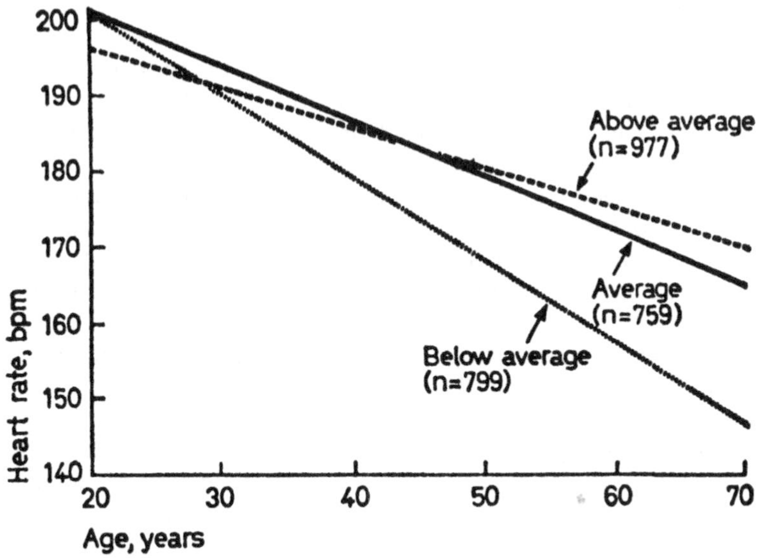

FIGURE 8–7. Maximum heart rates achieved according to fitness and age. (From Cooper et al,[43] with permission.)

Lester and coworkers[40] studied normal men ranging in age from 40 to 75 with a near-maximum graded test and also with the Master's step test. The submaximum test resulted in positive findings characterized by 1.0-mm horizontal or downsloping ST-segment depression in one subject. Five more abnormal tracings were recognized with the maximum test. In the analysis of 1000 tests in our laboratory, 19% of the men with abnormal findings manifested ST-segment changes in our fourth stage at 5 mph at a 10% grade. Most subjects will be very near their peak heart rate at this level. Twenty-one percent of the women with abnormal tracings were also detected at this stage. This suggests that pushing the patient to maximum effort is feasible. However, a higher yield of abnormal tests in so-called normal patients with the maximum stress test might cause an increased false-positive response.[28,44]

In our series of tests on healthy executives, 14% had abnormal ST-segment depression of 1.5 mm or more and almost all developed near-peak heart rate.[45] We have no information on how many of these had CAD. Strandell[46] reported a relatively high prevalence of abnormal responders in apparently normal men that increases with age. Aronow[47] found 13% abnormal maximum tests in normal men with a mean age of 51. It is interesting to note that none of the executives we tested with positive ST-segment depression had chest pain of any type when the changes were recorded near maximum capacity. The clinical significance of ST-segment depression discovered at maximum exercise levels is yet to be clarified, although our study of the time course of ST depression sheds some light on the subject.[48]

Blomqvist[49] has published data on ST depression in normal persons at high workloads (see Chapter 14). Kasser and Bruce[50] believe these changes represent some abnormality in myocardial function, but not always coronary ischemia. The relative absence of such changes in young persons and in a significant number of older people indicates that they are probably correct. On the other hand, the belief that late-onset, early-offset ST changes are always false-positives has been disproved.[48] During heart catheterization, we have found that many patients with left-ventricular dysfunction have exercise-induced ST-segment depression in spite of normal coronary arteries.

Bruce[50] reported more than 10,000 maximum stress tests without a fatality. In our series of about 30,000 tests, we have had four deaths, but two of the three developed trouble much before reaching their maximum heart rate.

Our survey of stress testing facilities suggest that the mortality has decreased in the face of increased use of maximum stress testing.[6] It has been our practice to suggest to patients that they may stop the test once their maximum predicted heart rates have been reached (Table 8–5), but that they may continue if desired. This maximum is rarely exceeded by more than 5 to 10 beats per minute, even in those who are pushed to exhaustion. On the other hand, those who voluntarily elect to continue and achieve heart rates 10 or 20 beats higher than the mean for their ages may be physiologically younger than their chronological age.

Table 8–5. **Ages and Maximal Heart Rate (MHR)***

Age	MHR	Age	MHR	Age	MHR
20	200	37	185	54	171
21	199	38	184	55	171
22	198	39	183	56	170
23	197	40	182	57	170
24	196	41	181	58	169
25	195	42	180	59	168
26	194	43	180	60	168
27	193	44	180	61	167
28	192	45	179	62	167
29	191	46	177	63	166
30	190	47	177	64	165
31	190	48	177	65	164
32	189	49	176	66	163
33	188	50	175	67	162
34	187	51	174	68	161
35	186	52	173	69	161
36	186	53	172	70	160

*Mean maximum heart rates used as a guide for determining approximate end-point of stress in our laboratory.

In summation, when maximum stress is used, there will be an increase in the number of subjects identified as having abnormal hearts if the ST segments alone are used as a marker for disease. As data are developed to validate other findings, the exact significance of ST depression at high workloads will probably be clarified. Patients who have abnormalities identified at the higher workloads will obviously have less serious disease than those identified early in the procedure or by submaximal tests.

PROTOCOL FOR EARLY STRESS TESTING (AFTER MI)

It was common before thrombolysis and angioplasty became popular to use exercise tests to evaluate patients who are ready to leave the hospital after acute MI.[51] This testing has proved useful in predicting the subsequent course of the disease and in analyzing arrhythmias. The clinical utility of post infarction exercise testing has not been well-studied in patients who have had primary revascularization. However, a less demanding protocol is usually used. Figure 8–8 illustrates the protocol used in our laboratory. Most investigators terminate exercise at heart rates near 120 to 130 beats per minute, but some have used maximum testing as early as 3 weeks[52] (see Chapter 10).

ISOMETRIC TEST

The isometric procedure consists of squeezing a dynamometer at from 25% to 75% of maximum hand strength and sustaining this for as long as possi-

STAGE	SPEED	GRADE	TIME	METS	TOTAL TIME	VO_2 ml/mm/Kg
1	1.5	0	3 min	2.8	3	6
2	1.5	4	3	3.2	6	9
3	1.5	8	3	3.7	9	12
4	1.7	10	3	4.0	12	15
5	2.0	12	3	5.0	15	20

FIGURE 8–8. Submaximal treadmill protocol used when patients are tested just before discharge after an MI (1–2 weeks following infarction). A heart rate of 120 beats per minute is now used as a target, but this may finally be less than desirable.

ble. The resultant increase in myocardial oxygen consumption is mainly due to the rise in systolic blood pressure, although there is also an increase in heart rate. If one measures the pulse pressure product at the end-point of angina or of ST-segment depression, such a heart rate is reasonably reproducible. The increase in heart rate is probably due to the withdrawal of vagal influence. The cardiac output increases, but the stroke volume usually remains constant until the grip is increased at more than 50% of the individual's total capacity, at which it may then decrease.[53] In spite of the rise in blood pressure, the blood flow to noncontracting muscles does not increase, probably because of reflex vasoconstriction. LVEDP rises and abnormal heart sounds such as S_4 or S_3 may be accentuated. The murmurs of aortic and mitral regurgitation are also accentuated. Thus, the isometric test may be useful to do at the bedside for subjects who are unable to walk. Isometric exercise can produce arrhythmias and the other hazards of exercise stress testing; therefore, continuous ECG and blood pressure monitoring should be routinely carried out. The test result cannot be correlated to aerobic capacity, so it is difficult to relate it to other types of activity. The isometric test would seem to have a limited application, but it is useful in certain situations.

Isometric Combined with Isotonic Exercise

Kerber and colleagues[54] have studied the relative relationship of isometric to dynamic exercise in CAD patients. They reported an isometric test to be an inefficient way of initiating ischemia. They also found that when isometric exercise was combined with treadmill exercise in patients carrying a briefcase, more CAD patients failed to have ST depression than those walking without carrying a briefcase. Systolic and diastolic pressures (thus, the double product) were increased by the isometric load, but the investigators postulated that the higher diastolic pressure improved perfusion enough to compensate for the increase in myocardial oxygen demands. Sheldahl and associates[55] found that a high percentage of post-MI patients carrying weights up to 50 lb had diastolic hypertension (greater than 120 mm Hg) but little ischemia.

EMOTIONAL STRESS TEST

It has long been recognized that fear, anger and other emotional stimuli can initiate ischemia and may result in mortality in patients with coronary artery disease.[56] The Northridge earthquake in 1994 resulted in an increase in deaths from the daily average of 36 to 101.[57] When Iraqi missile attacks on Tel Aviv and Haifa started in 1991 there was an increase in patients presenting to the Emergency Room with myocardial infarctions.[58] Ischemia associated with driving in traffic, parachute jumping and other emotionally disturbing interventions are well recognized.

A number of studies using standard emotional stimuli to initiate ischemia in patients with coronary artery disease have been performed and an excellent review by Goldberg has recently been published.[59] The most common stimuli have been public speaking, mental arithmetic and more recently, computer games (Stroop Test).[60] Markers of ischemia following these stimuli have been angina, ST depression and changes in left ventricular volume detected by a MUGA.[61]

In most studies, where the stimuli have been compared with exercise in patients with known coronary narrowing, the sensitivity has been less than 50%.[62] The use of a noninvasive impedance device to track peripheral vascular resistance has been tried with limited benefit.[63] During a multicenter test supported by the NIH about 60% of the ischemic responses were reproducible when the computer Stroop Test or the speech tests were used. It might seem advisable to combine exercise and emotional stimuli but at this time there is no satisfactory data reporting on this approach.[63] It would appear that inducing ischemia emotionally still needs further study before it becomes a routine approach to make a diagnosis in patients with suspected coronary artery disease.

CIRCADIAN INFLUENCE

A word about the timing seems in order. Yasue[64] has found that patients with vasospastic angina, even those with fixed lesions, are more likely to have changes in the morning. Joy and associates,[65] on the other hand, report that patients with stable angina have more ST depression in the afternoon. Autonomic changes for these phenomena are still poorly understood, and at this time it appears that testing can be performed whenever convenient without compromising the results.

SUMMARY

This chapter has described various protocols being used to evaluate patients with suspected CAD. There are many protocols that are not listed and many yet to be described. The reader is urged to examine the evidence available and select a method or methods best suited to the patient or to his or her own understanding of exercise physiology. There are numerous advantages, however, in selecting one or two methods and using them enough to become familiar with the response of normal and abnormal subjects alike. Using a protocol for which there is ample clinical experience makes it possible to better categorize each individual's performance. Consistency will also make it easier to compare the patient's performance from year to year and to compare one patient with another patient. The details of the protocol should also be clearly outlined when data are sent to other physicians.

REFERENCES

1. Garber, CE, Carleton, RA, and Camaione, DN: The threshold for myocardial ischemia varies in patients with coronary artery disease depending on the exercise protocol. J Am Coll Cardiol 17:1256–262, 1991.
2. Carleton, RA, Siconolfi, SF, and Shafique, M: Delayed appearance of angina pectoris during low level exercise. J Cardiac Rehab 3:141–148, 1983.
3. Grollman, A: Physiological variables in the cardiac output of man: The effect of the ingestion of food. Am J Physiol 89:366–370, 1929.
4. Niazi, K, et al: Negligible effects of moderate fluid intake and meal consumption on exercise performance. J Am Coll Cardiol 19:246A, 1992.
5. Master, MA: Two-step test of myocardial function. Am Heart J 10:495, 1934.
6. Stuart, RJ and Ellestad, MH: National survey of exercise testing facilities. Chest 77:94–97, 1980.
7. Hellerstein, HK and Hornsten, TR: The coronary spectrum: Assessing and preparing a patient for return to a meaningful and productive life. J Rehabil 32:48, 1966.
8. Arstila, M: Pulse conducted triangular exercise ECG test: A feedback system regulating work during exercise. Acta Med Scand 529(suppl):9, 1972.
9. Mitchell, JH, Sproule, BJ, and Chapman, CB: The physiological meaning of the maximal oxygen intake test. J Clin Invest 37:538, 1958.
10. The Committee on Exercise. Exercise testing and training of apparently healthy individuals. American Heart Association, Dallas, 1972.
11. Astrand, I: The physical work capacity of workers 50–64 years old. Acta Physiol Scand 42:73, 1958.
12. Lance, Vo and Spodich, DH: Constant load vs. heart rate targeted exercise: Responses of systolic time intervals. J Appl Physiol 38:794, 1975.
13. Fox, SM, Naughton, JP, and Haskell, WL: Physical activity and the prevention of coronary heart disease. Ann Clin Res 3:404, 1971.
14. Rainer, PH, et al: Greater diagnostic sensitivity of treadmill vs cycle exercise testing of asymptomatic men with coronary disease. Am J Cardiol 70:141–146, 1992.
15. Koyal, SN, et al: Ventilatory responses to the metabolic acidosis of treadmill and cycle ergometry. J Appl Physiol 40(6):864–867, 1976.
16. Bonzheim, SC, et al: Physiological responses to recumbent versus upright cycle ergometry, and implications for exercise prescription in patients with coronary heart disease. Am J Cardiol 69:40–44, 1992.
17. Currie, PJ, Kelly, MJ, and Pitt, A: Comparison of supine and erect bicycle exercise electrocardiography in coronary heart disease: Accentuation of exercise-induced ischemic ST depression by supine posture. Am J Cardiol 52:1167–1173, 1983.

18. Vellinga, T, Krubsack, A, and Sheldahl, L: Does posture affect exercise induced ischemia? Circulation (abstract) November 1989.
19. Taylor, HL, Buskirk, E, and Mitchell, A: Maximum oxygen intake as an objective measure of cardiorespiratory performance. J Appl Physiol 8:73, 1958.
20. Bruce, RA, et al: Exercise testing in adult normal subjects and cardiac patients. Pediatrics 32(suppl):742, 1963.
21. Kassebaum, DG, Sutherland, KO, and Judkins, MP: A comparison of hypoxemia and exercise electrocardiography in coronary artery disease. Am Heart J 7:371, 1932.
22. Naughton, J, Blake, B, and Nagle, F: Refinements in methods of evaluation and physical conditioning before and after myocardial infarction. Am J Cardiol 14:837, 1964.
23. Balke, B and Ware, RW: An experimental study of physical fitness of Air Force personnel. US Armed Forces Med J 10:675, 1959.
24. Astrand, PO: Principles in ergometry and their implications in sports practice. Sports Med 1:1–5, 1984.
25. Bruce, A: Comparative prevalence of segment S-T depression after maximal exercise in healthy men in Seattle and Taipei. In Simonson, E (ed): Physical Activity and the Heart. Charles C Thomas, Springfield, IL, 1967.
26. Astrand, I: The physical work capacity of workers 50–64 years old. Acta Physiol Scand 42:73, 1958.
27. Astrand, PO and Rudahl, K: Textbook of Work Physiology. McGraw-Hill, New York, 1970.
28. Sheffield, LT, Holt, JH, and Reeves, TJ: Exercise graded by heart rate in electrocardiographic testing for angina pectoris. Circulation 32:622, 1965.
29. Hellerstein, HK: Exercise therapy in coronary heart disease. Bull NY Acad Med 44:1028, 1968.
30. Froelicher, VF, et al: A comparison of the reproducibility and physiological response to 3 maximal treadmill exercise protocols. Chest 65:512, 1974.
31. Taylor, HL, et al: The standardization and interpretation of submaximal and maximal tests of working capacity. Pediatrics 32:703, 1963.
32. Pollock, MI: A comparative analysis of 4 protocols for maximal exercise testing. Am Heart J 93:39, 1977.
33. Redwood, DR: Importance of the design of an exercise protocol in the evaluation of patients with angina pectoris. Circulation 63:618, 1971.
34. Okin, PM, Ameisen, O, and Kligfield, P: A modified treadmill exercise protocol for computer assisted analysis of the ST segment/heart rate slope. J Electrocardiol 19(4):311–318, 1986.
35. Froelicher, VF, et al: Nomogram for exercise capacity using METS and age. Learning Center Highlights 8(2):1–5, 1992.
36. Blackburn, H, et al: The standardization of the exercise electrocardiogram: A systematic comparison of chest lead configurations employed for monitoring during exercise. In Simonson, E (ed): Physical Activity and the Heart. Charles C Thomas, Springfield, IL, 1967.
37. Bruce, RA, Kusumi, F, and Hosmer, D: Maximal oxygen intake and nomographic assessment of functional aerobic impairment in cardiovascular disease. Am Heart J 85:546, 1973.
38. Froelicher, VF, et al: A comparison of the reproducibility and physiological response to 3 maximal treadmill exercise protocols. Chest 65:512, 1974.
39. Givoni, B and Goldman, RF: Predicting metabolic energy cost. J Appl Physiol 30(3):429, 1971.
40. Lester, FM, et al: The effect of age and athletic training on the maximal heart rate during muscular exercise. Am Heart J 76:370, 1968.
41. Scandinavian Committee on Electrocardiogram Classification: The Minnesota code for ECG classification. Acta Med Scand 183(suppl 48)11, 1967.
42. Gibbons, L, et al: The value of maximal versus submaximal treadmill testing. J Cardiac Rehab 1(51:362–368), 1981.
43. Cooper, KH, et al: Age-fitness adjusted maximal heart rates. Med Sport 10:78, 1977.
44. Bellet, S and Muller, OF: Electrocardiogram during exercise: Value in diagnosis of angina pectoris. Circulation 32:477, 1965.
45. Ellestad, MH, et al: Maximal treadmill stress testing for cardiovascular evaluation. Circulation 39:517, 1969.
46. Strandell, T: Circulatory studies on healthy old men, with special reference to the limitations of the maximal physical work capacity. Acta Med Scand 175(suppl 414):1, 1964.

47. Aronow, WS: Thirty month follow-up of maximal treadmill stress test and double Master's test in normal subjects. Circulation 47:287, 1973.
48. Ellestad, MH, et al: The predictive value of the time course of ST segment depression during exercise testing in patients referred for coronary angiograms. Am Heart J 123:904–908, 1992.
49. Blomqvist, CG: Heart disease and dynamic exercise testing. In Willerson, JT and Sanders, CA (eds): Clinical Cardiology. Grune & Stratton, New York, 1977, p 218.
50. Kasser, IS and Bruce, RA: Comparative effects of aging and coronary heart disease on submaximal and maximal exercise. Circulation 39:759, 1969.
51. Ericsson, M, et al: Arrhythmias and symptoms during treadmill 3 weeks after myocardial infarction in 100 patients. Br Heart J 35:787, 1973.
52. Styperek, J, Ibsen, H, and Kjoller, E: Exercise ECG in patients with acute myocardial infarction before discharge from the CCU [abstract]. Am J Cardiol 35:172, 1975.
53. Nutter, DO, et al: Isometric exercise and the cardiovascular system. Mod Concept Cardiovasc Dis 41:11, 1972.
54. Kerber, RE, et al: Myocardial ischemic effects of isometric, dynamic, and combined exercise in coronary artery disease. Chest 67:388, 1975.
55. Sheldahl, LM, et al: Response of patients after myocardial infarction to carrying a graded series of weight loads. Am J Cardiol 52:698, 1983.
56. Barry, J, et al: Frequency of ST-segment depression produced by mental stress in stable angina pectoris from coronary artery disease. Am J Cardiol 61:989, 1988.
57. Leor, J, et al: Sudden cardiac death triggered by an earthquake. N Engl J Med 334:413, 1996.
58. Kark, JD, et al: Iraqi missile attacks on Israel: the association of mortality with a life-threatening stressor. JAMA 273:1208, 1995.
59. Goldberg, AD. Should we use emotional stress testing to identify ischemia? In Ellestad, MH and Amsterdam, EA (eds): Exercise Testing: New Concepts for the New Century. Kluwer Academic Publishers, Boston, Dordrecht, London, 2002, p. 163.
60. Yeung, AC, et al: The effect of atherosclerosis on the vasomotor response of coronary arteries to mental stress. Am Heart J 325:1551, 1991.
61. LaVeau, PJ, et al: Transient left ventricular dysfunction during provocative mental stress in patients with coronary artery disease. Am Heart J 118:1, 1989.
62. Specchia, G, et al: Mental arithmetic stress testing in patients with coronary artery disease. Am Heart J 108:56, 1984.
63. Goldberg, AD, et al for the PIMI investigators: Ischemic, hemodynamic and neurohormone responses to mental and exercise stress: experience from the psychophysiological investigations of myocardial ischemia (PIMI). Circulation 94:2402, 1996.
64. Yasue, H: Circadian variation in response to exercise: An important variable in interpretation of the exercise stress test. Pract Cardiol 9:43, 1983.
65. Joy M, et al: Diurnal variation in exercise responses in angina pectoris. Br Heart J 48:156, 1982.

9
Memorial Heart Institute Protocol

Timing
Questionnaire and Informed Consent
Clothing
Skin Preparation for Electrodes
Electrode Positions and Attachments
Examination and Explanation
Exercise
Handrail Support
Reassurance
Monitoring
Exercise Duration
Termination of Test
Recovery Period
Record Preparation
General Discussion

The description of the methodology used in our laboratory can be used as a lesson in "How to do it." For this reason, it will be described in considerable detail.

The protocol has been structured to obtain a maximum amount of information in as short a time as possible.[1] It is used for testing normal subjects who have a sedentary lifestyle or for the evaluation of cardiac patients. By extending the time and the exercise load, one can evaluate trained athletes. By establishing a standard protocol for almost all patients, we have been able to compare the responses of individuals with their previous tests and with the tests of other subjects. Although this has been a practical and useful routine, there is nothing absolute about its design. Most laboratory staffs doing stress testing today use some type of graded continuous system, Bruce being the most popular. The advantages of using an already established protocol will be obvious as we review the procedure.

TIMING

Although it would be best to test each patient the first thing in the morning before breakfast, the volume of tests makes this impractical. Therefore, we do tests at any time of the day and suggest only that patients eat lightly prior to the test.

QUESTIONNAIRE AND INFORMED CONSENT

When the patient arrives at the laboratory, he or she is asked to read a description of the procedure and then to sign a consent form that includes the statement that the patient has read and understood the description. The technician then fills out a questionnaire that includes statements about previous myocardial infarction, anginal pain, smoking, and exercising and present medications. It is often necessary for the technician to explain the meaning of some of the questions.

CLOTHING

The subject should be lightly clothed. We often dress men and women alike in hospital surgical scrub pants. The men go without a top, and a standard hospital gown is placed backward on the women so that it opens in the front. Patients should be advised to bring appropriate footwear such as tennis or running shoes.

SKIN PREPARATION FOR ELECTRODES

The quality of the recording depends greatly on good electrode contact. The discovery of this simple fact has had more to do with the good quality of exercise records than all the advances of electronic engineering up to this time. The elimination of the horny layer of the epidermis is the most important factor. This may be accomplished by superficial cleansing and application of electrode paste. Men who are very hirsute may need to be shaved. A number of lightweight liquid-contact, relatively nonpolarizing, silver chloride electrodes are now available. They have a plastic housing and light flexible cable with an immensely improved tracing quality. Disposable electrodes are now available from many suppliers. We have experimented with a number of these electrodes and are presently using the ones from CONMED, manufactured by CONMED Andover Medical, which are very satisfactory and in the middle price range. They have a plastic ring with a spongelike middle, are prefilled with paste, and have a good silver chloride core (Fig. 9–1).

ELECTRODE POSITIONS AND ATTACHMENTS

The 12-lead Mason-Likar[2] system with electrodes as demonstrated in Figure 9–2 is attached in the appropriate positions. The plastic adhesive electrodes have self-contained electrode jelly in the cap and need only to be stuck on and attached to the lead wires. A few minutes' delay between application and exercise allows for better contact and therefore less battery effect at the skin contact point. This minimizes the baseline wandering. It is very important that the right and left arm electrodes be placed laterally rather than in the midclavicular line as is sometimes done.

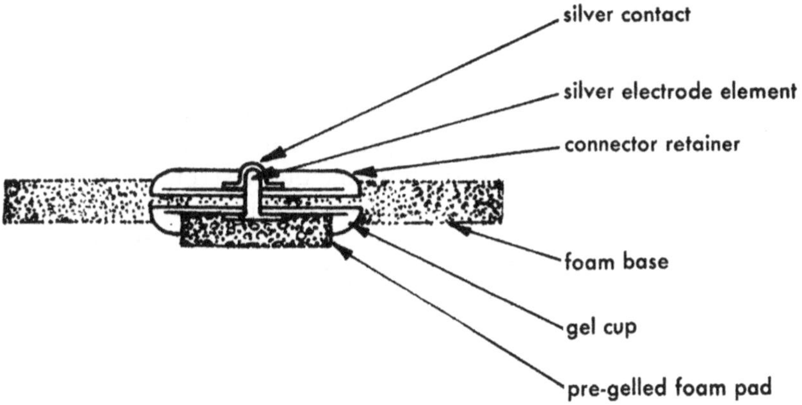

FIGURE 9–1. Diagram of disposable electrode used in our laboratory.

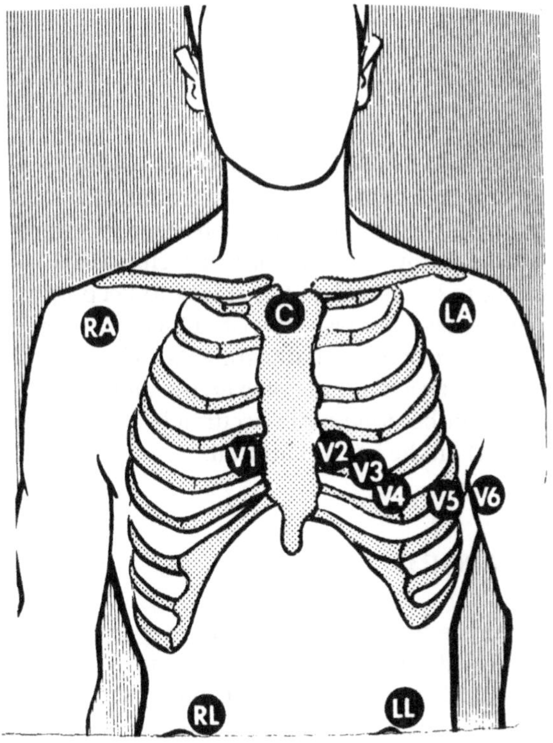

FIGURE 9–2. Lead positions adapted from Mason and Likar[2] with a "C" as location for negative electrode for CM_5 if it is being recorded. It is very important that the right and left arm electrodes not be placed medially near the sternum.

EXAMINATION AND EXPLANATION

During the time that the technician is applying the electrodes to the chest and the blood pressure cuff to the arm, the technician is explaining the test and reassuring the patient about the safeguards available. The technician also demonstrates how to mount the treadmill and the most comfortable gait. The physician then reviews the patient's questionnaire and asks the patient about possible pain patterns, exercise capacity, and cardiac history, and reviews the resting ECGs. Careful attention is given to determine what drugs might have been taken and when. The physician then listens to the patient's heart and lungs, especially noting third or fourth heart sounds and murmurs. We have found it to be especially important to inquire about recent chest pain patterns and recently recorded ECG. They should be reviewed if available. The blood pressure is recorded when the patient is sitting and standing while simultaneous ECGs are recorded. The physician should discuss the type of pain used for an end-point for termination if the patient has been subject to angina in the past. The method for terminating the test is also explained and the patient is given the option to terminate if he or she feels unable to continue.

EXERCISE

The treadmill is elevated to a 10% grade, then started at 1.7 mph and the patient is asked to step on. Some treadmills start out very slowly; in this type of treadmill, the patient can stand on the belt when it is started. If necessary, the patient is supported by the physician or technician during the first few seconds of walking to be certain of the ability to keep up with the moving belt. It is often necessary to advise the patient as to the length of stride, the position on the belt, and postural adjustments to walking up a 10% grade (Fig. 9–3). At the end of each minute of exercise, an ECG and blood pressure are recorded. This can be done more accurately if the patient lets the arm hang rather than rest on the bar or handrail.

HANDRAIL SUPPORT

Many patients who are weak, fearful, or short of breath find it essential to hold tightly to the handrail while walking. If accurate aerobic information is to be obtained, handrail support must be prohibited. On the other hand, we feel it is better to get some information than to get none at all, so we do not insist on total absence of support. The heart rate and pulse pressure product are good estimates of the magnitude of coronary flow and aerobic capacity as well as the time on the protocol.

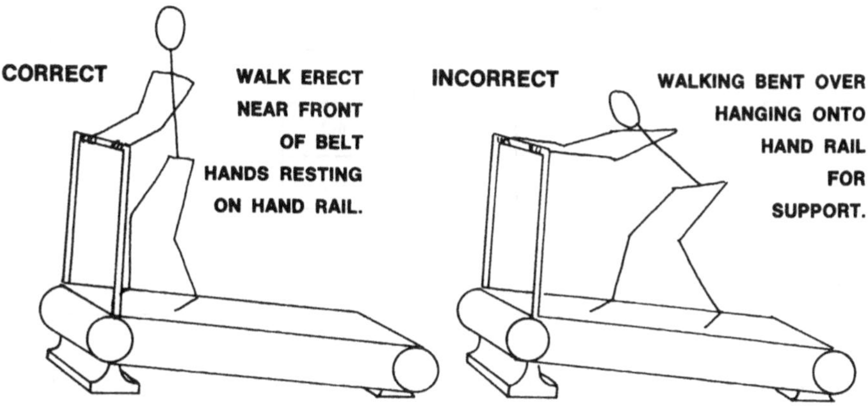

FIGURE 9–3. Correct and incorrect posture for treadmill walking. It is very important to instruct the patient in the proper technique. Erect posture is all important.

REASSURANCE

The physician should talk intermittently to the patients while they are being tested, reassuring them as to their progress and asking how they feel. When it is time to increase the speed of the treadmill, patients are notified and asked if they think they can go faster for a short time. We believe this continuous discussion is particularly important for those who are fearful and especially for those who are being tested for the first time.

MONITORING

The oscilloscope is under constant observation by both the technician and the physician doing the test. At the end of each minute, the blood pressure and ECG are recorded, and the heart rate is noted on the worksheet. Premature ventricular contractions (PVCs) or other arrhythmias are noted on the worksheet, recorded in the strip chart, and reported by the technician to the physician. The technician reminds the physician of the heart rate at the end of each minute. At the end of the third minute, after the blood pressure and ECGs are recorded, the treadmill speed is increased to 3 mph and thereafter increased according to the protocol in Figure 9–4.

If ST-segment depression is noted on the monitor or on the recorder, the patient is frequently questioned as to the presence of pain or tightness in the chest. The ability or propensity to report discomfort varies a great deal from patient to patient. Patients are asked to grade the intensity of the pain from 1 to 4 with 4 being the most severe in the patient's experience. Men are less likely to report pain than women.

After the patient is walking or jogging 4 mph or more, it is often difficult

STAGE	SPEED	GRADE	TIME	METS	TOTAL TIME	VO_2 ml/mm/Kg
1	1.7	10%	3	4	3	15
2	3	10%	2	6-7	5	25
3	4	10%	2	8-9	7	35
4	5	10%	2	10-12	9	45
5	5	15%	2	13-15	11	55
6	6	15%	2	16-20	13	65

FIGURE 9–4. The Memorial Hospital maximal treadmill protocol. More than 95% of our subjects are unable to progress past the fourth stage. (See Fig. 8–8 for submaximal treadmill protocol.)

or impossible to obtain an accurate blood pressure. Therefore, the general appearance in terms of skin color, facial expression suggesting anxiety, and the apparent strength and vigor of the patient's walk will give clues as to the adequacy of the circulatory system. The blood pressure tends to increase moderately with exercise until the maximum aerobic capacity is reached (see Chapter 18). After this, if the patient continues to exercise, the blood pressure begins to drop. If this drop is not detected by the technician, the patient may faint. Most patients, however, refuse to continue past their peak capacity and voluntarily decide to terminate exercise long before fainting occurs. If the peak heart rate has been reached, it can be predicted that patients will elect to terminate the exercise within a minute or so unless they are very well conditioned. Our practice has been to encourage them to continue if they feel like it. Peak exercise heart rate is quite variable and probably has predictive power.

EXERCISE DURATION

Most of our subjects reach their peak predicted heart rate response or have been terminated for other reasons within 8 to 10 minutes. For selected cases in which the subjects are well-conditioned athletes, we continue as long as necessary at an increased grade of 15%, and we increase the speed of the belt 1 mph every 2 minutes. This usually results in the subject reaching peak heart rate response and maximum capacity within a total exercise time of 12 to 15 minutes.

TERMINATION OF TEST

Although the indications for termination have been discussed in Chapter 5, it is appropriate to review them here. It is generally agreed by most workers in the field that the test should be terminated when:

1. PVCs develop in pairs or with increasing frequency or when ventricular tachycardia develops (runs of four or more PVCs).
2. Atrial tachycardia or atrial fibrillation supervenes.
3. There is onset of heart block—either second or third degree.
4. Anginal pain is progressive (grade 3 pain, if grade 4 is the most severe in patient's experience).
5. ST-segment depression has become severe, that is, 3 to 4 mm or more in vigorous asymptomatic subjects. If the patient is known to have severe CAD or angina at low workloads or if the the patient has ST-segment depression at rest, exercise should be terminated with only minor increases in ST-segment depression over the baseline tracing. One should also terminate exercise when ST-segment depression exceeds 2 mm if the onset of ischemia is at low workloads.
6. The heart rate or systolic blood pressure drops progressively with continuing exercise.
7. The patient is unable to continue because of dyspnea, fatigue, or feelings of faintness.
8. Musculoskeletal pain becomes severe, such as might occur with arthritis or claudication.
9. The patient looks vasoconstricted, that is, pale and clammy.
10. Extreme elevations in systolic and diastolic blood pressures.
11. The patient has reached or exceeded the predicted maximum pulse rate.
12. The physician is in doubt. We have found that it takes experience to determine how far to push a sick patient. The test can always be repeated another day. On the other hand, there are times when a few more seconds on the treadmill can result in a more certain diagnosis with no significant increase in risk.

RECOVERY PERIOD

At the instant exercise is discontinued, the ECG recorder is turned on and left running for a few seconds while the blood pressure is recorded, and the patient lies down. The evaluation of the ST segments and other ECG changes in the first few seconds is often very important. Occasionally, a more stable baseline can be obtained by asking the patient to hold his or her breath for a few seconds. Blood pressure is often low at the period just after the exercise, only to rise temporarily again about 1 minute later. This drop in blood pressure may be due to the temporary inadequacy in cardiac pumping capacity in relation to metabolic demand, or it may be due to the vasodilatation associated with increasing the lactic acid concentrations at peak stress. The blood pressure and ECG are then recorded at 1-minute intervals for 6 minutes while the patient is supine. ECG changes during exercise and recovery are

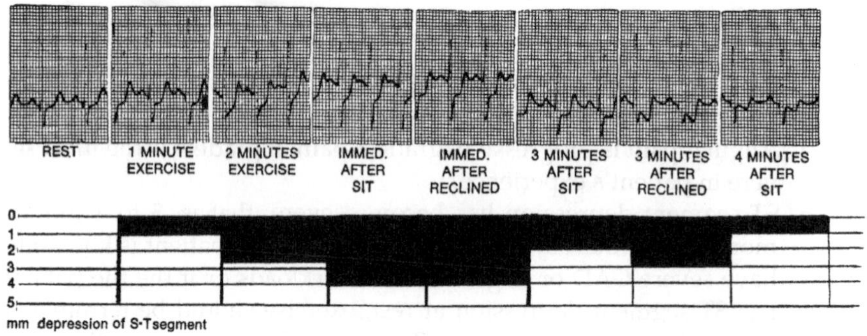

FIGURE 9–5. The ST-segment depression recorded in a patient with classic ischemic heart disease subjected to a treadmill stress test. Note the tendency of the ST segments to flatten when the patient is placed in the horizontal position. After sitting the patient up, the ST segments began to improve but became more pathological when the patient is again placed in the horizontal position in the third minute. We believe that the increased venous return in the horizontal position produces a higher LVEDP and therefore promotes more ST-segment depression.

entered on the worksheet. Special attention is paid to the blood pressure at 3 minutes into recovery.

It is common for the ECG pattern to be equivocal immediately after exercise. If this is so, elevating the patient's legs will increase the venous return at a time when the ventricular compliance is most likely to be reduced and the peripheral resistance is still elevated. This may result in an increased left-ventricular end-diastolic pressure (LVEDP) and a resultant increase in ST-segment depression (Fig. 9–5). The decrease in heart rate from that maximally achieved to 1 minute into recovery should be noted.

Late ST-segment depression and T-wave inversion should also be noted as well as the absence or presence of arrhythmias. At the end of the 6-minute observation period, if the patient is stable and comfortable, the physician doing the test reassures the patient and explains that the data will be forwarded to the patient's personal physician.

Patients should be monitored until the ECG has returned to baseline. As mentioned in Chapter 5, if the ST depression does not return to normal within 3 or 4 minutes, we recommend giving nitroglycerin. If the ST changes are equivocal, the response to this drug often helps with the interpretation.

RECORD PREPARATION

After termination of the test, the patient's heart rate is compared with the normal rate for age. Our practice has been to mount and send out copies of the averaged beats for each minute of the test. Most of the treadmill systems now provide examples of the averaged beat for each stage or minute, which are convenient to send out to the referring doctor. The total record is kept on file in the laboratory for review, if necessary. The appropriate computer codes designating the phrases to be printed out and the diagnostic implications are entered on the worksheet. The diagnostic computer code phrases are designed to represent the overall final diagnostic conclusion. The items listed under abnormalities constitute the events observed that influence the final diagnosis. It is important to enter the maximum ST depression if it is 0.5 mm or more and the R wave amplitude on the same lead.[3]

Comments are also added if indicated. The worksheet is given to the secretary, who enters it on the computer keyboard and sends the printout to the referring physician and for filing with the ECG strips.

GENERAL DISCUSSION

Various parts of the protocol procedure need special emphasis. In Chapter 8, a number of idealized standards were listed and discussed. It was stated that the protocol should provide:

1. Continuous ECG monitoring.
2. ECG recording when desired and preferably several simultaneous leads before, during, and after exercise. A minimum of muscle artifact is essential to good recording.
3. A type of stress that can be performed by the sedentary, poorly developed, and underconditioned subject as well as the trained athlete.
4. A workload that can be varied according to the capacity of the individual but is sufficiently standardized to be reproducible and to allow comparison with other subjects tested.
5. Repeated and frequent blood pressure measurements.
6. A way of estimating the aerobic requirements of the individual.
7. Maximum safety and minimum discomfort for each subject.
8. The highest possible specificity, sensitivity, and discrimination between health and disease.
9. A sufficient body of available information so that the response of both patients and normal subjects can be compared with those previously examined.
10. An initial stage of exercise long enough for a warm-up to occur.
11. Practicality with respect to the amount of time involved.

Our protocol is designed as a practical approach to day-to-day stress testing. Our experience has led us to believe that it has some unique advantages and fulfills most of the previously mentioned requirements. On the other hand, any well-established protocol can give the same information if the latter items are included.

MEMORIAL HEART INSTITUTE
EXERCISE STRESS TEST REPORT

Test Date: **8/8/01** FF#: **07-90-3**
MR#: M00057288-005 **OP**
Name:
Age: **75**
K#: **K220-0030**

Cardiologist: Ellestad Referring MD: Ellestad, Myrvin
Report To: Linderman, Lisa
Indication: Eval CAD risk factors

On 08/08/2001 the risks and benefits of the test were explained to the patient and he agreed to proceed. The patient was exercised on an Ellestad protocol for a total of 7 minutes achieving a maximum heart rate of 117, which is 81 percent of the predicted maximal heart rate, with a peak systolic BP of 154, at a 8 METS work load. The calculated maximum VO2 = 28.91. The test was terminated because of completion of protocol.

A Kligfield Index greater than 1.6 indicates ischemia. A Duke Score of -11 or less = high risk (5 year survival = 72%). A Duke Score of -10 to +4 = moderate risk (5 year survival = 91%). A Duke Score of +5 or more = low risk (5 year survival = 97%). A lead strength value of 0.1 or greater suggests ischemia.

Impression: Abnorm test typ. of ischemia ECG Code:

Abnormalities:
No angina, ST dep w/out pain, atrial extrasyst. w/ex.

Comments:
Onset of ST depression at 3 minutes. Prolonged ST depression in recovery.

Detail data:

Stage	Minutes	Grade %	MPH	Mets	HR	SYS	DIAS
Supine				1	56	138	74
Stand				1	64	150	80
Stage 1	1	10	1	4	77		
Stage 1	2	10	1	4	82	130	72
Stage 1	3	10	1	4	86	146	70
Stage 2	4	10	3	6	99	146	70
Stage 2	5	10	3	6	107	154	80
Stage 3	6	10	4	8	117		
Stage 3	7	10	4	8	117	142	78
Recovery					117	142	78
Recovery	1				83		
Recovery	2				76	148	68
Recovery	3				69	144	70
Recovery	4				67		
Recovery	5				68		
Recovery	6				68	134	78
Recovery	7				68	144	80

Kligfield Index: .05 Duke Score: - 8 Lead Strength: .13

FIGURE 9–6. Memorial Heart Institute Exercise Stress Test Report.

The printout contains some calculations that can easily be done by computer (Fig. 9–6). I believe one of the clinically validated treadmill scores, such as the Duke score[3] as well as the Kligfield index[4] and the lead strength fraction[5] should be included in the printout of the final report:

1. Percent predicted maximal heart rate.
2. METS achieved.

3. Physician's diagnosis. After thoroughly considering all the findings, the physician codes in his or her best impression. The cardiologist may qualify this with appropriate comments if desired.
4. Heart rate, blood pressures, measured ST changes, and arrhythmias according to their time on the protocol.

SUMMARY

This protocol has shorter exercise times than most and therefore allows completion in less than 10 minutes except for highly trained runners. We have found it to be satisfactory for clinical use as well as for research. Our long experience provides data on large populations that allow comparisons that are useful in clinical practice. Some reports show that when using the ST/HR slope, a protocol that accelerates slower than ours—such as the Cornell—gives better discrimination.[4] If this is confirmed in other centers and the use of this method becomes widespread, it may be advisable to consider such a modification.

REFERENCES

1. Ellestad, MH, et al: Maximal treadmill stress testing for cardiovascular evaluation. Circulation 39:517, 1969.
2. Mason, RE and Likar, I: A new lead system of multiple-lead exercise electrocardiography. Am Heart J 71:196–204, 1966.
3. Shaw, LJ, et al: Use of prognostic treadmill score in identifying diagnostic coronary subgroups. Circulation 98:1622, 1998.
4. Kligfield, P, Ameisen, O, and Okin, PM: Heart rate adjustment of the ST segment for improved detection of coronary artery disease. Circulation 79:245, 1986.
5. Ellestad, MH, et al: The significance of lead strength on ST changes during Treadmill stress tests. J Electrocardiol 25:31, 1993.

10
Stress Testing After Myocardial Infarction

Advantages and Benefits
Safety and Patient Selection
Protocols
Abnormal Stress Test Responses
ST-Segment Depression
Angina
Exercise-Induced Ventricular Arrhythmias
Hemodynamic Responses
ST-Segment Elevation
Reliability of Abnormalities
Estimating the Extent of Coronary Disease
Findings Predictive of Events
Extended Follow-up

This is probably the time to reevaluate the previously established beliefs about management of an acute myocardial infarction. The overall mortality is decreased significantly due to the use of thrombolysis and emergency angioplasty.[1] The national mortality reported by the NRMI Registry is approximately 11% but in centers where emergent PTCA with stenting is frequently applied, mortality is between 4 and 6%.[2] Even in hospitals where this treatment is common however, there are a significant number of patients who, because of late arrival or other reasons, are not treated with reperfusion.[3] Thus, there is a marked variation in the coronary status as well as the myocardial function in what is a very heterogeneous cohort of patients. Some patients who have very early angioplasty or thrombolysis have very little myocardial necrosis but may be left with a great deal of myocardium still at risk. Others have large scars but may not have significant areas threatened. So in many of these patients an exercise test can be very useful in planning the patient's future. It may even help to identify some who have hibernating myocardium, who would benefit from revascularization.

ADVANTAGES AND BENEFITS

Many postinfarction deaths are sudden and occur within the first 6 months after infarction.[4–7] Indices that determine patients at risk have been identified by reviewing the complications that develop during convalescence. The presence of pulmonary edema or heart failure, renal failure, ventricular arrhythmias, and angina are but a few of the problems imparting a poor prognosis.[8,9] Most of the indices identified as prognostically significant relate to residual ischemia, left-ventricular dysfunction, and electrical instability.[10] However, a large number of patients with MI have an uncomplicated convalescence.

An MI almost always indicates the presence of coronary artery disease (CAD) but does not imply its severity. Patients who are clinically stable, regardless of the size of infarction, commonly have severe CAD.[11]

However, up to one third of patients with an MI may have single-vessel disease, and if the tissue at risk has undergone necrosis, these patients may remain stable for long periods.[10] Aggressive medical therapy with beta-blockers and statins has been shown to significantly improve progress, as have both PTCA and thrombolysis.[12–14] Although routine invasive diagnostic procedures cannot be universally recommended, nonetheless, in selected patients with two- and three-vessel disease, coronary artery bypass probably prolongs survival, especially in left main coronary artery and three-vessel disease.[5] Moreover, medical therapy such as antiplatelet and beta-blocker drugs as well as ACE inhibitors also appears to reduce mortality.[14,15]

Exercise testing from 10 days to 3 weeks after an MI is an efficient and established way to detect those at high risk.[16,17] Although the risks of doing exercise testing have probably been underreported, at this point, it seems reasonably safe. The post-MI stress test, then, emerged to provide us with a means of selecting patients at high risk among those who are asymptomatic and have an uncomplicated convalescence, permitting the implementation of aggressive management that might reduce mortality and morbidity. After thrombolysis and angioplasty became commonly used with early hospital discharge, often in 2 to 3 days, the exercise test was usually delayed until a few weeks later, and usually done on an outpatient basis.

Stratification of patients soon after an MI with exercise stress testing offers several other benefits. Patients at low risk may be spared needless invasive and costly studies. Exercise testing defines the patient's functional cardiac capacity by which activity level and rehabilitation can be rationally prescribed. It provides a safe basis to advise patients regarding return to normal activities and work. Psychologically, the test promotes self-confidence and reassures both patient and physician that routine daily tasks can be performed safely, thereby avoiding unnecessary restrictions. Even if the convalescent cardiac patient is subject to ischemia or arrhythmias during exercise testing, the patient is best served by exposing these problems under supervision.

SAFETY AND PATIENT SELECTION

A sizable experience with post-MI stress testing has demonstrated its safety. Several thousand predischarge and post-MI exercise tests have been reported with only a few serious complications.[11] The major determinant of risk is probably patient selection. Generally, post-MI patients with clinical heart failure, recent angina, uncontrolled high-grade ventricular ectopy, unstable ECG, and severe hypertension are excluded from stress testing. If the patient had an angiogram while in the hospital this information will contribute to following clinical decision-making and how aggressive therapy should be applied.

PROTOCOLS

Most early treadmill stress tests performed either at discharge or within 1 to 2 weeks of an MI are terminated with the attainment of a specific heart rate, usually 70% of the maximum predicted heart rate for age (normally 120 to 130 beats per minute) or when a workload of 3 to 5 MET (multiples of resting energy expenditure) has been achieved. This response is indicated if reperfusion therapy is not utilized. These modified protocols begin with a low initial workload and are advanced in small increments. Figure 8–9 is an example of such a protocol. Modified heart-rate–limited or workload-limited tests are referred to as submaximal treadmill stress tests and impose a stress equivalent to that encountered during routine daily activity.[18] Some studies, however, include symptom-limited or sign-limited tests using greater workloads.

These protocols are generally recommended for patients in the later post-MI period, that is, more than 2 weeks after infarction. Symptom-limited tests are terminated with the onset of angina, dyspnea, or fatigue, regardless of the magnitude of ST-segment depression. Sign-limited protocols are concluded at the onset of significant ST-segment depression, ventricular arrhythmias, or hypotension.

DeBusk and Haskell[18] compared symptom-limited and heart-rate–limited modified treadmill protocols at 3 weeks after an MI and found both equally safe and effective in provoking ischemic abnormalities and identifying patients at risk of subsequent coronary events. Higher peak heart rates and workloads were achieved with the symptom-limited protocol, yet the prevalence of ischemic test abnormalities was similar with both protocols, with the abnormalities usually occurring at heart rates of 130 beats per minute or less. However, a similar study by Starling and colleagues[19] demonstrated a greater yield with a symptom-limited modified test. At 6 weeks, a standard maximum symptom-limited stress test protocol appears superior to a modified symptom-limited test, but at 10 days to 2 weeks, I still believe a low-level modified protocol is more appropriate in the first two or three weeks, especially if the patient has not had an angiogram (see Fig. 8–9).

ABNORMAL STRESS TEST RESPONSES

ST-Segment Depression

The development of ST-segment depression with exercise is probably the most reliable sign of a myocardial ischemia and appears to be the most useful parameter of prognostic importance. In post-MI patients, the incidence previously reportedly varies from 15% to 40%.[16,17,20] Theroux and coworkers[16] found that exercise-induced ST-segment depression of 1 mm or greater on a submaximal treadmill protocol was highly predictive of subsequent mortality during a one-year period. These data were reported before the advent of reperfusion therapy.

Sami and colleagues[20] similarly noted an eightfold increased risk of cardiac arrest and recurrent infarction in patients with ST-segment depression of 2 mm or greater on a modified symptom-limited treadmill test. In this study, there was a tendency toward increased risk with greater ST-segment depression. Although the number of patients was small, the risk of a cardiac event doubled between ST-segment depression of 1 to 2 mm and ST-segment depression of 2 mm or greater. I would suspect that this would apply today.

Ischemic ST-segment changes alone or in conjunction with other stress test abnormalities predict a group of patients at risk of subsequent cardiac events such as stable and unstable angina,[21] serious ventricular arrhythmias,[22] heart failure,[23] and coronary artery bypass surgery.[20]

The accuracy of exercise-induced ST-segment depression in providing prognostic information can be influenced by several factors. Early termination of the stress test at a predetermined level of exercise may result in underestimating the incidence of ischemic ST changes. Resting ST-segment abnormalities, digitalis effect, myocardial hypertrophy, and conduction abnormalities make interpretation of exercise-induced ST-segment changes difficult.

Recent MIs may increase the number of false-negative responses with exercise testing. Castellanet and associates[24] found that ischemia after an anterior MI was less apparent than with the same process following an inferior MI. This is because an anterior wall akinetic segment and scar tissue in the myocardial wall appears to mask or alter significant ST depression in most leads.

Angina

Few studies have investigated exercise-induced angina as an isolated prognostic factor, although it occurs in a significant number of patients undergoing post-MI exercise testing.[25,26] Although Theroux and coworkers[16] could not demonstrate that angina predicts mortality or morbidity, they found it does correlate with the development of stable angina within 1 year.

Davidson and DeBusk[26] found that angina in the absence of ST-segment depression was not predictive of future medical events except that it was predictive of eventual coronary bypass surgery. Angina reflects the subjective status of patients and provides an incentive to intervene therapeutically.

Exercise-Induced Ventricular Arrhythmias

The prognostic significance of ventricular ectopy provoked by stress testing after an MI is controversial. Complex ventricular arrhythmias detected by ambulatory ECG monitoring during the late hospital phase of an infarction have been reported to adversely affect prognosis.[27,28] Reports of the incidence of ventricular ectopy with post-MI exercise tests range from 20% to 60%.[16,17,20] Some investigators have found that ventricular ectopy during post-MI exercise tests is predictive of mortality.[29,30] Other studies have found it of little prognostic significance for predicting subsequent coronary events, even if high-grade ventricular arrhythmias or a high frequency of premature beats are observed.[19,22,26] Rarely in this population is there a relationship between arrhythmias and ST-segment depression.

It is well established, however, that ventricular ectopy associated with left-ventricular dysfunction is more onerous.[30,31] Schultz and coworkers,[30] using Holter monitoring, demonstrated that only patients with an ejection fraction of less than 40% and complex ventricular activity had sudden death within 6 months after an MI. Borer and colleagues[32] noted a relationship between impaired ejection fraction, determined by nuclear studies, and ventricular ectopy frequency and complexity. They found that ventricular ectopy provided no more predictive information than ejection fraction alone.

Ambulatory ECG monitoring is superior to exercise testing in detecting ventricular arrhythmias[14,33] although there is some evidence that the arrhythmias may have somewhat different mechanisms. Also, exercise testing may demonstrate advanced grades of ventricular ectopy not detected by ambulatory monitoring, and it would appear that both tests may be complementary.[34]

Hemodynamic Responses

Certain hemodynamic responses to predischarge treadmill stress testing are also important. Reduced exercise capacity roughly reflects impaired left-ventricular function and may attribute its prognostic value to this association.[35] Performing modified workload-limited stress tests at 2 weeks post-MI, Weld and associates[36] found that exercise duration provided the most useful variable for predicting mortality. Completing a workload of at least 3 MET implied a favorable prognosis even if ST-segment depression or ventricular arrhythmias occurred.

Excluding patients with clinical heart failure, Davidson and DeBusk[26] found a maximum workload of less than 4 MET at 3 weeks after infarction to be a risk factor for future cardiac events.

Inadequate blood pressure response (defined as an increase of 10 mm or less in systolic blood pressure with a peak systolic pressure of 140 mm or less, or a fall of greater than 20 mm in systolic pressure from peak systolic blood pressure) also appeared predictive of coronary events and seemed to correlate with exercise duration.[21] Granath and colleagues[29] and Lundvall and Kaijser,[37] exercising patients on a bicycle ergometer, found that heart rates of greater than 125 to 130 beats per minute at workloads of 33 to 50 W (2.6 to 4 MET) constituted a significant prognostic factor. As far as I know, chronotropic incompetence has not been studied in a cohort of patients with a previous MI but its predictive value in large populations has been well established.[38]

ST-Segment Elevation

Exercise-induced ST-segment elevation is common in subjects with post-MI stress tests in leads where Q waves are present.[31] It has been correlated with abnormal wall motion in the area of infarction; however, approximately 50% of the ST-segment elevations observed initially with predischarge stress tests will be absent on retesting at 6 weeks, which may reflect improvement of abnormal wall motion with fibrosis and scarring,[10] or it may be due to recovery of hybernating myocardium. It rarely occurs with inferior infarction, and the ejection fraction is significantly lower in patients demonstrating ST-segment elevation. Thus, when the ST-segment elevation is noted on post-MI stress testing that becomes more marked with exercise it may indicate viable myocardium in the region of the infarct. (See Chapter 12.) Gerwirtz and colleagues,[39] using thallium perfusion scans, found that these changes correlate with the size of the scar and the increase in heart rate during the test. They found no evidence that ischemia was a consistent finding when ST elevation was present, and furthermore their patients with the most marked ST elevation (4 mm) had no ischemia detected by thallium. Their findings have been supported by a recent study from Greece.[39a] It may be that changes in QT interval will help us determine the significance of these changes.[40]

RELIABILITY OF ABNORMALITIES

Knowledge of the consistency of post-MI exercise test abnormalities is important in assessing the validity of its prognostic value. Different timing in the performance of stress tests with relation to the infarction may alter the ability to provide prognostic information.

Starling and coworkers[34] compared modified symptom-limited treadmill tests performed at 2 weeks and 6 weeks post-MI. The frequency of ST-segment depression was a similar result on both stress tests and exhibited a high reproducibility. The frequency of angina, inappropriate blood pressure response, and ventricular arrhythmias for the group were also similar; however, these abnormalities demonstrated limited reproducibility and substantial variation in individual patients. Furthermore, almost one fourth of abnormal 2-week tests were normal at 6 weeks, and nearly one third of abnormal tests became normal. Also, the patients who had an intervening cardiac event between 3 and 6 weeks had abnormal 2-week stress tests.

Therefore, early or predischarge stress tests identify a group of patients at early risk, in addition to determining the exercise capacity, ischemic ST response, and ventricular arrhythmias that aid in predicting long-term prognosis. A second test performed several weeks after an MI is important to further identify patients who had previously normal early stress tests and may still be at risk for subsequent cardiac events. This is of most benefit in those who have not had reperfusion therapy.

ESTIMATING THE EXTENT OF CORONARY DISEASE

Because the severity of coronary artery disease (CAD) has been demonstrated to be an important determinant of survival,[41,42] and because multivessel disease has been demonstrated angiographically in as many as 50% to 75% of patients soon after an MI,[10,11,31,38] it would be helpful if testing would predict the severity of disease in those who have not had an angiogram. Although symptomatic patients appear to have a higher prevalence of multivessel involvement, symptoms or complications are relatively insensitive discriminating factors.[43,44]

It would be desirable if the absence of exercise-induced ischemic ECG responses signified no further CAD, that is, single-vessel disease. If a positive stress test response reflected ischemia at sites adjacent to or remote from the infarction where viable myocardium is supplied by stenotic vessels, it would predict multivessel involvement.

Two studies, Fuller and colleagues[45] and Schwartz and associates,[11] found that ST-segment depression of 1 mm or greater, angina, or both correctly identified most patients with multivessel disease. Hemodynamic parameters such as achieved workload or double product, however, did not assist in predicting patients with multivessel involvement. Both studies found that a positive ischemic response was of moderate sensitivity, approximately 55% to 67% in detecting multivessel disease, and had a high specificity of about 90% with a predictive value also near 90%. Fuller and associates[45] found that 73% of negative responses on exercise tests identified single-vessel disease. However, Schwartz and colleagues found that a negative exercise test could not reliably indicate single-vessel disease because more than 50% of the patients with negative responses had multivessel disease. Therefore, an abnormal post-MI stress test identifies most patients with multivessel disease, but a negative test does not necessarily preclude multivessel involvement.

Findings Predictive of Events

1. ST-segment depression
2. Short exercise duration
3. High heart rate at low workload
4. Failure to increase blood pressure or fall below control
5. Complex premature ventricular contractions with poor left-ventricular function

EXTENDED FOLLOW-UP

Most of the follow-up data reported cover fairly short periods. Theroux and associates[46] report a 5-year follow-up that is of special interest. They found that the usual markers—ST-segment depression, decreasing blood pressure, and short exercise duration—were excellent predictors for events in the first year after MI, but thereafter factors that were markers for decreased ventricular function, such as size of infarct from the ECG, history of previous infarctions, and ventricular arrhythmias, were more important. Thus, when making a short-term determination, the decision-making process is different from when the first year is behind us and we are going for the long haul. Taylor and associates[47] report that the results of the exercise test can be used to reassure wives as to their husbands' capacity for activity.

SUMMARY

Although statistical data suggest that the clinical approach recommended makes sense at this time, individual patients often present individual problems, and our responsibility is to try to do what is best for each person. The mark of a good clinician is not only to know the statistics, but to be able to apply their probabilities to each patient. Many exceptions will occur, and our ability to deal effectively with each complex situation will be the true test of our mettle.

REFERENCES

1. Canto, JG, et al: The volume of primary angioplasty procedures and survival after acute myocardial infarction. New Engl J Med 342:1573, 2000.
2. Rogers, WJ, et al: Treatment of myocardial infarction in the United States (1990 to 1993): Observations from the National Registry of Myocardial Infarction. Circulation 90:2103, 1994.
3. Every, NR, et al: A comparison of the National Registry of Myocardial Infarction with the Cooperative Cardiovascular Project. J Am Coll Cardiol 34:1886, 1999.

4. Marginato, A, et al: Exercise-induced ST elevation on infarct- related leads: A marker of residual viability [abstract]. Circulation 86(suppl 1): I-138, 1992.
5. Moss, AJ, et al: The early posthospital phase of myocardial infarction: Prognostic stratification. Circulation 54:58, 1976.
6. Weinblatt, E, et al: Prognosis of men after first myocardial infarction: Mortality and first recurrence in relation to selected parameters. Am J Public Health 58:1329, 1968.
7. Moss, AJ, et al: Cardiac death in the first 6 months after myocardial infarction: Potential for mortality reduction in the early posthospital period. Am J Cardiol 39:616, 1977.
8. Bigger, JT, et al: Risk stratification after acute myocardial infarction. Am J Cardiol 42:202, 1978.
9. Kannel, WB, et al: Prognosis after initial myocardial infarction: The Framingham Study. Am J Cardiol 44:53, 1979.
10. Miller, RR, et al: Chronic stable inferior myocardial infarction: Unsuspected harbinger of high-risk proximal left coronary arterial obstruction amenable to surgical revascularization. Am J Cardiol 39:954, 1976.
11. Schwarts, KM, et al: Limited exercise testing soon after myocardial infarction: Correlation with early coronary and left ventricular angiography. Ann Intern Med 94:727, 1981.
12. Kennedy, HL and Rosenson, RS. Physician use of beta-adrenergic blocking Therapy: A changing perspective. JACC 26(2):547, 1995.
13. Rosenson, RS and Tangney, CC: Antiatherothrombotic properties of statins. JAMA 279(20):1643, 1998.
14. Waldecker, B, et al: Long-term follow-up after direct percutaneous transluminal coronary angioplasty for acute myocardial infarction. J Am Coll Cardiol 32:1320, 1998.
15. Miller, DH and Borer, JS: Exercise testing early after myocardial infarction: Risks and benefits. Am J Med 72:427, 1982.
16. Theroux, P, et al: Prognostic value of exercise testing soon after myocardial infarction. N Engl J Med 301:341, 1979.
17. Smith, JW, et al: Exercise testing three weeks after myocardial infarction. Chest 75:1216, 1979.
18. DeBusk, RF and Haskell, W: Symptom-limited vs. heart rate-limited exercise testing soon after myocardial infarction. Circulation 61:738, 1980.
19. Starling, MR, et al: Superiority of selected treadmill exercise protocols predischarge and six weeks post-infarction for detecting ischemic abnormalities. Am Heart J 104:1054, 1982.
20. Sami, M, et al: The prognostic significance of serial exercise testing after myocardial infarction. Circulation 60:1238, 1979.
21. Starling, MR, et al: Exercise testing early after myocardial infarction: Predictive value for subsequent unstable angina and death. Am J Cardiol 46:909, 1980.
22. Markiewiez, W, et al: Exercise testing soon after myocardial infarction. Circulation 56:26, 1977.
23. Koppes, GM, et al: Response to exercise early after uncomplicated acute myocardial infarction in patients receiving no medication: Long term follow-up. Am J Cardiol 46:764, 1980.
24. Castellanet, M, et al: Comparison of 57 segment changes on exercise testing of angiographic findings in patients with prior myocardial infarction. Am J Cardiol 42:24, 1978.
25. Ericsson, M, et al: Arrhythmias and symptoms during treadmill testing three weeks after myocardial infarction in 100 patients. Br Heart J 35:787,1973.
26. Davidson, DM and DeBusk, RF: Prognostic value of a single exercise test 3 weeks after uncomplicated myocardial infarction. Circulation 61:236, 1980.
27. Moss, AJ, et al: Ventricular ectopic beats and their relation to sudden and non-sudden cardiac death after myocardial infarction. Circulation 60:998, 1979.
28. Bigger, T, et al: Prevalence, characteristics and significance of ventricular tachycardia (three or more complexes) detected with ambulatory electrocardiographic recording in the late hospital phase of acute myocardial infarction. Am J Cardiol 48:815-823, 1981.
29. Granath, A, et al: Early workload tests for evaluation of long term prognosis of acute myocardial infarction. Br Heart J 39:758, 1977.
30. Schultz, RA, et al: Sudden death in the year following myocardial infarction: Relation to ventricular premature contractions in the late hospital phase and left ventricular ejection fraction. Am J Med 62:192, 1977.
31. DeFeyter, PJ, et al: Prognostic value of exercise testing coronary angiography and left ventriculography 6-8 weeks after myocardial infarction. Circulation 66:527, 1982.

32. Borer, JS, et al: Sensitivity, specificity, and predictive accuracy of radionuclide cineangiography during exercise in patients with coronary artery disease: Comparison with exercise electrocardiography. Circulation 60:572, 1979.
33. Weiner, OA, et al: S-T segment changes post-infarction: Predictive value for multivessel coronary disease and left ventricular aneurysm. Circulation 58:887, 1978.
34. Starling, MR, et al: Treadmill exercise tests predischarge and six weeks post-myocardial infarction to detect abnormalities of known prognostic value. Ann Intern Med 94:721, 1981.
35. Paine, TD, et al: Relation of graded exercise test findings after myocardial infarction to extent of coronary artery disease and left ventricular dysfunction. Am J Cardiol 42:716, 1978.
36. Weld, FM, et al: Risk stratification with low-level exercise testing 2 weeks after acute myocardial infarction. Circulation 64:306, 1981.
37. Lundvall, K and Kaijser, L: Early exercise tests after uncomplicated acute myocardial infarction before early discharge from hospital. Acta Med Scand 210:257, 1981.
38. Lauer, MS, et al: Impaired heart rate response to graded exercise: prognostic implications of chronotropic Incompetence in the Framingham Heart Study. Circulation 93:1520, 1996.
39. Gewirtz, H, et al: Role of myocardial ischemia in the genesis of stress-induced ST segment elevation in previous anterior myocardial infarction. Am J Cardiol 51:1289, 1983.
39a. Hahalis, G, et al: Contribution of the ST elevation/T-wave normalization in Q-wave leads during routine, pre-discharge treadmill exercise test to patient management and risk stratification after acute myocardial infarction. JACC 40:62, 2002.
40. Bertella, M: Defining the meaning of exercise-induced S-T segment elevation in Q wave leads in postinfarction patients using a new ECG parameter of transmural ischemia: The stress-induced Q-Tc interval shortening. Cardiology 95:51, 2001.
41. Humphries, JO, et al: Natural history of ischemic heart disease in relation to arteriographic findings: A twelve year study of 224 patients. Circulation 49:489, 1974.
42. Reeves, TJ, et al: Natural history of angina pectoris. Am J Cardiol 33:423, 1974.
43. Turner, JD, et al: Coronary angiography soon after myocardial infarction. Chest 77:58, 1980.
44. Rigo, P, et al: Value and limitations of segmental analysis of stress thallium myocardial imaging for location of coronary artery lesion. Circulation 61:973, 1980.
45. Fuller, CM, et al: Early post-myocardial infarction treadmill stress testing: An accurate predictor of multivessel coronary disease and subsequent cardiac events. Ann Intern Med 94:734, 1981.
46. Theroux, P, et al: Exercise testing in the early period after myocardial infarction in the evaluation of prognosis. Cardiol Clin 2(1):71, 1984.
47. Taylor, CB, et al: Exercise testing to enhance wives' confidence in their husbands' cardiac capability. Am J Cardiol 55:635, 1958

11 Stress Testing After Surgical Intervention and Coronary Angioplasty

Questions
Coronary Artery Bypass Graft Surgery
Prediction of Postoperative Results from Preoperative Stress Testing
Prediction of Ischemia and Postoperative Testing
Preoperative and Postoperative ST-Segment Depression
Diagnostic Value of Angina
Postoperative Exercise Performance
Serial Postoperative Exercise Testing
Angioplasty

Most patients, prior to undergoing coronary artery bypass graft surgery, have experienced a major decrease in function, especially during exercise, and the aim of surgery is to improve their performance. The expected improvement as measured by stress testing includes an increase in aerobic capacity and an ability to exercise without undue dyspnea and without significant chest pain or discomfort. Because it is common for most cardiac patients to be asymptomatic at rest, a test of functional capacity before and after a treatment is important in evaluating the benefit derived from the intervention.

Stress testing is one of the most useful ways to measure the response to surgery or catheter-based revascularization and to evaluate progress or the lack of it immediately after the procedure and in the ensuing years. It has been used in valvular surgery, coronary bypass surgery, and recently in angioplasty. It is often used to measure changes expected from medical therapy as well.

QUESTIONS

Questions we would like to answer in the evaluation of angioplasty or bypass patients are as follows:

1. Can we predict the result from the preprocedural stress test?

2. Does postprocedural ST depression depict graft closure or restenosis or residual or new myocardial ischemia? Is it as reliable as the preoperative stress test?
3. Does comparison of the preoperative and postoperative exercise tests have more value in assessing graft patency than the postoperative test alone?
4. Does angina or its lack during stress testing postoperatively predict the presence or absence of myocardial ischemia?
5. Does the postoperative exercise tolerance correlate with ischemia or graft patency?
6. Does serial postoperative testing aid in patient evaluation and follow-up?

CORONARY ARTERY BYPASS GRAFT SURGERY

Prediction of Postoperative Results from Preoperative Stress Testing

Stuart and I[1] conducted a study of 387 postoperative patients, 196 of whom had completed preoperative and postoperative exercises tests. We compared age, sex, workload at onset of ischemia, and the presence of anginal pain during testing and found that none of these helped to distinguish those who would have a good result from those who would have a poor result; thus, the study appeared to fail as an adjunct in determining the need for surgery. We had believed angina manifested on the preoperative treadmill would be a predictor for both ultimate survival and relief of ischemia. This was because we knew that generalized scarring of the myocardium, which is more common in coronary disease patients without angina, should carry a poor prognosis, whereas exercise pain, signaling a viable myocardium, should predict a better result after bypass. However, we found no evidence to confirm this hypothesis in our data.

On the other hand, Weiner and colleagues,[2] when analyzing the nonrandomized patients in the CASS registry, found those with a high-risk exercise test (ST depression greater than 1 mm and a short exercise time (Bruce first stage only) had better survival with surgery than if treated medically. Those reaching Bruce stage IV, regardless of the ST changes, also did better with surgery than those with limited exercise capacity. The CASS study[3] also found that those who had angina during the preoperative exercise test did better when treated surgically than medically (5-year survival rate of 94% for surgery compared with 87% for medical therapy). It is also well known that the high crossover from medical to surgical treatment (23%) in the CASS study favors good results in the medical cohort, so that if these patients were counted as poor results, the data would force surgery even more.

The so-called high-risk treadmill patients also had an improved quality of life, characterized by less angina and a longer exercise time if they had had bypass surgery. This is also compatible with the findings of the European coronary surgery randomized trial.[4]

Thus, when comparing operated with nonoperated patients, our original thesis was confirmed; that is, the exercise test is useful in deciding who should have surgery. The best predictor is a short exercise time.

Prediction of Ischemia and Postoperative Testing

Several studies found that complete disappearance of ST depression was usually associated with complete revascularization.[5–9] However, Siegel and associates[9] reported that 30% of their patients with complete revascularization continued to have ST depression after surgery. When some of the bypass grafts are open and some are closed, there is also a high probability of a normal ST response. Although the postoperative ST response is helpful, a significant number of those with all grafts closed will have normal ST segments.[10] Our experience has been similar to that of Siegel and coworkers[9] in that some patients with open grafts continue to have ST depression. Although it is somewhat difficult to document, postoperative ST-segment depression is probably not as reliable as preoperative ST-segment depression in predicting the presence or absence of ischemia. This is even more apparent in patients who have angioplasty.[11]

Assad-Morell[8] reported an excellent correlation between graft patency postoperatively and exercise-induced ST depression. When all grafts were patent, only 9% had ST depression, and none of their patients with total failure to be revascularized had normal ST segments. However, no other study has been reported in which the exercise test provides as good discrimination (Table 11–1). Nevertheless, we might conclude that reversion

Table 11–1. **Postoperative Treadmill Exercise Response by Number of Vessels Left Ungrafted (VLU)**

	No VLU	One VLU	Two VLU	Three VLU
Total patients (no.)	23	33	24	5
Treadmill exercise response:				
Positive	2 (9%)	23 (70%)	23 (96%)	5 (100%)
Negative	21 (91%)	10 (30%)	1 (4%)	0 (0%)
Patients by vessels diseased (no.):				
One vessel	10	2	0	0
Two vessels	11	18	7	0
Three vessels	2	13	17	5
Total grafts*	38	56	46	9
Grafts patent:				
No.	38	42	23	0
%	100	75	50	0

*Total number of grafts in group.
(From Assad-Morell et al.[8] with permission.)

of postoperative ST segments to normal usually indicates complete revascularization, with many exceptions. It almost always indicates improved perfusion.

Preoperative and Postoperative ST-Segment Depression

When preoperative and postoperative ST segments are compared, most investigators report that the conversion from abnormal to normal is associated with a high probability of total revascularization. Hartman and associates[10] reported this in 88% of patients. They also found that in those with improved coronary flow, but less than total revascularization, ST depression disappeared in 79%. Even in those who were shown to be unimproved by angiography, 50% lost their ST depression postoperatively.

From the data available, it appears that when an abnormal ST pattern converts to normal, there is a high probability of total revascularization.[5,12] On the other hand, a significant number of patients with total revascularization will continue to have ST depression, and there will also be some with failed grafts who have a normal ST response.[13] Postoperative testing can be interpreted with much more reliability when the preoperative test is available.

Diagnostic Value of Angina

The diagnostic value of angina during postoperative testing has been studied by a number of authors.[5,7,9] Almost all patients with complete revascularization are free of exercise-induced angina; in fact, over 90% of those who have had bypass surgery lose their angina. The loss of angina, however, is a weak predictor of graft patency. Anginal relief occurs with improvement of perfusion in almost every case, but may also occur in patients with little or no change in myocardial blood flow. Of patients with at least one patent graft in the early postoperative period, 79% fail to have angina, and Hartman and colleagues[10] found that 50% of those without any revascularization became free of angina. It is important to remember that 38% of patients either lost or had marked improvement in their angina after the discarded Vineberg operation, which may have improved collateral flow a little, but was by no means a complete revascularization.[14]

Postoperative Exercise Performance

Exercise performance may be very bad in patients with normal function and very good in those with severely compromised cardiac output.[15] Therefore, it is not surprising that total exercise time, maximum achieved heart rate, and maximum achieved double product have not been shown to have much validity in predicting the degree of revascularization.[16,17] Although most patients with good anatomical results improve their exercise capacity after surgery, as an individual predictor, exercise fails to stand up. This may be because pain, which determines the exercise end-point in many cases, is commonly lost even in those with failed revascularization. We know that in the absence of angina, patients often exercise longer and may reach an increased double product. Therefore, there is fairly good correlation between the loss of induced angina and increased functional capacity. The paper by Block and coworkers[18] demonstrates this concept. They studied 23 patients following unsuccessful revascularization and reported a statistically significant improvement in maximum heart rate and lesser improvement in functional aerobic impairment, absolute duration of exercise, and pressure–rate product (Fig. 11–1).

On the other hand, when patients fail to have pain relief after coronary bypass surgery, they almost invariably have a significant amount of ischemic myocardium, unless they have vasospastic angina.[9] Although there is still inadequate confirmation by other authors, I believe that the double product at the onset of ischemic ST depression is the most reliable stress testing measure of change in the degree of ischemia over time or as a result of an intervention. We found this index to be improved in 61% of our patients after coronary bypass surgery.[2]

Serial Postoperative Exercise Testing

Although in clinical practice it is common to use the exercise test in following up and reevaluating postoperative coronary bypass patients, there is not much documentation of its usefulness. Guttin's group[19] in Houston found

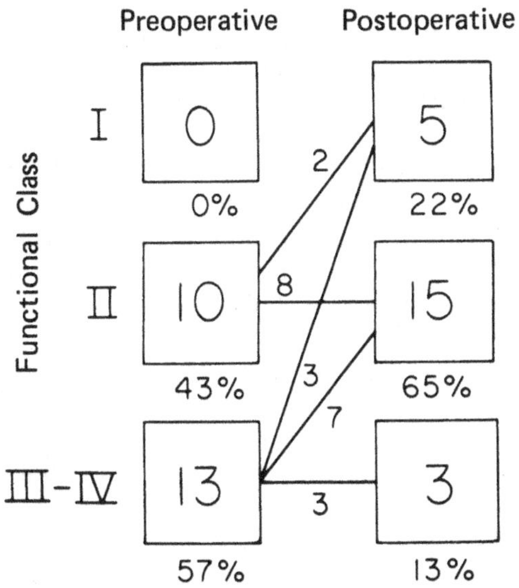

FIGURE 11–1. Changes in functional class in 23 patients after unsuccessful revascularization. Note the improvement despite the lack of functioning grafts. (From Block et al,[18] with permission.)

that 20% of those who had negative findings after coronary bypass surgery converted to an abnormal test in 23 months. Many of these had progression of disease or graft failure. In our experience, the onset of ST depression or angina at a lower workload or lower double product has usually led us to the discovery of progressive ischemia. Postoperative testing thus is a useful and practical approach to patient evaluation and should be used as an aid in following coronary bypass patients.

ANGIOPLASTY

It might be assumed that the concepts presented in postoperative coronary bypass patients would hold for those who have undergone angioplasty. Because many patients undergoing coronary angioplasty have only one vessel opened, one might suspect some variations in findings compared with those of coronary artery bypass patients. Marco and colleagues[20] followed up 62 patients with successful angioplasty and found that exercise testing within 2 days of the procedure reliably predicted the 32% who developed restenosis. In my experience, anginal pain is a reliable predictor of restenosis or progression of disease in another vessel in angioplasty patients. Also, postangioplasty resolution of ST depression has been a reliable indicator of a successful result. el-Tamimi, however, has reported that exercise-induced ST depression shortly after PTCA is often obliterated by isosorbide dinitrate and is due to small-vessel constriction produced by the procedure.[22] Downstream emboli of small fragments occur in a high percentage of patients who undergo this therapy.[21] Meier and associates[23] used bicycle ergometry on those with successful angioplasty and found that their work capacity increased from 72 to 122 W. Rosing and colleagues[24] reported on 66 patients from the National Heart, Lung, and Blood Institute Registry who had undergone successful angioplasty. Only 33% had ST depression prior to the procedure, and 7% of these were abnormal afterward. If angina was used as an indicator of abnormality, 68% were abnormal before and 7% afterward. The low sensitivity of ST depression in this group probably reflects the original restrictions of this procedure to single-vessel disease. It is of interest that those patients who had an abnormal thallium test after the procedure had a higher risk of restenosis.

Several reports of sudden closure shortly after an exercise test of the vessel that had undergone angioplasty raise some concern.[25–29] Several cases have been reported in the literature, most of whom were tested on the second postoperative day. The incidence of this complication has been quoted as 0.08% in a series of 1264 tests. Sheer stress, coronary spasm, hyperaggregable platelets, and possible flaps caused by the increased flow velocity have been postulated as the mechanisms. Because of these reports, most centers have abandoned exercise testing prior to discharge, believing it will be safer to test the patients a few weeks afterward. During the postangioplasty period (3 to 6 months), patients who have exercise-induced ST depression or angina have been shown to have a significantly higher incidence of coronary events as might be expected.[30]

DISCUSSION AND SUMMARY

The reason why ST depression may be absent in patients with failed bypass surgery remains obscure. Fibrosis or injury of the subendocardium, the origin of the ST changes, may be a cause.

Some patients with angiographic evidence of total revascularization continue to have ST depression in the postoperative period. The measurement of coronary flow as generated by digital angiography by Bates and coworkers[31] may give an explanation. They found that the reactive hyperemia associated with contrast media increased velocity in normal coronaries to about 1.8 times normal. This reactive increase is reduced, depending on the severity of the coronary lesion. When the investigators studied normal-appearing bypass grafts, the increased flow was about 50% of that seen in normal vessels. It may be that even though the graft is patent, the rigid tube almost universally found after a year or so cannot deliver the magnitude of flow increase necessary to supply myocardial needs during exercise.

The work of Ribeiro and colleagues[32] is of special interest. They found some patients with bypass surgery who had open grafts, yet had ischemia documented by Holter monitor, exercise testing, and positron emission tomography using rubidium 82. Their work supports that of Bates and associates[31] in that ischemia can be present in areas of the myocardium that one would expect to be adequately perfused when viewing the angiogram. Mechanisms responsible for this are better understood. Coronaries that have nonocclusive plaques do not have healthy endothelium and probably constrict rather than dilate with exercise.[33] If they are aggressively treated with statins this may improve.[34]

Even though the exercise test has limitations in the postoperative patient, it can be very useful. The aerobic capacity, blood pressure, heart rate response, initiation of arrhythmias, and other findings are probably as valuable as the detection of ST-segment depression when considered as a whole and with knowledge of the patient's previous performance.

REFERENCES

1. Stuart, RJ and Ellestad, MH: The value of exercise stress testing in predicting benefits from aorto-coronary bypass surgery. Angiology 30:416, 1979.

2. Weiner, DA, et al: Value of exercise testing in identifying patients with improved survival after coronary bypass surgery [abstract]. Circulation II(70):771, 1984.
3. Ryan, TJ, et al: The role of exercise testing in the randomized cohort of CASS [abstract]. Circulation 70:78, 1984.
4. European Coronary Study Group: Long-term results of prospective randomized study of coronary artery bypass surgery in stable angina pectoris. Lancet Oct–Dec: 1173, 1982.
5. McConahay, DR, et al: Accuracy of treadmill testing in assessment of direct myocardial revascularization. Circulation 56(4):548–522, 1977.
6. Knobel, SB, et al: The effect of aortocoronary bypass grafts on myocardial blood flow reserve and treadmill exercise tolerance. Circulation 50:685–693, 1974.
7. Bode, RF Jr and Zajtchuk, R: Evaluation of saphenous vein bypass surgery with multistage treadmill test and ventricular function studies. J Thorac Cardiovasc Surg 74(1):44–46, 1977.
8. Assad-Morell, JL, et al: Aorto-coronary artery saphenous vein bypass surgery: Clinical and angiographic results. Mayo Clin Proc 50:379, 1975.
9. Siegel, W, et al: The spectrum of exercise test and angiographic correlations in myocardial revascularization surgery. Circulation II (suppl 1):51–52, 156–162, 1975.
10. Hartman, CW, et al: Aortocoronary bypass surgery: Correlation of angiographic, symptomatic and functional improvement at 1 year. Am J Cardiol 37:352–357, 1976.
11. Bech, GJW, et al: Fractional flow reserve to determine the appropriateness of angioplasty in moderate coronary stenosis: A randomized trial. Circulation 103:2928, 2001.
12. Glasser, SP and Clark, PI: The Clinical Approach to Exercise Testing. Harper & Row, New York, 1980.
13. Dodek, A, et al: Stress electrocardiography in the evaluation of aortocoronary bypass surgery. Am Heart J 86:292, 1973.
14. Kassebaum, DG, et al: Stress electrocardiography in the evaluation of surgical revascularization of the heart. Circulation 40:297, 1969.
15. Block, T, et al: Changes in exercise performance following unsuccessful coronary bypass grafting [abstract]. Am J Cardiol 37:122, 1976.
16. Lapin, ES, et al: Changes in maximal exercise performance in the evaluation of saphenous vein bypass surgery. Circulation XLVII:1164, 1973.
17. Merrill, AJ Jr, et al: Value of maximal exercise testing in assessment of results. Circulation II:(suppl 1)51, 173, 1975.
18. Block, TA, et al: Improvement in exercise performance after unsuccessful myocardial revascularization. Am J Cardiol 40:673, 1977.
19. Guttin, J, et al: Longitudinal evaluation of patients after coronary artery bypass by serial treadmill testing [abstract]. Am J Cardiol 35:142, 1975.
20. Marco, J, et al: Two years or more follow-up after successful percutaneous transluminal-coronary angioplasty [abstract]. Eur Heart J 5(suppl 1):76, 1984.
21. Tamimi, H, et al: Inappropriate constriction of small coronary vessels as a possible cause of a positive exercise test early after a successful coronary angioplasty. Circulation 84: 2307, 1991.
22. Meier, B, et al: Long-term exercise performance after percutaneous transluminal coronary angioplasty and coronary artery bypass grafting. Circulation 68(4):796, 1983.
23. Ricciardi, MJ, et al: Visualization of discrete microinfarction after percutaneous coronary intervention associated with mild creatinine kinase-MB elevation. Circulation 103:2780, 2001.
24. Rosing, DR, et al: Exercise, electrocardiographic and functional responses after percutaneous transluminal coronary angioplasty. Am J Cardiol 53:36C, 1984.
25. Dash, TW: Delayed coronary occlusion after successful percutaneous transluminal coronary angioplasty: Association with exercise testing. Am J Cardiol 52:1143, 1982.
26. Nygaard, TW, et al: Acute coronary occlusion with exercise testing after initially successful angioplasty for acute myocardial infarction. Am J Cardiol 57:687, 1986.
27. Schweiger, MJ, et al: Acute coronary occlusion following negative exercise testing after successful coronary angioplasty. J Invas Cardiol 4:199, 1992.
28. Sionis, D, et al: Early exercise testing after successful percutaneous transluminal angioplasty: A word of caution. Am Heart J 123(2):530, 1992.
29. Goodman, SG, et al: Acute coronary thrombotic occlusion following exercise testing 6 weeks after PTCA. Cathet Cardiovasc Diagn 27:40, 1992.

30. Kaul, U, et al: Silent myocardial ischemia after PTCA and its prognostic value. Clin Cardiol 14:563, 1991.
31. Bates, ER, et al: The chronic coronary flow reserve provided by saphenous vein bypass grafts as determined by digital coronary radiography. Am Heart J 106:462, 1984.
32. Ribeiro, P, et al: Different mechanisms for the relief of angina after coronary bypass surgery. Br Heart J 52:502, 1984.
33. Hijmering, ML, Stroes, ESG, Olijhoek, J, et al: Sympathetic activation markedly reduces endothelium-dependent, flow-mediated vasodilation. J Am Coll 39:683, 2002.
34. Brown, BG, et al: Simvastatin and niacin, antioxidant vitamins, or the combination for the prevention of coronary disease. N Engl J Med 345:1583, 2001.

12
ECG Patterns and Their Significance

Introduction
Conventional Elecrocardiographic Changes
- Normal Exercise Electrocardiographic ST and J Point
- Upsloping ST Segments
- Horizontal versus Downsloping ST Segments
- Downsloping ST Segments
- ST Depression in Recovery Only
- ST Integral and Slope
- Time Course of ST Depression
- Magnitude of ST Depression
- Intraobserver Agreement
- Distribution of ST Depression

ST Elevation
- ST Elevation in Leads without Q Waves
- ST Elevation in Leads with Q Waves
- ST Elevation at Rest (Early Repolarization)

Unconventional Electrocardiographic Changes with Exercise
- Lead Strength (ST/R)
- ST-Heart Rate Slope
- ST-Heart Rate Index (Kligfield Index)
- ST Evolving toward Normal with Exercise
- Intermittent ST Depression
- ST Depression with Long Diastolic Filling
- ST Hysteresis (HR Recovery ST Loop)
- Rounded ST Depression
- ST Depression with Nodal Premature Contractions

QRS Changes
- R Wave Amplitude
  - *Decreased R + ST Depression*
  - *Increased R Wave with Atrial Extra Systoles*
- Increased QRS Duration
- ATHENS Score
- Changes in QRS Axis
- Changes in S Waves

Q Wave and QT Intervals
- QX/QT Ratio
- Septal Q Waves
- QT Dispersion
- Prolonged QT
- Congenital Long QT Syndrome

T Wave Alterations
- Normalization of Inverted T Waves
- Peaked T Waves
- Deep T Wave Inversions
- Tall T Waves

P Wave Changes
False-Positive ST Changes
- Sloping PQ Segment (Sapin)
- Digitalis
- Hypokalemia
- ST Depression in Inferior Leads Only
- False-Positive Tracings Due to Computer Averaging
- Increased Sympathetic Tone (Vasoregulatory Asthenia)
- Hyperventilation and Orthostatic Changes
- Short PR Interval
- Convex ST-Segment Depression—"Hump Sign"
- ST Segment Variability
- Localization of Ischemia by Electrocardiographic Patterns
- ST Elevation Due to Transmural Ischemia
- ST Elevation in AVR
- ST Depression in V1
- Peaked T Waves in V2
- Localization of Proximal or Distal LAD
- Localization with Right Precordial Leads

U Waves

INTRODUCTION

It is truly remarkable that although electrocardiographic (ECG) changes were first recognized as markers for ischemia about 1918,[1] here more than 80 years later we are still discovering that there is more to learn in this area. In the last few years numerous papers point out new ECG markers that have utility[2–5] and I predict this trend will continue into the future. This chapter has been revised to present the more commonly used (conventional) electrocardiogram exchanges separately from the less commonly recognized changes (unconventional).

Although computers are being used more to evaluate the ECG changes associated with exercise,[6,7] it is still essential to carefully scrutinize the ECG visually, since computer measures are far from error-free. Also, technical writers of computer programs are always years behind the latest knowledge base. This chapter presents many ways of evaluating the exercise ECG that have not been incorporated into a computer program and may never be. Careful inspection of tracings from appropriate lead systems, using properly applied electrodes and recording systems with a good frequency response, can usually result in accurate evaluation of changes now known to be clinically significant. If you want to be an expert in the evaluation of exercise tests, you will find many concepts mentioned here that will set you apart from those who examine only the ST segment.

CONVENTIONAL ELECTROCARDIOGRAPHIC CHANGES

Normal Exercise Electrocardiogram ST and J Point

As the heart rate increases with exercise, a number of predictable changes occur in a normal ECG tracing. The PR interval is shortened after 1 minute of exercise.[8] The P wave becomes taller[9] and the Ta wave (wave of repolarization) increases, resulting in a downward displacement of the PQ junction. This is particularly important because the so-called baseline, for terms of evaluating ST-segment change, is below that usually considered to be isoelectric in the resting tracing (Fig. 12–1). With exercise, the Ta wave tends to extend through the QRS and may influence the junction between the ST segment and T wave. Lepeschkin[9] believed that this alteration in baseline extends well into the ST segment and may cause fictitious ST-segment depression (Fig. 12–2).

Recently Sapin and colleagues[10] have reemphasized the importance of the Ta wave as a cause of false-positive ST depression and have proposed that the PQ-segment slope can alert us to this possibility (See Figure 12–3). When the slope is steep, they found the likelihood of false-positive ST depression to be greatly increased. This depression is also more likely

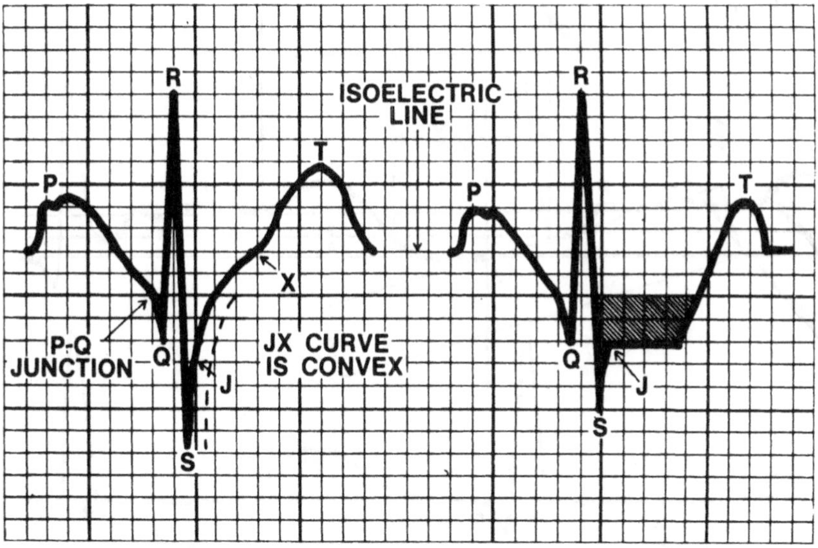

FIGURE 12–1. *(Left)* The normal exercise ECG complex. It can be noted that the PQ segment is deflected below the isoelectric line. This point is considered to be a baseline for determining ST-segment abnormalities. *(Right)* A horizontal ST-segment depression of 2 mm as measured from the PQ segment.

when the P waves are taller than normal and is more common in leads 2 and 3.

It has become standard practice to use the line marked 2 in Figure 12–2, or the PQ or PR junction, indicated in Figure 12–1, as a marker for the baseline, rather than to use line 3 (see Fig. 12–2). The excellent computer analysis of this problem, performed in the laboratory of Bruce and colleagues[11] has been followed by the study of Blomqvist,[12] indicating the appearance of progressive depression of the J-junction. When the ST segment is measured at one-fourth the distance between the QRS and peak T in left-to-right leads, considerable depression is usually seen. The anterior-posterior lead changes (V1 to V2) are less prominent than those in the lateral and vertical leads. Figure 12–4 illustrates the findings in the orthogonal leads at the various heart rates. Depression in the Y, or vertical, lead gives a clue as to why this lead has a high incidence of so-called false-positive ST-segment changes.[13] It can be seen that the changes are less significant in the frontal, or transverse, lead X.

The absence of significant ST-segment depression in young, vigorous boys and in athletic, middle-aged men exercised in our laboratory suggests that the effect of the Ta wave can usually be recognized because of the short duration (usually 0.04 second) of the J-point depression.

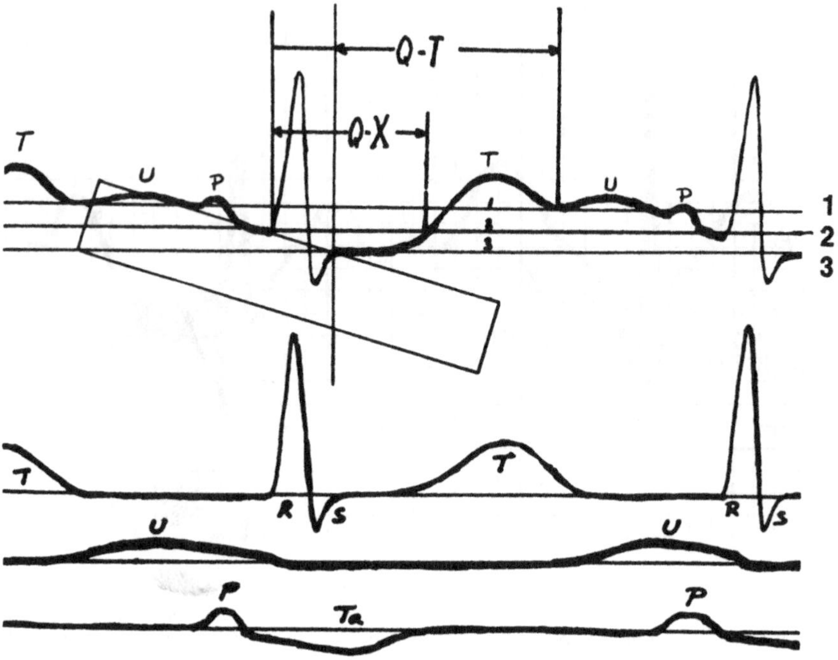

FIGURE 12–2. Deviation of ST segments associated with exercise. Lepeschkin's premise was that the repolarization wave of the U wave and the repolarization wave of the P wave combined to depress the ST segment to the line marked "3" in the illustration. For practical purposes, most workers in the field use the line marked "2" as the point of measurement for the evaluation of ST-segment depression. (From Lepeschkin,[9] with permission.)

Upsloping ST Segments

There is no subject in exercise literature that has generated more controversy than the significance of upsloping ST segments. Froelicher,[14] one of the recognized experts in the field taught that the upsloping ST depression did not indicate ischemia until his latest book when he conceded that this pattern was associated with an increased risk of coronary artery disease.

From our material,[15] the upsloping ST segment is considered to indicate ischemia if, at 80 msec after the J point, the segment is 1.5 mm below the baseline level of the PQ junction (Fig. 12–5). Of 70 subjects with these changes who were catheterized in our laboratory, 57% had either two or three-vessel disease. Bruce and Blackman[16] and others[42] concede that upsloping ST segments may be indicative of ischemia. Brody[17] found what he called junctional ST-segment depression of 1.5 mm or more in 756 business executives tested with a double Master's test. Twenty-one percent of these men developed coronary artery disease (CAD). Brody also found that patients with junctional changes from 0.5 to 1.4 mm had a 2.5% occurrence of CAD. This incidence of CAD is similar to that of subjects with completely normal exercise tracings. Kurita and Chaitman[18] also found a strong correlation between angiographically demonstrated stenosis and Upsloping ST changes

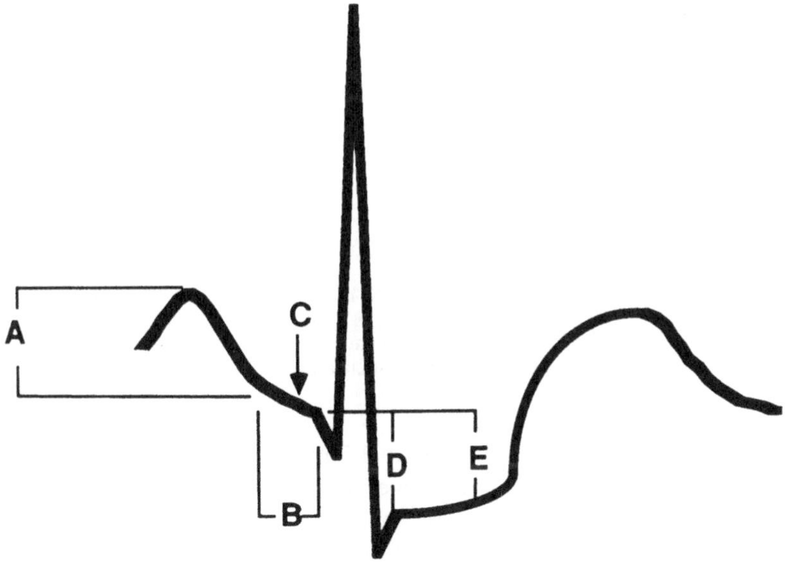

FIGURE 12–3. ST depression due to the Ta wave. Sapin and colleagues[6] believe that the slope of the PQ segment (C) can predict how much the Ta wave will suppress the ST segment. The magnitude of the P voltage (A) may determine the magnitude of the ST depression (D, E). PQ slope is measured during the interval designated as B.

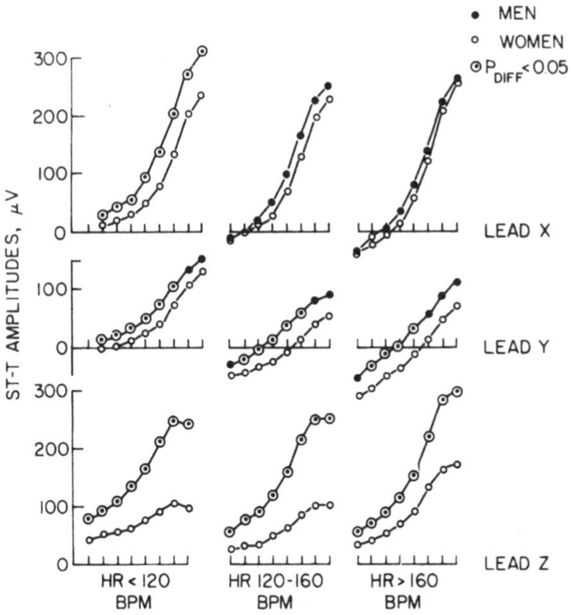

FIGURE 12–4. Variations in measurements of the ST segment, divided into eight equidistant points between Q and peak T wave, in normal men and women. Note that the deviations, even at high heart rates, are less pronounced in lead X than in other leads, as are the differences between men and women. (From Blomqvist,12 with permission.)

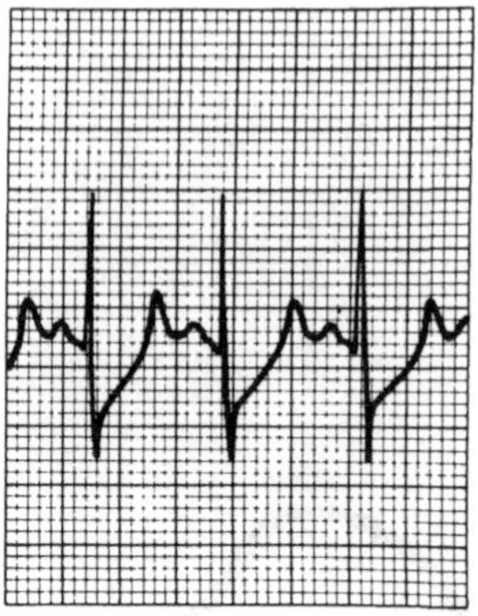

FIGURE 12–5. The upsloping ST segment depicted here is at an angle of 508. Although some would label this J-point depression, we have called this "upsloping ST segment," and it is usually associated with ischemia.

when the depression was greater than 1.5 mm at 80 msec after the J-point. Goldschlager and associates,[19] however, found the Upsloping pattern to be somewhat less sensitive than horizontal or Downsloping patterns, and Froelicher and colleagues[14] until recently maintained that only horizontal or Downsloping patterns indicate ischemia.

The evidence demonstrates that upsloping ST-segment changes should be considered abnormal when the degree of depression at 80 msec from the

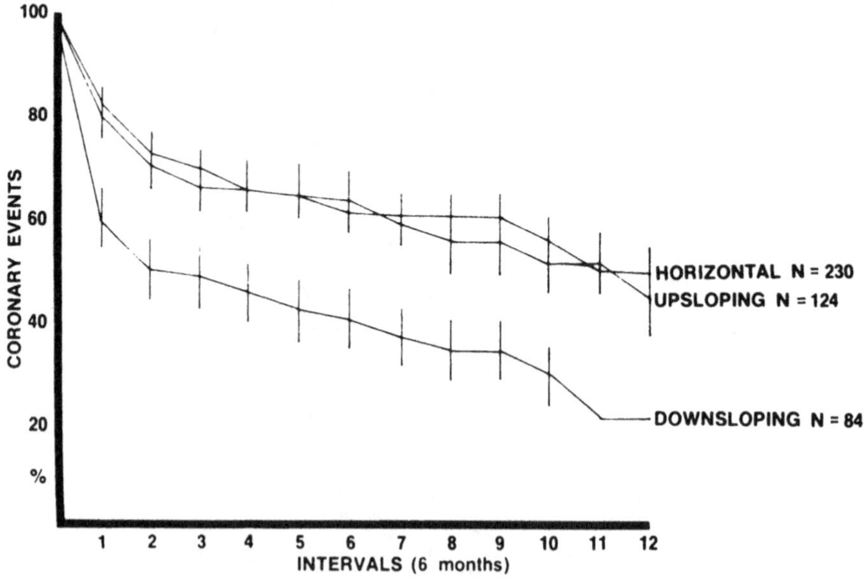

FIGURE 12–6. Life table analysis of new coronary events (progression of angina, myocardial infarctions, and death) in patients manifesting horizontal, upsloping, and downsloping ST-segment depression with exercise. The incidence of coronary events in patients with upsloping ST-segment depression is the same as in those with horizontal ST-segment depression. Those with downsloping ST-segment depression have a higher incidence of events.

J-point is down 1.5 mm or more. Figure 12–6 illustrates that the frequency of new coronary events on follow-up in patients with upsloping ST segments is the same as in those with flat ST segments. On the other hand, junctional changes with very steep upsloping ST segments are probably not pathological.

Bruce and colleagues[11] have claimed that J-point and ST-segment changes in normal subjects can be in some cases a normal result of exercise. Observing Blomquist's Figure 12–4 will help to distinguish the abnormal from the normal.[12]

TAKE-HOME MESSAGE

Slowly Upsloping ST depression usually indicates ischemia.

Horizontal versus Downsloping ST Segments

It is ironic that 70 years after the significance of depressed ST segments was first recognized, the criteria for identification of these changes are still not totally agreed upon. The physiological basis for the observed ECG abnormalities is complex and may be multifactorial. One reason for so much confusion is that investigators have attempted to correlate ST-segment depression with the degree of anatomical CAD. The electrical changes in the muscle producing abnormalities in the ECGs are obviously the result of many influences, including those caused by electrolytes, hormones, and hemodynamic and metabolic, as well as anatomical, changes (see Chapter 3).

The magnitude of the stenosis in an artery, estimated by angiography, may not accurately predict the amount of restriction in flow, especially when spasm may be induced by exercise. There has been general agreement, however, that an increased magnitude of ST-segment depression usually denotes an increased degree of ischemia. Robb and associates[15] reported this from their follow-up studies of subjects using the Master's protocol. Recent work, however, has challenged this concept. We and others[20,21] have been unable to correlate the ischemia estimated from the magnitude of the ST-segment depression in any lead or from the sum of the ST changes in all leads with either the number of diseased coronary arteries or the size of the area of reversible ischemia observed on the thallium scintigram. This disagrees, however, with our survival data[22] and with Ekelund,[23] who reported almost a threefold increase in cardiac events in patients with the so-called strongly positive exercise test (ST depression of 2 mm or more).[24]

In the early days of our stress testing program, we were most anxious not to affix a diagnosis of CAD to a healthy person, so we selected 2.0 mm of depression with a horizontal or downsloping ST segment as the only definite criterion for an abnormal finding. Careful follow-up of our patients has convinced us that we were being too stringent. Our criteria were later modified to accept 1.5 mm of depression at 0.08 second from the J-point even if the ST

Table 12–1. **ST Measurements 50 to 59 msec After Nadir of S Wave**

HR	Normal	Abnormal
75	+0.5	+0.5
100	0.0	−0.25
125	−0.5	−1.0
150	−0.7	−1.5
175	−1.0	−2.0
	N=48	N=22
	−0.4 ± 0.52	−1.36 ± 0.52

segment slopes upward. I believe that 1.0 mm is probably the best available minimum level to use in horizontal ST-segment changes (Table 12–1). The problem of marginal or equivocal findings can sometimes be resolved by urging the patient to exercise a little longer and therefore increase the metabolic load on the heart. This often causes apparently equivocal tracings to evolve into a diagnostic pattern.

If ST-segment depression of 0.5 to 1.0 mm is accepted as abnormal, as recommended by Master and Jaffe,[25] the number of false-positive tests will increase but the number of false-negative tests will decrease. Examination of our follow-up data revealed that the increased incidence of coronary abnormalities in our tests rated equivocal (ST-segment depression of 0.5 to 1.4 mm) indicated that a significant number of patients with CAD or decreased ventricular function were included in this group (Fig. 12–7). Mason and associates,[26] in a study of correlation with coronary angiography, found that the

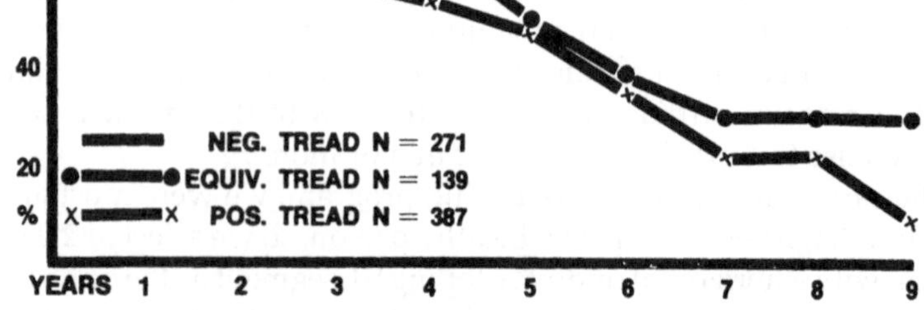

FIGURE 12–7. The incidence of coronary events in patients with equivocal ST-segment depression (0.5–1.4 mm marked "52") is so close to that of patients with positive test results that it must be assumed that many of them have CAD.

sensitivity when using 0.5 mm ST-segment depression was 83% and the specificity was 60%. On the other hand, when 1.5 mm was used, the sensitivity dropped to 44%, but the specificity rose to 90%. (See "Sensitivity" and "Specificity", Chapter 14.) Martin and McConahay[27] found that using 1.0 mm of depression in correlation with angiographically demonstrated narrowing of 50% or more yielded a specificity of 89% and a sensitivity of 62%. Also, in the series by Mason and colleagues,[26] reducing the depression of the ST segment to 0.5 mm increased the sensitivity to 84% but decreased the specificity to 57%. They found that the ST segments alone at maximum exercise levels correlated best with an increased left-ventricular filling pressure in 90% of patients. In our laboratory, we have measured ST-segment depression as illustrated in Figure 12–8.

Downsloping ST Segments

The long term follow up information suggests that patients who's ST depression evolves to downsloping have more severe disease than those that do not.

Recently Bertella[28] has reported that downsloping ST depression indicates that a larger area of myocardium is involved and that when the subepi-

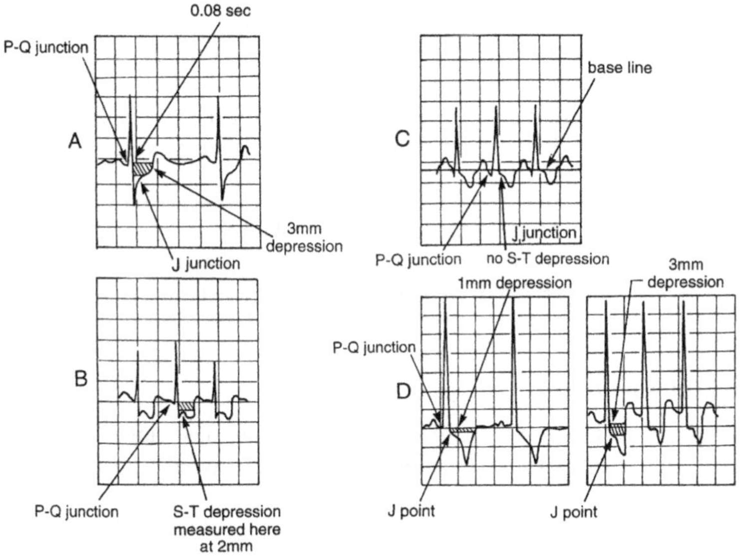

FIGURE 12–8. (A) Horizontal ST-segment depression is measured from a point 0.08 second from the J-point. (B) If the ST segment is convex, the depression is measured from the top of the curve to the level of the PQ junction. (C and D) With downsloping ST segments, the depression is measured at the point where the ST-segment changes slope, which is very close to the point usually called the "J junction."

cardial muscle, as well as the subendocardium is also ischemic, it is usually due to multivessel disease.

He believes that the downsloping pattern in V3 and V4 may be due to the additive effects of anterior wall subendocardial ischemia, superimposed on transmural posterior wall ischemia. We know that anterior transmural ischemia results in ST elevation and would expect transmural posterior wall ischemia would produce a vector in the same direction as the anterior subendocardial ischemia process.

TAKE-HOME MESSAGE
Downsloping ST depression in V3 and V4 probably represents more severe ischemia than horizontal. It may be a marker for multivessel disease.

ST Depression in Recovery Only

Although ST depression during exercise often persists into recovery, it may not manifest until exercise has been terminated. The reasons for this are still not clear but the phenomena have been studied by several investigators. Lacterman[30] reported on 168 subjects with ST depression, 15% of whom only occurred during the recovery. They concluded that it had the same predictive power as exercise ST changes occurring during exercise. Bywik et al,[31] also found that recovery-only ST depression has the same significance as exercise-induced ST changes in healthy volunteers (Figure 12–9).

Our experience has been similar to that published by Lachterman and Fleg, that the ECT changes occurring only during recovery have the same predictive power (85%) as those occurring only during exercise.

TAKE-HOME MESSAGE
ST depression during recovery is as reliable as that occurring during exercise in predicting coronary artery disease.

ST Integral and Slope

The use of computers to record the voltage changes associated with the ECG complex lends itself to measurements that are otherwise laborious. Two that have been used in several centers are the slope of the ST segment in the area subtended by the negative deviation and the integral (Fig. 12–10). Empirical correlations with coronary narrowing have been published.[32]

Most of the measurements of the slope are combined with a measurement of the ST depression in order to predict ischemia, because the slope could be flat when the deflection below the baseline is minimal. This results in a pattern that usually at least looks normal. In 1968, McHenry and col-

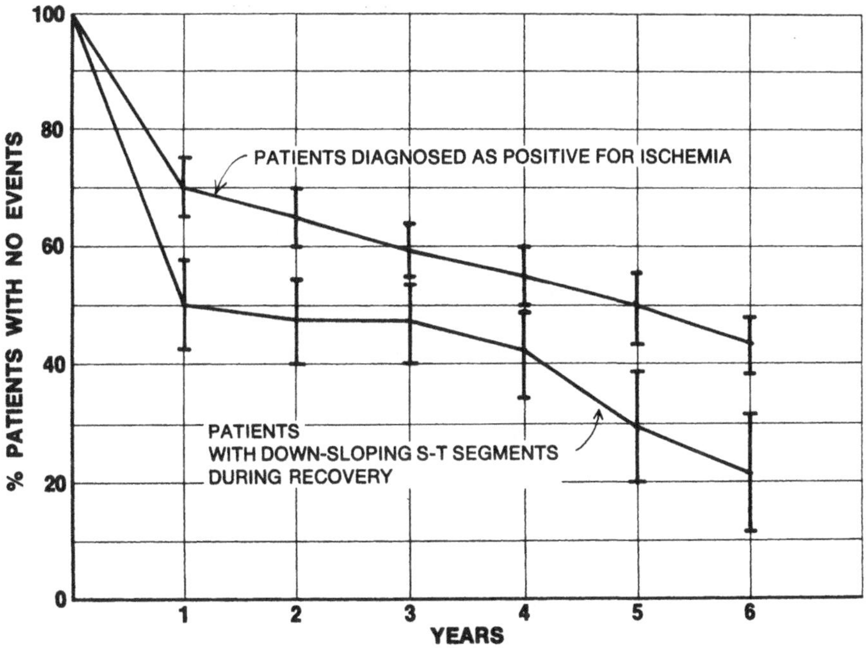

FIGURE 12–9. Incidence of coronary events in patients with ST-segment depression. Those patients who have horizontal or upsloping ST segments immediately after exercise, but which evolve into a downsloping pattern, have a higher prevalence of coronary events than all positive responders as a group.

leagues[32] reported an analysis of the ST interval by combining a computerized slope and ST measurement and indicated its usefulness in analysis of exercise tracings. Shortly afterward, Sheffield and associates[33] reported on both the slope and the integral. Ascoop and coworkers[34] measured the slope during the first 50 msec (0.05 sec) after the J-point and used a slope of no greater than 180 μV/msec as the upper limit for an abnormal value. The sensitivity increased to 70% without much loss in specificity. Forlini and colleagues[35] used the slope and integral, but isolated the integral by extending the slope through the T wave. They reported a sensitivity of 79%, somewhat better than the results previously cited by Ascoop and associates.[34] The calculation of slope and integral is standard on a number of commercially available computerized stress testing systems and seems to improve the analysis of the ST segment, especially when the ST is marginal. One of the best evaluations of the integral was done by Sketch and coworkers,[36] who were able to correlate the integral with severity of disease and found that it improved predictive value.

I believe the ST-integral and slope method shows promise, even though enthusiasm is still limited more than 20 years after the measurements have become technically practical.

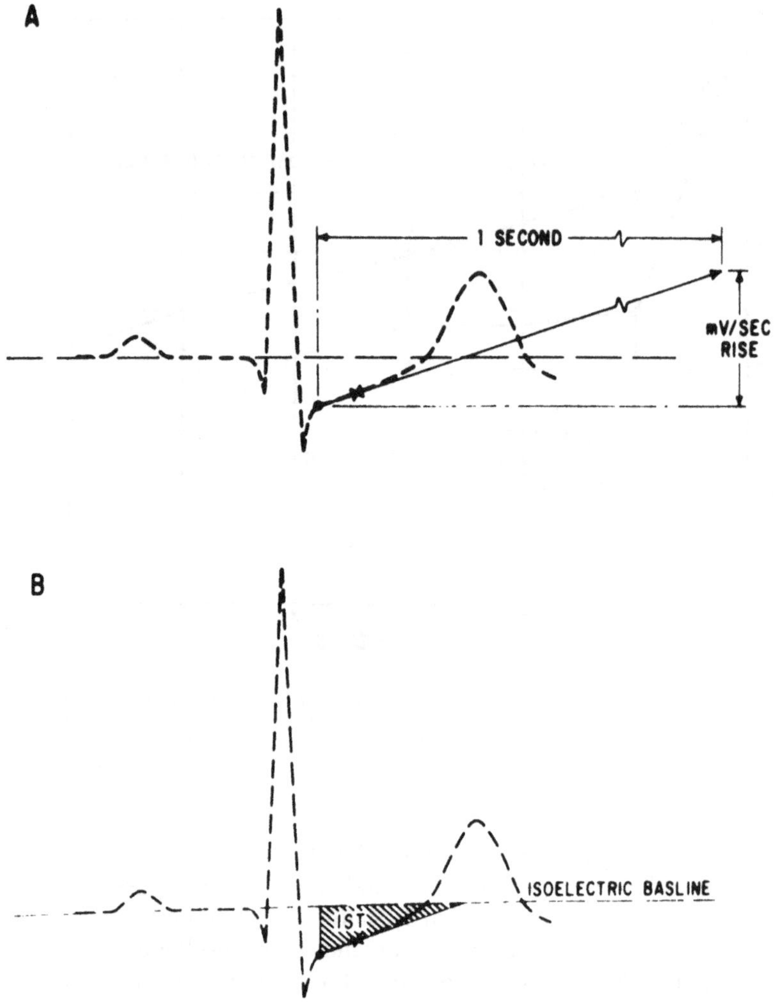

FIGURE 12–10. ST slope and integral. (A) The slope of the ST segment. It is usually measured in millivolts per second, a positive number if upsloping and a negative one if downsloping. (B) The shaded area under the isoelectric line subtended by the ST segment defines the integral. The area will increase as the depression increases and the slope decreases.

Time Course of ST Depression

It has long been recognized (and is logical) that when ST depression comes on early at low workloads, the degree of ischemia is likely to be more severe. In an attempt to analyze the significance of the time of onset of ST depression, we stratified a group of patients according to the onset and offset of ST depression and compared the results with angiographic findings.[37] The var-

Table 12–2. **Distribution of Coronary Disease According to Time Course Type**

Type	0 Vessels	3 Vessels	2 & 3 Vessels	1, 2, & 3 Vessels	MI	Total
0	96 (56%)	16 (9%)	61 (35%)	77 (44%)	21 (12%)	173
1	17 (31%)	15 (27%)	25 (45%)	38 (69%)	5 (9%)	55
2	10 (26%)	13 (33%)	21 (54%)	29 (74%)	6 (16%)	39
3	9 (21%)	21 (50%)	28 (67%)	33 (79%)	8 (19%)	42

MI, Myocardial infarction. From Ellestad et al: The predictive value of the time course of ST segment depression during exercise testing in patients referred for coronary angiograms. Am Heart J 123:906, 1992, with permission.

ious categories are illustrated in Figure 12–11 and the magnitude of their CAD is presented in Table 12–2.

Late Onset, Early Offset

It has long been taught that when ST depression comes on at high workloads but resolves very quickly after exercise, it constitutes a false-positive ST depression; in many centers the test is called negative. We found, however, that significant CAD was more common than not, at least in those who were referred for angiography.

Early Onset, Late Offset

As might be expected, patients with early-onset, late-offset ST depression usually had severe disease.

Resting ST Depression Increased with Exercise

This group was found to have severe disease. It has often been stated that these patients should not be tested because the results would include a large number of false-positives. This might be true if the patients are asymptomatic, but certainly does not pertain to those who have anginal chest pain. This finding has been confirmed by Miranda and associates. [38]

TAKE-HOME MESSAGE

Not *all* patients with rapid resolution of ST depression during recovery have normal coronary arteries.

Magnitude of ST Depression

It is intuitive that the magnitude of ST depression should correlate with the degree of the ischemia. Several reports originally seemed to confirm this finding. Bogaty[39] reported that in patients with left main or left main

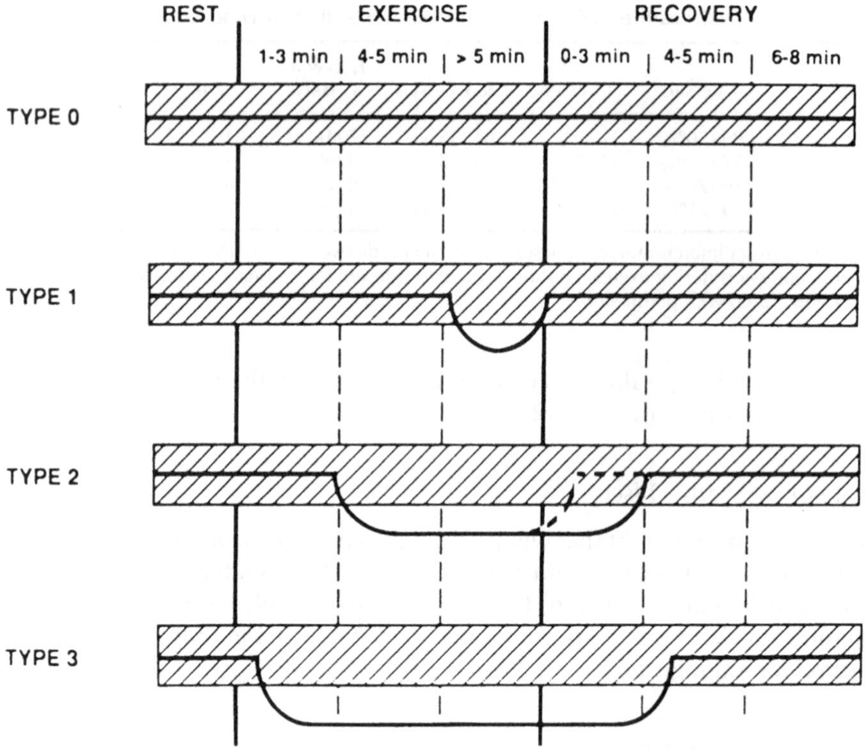

FIGURE 12–11. Time course of ST depression. The dark line in the hatched bar illustrates the ST voltage. When this line goes below the hatched bar, the ST segment is at least 1 mm below baseline. Note the times of the ST measurements above the bar. The various patterns have relevance in the evaluation of the exercise test.

equivalent angiographic changes or with other severe degrees of the ischemia, they found the magnitude of ST depression was greater. It has also been reported that when 2 mm or more of ST depression is present the probability of left main disease increases. On the other hand, we have been unable to confirm this.[40] We found no correlation with the magnitude of ST depression or the number of leads with ST depression and the coronary anatomy. The degree of ST depression at higher workloads depends on what is used for the indication to terminate exercise. If patients are pushed enough, or if they have some degree of left ventricle hypertrophy (LVH) they may have severe ST depression. If patients with single vessel disease are encouraged to exercise strenuously or if they have some degree of LVH, they may have very severe ST depression. Bogaty found that in patients with 2 mm or more of ST depression, survival was determined by the time on the Bruce protocol, not on the magnitude of depression.

> **TAKE-HOME MESSAGE**
> The magnitude of ST depression at maximum workload may not indicate the severity of coronary artery disease. Major ST depression at low workloads indicates severe disease.

Intraobserver Agreement

The analysis of ST-segment depression by a group of 14 experts from 7 medical centers was correlated by Blackburn,[37] who reported that the accuracy of positive responses with undefined criteria varied from 5% to 55% for each physician. Agreement among all 14 observers was obtained on only 7 normal patients and one abnormal patient. The mean estimation of accuracy was only 10.8%. Although agreement was poor in this study, Blackburn believes that it can be improved by following strict criteria.

Hornsten and Bruce[42] analyzed 100 tracings by computer, which identified 0.10 mV (equivalent to 1.0 mm) depression at 40 to 70 msec after the nadir of the S wave. This gave a specificity for true-negatives of 91% and a sensitivity for true-positives of 85% when averaging 20 complexes with the computer; however, transient ischemia was averaged out. The investigators concluded that this degree of depression was the most reliable in predicting ischemia. They also found some degree of ST-segment depression in the so-called normal patients as a result of tachycardia.

Although the criteria previously described are generally useful, especially in men, more and more exceptions are now recognized. Simoons[43] has suggested that the ST be corrected for heart rate, a concept that would fit with the observations of Blomqvist.[12] There is little doubt that a computer can measure changes in voltage better than can be done by visual inspection, but it misidentifies the baseline often enough that it is necessary to check the measurements to ensure their accuracy. As emphasized several times throughout this book, the patient must be considered as a whole, including factors such as age, sex, and blood pressure, as well as other findings.

Distribution of ST Depression

Although it has been recognized for years that lead V4, V5, and V6 are most likely to demonstrate ischemia, they are by no means the only changes of importance. Exercise-induced ischemia may occur in almost any lead and the common tendency to ignore changes in leads other than the lateral precordium should be discouraged. Viik et al[40] from Finland has published an excellent review of the subject and Figure 12–12 summarizes their findings in 201 patients, half of whom had coronary artery disease. One should note they have used a negative AVR so that on the conventional electrocardiogram the ischemic patients have ST elevation. AVR showed the best receiver operating characteristic (ROC) curve of the limb leads and V5 and V6 were

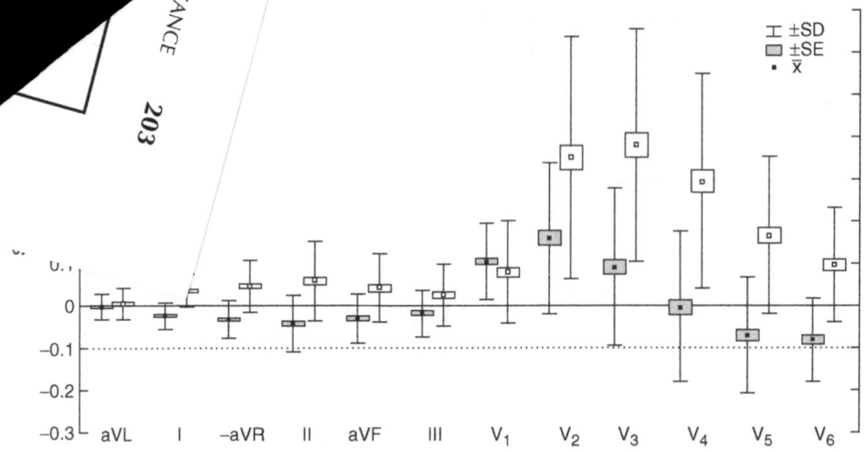

FIGURE 12–12. The mean values of ST segment deviation by lead at peak exercise of 101 coronary artery patients (*shaded symbols* = CAD, *open symbols* = normals). Note that AVR is negative and that ischemia causes ST elevation in V1 to V3 from VIC. (From Viik et al,[44] with permission.)

about the same using chest leads. Their data suggest the best diagnostic group was lead 1, AVR, V4, V5, and V6.

The inferior leads, 2, 3 and AVR, while often positive in ischemia are most likely to be false positive, probably due to the distortion by atrial repolarization.

TAKE-HOME MESSAGE
For the best diagnosis—leads 1, AVR, V4, V5 and V6.

ST ELEVATION

ST Elevation in Leads without Q Waves

ST elevation in leads without Q waves can occur in two very different situations, both of which are fairly uncommon.[45] The first is when patients have a very high-grade proximal LAD stenosis or a high-grade stenosis of a large right coronary artery. We believe that ischemia associated with ST depression is subendocardial, whereas ischemia producing ST elevation is transmural, affecting the full thickness of the heart. It follows that full-thickness ischemia is rare during exercise even with high-grade proximal stenosis.

The second cause of ST elevation is coronary spasm that is so severe that it completely obliterates antegrade flow through epicardial arteries. This has been termed Prinzmetal's angina and is most commonly seen at rest, but very occasionally occurs with exercise.[46] It is common for arrhythmias to accompany this process (Fig. 12–13).

Detry and colleagues[47] have reported ST elevation with exercise in variant angina, as have others.[28,93] It appears that patients with angiographically normal coronary arteries and Prinzmetal's syndrome due to spasm, as described by MacAlpin and colleagues,[48] usually have no change during exercise. If they have CAD, with or without spasm, ST elevation as well as depression may be seen. Exercise-induced ST elevation in a subject with variant angina probably indicates hemodynamically significant coronary atheroma. Belik and Gardin[49] report a case with alternating ST elevation, ST depression, ventricular conduction abnormalities, and U-wave inversion most of the classic signs of ischemia.

Occasionally, we have seen ST depression occur during stress testing and then elevation develop when exercise is continued.

TAKE-HOME MESSAGE

ST elevation in V2, V3, V4 = severe anterior wall ischemia. ST elevation in lead II, III, AVF = severe inferior wall ischemia.

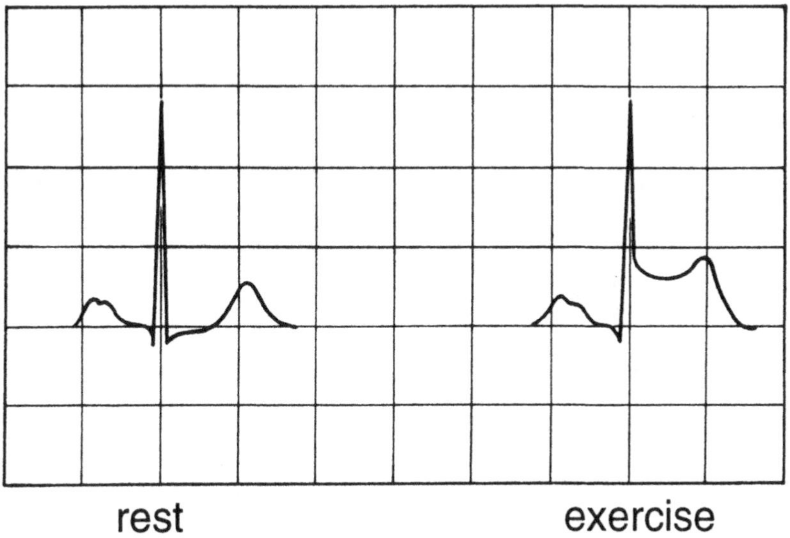

FIGURE 12–13. ST elevation in leads with R waves. When this occurs, very high-grade stenosis can be predicted in the appropriate artery (in the LAD when it occurs in leads V2 to V4, and in the right coronary artery when it occurs in leads III and aVF).

ST Elevation in Leads with Q Waves

When ST-segment elevation occurred during exercise in leads with Q waves, we originally believed that it was due to a ventricular akinetic or dyskinetic segment in most of the cases studied by angiography in our laboratory.[50] There seemed to be an area of scar producing the ST elevation, but it did not make sense that ST elevation, which is experimentally clearly a current of injury, would come from scar tissue in the absence of injured cells. In recent reports, thallium scintigrams in areas of myocardium-producing ST elevation suggest that there is usually an area of ischemic muscle, usually adjacent to the scar.[51,52] Thus, exercise-induced ST elevation in areas of Q waves probably identifies ischemia and may also be a way of identifying hibernating myocardium (Fig. 12–14). Bertella reports that if the QTc shortens 10 m/sec with exercise there is definitely viable myocardium.

ST Elevation at Rest (Early Repolarization)

Although a stable left-ventricular aneurysm may often manifest ST-segment elevation in the precordial leads at rest, some subjects with normal hearts show a degree of elevation in the anterior precordial leads and also frontal leads (Fig. 12–15). This phenomenon, termed early repolarization, is most

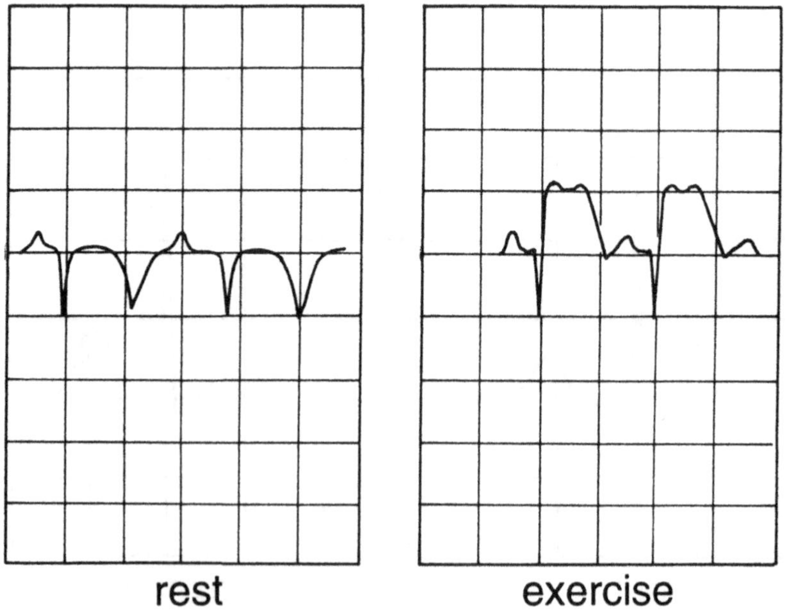

FIGURE 12–14. ST elevation in a patient with a previous infarct. Exercise ST elevation in leads with Q waves was originally believed to be due to a dyskinetic myocardial segment but has recently been shown to indicate peri-infarction ischemia.

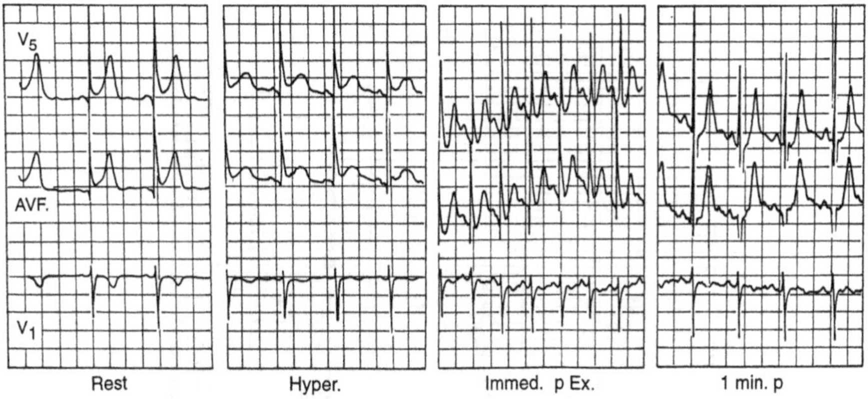

FIGURE 12–15. Note resting ST elevation increased with hyperventilation and resolved with exercise. This is typical of early repolarization.

commonly seen in young black men[53] but is by no means limited to this group. Kambara and Phillips[54] have reviewed this syndrome and report that 26% of affected patients have eventual disappearance of the characteristic findings as they get older. We have found it to be very common in well-conditioned athletes. If this type of ST-segment elevation returns to normal during exercise, it is usually associated with a normal heart. Figure 12–15. When measuring for significant ST depression in these patients, we do not use the resting ST level as baseline, as in those with normal ST segments. Any exercise-induced ST depression seen should be analyzed as if the resting ST were isoelectric. Other reports describing this syndrome have also been published.[53,54] It has been correlated with the degree of aerobic fitness. It has also been compared with the Brugata syndrome, where a similar pattern indicated the likelihood of severe, sometimes lethal, arrhythmias. Excellent reviews of this concept have been recently published.[55,56]

UNCONVENTIONAL ELECTROCARDIOGRAPHIC CHANGES WITH EXERCISE

Lead Strength (ST/R)

When the R wave in the lateral precordial leads is less than 10 mm, the sensitivity of ST depression is very low if 1 mm of ST depression is used as a standard.[57] We have corrected the ST for R-wave amplitude by simply dividing the ST by the R amplitude.[58] When using 0.1 as a cutoff for an abnormal test, the sensitivity is increased markedly, especially in those with R waves less than 10 mm. When applying this method to patients with tall R waves, the specificity is increased but, as might be expected, the sensitiv-

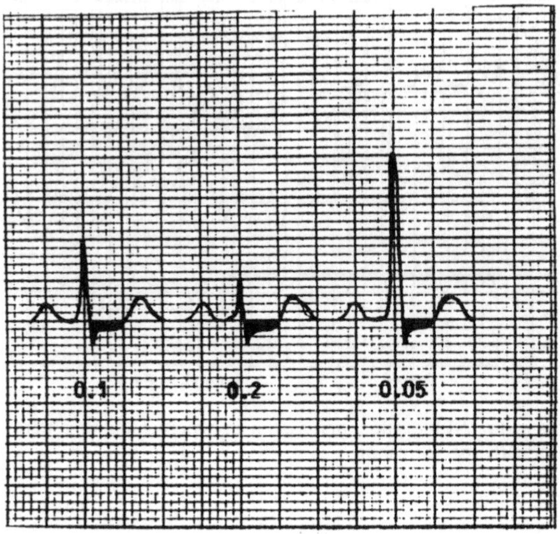

FIGURE 12–16. Lead strength. The complex with a 10-mm R wave illustrates the calculation of the ST/R ratio (1/10 = 0.10). If the R wave is only 5 mm, an ST depression of 1 mm results in a ratio of 0.2. This is equivalent to 2 mm of ST depression in a patient with a 10-mm R wave. When the R wave is 20 mm and the ST depression is 1 mm, the ratio is 0.05, which is nonsignificant for ischemia. (From Ellestad,58 with permission.)

ity is decreased. I believe this type of correction should become standard practice in the future (Fig. 12–16). However, at this point in time it's value is rarely appreciated.

ST-Heart Rate Slope

Correcting ST depression for heart rate seems to be based on sound physiological principles and has been proposed by a number of investigators. Simoons[59] reported on this in 1977, and was followed by Elamin and associates,[60] who reported that he could achieve 100% sensitivity and specificity in the discrimination of CAD and also could separate with perfect accuracy one-vessel, two-vessel, and three-vessel disease. Unfortunately, no one else has been able to confirm his findings. Kligfield et al have done extensive studies using the ST/HR slope and believe it adds a good deal to diagnostic accuracy.[61]

Some of the studies disagreeing with Kligfield et al's work are due to the population studied and the treadmill protocol.[62] I believe that when their methodology is applied according to their guidelines, the calculation of the ST heart rates slope can improve significantly the discrimination of exercise testing in patients with coronary disease. Kligfield et al use a slope of 2.4 microvolts/r/beat minute as a threshold for the presence of ischemia.[61]

ST Heart Rate Index (Kligfield Index)

This index is a byproduct of the studies of ST heart rate slope by Kligfield et al.[61] To calculate the index, the maximum ST depression is divided by the Delta heart rate (difference between resting and maximum heart rate). Because the calculation is very simple and not so dependent on a more gradual protocol, it has a considerable utility. It is important to remember that ST depression should be measured in fractions of a millimeter. When using an index of greater than 1.6 to identify ischemia they report a sensitivity of 90% and a specificity of 95%.

TAKE-HOME MESSAGE

The simple ST heart rate index should be calculated in all exercise tests where there is at least 0.5 mm of ST depression.

ST Evolving Toward Normal with Exercise

Patients with abnormal autonomic drive have demonstrated ST-segment depression after hyperventilation as well as after exercise. In our experience, patients who display ST-segment depression at rest or an increased ST-segment depression after hyperventilation, in whom the depression tends to return to normal with exercise, usually do not have epicardial CAD. Jacobs and coworkers[63] also report that changes associated with hyperventilation are usually associated with normal coronary arteries. Propranolol and other beta blockers have been shown to block the ST changes associated with hyperventilation, suggesting an autonomic etiology.[64,65] The common finding that body position may produce similar changes tends to support this concept. These types of changes are common in patients with mitral prolapse.[66]

Intermittent ST Depression

We have seen several patients who progressed from variable ST-segment depression, often associated with respiration, to the classic ST-segment changes typical of ischemia. We examined a 59-year-old man who had never experienced cardiac symptoms of any type, but who underwent a stress test as a routine screening procedure. Two years after a tracing similar to the one illustrated in Figure 12–17, he had evolved from the variable ST-segment depression into a classic ischemic pattern, but still exhibited moderate variability. Subsequent coronary angiography studies disclosed advanced two-vessel disease. The mechanism of this condition seems to be related to the fact that inspiration and expiration are associated with different rates of left-ventricular filling. If the compliance of the left ventricle is slightly decreased, the increased rates of the filling may produce an elevation in the end-diastolic pressure and therefore ST-segment depression for only a few beats. This is almost always seen near maximum stress levels, when compli-

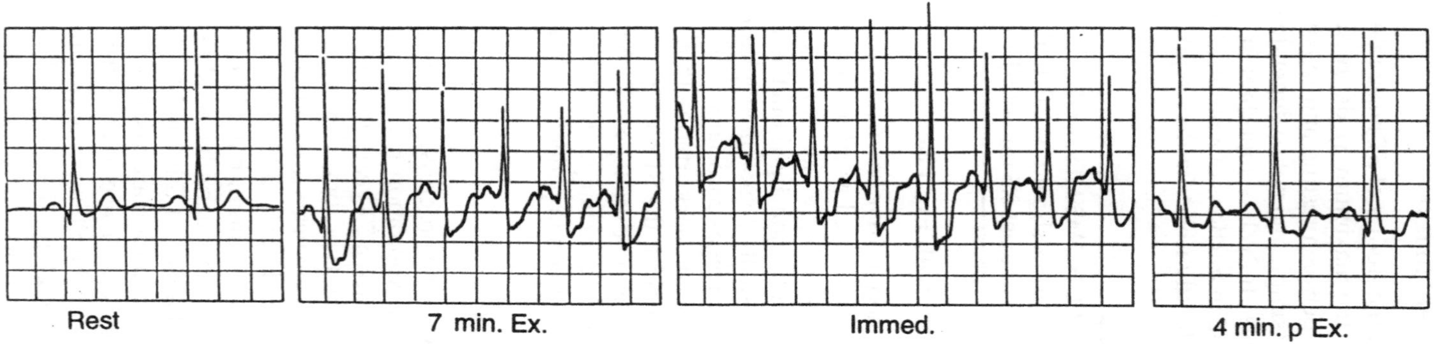

FIGURE 12–17. Exercise-induced variations in R wave and ST segments in a 59-year-old man. The R-wave amplitude and ST-segment depression were related to respiration. Coronary angiography revealed a complete obstruction of the right coronary artery, 90% obstruction of the left anterior descending artery, and

ance of the ventricle would be expected to be decreased the most and when the thoracoabdominal pump would be returning the blood to the heart at the greatest velocity.

In an effort to understand this phenomenon, left-ventricular pressures have been recorded during deep respiratory cycles in subjects with poor left-ventricular function. The left-ventricular end-diastolic pressure (LVEDP) fluctuates and seems to increase near the end of inspiration and decrease late in expiration. The ST-segment depression follows this same pattern, with a drop in ST segments at the same time the LVEDP is rising. The changes described here have never been recorded in patients with completely normal ventricles and are usually seen only in those with some degree of dysfunction. The amplitude of the R waves also increases at the same time that the ST segment is depressed, so that the respiratory pattern is evident both in terms of the increased amplitude of the R waves and in the depth of the ST-segment depression (Fig. 12–18).

ST Depression with Long Diastolic Filling

For the person with a slow heart rate and a long period of diastole after a premature ventricular contraction, the next beat is often associated with ST-segment depression. It is well established that the individual has overfilling

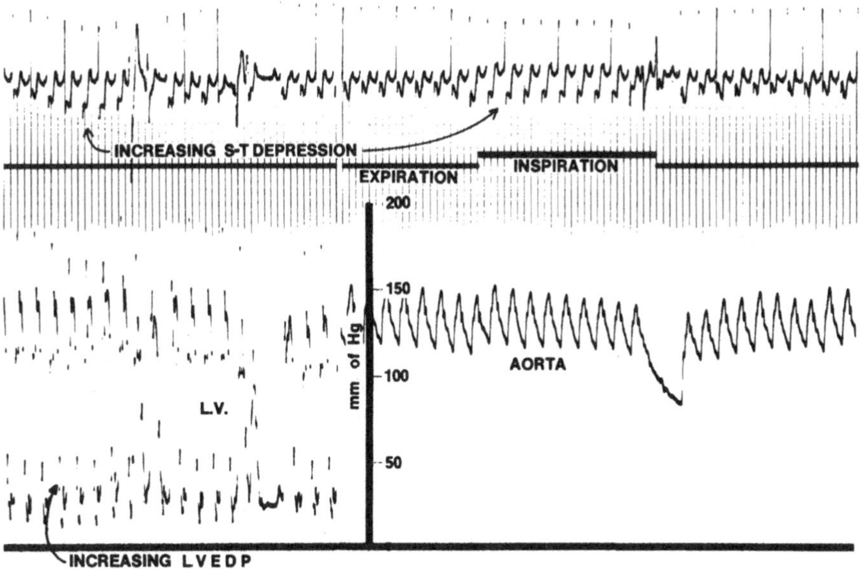

FIGURE 12–18. Recordings taken during a heart catheterization illustrating an increase in the LVEDP and in the amount of ST-segment depression associated with respiration. It can be seen that with inspiration, there is a tendency for the LVEDP to rise and the ST-segment depression to increase.

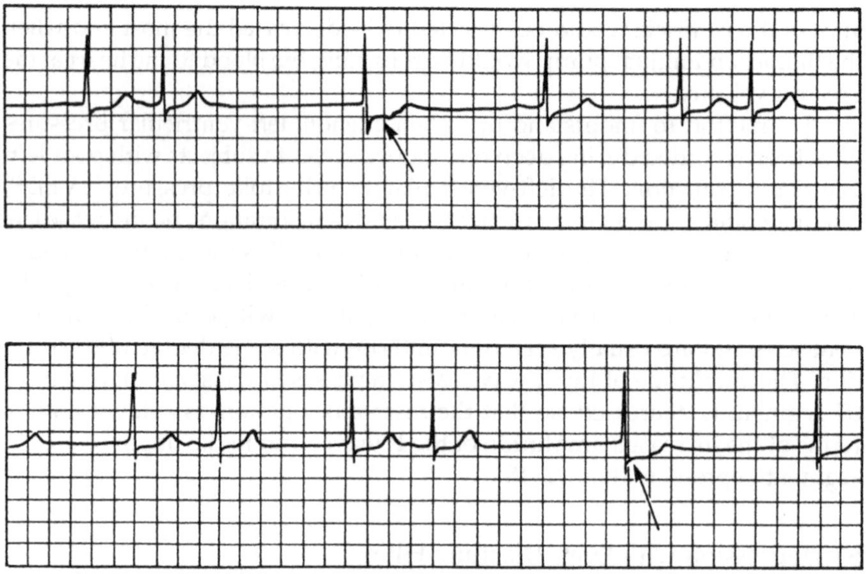

FIGURE 12–19. Tracings recorded shortly after exercise. The complexes marked by the arrow represent a nodal escape with a retrograde P wave. Note the increased ST-segment depression in these complexes.

of the ventricle, and if the compliance is compromised, the increased diastolic pressure may be associated with ST-segment depression.

This is seen repeatedly and correlates well with the diagnosis of clinical ischemia. It is most commonly recorded immediately after the exercise is terminated. This type of ST-segment depression has not been recognized in our laboratory in very young people with sinus arrhythmia or with congenital heart block (Fig. 12–19).

ST Hysteresis (HR Recovery ST Loop)

Although the rate of recovery of ST depression has been recognized as a measure of ischemia severity for many years it remained for Sheffield et al[67] to formalize an approach to quantitative these changes in the analysis of the exercise testing. This was followed by Simoons in 1975[68] and later by Okin et al.[69] When comparing the magnitude of ST depression during recovery according to the time, with that just before termination of exercise, it has little discriminatory power. When recovery ST depression is plotted according to heart rate and compared to ST depression during exercise at similar heart rates, the result becomes more useful. A clockwise plot is common in normals who have ST depression whereas a counterclockwise plot depicts the ischemia. The figure in edition 4 from Bruce plotted ST depression in the opposite direction so that a positive ST loop would be clockwise not counterclockwise (Fig. 12–20). Some of the commercial treadmill systems have automated this function, which is somewhat laborious to do manually. The

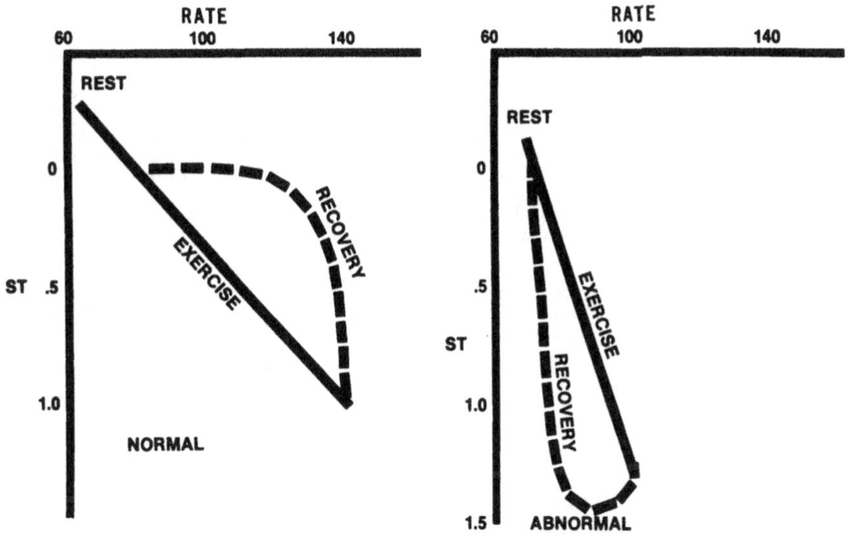

FIGURE 12–20. The heart rate is presented on the abscissa and the magnitude of the ST-segment depression on the ordinate. The normal subject tends to immediately correct the minor ST-segment depression associated with exercise when recovery begins. The abnormal subject may actually increase the ST-segment depression somewhat during the early periods of recovery, even though the heart rate is slowing. (Adapted from Bruce et al.[72])

mechanisms related to post exercise ischemic changes are discussed in detail by Gullestad et al[70] and should be reviewed by those who would like to understand more about this process.[70] Several investigators have reported sensitivity and specificity near 95%.[66] I doubt that in most centers these numbers will be duplicated. This certainly outperforms conventional ST measurements. We have found however that in some patients with abnormal coronary angiograms the ST depression recovers but so rapidly after exercise that it is impractical to construct an ST recovery loop.[69] If these patients are labeled "normal," the sensitivity will be reduced significantly (See Time Course of ST Depression, Fig. 12–20).

Rounded ST Depression

A rounded ST-segment depression pattern in the CM5 lead, as well as in other leads, is common and is often associated with ischemia. Figure 12–21 depicts the ECG of a 48-year-old physician who was experiencing classic anginal pains. Substernal pressure developed during the test, and 1 year later he sustained a myocardial infarction. This pattern is somewhat difficult to evaluate if the duration of the ST-segment sagging is very short, but it usually reflects ventricular dysfunction. Stuart and I[71] found this pattern to be associated with a slightly increased incidence of subsequent coronary events

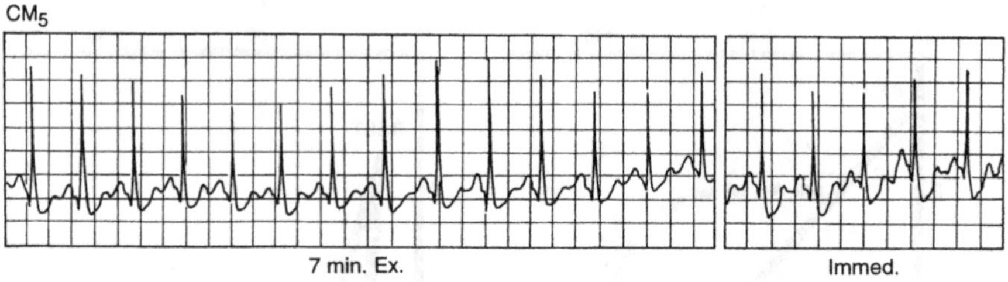

FIGURE 12–21. A tracing taken during and immediately after exercise in a 48-year-old physician who had typical angina and severe two-vessel disease on angiography. Note the rounded ST segments and the variable R-wave amplitude.

in a follow-up study. Patients with a rounded pattern had a 5.8% per year incidence of coronary events, compared with 8.3% per year for those with a horizontal pattern (Fig. 12–21).

ST Depression with Nodal Premature Contractions

ST-segment depression is often associated with the wide complex of a premature ventricular contraction (PVC) or a left bundle branch block (LBBB) pattern. These changes are thought to be secondary to the abnormal conduction pathway and may not be a sign of abnormal left-ventricular function. On the other hand, nodal or atrial premature contractions, when seen in the so-called normal heart, are not usually associated with ST-segment depression.

A number of patients with significant CAD demonstrated by angiography have exhibited ST-segment depression with nodal or atrial extrasystoles during or immediately after exercise. These same patients, when having nodal or atrial extrasystoles at rest, did not have ST-segment depression. As a result, we consider such a finding to be presumptive evidence of ischemic heart disease. Michaelides and associates[73] have reported that ST depression after premature atrial contractions is also useful (see Chapter 13). In Figure 12–22, note that the nodal premature contractions at rest demonstrate only slight ST-segment depression, but during exercise it evolved to at least 3.0 mm. Again this same beat presents almost no ST-segment depression during the recovery period. No significant ST-segment depression is present in either the sinus or the paced beats. It is possible that the degree of muscle relaxation is incomplete, resulting in a decreased compliance even with a shorter diastolic filling period and thus decreased subendocardial perfusion (Fig. 12–22).

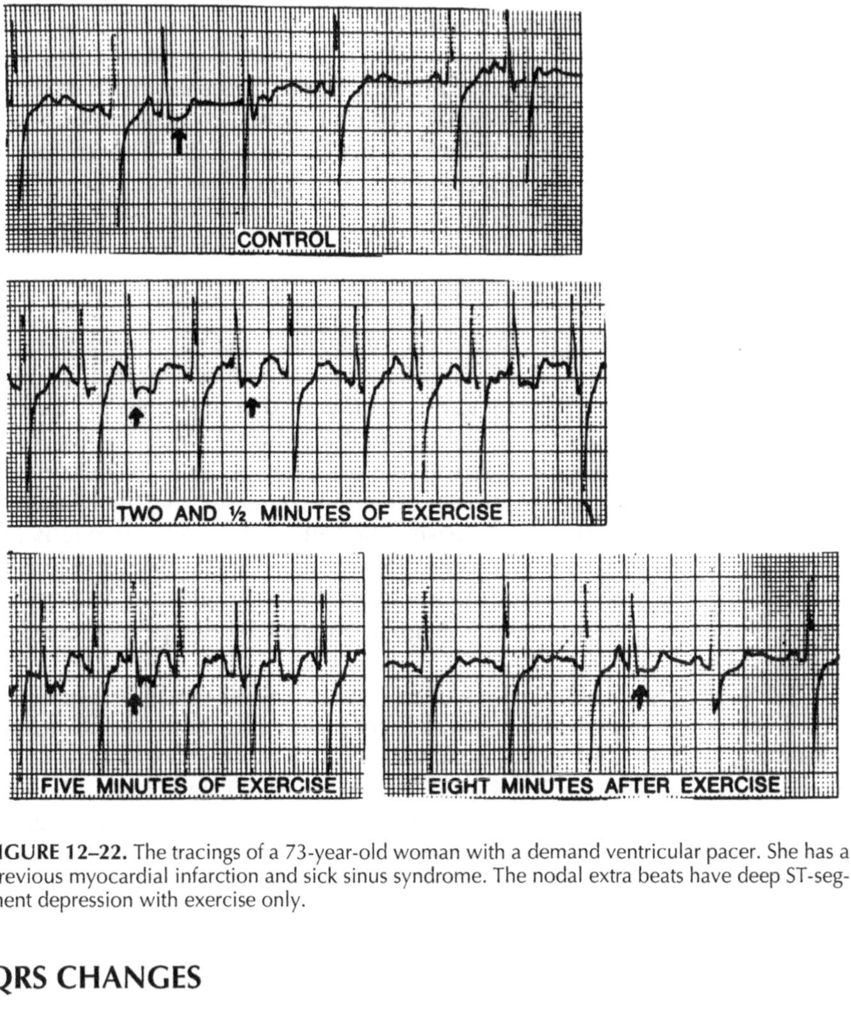

FIGURE 12–22. The tracings of a 73-year-old woman with a demand ventricular pacer. She has a previous myocardial infarction and sick sinus syndrome. The nodal extra beats have deep ST-segment depression with exercise only.

QRS CHANGES

The total amplitude of the QRS complex with exercise usually decreases near peak workload, as does the T-wave amplitude, and there is a tendency toward right-axis deviation. The QRS duration does not change significantly. If the stroke volume increases, the T wave may actually increase, which occurs early in exercise with moderate workloads. A decrease in R wave is more likely to be seen immediately after the exercise period, however, rather than during it. When considering the QRS in the various leads during maximum exercise, there is a tendency toward a reduction in R-wave or S-wave amplitude; this is more marked in normal than in abnormal subjects. The decreased amplitude following a peak exercise period may be due to a decrease in systolic and possibly diastolic volumes,[74] that often develops after peak cardiac output is attained. A study of this phenomenon was done by Brody[75] in 1956, and Pipberger and coworkers,[76] in 1971. The latter investigators have termed this the Brody effect and found that left-ventricular forces decreaseas stroke volume decreases and that right-ventricular forces usually increase at the same time. In ischemia, the systolic volume increases, stroke volume decreases, and the left-ventricular R waves may become taller. This correlates with our experience in the observation of respiratory-related R-wave and ST-segment amplitude changes.

R-Wave Amplitude

The R-wave amplitude in the lateral precordial leads usually decreases more in normal than in abnormal subjects and correlates with left-ventricular function. In our laboratory, Bonoris and coworkers[77] demonstrated the usefulness of observing changes in R-wave amplitude during stress testing. They reported that patients with severe CAD are likely to have an increase in R-wave amplitude with exercise. As exercise progresses and the heart rate increases, R-wave amplitude increases normally until the heart rate is approximately 120 or 130 beats per minute, and then the amplitude begins to decrease. This suggests that for the R wave to have significance, an increase in amplitude should be at a heart rate greater than 120 beats per minute (Fig. 12–23).

Three basic types of patterns were recognized, as shown in Figure 12–24. The changes seen in panel C are more likely to illustrate patients with severe three-vessel disease and global ischemia. Some of these patients have no ST depression or may have a 3 or 4 mm ST depression. We have found the sensitivity of an R-wave increase to be rather poor but the specificity can be good if the patient reaches high heart rates.

The application of R-wave criteria to patients with LBBB was investigated by Orzan and associates,[78] who report that these criteria will not help

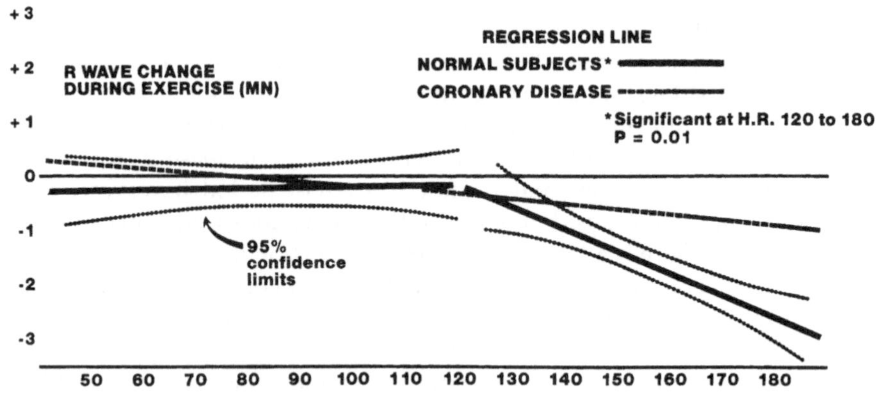

FIGURE 12–23. R-wave responses to exercise.

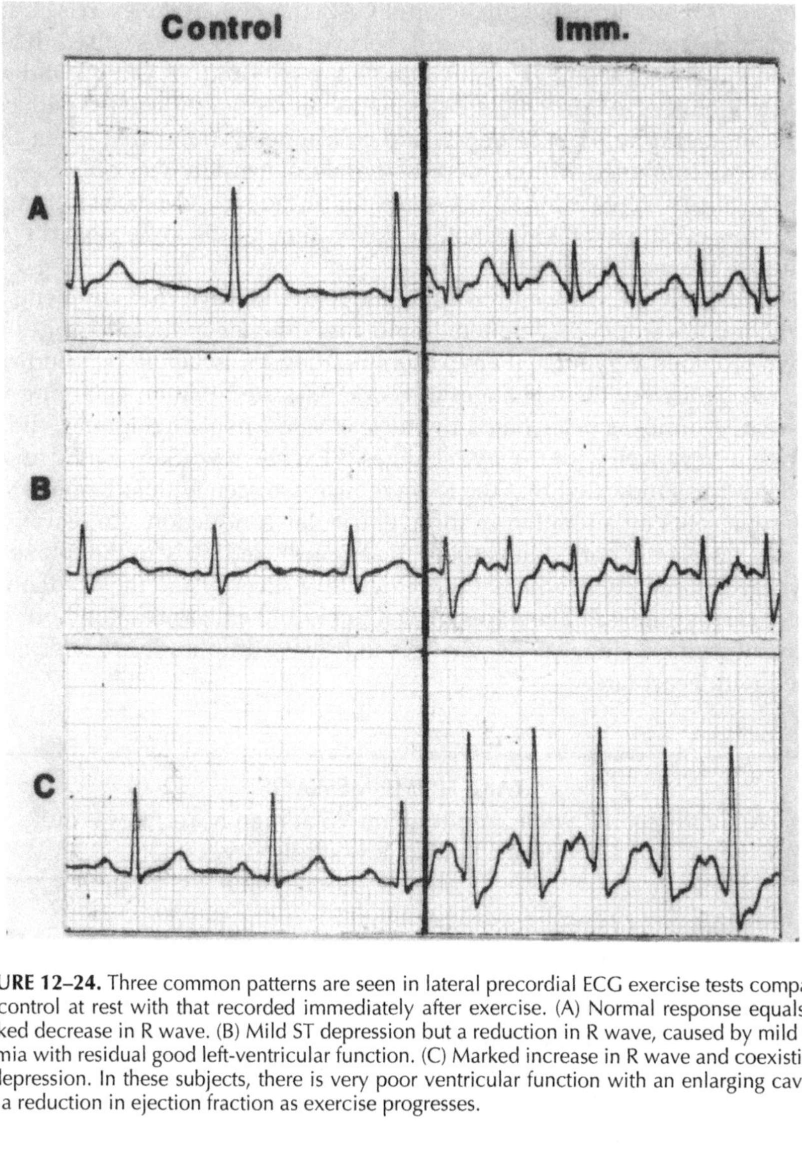

FIGURE 12–24. Three common patterns are seen in lateral precordial ECG exercise tests comparing control at rest with that recorded immediately after exercise. (A) Normal response equals a marked decrease in R wave. (B) Mild ST depression but a reduction in R wave, caused by mild ischemia with residual good left-ventricular function. (C) Marked increase in R wave and coexisting ST depression. In these subjects, there is very poor ventricular function with an enlarging cavity and a reduction in ejection fraction as exercise progresses.

to identify those with CAD compared with those with conduction abnormalities from other causes. On the other hand, Lee and colleagues[79] reported that R-wave changes in 23 patients with LBBB had a 93% sensitivity, 88% specificity, and 93% predictability. Our experience tends to support Lee in that a reduction in amplitude helps to predict normal coronary arteries and good left-ventricular function in LBBB, but we do not find the reliability of a change in amplitude to be nearly as good. Morris and coworkers[80] have determined that the trend in amplitude changes in the first few minutes after exercise is a more reliable predictor of CAD than when the exercise tracing is compared with that of the control. Berman and associates[81] used the sum of the R waves in aVL, aVF, and V3 and V4, plus S and V1 and V2, and were able to identify CAD in 93% of 230 patients subsequently studied with coronary angiography. Van Tellingen and colleagues[82] found that when the R wave was combined with ST depression, the sensitivity was only 51%, but the specificity increased to 93%. R-wave amplitude has also been reported to be useful in patients taking digitalis, given that it fails to be altered by the drug, unlike the ST segment.[83]

Although we were enthusiastic about the R-wave measurements initially, reports from other centers found that exercise-induced changes in R wave provided very little, if any, discrimination for ischemia.[84,85] Studies on the mechanism of these changes also demonstrated that an enlarging ventricular volume, as determined by nuclear blood pool angiograms, did not correlate very well with R-wave changes.[86] Excellent work by David and associates[87] has indicated that the R-wave increase seen with ischemia probably represents an alteration in intraventricular conduction. An R-wave increase has been reported in vasospastic angina[88] and early in the course of a myocardial infarction, where it is predictive of severity and the likelihood of severe arrhythmias.[89] The paper by DeCaprio and colleagues[90] and our subsequent studies[91] suggest that changes in R-wave amplitude are often correlated with heart rate.

TAKE-HOME MESSAGE

An increase in R wave amplitude in V5 at high heart rates is quite specific but has low sensitivity.

Decreased R + ST Depression

In an effort to reevaluate R wave changes Cheng-Le reported that when ST depression occurs in the lateral precordial leads in conjunction with R wave decrease the identification of ischemia can be improved.[92] Using a cut off of 0.5 mm of ST depression and a reduction in R wave amplitude of 1 mm "the sensitivity was 76 and the specificity was 83%." He also reported that the combination held up in patients with hypertension who did not have LVH.

Increased R Wave with Atrial Extra Systoles

Michaelides,[88] an outstanding expert in exercise testing has reported that in patients who were not ischemic, the R wave amplitude of the atrial premature contractions is the same as the regular beat. When the patient is ischemic the R wave of the etopic beat is taller (See Chapter 13).

Increased QRS Duration

The duration of the QRS is usually reduced slightly during exercise because catecholamines increase conduction velocity in the Purkinje fibers and through ventricular muscle.[13] A number of studies have shown that ischemia decreases conduction velocity[14,15]; thus, we should be able to use this in diagnosis. Efforts by us and by others[15] to detect this phenomenon have had mixed results, although we have seen occasional examples in which severe global ischemia has been associated with a clear-cut increase in the duration of the QRS without developing a classic bundle branch block pattern. Michaelides and coworkers[94] recently reported QRS prolongation in exercise ischemia measured in V5 by using a 50 mm paper speed. They analyzed 330 patients with coronary angiograms and exercise tests and found QRS duration prolonged by exercise in CAD patients. The greatest prolongation was found in those with three-vessel disease. Variations around the mean value were so large that the investigators made no attempt to use it in individuals to diagnose the presence or absence of ischemia. As automated computer programs are developed to measure QRS duration I would expect that it may become more useful clinically. Takaki, using a computerized analysis of QRS duration found that exercise induced increase was diminished after PTCA.[95]

ATHENS Score

Changes in R waves, S waves, and Q waves have all shown some usefulness, but each is a weak predictor of CAD. Therefore Michaelides and colleagues[96] have proposed an index or score to combine these factors. By combining the amplitude changes of the three waves in the formula:

$$\text{mm} = (\text{DR-DG-DS})\ \text{aVF} + (\text{DR-DQ-DS})\text{V5}$$

and using a cutoff of less than 5 mm, they were able to obtain a sensitivity of 75% and a specificity of 73% (Fig. 12–25). This was better than using ST depression alone. We attempted to confirm their work and found it to have diagnostic power similar to, but not superior to, ST depression.[97]

Changes in QRS Axis

As exercise progresses in normal subjects the QRS Axis rotates to the right. When patients have single significant LAD narrowing, exercise results in a leftward rotation of the frontal axis. Patients with single vessel right coronary artery disease rotate to the right and thus are indistinguishable from normals.

> **TAKE-HOME MESSAGE**
> When exercise causes the frontal plane axis to rotate to the left the patients is usually ischemic. Usually due to LAD disease.

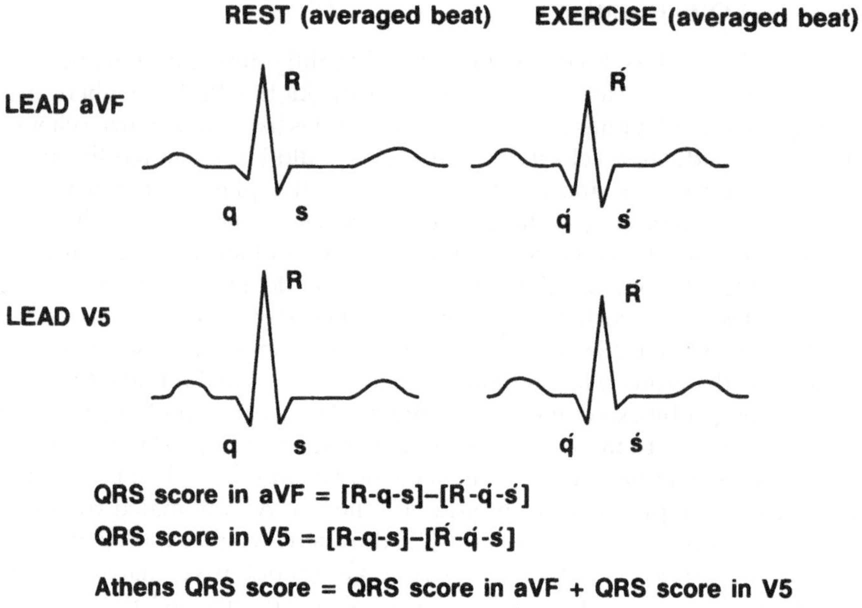

FIGURE 12–25. Calculations for the Athens QRS Score. In aVF, the Q and S amplitude are subtracted from the R, and the same measurements during exercise are subtracted from the resting tracing. This value is then added to the same measurements taken from V_5.

Changes in S Waves

Glazier and colleagues[98] reported that the S wave increased with ischemia, especially when patients also had ST-segment depression. They also found an S-wave increase in normals and in ischemic patients occasionally in the absence of ST depression. The investigators thought the finding might be useful but had a poor specificity. Michaelides and colleagues[99] reported a prolonged S wave with exercise in patients with left anterior descending (LAD) lesions, especially if they also had anterior hemiblock and right bundle branch block.

Q WAVE AND QT INTERVALS

QX/QT Ratio

The concept of measuring the QX/QT ratio was introduced by Lepeschkin and Surawicz[100] as a method of evaluating ST-segment depression to separate moderate J-point changes from true ischemic abnormalities (Fig. 12–26). The assumption was that the ST-segment depression due to ischemia would persist longer than that associated with tachycardia or changes in the ventricular gradient. It was proposed that a QX/QT ratio of 50% or more would be a relatively reliable point of differentiation. They reported, however, that the QX/QT was greater than 50% in 13% of their normal control subjects. This was later studied by other authors, including Roman and Bellet,[101] who reported on 150 supposedly normal subjects. They found that 61% had a negative test by the QX/QT criterion, but that the remainder would have been classified as abnormal. Their conclusion was that this measurement was not valid in determining the presence or absence of ischemic heart disease. Master and Rosenfelt[102] and Robb and Marks[15] supported their position. Our study of QX/QT led us to believe that it is a weak predictor of disease (see Fig. 12–26).[102]

Septal Q Waves

For a number of years, we had noted an increase in septal Q waves in normals and a lack of this response in subjects with significant ischemic ST depression. Remembering the work of Burch and DePasquale[103] on the loss of septal Q waves in the resting ECG, we postulated that the disappearance was due to the loss of contractility secondary to ischemia. Morales-Ballejo and associates,[99] working in our laboratory, correlated this change with angiographic findings. Since then, we have shown a high correlation with LAD disease when the septal Q waves decrease. Our work has been confirmed by O'Hara and colleagues.[105] Although Q waves in the anterior precordial leads are often missing, when they are present, they may aid in the differentiation between true-positive and false-positive ECGs. When ST depression is associated with an enlarging septal Q, it is rarely due to ischemia, or at least not due to LAD narrowing (Fig. 12–27).

QT Dispersion

QT dispersion is the difference between the QT interval measured from one part of the heart and the QT interval measured from another part of the heart. The QT interval must be measured in each lead, corrected for heart rate, and compared with all the other leads. The difference between the longest QT and the shortest is the dispersion. QT dispersion has been studied extensively in patients with myocardial injury and has been found to correlate

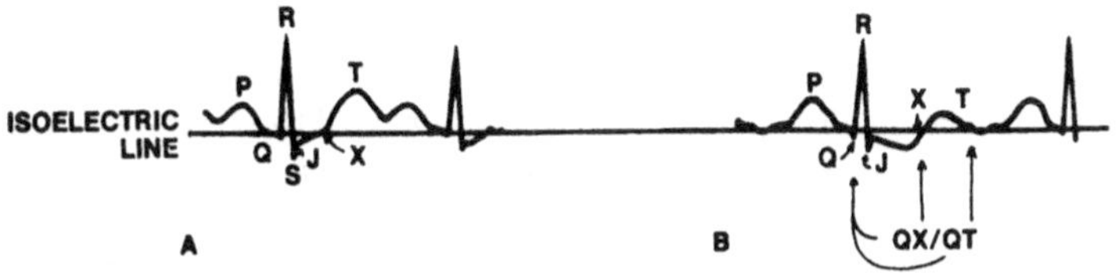

FIGURE 12–26. When the QX interval exceeds 50% of the QT interval, it has been inferred that ischemia is present.

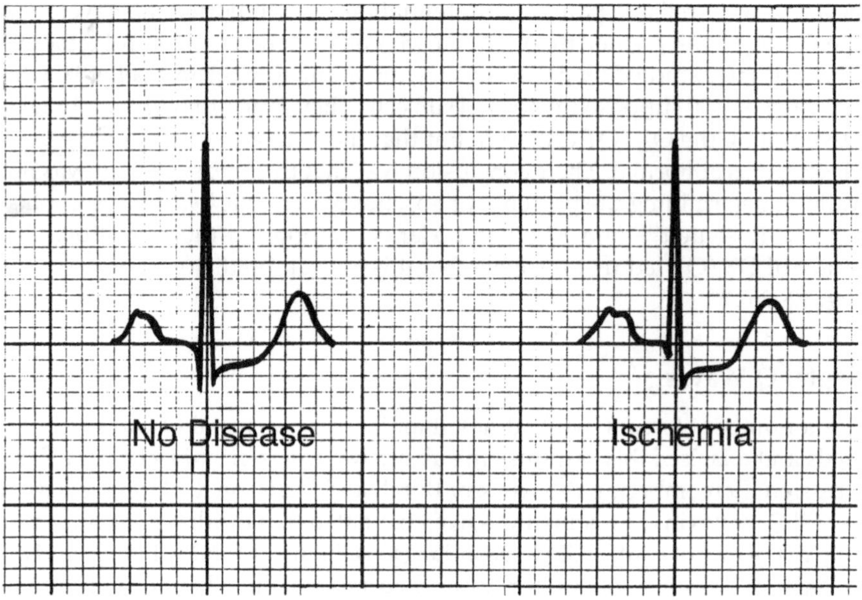

FIGURE 12–27. Septal Q waves: When ST-segment depression occurs in conjunction with a deep septal Q wave, it usually does not indicate CAD. When ischemia is present, the septal Q wave gets shorter than at rest or disappears altogether.

with the risk of serious ventricular arrhythmias[106,107] and has also been measured before and after exercise.[107] Patients who have the maximum QT dispersion increase with exercise are more likely to have ischemia. We have found that when an increase in QT dispersion of greater than 20 msec is combined with ST depression, the specificity is 87%. The measurements necessary to calculate dispersion however are tedious and time consuming. Aufderheide[108] recently reported on an automated method to measure dispersion. If this proves to be accurate and commonly available it may add to the parameters available to identify ischemia.

Prolonged QT

In the early 1950s, Yu and coworkers,[109] studied QT intervals and their relationship to ischemia. They found a definite prolongation in corrected QT intervals (QT_c) in patients with ischemic and hypertensive heart disease. They also correlated the prolongation with the severity of the disease as measured by the patient's endurance and the presence of ST-segment depression. The QT interval correlates well with the carotid ejection time, which is also prolonged when patients with ischemic disease exercise (see Chapter 8). The interest in the analysis of the QT interval and its association with ischemia has diminished partly because it is difficult to measure accurately. As the rate in-

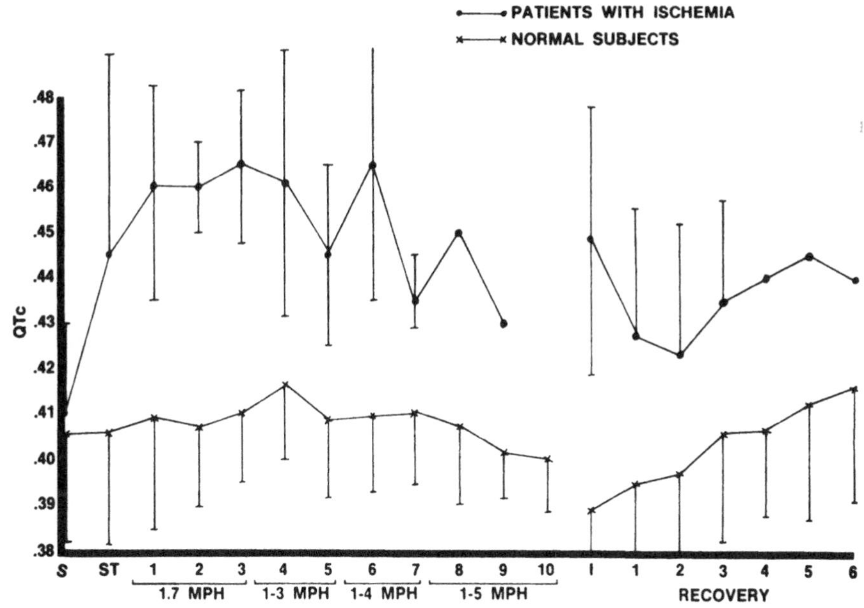

FIGURE 12–28. The corrected QT interval plotted for each minute of our exercise protocol in 10 normal subjects and 6 abnormal subjects with classic ischemic changes. Note that in the patients with ischemia, the QT interval tends to become prolonged quickly early in exercise as compared with the normal subjects.

creases, the T wave merges with the U wave and then finally with the P wave. Thus, the end of the T wave can be recognized only as a notch between the T wave and the P wave. Nevertheless, changes in the QT interval are often significant, and more research needs to be done on the subject .

The data in Figure 12–28 were assembled several years ago from a small group of patients with severe ST depression and suggest that there might be useful information in the QT interval. We studied the QT intervals, along with ST segments, R-wave changes, and QX/QT ratios, in 74 patients who had both stress tests and coronary angiograms.[111] The QT_c was found to be most useful in patients who have an upsloping ST pattern, but it was a weak predictor when used alone.

The most common method used to correct the QT interval for changes in heart rate is to use Bezett's formula.

$$QTC = QT \text{ msec } \sqrt{QT/60}.$$

Bertella has studied the response of the QT interval in a number of patients' subsets and reports that in patients with a resting ST segment elevation the QT_c duration will decrease if there is ischemic but viable myocardium in the region of the old infarction scar.[112] When this occurs he believes that it is because the ischemic epicardial cells activate potassium ATP channels. There is evidence that when ischemia is primarily subendocardial the QT interval will get longer and when the ischemia is transmural the QT will reduce because the subepicardial cells are involved.[113]

Congenital Long QT Syndrome

When a relatively young person has an unexplained syncope and a family history of unexplained sudden death, one should think of a congenital long QT syndrome.[114] If the QT is marginal the exercise test will frequently result in a marked prolongation that provides strong evidence that the patient has this rare but life-threatening anomaly. Along with prolongation of the QT (greater than 450 milliseconds), variations in T wave morphology and T wave alternans are often seen during exercise. These changes have been shown to be due to alterations in genes encoding cardiac ion channels. Treatment with beta blockers has been shown to minimize the tendency for exercise to prolong the QT and prevent the malignant ventricular tachycardia[115] (See Chapter 13.)

T WAVE ALTERATIONS

Normalization of Inverted T Waves

In patients with flat or inverted T waves at rest, the evolution to an upright T wave has been considered by some to be a sign of ischemia. This phenomenon has been labeled by some researchers as "pseudonormalization" of the T waves.[116] Bellet and colleagues[116] reported this evolution in patients with clear-cut angina and considered it to indicate ischemia. As mentioned with regard to tall T waves, however, this may be owing to changes in the potassium balance in the body or to other factors that are as yet poorly elucidated. Noble and colleagues[117] studied 38 patients with angiographically demonstrated ischemia and inverted T waves at rest. They found that angina that was exercise-induced or caused by intravenous isoproterenol caused the T wave to revert to upright in most cases. Aravindaksham and associates,[118] however, compared the T-wave response in both ischemic patients and asymptomatic subjects with primary R-wave abnormalities. They showed that 27% of those with ischemic heart disease had all T waves revert to normal with exercise, whereas 57% of those without disease reverted to normal. They excluded subjects with R-wave inversion due to hypertrophy, LBBB, and drugs, but included in their ischemic group those with a previous infarction. They found that complete T-wave normalization was associated with significant ST-segment depression in 90% of ischemic patients, and with a negative test in all patients without ischemic heart disease.

Many patients with inverted T waves on the basis of metabolic abnormalities will manifest upright T waves at the time of exercise. This is partic-

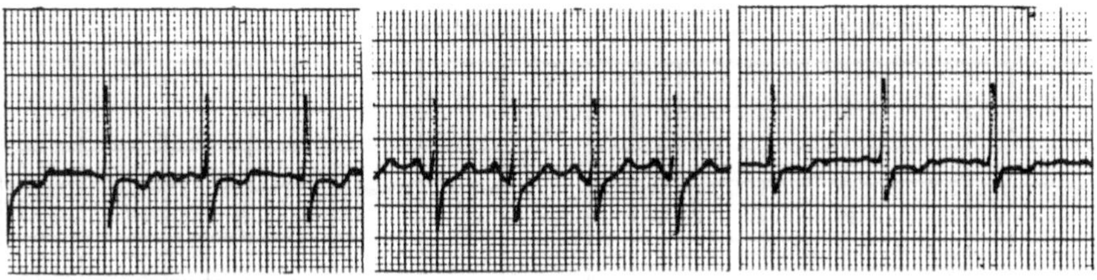

FIGURE 12–29. A 32-year-old asymptomatic woman with normal exercise tolerance whose inverted T waves became upright with exercise. History and physical examination failed to reveal any evidence of cardiac abnormality.

ularly true in women. Figure 12–29 is an ECG of a patient with no coronary symptoms and came in for a screening test. In our experience, this finding does not usually indicate ischemia. On the other hand, ischemia associated with coronary spasm has been shown to cause inverted T waves to become upright. When the patient is not exercising, this type of change has considerable significance.

Peaked T Waves

In our experience an exercise-induced increase of T wave amplitude in V2 is quite predictive of anterior wall ischemia. (specificity = 95%). It appears that this may be a form fruste of ST elevation in the same lead, which is believed to be due to transmural ischemia[119] (Fig. 12–30).[115]

Deep T Wave Inversions

T wave inversion induced by exercise is almost always associated with significant ST segment depression and has long been identified with a more severe degree of coronary disease. An excellent report by Chikamore[120] confirms previous reports that it is usually associated with 3-vessel disease and has been reported to have a specificity of 96%.

Tall T Waves

Scherf[121] and Scherf and Schoffer[122] have reported that tall T waves during or after exercise indicate inferior wall ischemia. From our experience, this is unusual. We have found that tall T waves in the lateral precordial leads after exercise are a normal result of an increased stroke volume and are usually seen in subjects with a normal myocardium. Figure 12–31 illustrates the test of a 23-year-old man with congenital heart block. Because he was unable to increase his heart rate as much as is normal, it has to be assumed that his

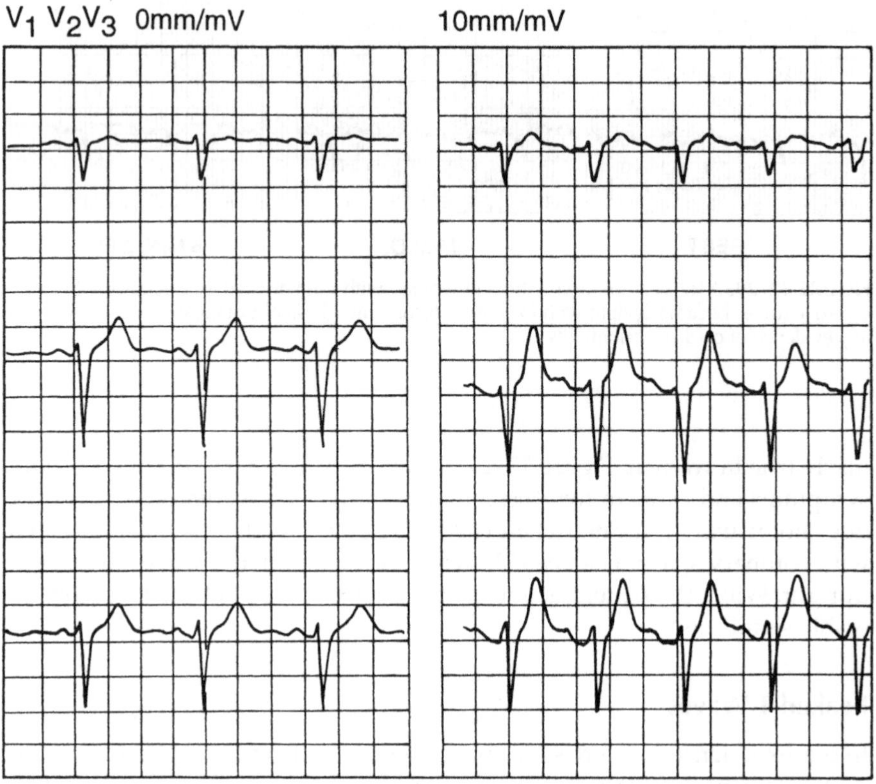

FIGURE 12–30. Leads V_1, V_2, and V_3 on left at rest and on right immediately after exercise. The increase in amplitude of the T wave is associated with proximal LAD disease.

stroke volume became larger to meet the increasing metabolic demands. The progressively increasing height of the T waves appears to correlate with the increasing stroke volume. This phenomenon is seen in many healthy teenage boys immediately after the exercise period. At this time, the pulse drops very

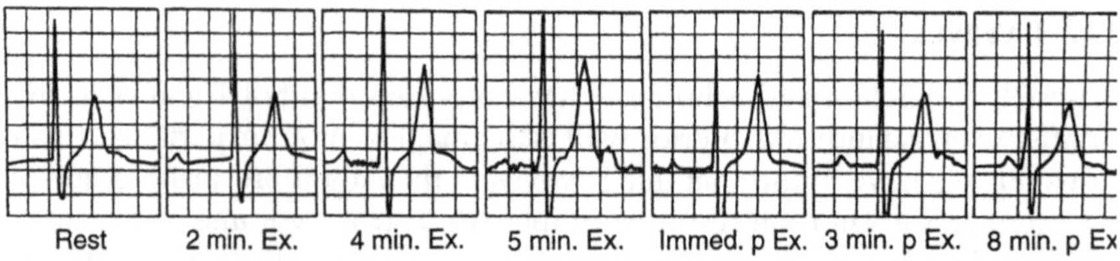

FIGURE 12–31. Tracings from a 23-year-old man with congenital heart block. The T-wave amplitude increases as exercise progresses.

rapidly, and it appears that the stroke volume must increase to make up for the lingering metabolic debt.

The increased prevalence of tall T waves in the younger age groups weighs heavily against its being an abnormal finding. Blomqvist[123] has postulated that tall T waves are due to a higher serum potassium level after exercise. We have found that when this T-wave pattern occurs with exercise, ischemia due to LAD artery narrowing is likely.

P WAVE CHANGES

Changes in P wave morphology have been well described in resting tracings and are very useful in identifying right- and left-sided hemodynamic alterations due to both volume and pressure load. We originally believed that as left ventricular end diastolic pressure increased with the ischemia, the left atrial component of the P wave should increase in amplitude. Careful study however revealed that it was P wave duration that was altered during ischemia. Myrianthiefs, working in our laboratory, demonstrated that prolongation of the wave duration with ischemia correlated with angiographically identified coronary artery disease.[124] As left ventricular end diastolic pressure increases with a loss of ventricular compliance, the left atrial wall is distended by increasing pressure, which apparently slows conduction through the atrium and thus prolongs the depolarization wave. The low amplitude of P waves however makes the measurements difficult, which probably accounts for the low sensitivity of this finding. We have found it quite useful however, when other signs of ischemia, for example, ST depression, are missing (Fig. 12–32).

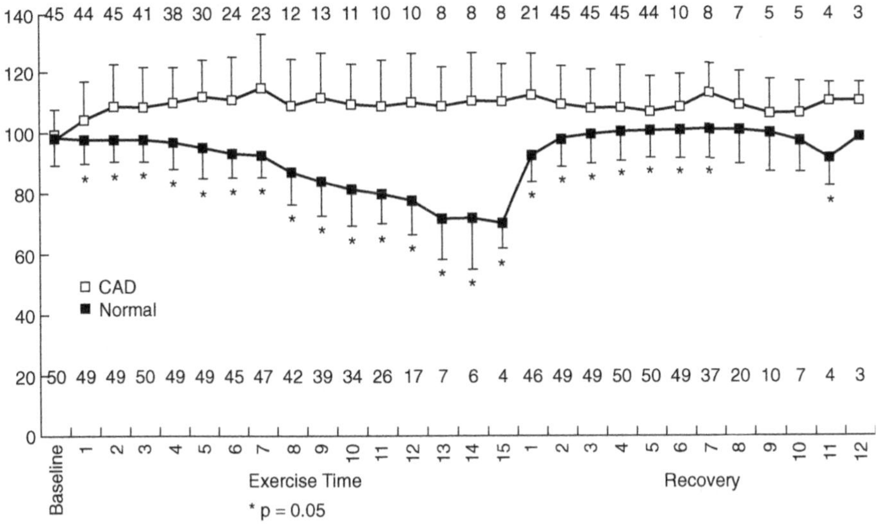

FIGURE 12–32. P-wave duration is plotted for each minute of exercise in ischemic patients (open symbols) and normals (solid symbols). P duration in normals shortens with exercise and prolongs with ischemia. Numbers represent the number of patients in each time slot.

TAKE-HOME MESSAGE
When other signs of ischemia are equivocal, measure the change in P duration from rest to exercise. (Best measured in lead 2). An increased duration of greater than 20 milliseconds provides a specificity of 64%.

FALSE-POSITIVE ST CHANGES

Sloping PQ Segment (Sapin)

Although Lepeschkin in 1969[9] published figures that illustrate the effect of atrial repolarization on the ST segment, the concept was revived by Sapin in 1991,[10] who emphasized that the slope of the PQ segment could help predict the magnitude of the influence of P wave repolarization and thus help predict which patient would have false-positive ST segments. This sign should be looked for especially in leads 2 and 3 and AVF and is most commonly seen when the P wave amplitude is increased (Fig. 12–33). It is believed that this is the reason ST depression, found only in these leads, is more likely to be a false-positive response.

TAKE-HOME MESSAGE
When the P waves are large in leads 2 and 3, look for a steep PQ slope and consider the possibility of false positive ST depression.

Digitalis

It has long been recognized that digitalis may cause ST depression, and that it is exaggerated by exercise. This is discussed in more detail in Chapter 23.

Hypokalemia

There are many causes of hypokalemia that may induce ST depression in patients with normal coronary arteries. This is discussed in more detail in Chapter 23.

ST Depression in Inferior Leads Only

As was mentioned in the paragraph on PQ Slope (see Fig. 12–3), ST depression is often manifested in only the inferior leads.[125] This should alert us to the possibility that these patients may not have ischemia.

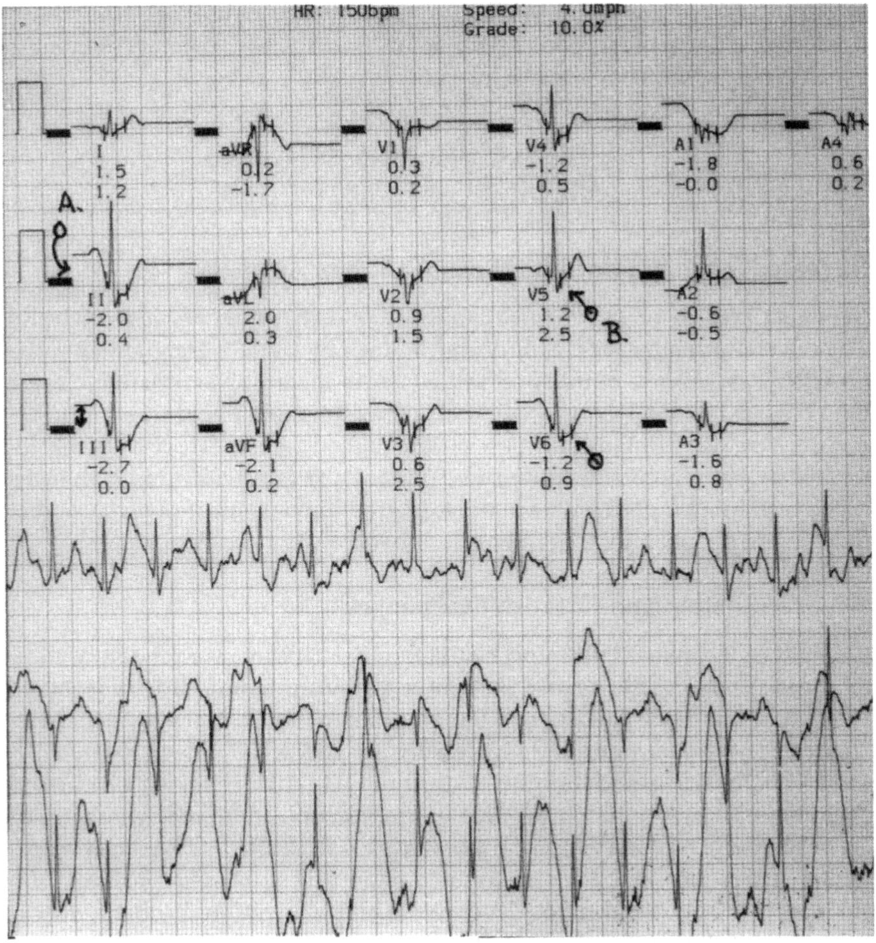

FIGURE 12–33. Computer Averaged Artifact in a Healthy 56-Year-Old Woman. This woman had atypical chest pain developing 2 days prior to the test. Six minutes into exercise the average beats show ST changes. Raw data show artifact probably due to loose lead wire. The error in baseline that produced ST depression in the average beats in lead 2 is marked *A*. A normal ST in V5 and a deep ST depression in V6 is physiologically impossible and is marked *B*.

False-Positive Tracings Due to Computer Averaging

All of us who work in the stress lab have seen frequent false measurements made by computer programs and numerous experts have labored over this problem but it has not gone away and I predict it may never. The most common is the failure of the computer to identify the PQ junction accurately. If using computer measurements for diagnosis or calculations, check the tick mark that identifies the PQ junction. When the tick does not fall on the proper PQ junction all other measurements are also in error. There are times when averaging algorithms result in errors, especially if there is a lot of muscle artifact or motion artifact. The careful analysis of the raw data is essential to avoid these errors. They are not infrequent.

TAKE-HOME MESSAGE
Always inspect the raw data carefully.

Increased Sympathetic Tone (Vasoregulatory Asthenia)

Yanowitz and associates[126] have demonstrated that many types of ST and T-wave abnormalities can be induced in dogs by stellate ganglion stimulation. We have seen a number of patients with increased sympathetic drive who have exhibited T-wave inversion and ST-segment depression upon exercising (Fig. 12–34). This may be a variant of the vasoregulatory asthenia described by Holmgren and colleagues.[127] Many patients with similar changes do not exhibit symptoms typical of Holmgren's syndrome, however, in that they do not show evidence of poor peripheral oxygen extraction.

Hyperventilation and Orthostatic Changes

Changes in T waves with hyperventilation or standing are relatively common and are thought to be mediated through the autonomic nervous system. When they are associated with ST-segment depression, the prevalence decreases; it has been reported to be less than 1% to 2%.[128] The mechanism is somewhat obscure and has been attributed to pH changes, electrolyte changes (especially potassium), changes in heart position, coronary arteriolar vasospasm, and excessive catecholamines. Because T waves can be reduced by beta blockers and accentuated by intravenous epinephrine,[129] the changes probably are due to asynchronous repolarization, probably mediated through the sympathetic pathway. Because the response of the autonomic system may be blunted in CAD, these changes have been labeled negative predictors for ischemia.[129]

More recently, it has been shown that mitral prolapse is commonly associated with ST-segment depression secondary to hyperventilation.[130] It is possible that some of Holmgren et al's[122] patients have unrecognized mitral prolapse. Bugiardini and colleagues[131] have described an increased magnitude of coronary narrowing in a cohort of patients with syndrome X and Prinzmetal's angina. Because alkalosis has been known to produce vasoconstriction, this enhanced tendency in some patients may well produce ischemia in the absence of CAD. It is now accepted that this syndrome is associated with major disturbances in autonomic balance, and exercise-induced ST depression with exercise is not uncommon.

Marcomichelakis and coworkers[132] believe that when exercise-induced ST depression is found in patients who are likely to have noncoronary causes, it can be identified if the changes are abolished by a beta blocker.

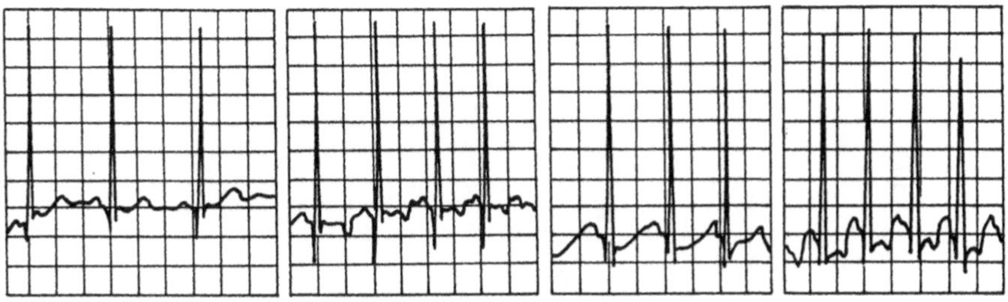

FIGURE 12–34. Note the shape of the early part of the ST segment, especially after hyperventilation, in a patient with increased sympathetic tone. We believe this pattern can be differentiated from classic ischemic ST-segment changes. Note deep septal Q waves.

They found that the drug did not eliminate the ST depression in any patients with significant CAD, but did correct the ST in those with normal coronary angiograms.

Hyperventilation, therefore, should be used at rest if there is clinical evidence that the ST changes are not due to ischemia.

Figure 12–35 is the tracing of a 28-year-old woman who suffered from chronic hyperventilation and a neurotic personality. The marked ST-segment depression after hyperventilation improved with exercise, but returned during the recovery period.

Short PR Interval

A short PR interval may favor ST depression due to atrial[134] repolarization. (See Chapter 13, page 243.)

Convex ST-Segment Depression—"Hump Sign"

Lepeschkin[9] reported that the prominent Ta wave (wave of atrial repolarization) and the superimposition of the U wave on the baseline adjustments tend to accentuate the depression of the proximal part of the ST segment and may lead to an erroneous diagnosis of ischemia. The tracings depicted in Figure 12–35 had normal coronary arteries and normal left-ventricular function. Pippin and colleagues[135] report that when the ST segment is convex, labeled the *hump sign*, it is very likely a false positive. Confirmation of this finding needs to be available, but I believe it may be valid.

ST Segment Variability

At peak exercise, modest QT segment depression is often associated with considerable lead to lead variation. When this occurs the possibility of a false

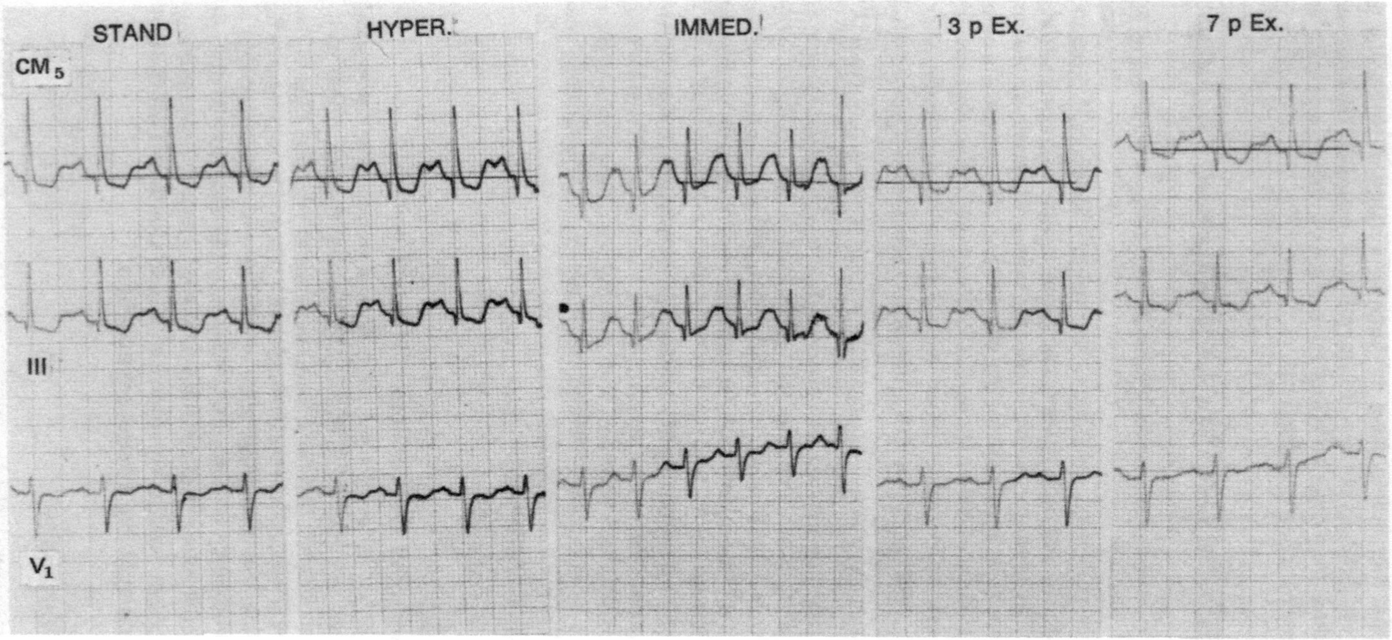

FIGURE 12–35. Exercise test of a 28-year-old woman with chronic hyperventilation and a neurotic personality. The resting ST-segment depression increased by hyperventilation tends to return almost to normal with exercise.

positive is increased. Michaelides et al report that 85% of patients with this finding are false positives.[138]

Localization of Ischemia by Electrocardiographic Patterns

Because exercise-induced ischemia is usually primarily a subendocaridal affair, resulting in what is believed to be a generalized process, it has long been believed that exercise testing cannot localize the culprit artery or arteries. There are several exceptions to this however, which will be described.

ST Elevation Due to Transmural Ischemia

When ST elevation occurs with exercise it usually identifies the LAD as the culprit artery. ST elevation in lead 2 and 3 in AVF, which is much less common, identifies right coronary disease and in V2 and V3 identifies LAD disease. (See page 205).

TAKE-HOME MESSAGE

ST elevation localizes the ischemic area, which is transmural.

ST Elevation in AVR

Lead AVR often develops ST elevation as a reciprocal of ST depression in lead V2 to V6 or to leads 2 and 3. It also may occasionally show ST elevation in the absence of significant changes in the other leads. AVR is positioned so that it reflects the left ventricular cavity and, when the right and left coronary beds are ischemic and cancel out, changes in the apex can be manifested. It has been suggested that ST elevation in AVR of .5 millimeter is significant for ischemia. It has been reported that this finding has a sensitivity of 89% but a specificity of only 44% for LAD disease.[136]

ST Depression in V1

Michaelides et al reported that 75% of patients with this finding had right coronary disease. Halon reported 94% had circumflex disease, with a sensitivity of 89%. It seems likely that it is a rare but reliable marker for inferior wall ischemia.[138]

Peaked T Waves in V2

Exercise-induced peaked T waves usually indicate LAD disease. (See page 226.)

Localization of Proximal or Distal LAD

When the narrowing is in the proximal LAD above the first diagonal, the following changes may be seen:

1. ST elevation in V1
2. Decreased T wave negativity in V1
3. ST depression in two of the three leads, 2, 3 or AVF
4. LAD below the diagonal

The above triad is missing but ST depression is usually present in V4, V5 and V6.[139]

Localization with Right Precordial Leads

The reduced sensitivity for identifying right coronary disease with the standard 12-lead system has been of concern for a long time. Braat et al,[137] in 1985, suggested using V4R as a way to deal with this problem. In spite of favorable reports, the use of these leads has not become commonplace. In 1999 Michaeledes reported on 245 patients where the standard precordial leads were supplemented by V3R, V4R, and V5R.[138] They reported an improvement in sensitivity for right coronary disease from 25% to 89%. They also found an increase overall sensitivity for any coronary disease from 66% to 92%. Although their work has not been replicated it suggests that an increased number of leads should be seriously considered. We have been using 15 leads for some time. We have not carefully analyzed our data at this time but hope to be able to report an improvement in sensitivity.

U WAVES

Lepeschkin[139] has published an excellent review of the significance of the U wave. The U wave is usually upright if the T is also upright and is highest at low heart rates. It generally follows the T wave at the same time ventricular relaxation is occurring. When the heart rate increases to more than 90, the U wave is rarely visible because it becomes merged with the end of the T wave and the ascending limb of the P wave. Most workers believe that it represents afterpotentials of the T wave. The U wave is accentuated by a larger diastolic volume, hypokalemia, and increased digitalis or calcium. Occasionally, in patients with very low potassium, the U wave can become so tall that it is mistaken for a tall T wave. Patients with inverted U waves may have an overload of central volume, and the tall U wave may represent a distended papillary muscle. Lepeschkin[139] reports that in patients with CAD, the incidence of inverted or diphasic U waves is about 30% at rest and 62% after exercise. If one makes an analysis of all patients with inverted U waves, LVH is the most common cause; angina is responsible for about 20% (Fig. 12–36).

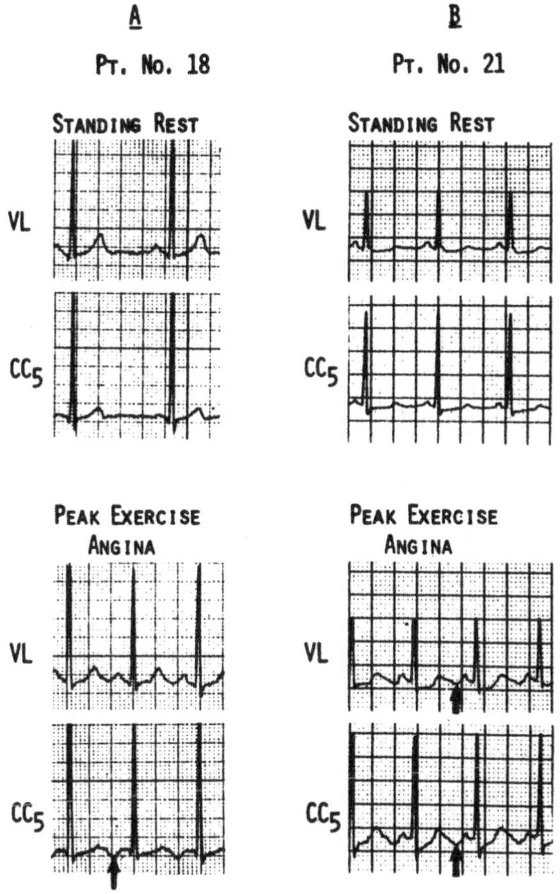

FIGURE 12–36. *(A)* Demonstration of simultaneously recorded vertical (VL) and modified CC_5 lead ECGs during standing rest and at peak exercise for patient 18. Marked U-wave inversion appeared in lead CC_5 at the time of exercise-induced angina pectoris. The exercise ST segment remained normal. *(B)* Patient 21 was taking digoxin, making the ST segment response to exercise difficult to interpret. However, during exercise-induced angina pectoris, this patient demonstrated marked U-wave inversion in both leads. The appearance of detectable U-wave inversion in the vertical lead was unusual in this study. (From Farris,[124] with permission.)

REFERENCES

1. Bousfield, G: Angina pectoris: Changes in electrocardiogram during paroxysm. Lancet 2:457, 1918.
2. Miranda, CP, et al: Correlation between resting ST segment changes, exercise testing, coronary angiography, and long term prognosis. Am Heart J 122:1617, 1991.
3. Michaelides, AP, et al: Exercise induced S wave prolongtion in left anterior descending coronary stenosis. Am J Cardiol 70:1407, 1992; 7:1299, 1995.
4. Pandya, A, et al: Time course of changes in P-wave duration during exercise. Cardiology 87:343, 1996.

5. Elliott, SE, et al: The use of the digital computer in the study of patients during exercise induced stress. Am Heart J 79:215, 1970.
6. Sheffield, LT, et al: On-line analysis of the exercise electrocardiogram. Circulation 40:935, 1969.
7. Kahn, KA and Simonson, E: Changes of mean spatial QRS and T vectors and of conventional electrocardiographic items in hard anaerobic work. Circ Res 9:629, 1957.
8. Bellet, S, et al: Radioelectrocardiographic changes during strenuous exercise in normal subjects. Circulation 25:686, 1962.
9. Lepeschkin, E: Physiological factors influencing the electrocardiographic response to exercise. In Blackburn, H (ed): Measurements in Exercise Electrocardiography. Charles C. Thomas, Springfield, IL, 1969, p 67.
10. Sapin, PM, et al: Identification of false positive exercise tests with the use of electrocardiographic criteria. J Am Coll Cardiol 18:127, 1991.
11. Bruce, RA, et al: Electrocardiographic responses to maximal exercise in American and Chinese population samples. In Blackburn, H (ed): Measurement in Exercise Electrocardiography. Charles C. Thomas, Springfield, IL, 1969, p 126.
12. Blomqvist, CG: Heart disease and dynamic exercise testing. In Willerson, JT and Sanders, CA (eds): Clinical Cardiology. Grune & Stratton, New York, 1977, p 126.
13. Froelicher, VF, et al: A comparison of two bipolar exercise ECG leads to V5. Chest 70:611,1976.
14. Froelicher, VF and Myers, JN: Exercise and the Heart, 4th ed. W.B. Saunders Co., Philadelphia, PA.
15. Stuart, R and Ellestad, MH: Upsloping ST segments in exercise testing. Am J Cardiiol 37:19, 1976.
16. Bruce, RA and Blackman, JR: Exercise testing in adult normal subjects and cardiac patients. Pediatrics 32(suppl):742, 1963.
17. Brody, AJ: Masters two-step exercise test in clinically unselected patients. JAMA 171:1195, 1959.
18. Kurita, A, et al: Significance of exercise-induced ST depression in evaluation of coronary artery disease. Am J Cardiol 40:492, 1977.
19. Goldschlager, N, et al: Treadmill stress tests as indicators of presence and severity of coronary artery disease. Ann Intern Med 85:277, 1976.
20. Hustead, R, et al: The failure of multi-lead ST depression to predict severity of ischemia (abstract). Am J Noninvas Cardiol 8:386, 1994.
21. Taylor, AJ and Beller, GA: Patients with greater than 2 mm of ST depression do not have a greater ischemic burden by thallium-201 scintigraphy. Circulation 86(suppl II):138, 1992.
22. Ellestad, MH and Halliday, WK: Stress testing in the management of ischemic heart disease. Angiology 28:149, 1977.
23. Ekelund, L, et al. Coronary heart disease morbidity and mortality in hypercholesterolemic men predicted from the exercise test. J Am Coll Cardiol 14:556, 1989.
24. Detry, JR: Exercise Testing and Training in Coronary Heart Disease. Williams & Wilkins, Baltimore, 1973.
25. Master, AM and Jaffe, HL: The electrocardiographic changes after exercise in angina pectoris. J Mt Sinai Hosp 7:629, 1941.
26. Mason, RE, et al: Correlation of graded exercise electrocardiographic response with clinical and coronary cinearteriographic findings. In Blackburn, H (ed): Measurements in Exercise Electrocardiography Charles C. Thomas, Springfield, IL, 1969, p 67.
27. Martin, CM and McConahay DR: Maximum treadmill exercise electrocardiography: Correlations with coronary arteriography and cardiac hemodynamics. Circulation 46:956, 1972.
28. Bertella, M, et al: Localizing the site of coronary artery obstructions in patients with stress-induced ST-segment depression in precordial leads by simple ECG parameters (abstract). Proceedings of the XXVII International Congress on Electrocardiology; 2000, June 27–July 1, Milan, Italy. Milan: MGR Srl—Congress Division.
29. Ellestad, MH, et al: The significance of lead strength on ST changes during treadmill stress tests. J Electrocardiog 25(suppl): 31, 1993.
30. Lachterman, B, et al: Comparison of ST segment/heart rate index to standard ST criteria for analysis of exercise electrocardiogram. Circulation 82:44, 1990.
31. Rywik, TM, et al: Independent prognostic significance of ischemic ST-segment response limited to recovery from treadmill exercise in asymptomatic subjects. Circulation 97(21):2117, 1998.

32. McHenry, PL, et al: Computer quantitation of the ST segment response during maximal treadmill exercise. Circulation 38:691, 1968.
33. Sheffield, LT, et al: On-line analysis of the exercise electrocardiogram. Circulation 40:935, 1969.
34. Ascoop, CA, et al: Clinical value of quantitative analysis of ST slope during exercise. Br Heart J 39:212, 1977.
35. Forlini, FJ, et al: St segment isolation and quantification as a means of improving diagnostic accuracy in treadmill stress testing. Am Heart J 90:431, 1975.
36. Sketch, MH, et al: Automated and nomographic analysis of exercise tests. JAMA 243:1052, 1980.
37. Ellestad, MH, et al: The predictive value of the time course of ST depression during exercise testing in patients referred for angiograms. Am Heart J 123:904, 1992.
38. Miranda, CP, et al: Correlation between resting ST segment changes, exercise testing, coronary angiography, and long term prognosis. Am Heart J 122:1617, 1991.
39. Bogaty, P, et al: Does more ST segment depression on the 12-lead exercise electrocardiogram signify more severe ischemic heart disease (Abstract). Circulation 88(suppl 2): 1, 1993.
40. Husted, R,et al: The failure of multilead ST depression to predict severity of ischemia. Am J Noninvas Cardiol 8:386, 1994.
41. Blackburn, H: The exercise electrocardiogram: Technological, procedural and conceptual development. In Simonson, E (ed): Physical Activity and the Heart. Charles C Thomas, Springfield, IL, 1967, p 39.
42. Hornsten, TR and Bruce, RA: Computed ST forces of frank and bipolar exercise ECG's. Am Heart J 78:346, 1969.
43. Simoons, ML: Optimal measurements for detection of coronary artery disease by exercise ECG. Comput Biomed Res 10:483, 1977.
44. Viik, J, et al: Correct utilization of exercise electrocardiographic leads in differentiation of men with coronary artery disease from patients with a low likelihood of coronary artery disease using peak exercise ST-segment depression. Am J Cardiol 81:964, 1998.
45. Cahahine, RA, et al: The clinical significance of exercise induced ST segment elevation. Circulation 54:209, 1976.
46. Prinzmetal, M, et al: Variant from angina pectoris. JAMA 174:1794, 1960.
47. Detry, JMR, et al: Maximal exercise testing in patients with spontaneous angina pectoris associated with transient ST segment elevation. Br Heart J 37:897, 1975.
48. MacAlpin, RN, et al: Angina pectoris at rest with preservation of exercise capacity: Prinzmetal's variant angina. Circulation 47:946, 1973.
49. Belik, N and Gardin, JM: ECG manifestations of myocardial ischemia. Arch Intern Med 140:1162, 1980.
50. Manvi, KN and Ellestad, MH: Elevated ST segments with exercise in ventricular aneurysm. J Electrocardiol 5:317, 1972.
51. Dunn, RF, et al: Exercise-induced ST elevation. Circulation 61:889, 1980.
52. Margonato A, et al: Exercise induced ST elevation on infarct related leads: A marker of residual viability (abstract). Circulation 86(suppl 1), 1992
53. Chelton, LG and Burchell, HB: Unusual ST segment deviations in electrocardiograms of normal persons. Am J Med Sci 230:54, 1955.
54. Kambara, H and Phillips, J: Long-term evaluation of early repolarization syndrome. Am J Cardiol 38:157, 1976.
55. Lloyd-Thomas, H: The effect of exercise on the electrocardiogram in healthy subjects. Br Heart J 23:260, 1961.
56. Gussak, I and Antzelevitch, C: Early repolarization syndrome: Clinical characteristics and possible cellular and ionic mechanisms. J Electrocardiol 33:299, 2000.
57. Hakki, AH, et al: R wave amplitude: A new determinant of failure of patients with coronary heart disease to manifest ST depression during exercise. J Am Coll Cardiol 3:1155, 1984.
58. Ellestad, MH, et al: The significance of lead strength on ST changes during treadmill stress tests. J Electrocardiog 25(suppl):31, 1993.
59. Simoons, ML: Optimal measurements for detection of coronary artery disease by exercise ECG. Comput Biomed Res 10:483, 1977.
60. Elamin, MS, et al: Accurate detection of coronary heart disease by new exercise test. Br Heart J 48:311, 1982.
61. Kligfield, P, et al: Heart rate adjustment of St segment depression for improved detection of coronary artery disease. Circulation 79:245, 1986.

62. Lachterman, B, et al: Comparison of ST segment/heart rate index to standard ST criteria for analysis of exercise electrocardiogram. Circulation 82:44, 1990.
63. Jacobs, WF, et al: False positive ST-T wave changes secondary to hyperventilation and exercise. Ann Intern Med 81:479, 1974.
64. Lary, D and Goldschlager, N: ECG changes during hyperventilation resembling myocardial ischemia in patients with normal coronary arteriograms. Am Heart J 87:383, 1974.
65. Wasserburger, RH, et al: The effect of hyperventilation on the normal adult ECG. Circulation 13:850, 1956.
66. Tommaso, CL and Gardin, JM: Pseudoischemic ST segment changes induced by hyperventilation. Prim Cardiol April 111, 1983.
67. Sheffield, LT, et al: On-line analysis of the exercise electrocardiogram. Circulation 40:935, 1969.
68. Simoons, ML: Optimal measurements for detection of coronary artery disease by exercise electrocardiography. Comput Biomed Res 10:483, 1977.
69. Okin, PM, et al: Recovery-phase patterns of ST segment depression in the heart rate domain. Circulation 80:533,1989.
70. Gullestad, L, et al: Post exercise ischemia is associated with increased neuropeptide Y in patients with coronary artery disease. Circulation 102:987, 2000.
71. Stuart, RJ and Ellestad, MH: Upsloping ST segments in exercise testing. Am J Cardiol 37:19, 1976.
72. Bruce, R and McDonough, JR: Stress testing in screening for cardiovascular disease. Bull NY Acad Med 45:1288, 1969.
73. Michaelides, AP, et al: Significance of ST depression in exercise induced superventricular extrasystoles. Am Heart J 117:1035, 1989.
74. Rerych, SK, et al: Cardiac function at rest and during exercise in normals and in patients with coronary heart disease. Ann Surg 186:449, 1978.
75. Brody, DA: A theoretical analysis of intracavitary blood mass influence on the heart lead relationship. Circulation 4:731, 1956.
76. Pipberger, HV, et al: QRS amplitude changes during heart filling and digitalization. Am Heart J 83:292, 1972.
77. Bonoris, PE, et al: Evaluation of R wave changes vs. ST segment depression in stress testing. Circulation 57:904, 1978.
78. Orzan, F, et al: Is the treadmill test useful for evaluating coronary artery disease in patients with complete LBBB? Am J Cardiol 42:36, 1978.
79. Lee, G, et al: Accuracy of left precordial R wave analysis during exercise testing in reliably detecting coronary disease in LBBB patients. Personal Communication, 1981.
80. Morris, SL, et al: Comparison of R wave and QRS amplitude during treadmill testing in normals and patients with coronary disease (abstract). Am Cardiol 43:353, 1979.
81. Berman, JL, et al: Multiple lead treadmill exercise tests. Circulation 61:53, 1980.
82. Van Tellingen, C, et al: On the clinical value of conventional and new exercise ECG criteria. Int J Cardiol 5:689, 1984.
83. Degre, S, et al: Analysis of exercise-induced R wave amplitude changes in detection of coronary artery disease in patients with typical or atypical chest pain under digitalis treatment. Cardiology 68(suppl 2):178, 1981.
84. Fox, K, et al: Inability of exercise-induced R wave changes to predict coronary artery disease. Am J Cardiol 49:674, 1982.
85. Fox, K, et al: Precordial electrocardiographic mapping after exercise in the diagnosis of coronary artery disease. Am J Cardiol 43:541, 1979.
86. Greenberg, PS, et al: Radionuclide angiographic correlation of the R wave, ejection fraction, and volume responses to upright bicycle exercise. Chest 80:459, 1981.
87. David, D, et al: Intramyocardial conduction: A major determinant of R wave amplitude during acute myocardial ischemia. Circulation 65:161, 1982.
88. Ekmekci, A, et al: Angina pectoris. Am J Cardiol April :521, 1961.
89. Madias, JE and Krikelis, EN: Transient giant R waves in the early phase of acute myocardial infarction: Association with ventricular fibrillation. Clin Cardiol 4:339, 1981.
90. Decaprio, L, et al: R wave amplitude changes during stress testing: Comparison with ST segment depression and angiographic correlation. Am Heart J 99:413, 1980.
91. Ellestad, MH: The mechanism of exercise induced R wave amplitude changes in coronary heart disease: Still controversial. Arch Internal Med. 142:963, 1982.

92. Cheng, S-L, et al: Significance of ST-segment depression with R-wave amplitude decrease on exercise testing. Am J Cardiol 83:955, 1999.
93. Michaelides, AP, et al: Exercise induced S wave prolongation in left anterior descending coronary stenosis. Am J Cardiol 70:1407, 1992.
94. Michaelides, AP, et al: Effect of number of coronary arteries significantly narrowed and status of intraventricular conduction on exercise-induced QRS prolongation in coronary artery disease. Am J Cardiol 70:1487, 1993.
95. Takaki, H, et al: Exercise-induced QRS prolongation in patients with mild coronary artery disease. J Electrocardiol 32(suppl):206, 1999.
96. Michaelides, AP, et al: New coronary disease index based on exercise-induced QRS changes. Am Heart J 120:292, 1990.
97. Herzog, J, et al: Analysis of the Athens score in the diagnosis of ischemia during exercise testing. J Noninv Cardio March/April:7, 1998.
98. Glazier, JJ, et al: Increase in S wave amplitude during ischemic ST segment depression in stable angina pectoris. Am J Cardiol 59:1295, 1987.
99. Michaelides, AP, et al: Exercise induced S wave prolongation in left anterior descending coronary stenosis. Am J Cardiol 70:1407, 1992.
100. Lepeschkin, E and Surawicz, B: Characteristics of true positive and false positive results of electrocardiographic exercise tests. N Engl J Med 248:511, 1958.
101. Roman, L and Bellet, S: Significance of the QX/QT ratio and the QT ratio (QTr) in the exercise electrocardiogram. Circulation 32:435, 1965.
102. Master, AM and Rosenfelt, I: Two-step exercise test: Current status after 25 years. Mod Concept Cardiovasc Dis 36:19, 1967.
103. Burch, GE and Depasquale, N: A study at autopsy of the relation of absence of the Q wave in leads 1, aVL, V5, and V6 to septal fibrosis. Am Heart J 60:336, 1960.
104. Morales-Ballejo, H, et al: The septal Q wave in exercise testing. Am J Cardiol 48:247, 1981.
105. O'Hara, NJ, et al: Changes of Q wave amplitude during exercise for the prediction of coronary artery disease. Int J Cardiol 6:35, 1984.
106. Kuo, CS, et al:. Characteristics and possible mechanisms of ventricular arrhythmia dependent on the dispersion of action potential durations. Circulation 67:1356, 1983.
107. Koide, Y, et al: Usefulness of QT dispersion immediately after exercise as an indicator of coronary stensosis and independent of gender or exercise-induced ST-segment depression. Am J Cardiol 86:1312, 2000.
108. Aufderheide, TP, et al: The added diagnostic value of automated QT-dispersion measurements and automated segment deviations in the electrocardiographic diagnosis of acute cardiac ischemia. J Electrocardiol 33:329, 2000.
109. Yu, PNG, et al: Observations on change of ventricular systole (QT interval) during exercise. J Clin Invest 29:279, 1950.
110. Yu, PNG and Soffer, A: Studies of electrocardiographic changes during exercise (modified double two-step test). Circulation 6:183, 1952.
111. Greenberg, PS, et al: Comparison of the predictive accuracy of ST depression, R wave amplitude, QX/QT and QTc during stress testing. Am J Cardiol 44:18, 1979.
112. Bertella, M, et al: Is the shortening of the QTc-interval in Q-waves leads showing ST-segment shift during exercise testing a new ECG marker of myocardial ischaemia and viability in patients with previous anterior myocardial infarction. G Ital Cardiol 29:647, 1999.
113. Bertella, M, et al: Assessment of QTc-interval variability in vasopspastic and nonvasospastic transmural ischemia: Possible clinical implications of a different behaviour. Cardiology 2000: Proceedings of the XXVII International Congress on Electrocardiology; 2000, June 17-July 1, Milan, Italy.
114. Nirula, A: Exercise testing in the congenital/idiopathic long QT syndrome. Symposium on Exercise Testing, Kluwer, (Ed) Ellestad, 2001.
115. Vincent, GM, et al: The inherited long QT syndrome: from ion channel to bedside. Cardiol Review 7:44, 1999.
116. Bellet, S, et al: The electrocardiogram during exercise as recorded by radioelectrocardiography: Comparison with the post-exercise electrocardiogram (Master's two-step test). Am J Cardiol 18:385, 1961.
117. Noble, J, et al: Normalization of abnormal T-waves in ischemia. Arch Intern Med 136:391, 1976.
118. Aravindaksham, V, et al: ECG exercise test in patients with abnormal T waves at rest. Am Heart J 93:706, 1977.

119. Lee, JH, et al: Significance of precordial T-wave increase during treadmill stress testing. Am J Cardiol 76:1297, 1995.
120. Chikamori, T, et al: Clinical and electrocardiographic profiles producing exercise-induced U-wave inversion in patients with severe narrowing of the left anterior descending coronary artery. Am J Cardiol 80:628, 1997.
121. Scherf, D: Fifteen years of electrocardiographic exercise test in coronary stenosis. NY State J Med 47:2420, 1947.
122. Scherf, D and Schoffer, AI: The electrocardiographic exercise test. Am Heart J 43, 1952.
123. Blomquist, CG: Use of exercise testing for diagnostic and functional evaluation. Circulation 44:1120, 1971.
124. Myrianthefs, MM, et al: Significance of signal-averaged P-wave changes during exercise in patients with coronary artery disease and correlation with angiographic findings. Am J Cardiol 68:1619, 1991.
125. Miranda, CP, et al: Usefulness of exercise-induced ST-segment depression in the inferior leads during exercise testing as a marker for coronary artery disease. Am J Cardiol 69:303, 1992.
126. Yanowitz, F, et al: Functional distribution of right and left stellate innervation to the ventricles: Production of neurogenic electrocardiographic changes by unilateral alteration of sympathetic tone. Circ Res 18:416, 1966.
127. Holmgren, A, et al: Electrocardiographic changes in vasoregulatory asthenia and the effect of training. Acta Med Scand 165:21, 1967.
128. Karjalainen, J: Function and myocarditis-induced T-wave abnormalities. Chest 83:6, 1983.
129. McHenry, PL: Treadmill exercise testing in the diagnosis and evaluation of coronary heart disease. J Contin Ed Cardiol 11:1425, 1978.
130. Tommaso, CL and Gardin, JM: Pseudoischemic ST segment changes induced by hyperventilation. Prim Cardiol April 111, 1983.
131. Bugiardini, R, et al: Vasotonic angina: A spectrum of ischemic syndromes involving functional abnormalities of the epicardial and microvascular coronary circulation. Am J Cardiol 22:417, 1993.
132. Marcomichelakis, J, et al: Exercise testing after beta-blockade: Improved specificity and predictive value in detecting coronary heart disease. Br Heart J 43:252, 1980.
133. Astrand, I, et al: ST changes at exercise in patients with short P-R interval. Acta Med Scand 185:205, 1969.
134. Myrianthiefas, MM, et al: False positive ST segment depression during exercise in subjects with short PR intervals and normal coronary arteries. J Electrography 31(13):203, 1998.
135. Pippin, JJ, et al: The St hump sign: A reliable indicator for false positive electrocardiographic response during treadmill exercise. Circulation 102(suppl 2):1917, 2000.
136. Ellestad, MH: Can the exercise electrocardiogram be used to determine the severity of ischemia and to localize the area of the myocardium at risk? ACC Educational Highlights 15-16, Summer 1998.
137. Braat, SH, et al: Value of lead V4R in exercise testing to predict proximal stenosis of the right coronary artery. J Am Coll Cardiol 5:1308, 1985.
138. Michaelides, AP, et al: Improved detection of coronary artery disease by exercise electrocardiography with the use of right precordial leads. New Eng J Med 340:340, 1999.
139. Lepeschkin, E: Physiological basis of the U wave. In Schlant RC and Hurst, JW (eds): Advances in Electrocardiography, Vol. 2. Grune & Stratton, New York, 1977, p. 172.
140. Farris, SV, et al: Concepts and applications of treadmill exercise testing and the exercise electrocardiogram. Am Heart J 95:102, 1978.
141. Yano, H, et al: Negative U wave during percutaneous transluminal coronary angioplasty. Clin Cardiol 14:232, 1991.

13

Rhythm and Conduction Disturbances in Stress Testing

Introduction
Sick Sinus Syndrome (Chronotropic Incompetence)
Short PR Interval
Supraventricular Arrhythmias
Atrial Extrasystoles
Atrial Fibrillation or Flutter
Paroxysmal Atrial Tachycardia
Ventricular Arrhythmias
Resting
Exercise-Induced Ventricular Arrhythmias
Ventricular Ectopy in Patients with Coronary Artery Disease
Abolition of Arrhythmias by Exercise
PVCs During Recovery
ST Segments in Exercise-Induced PVCs
Ventricular Tachycardia
Exercise-Induced Sustained VT
Exercise Testing to Evaluate Spontaneous VT
Arrhythrogenic Right Ventricular Dysplasia
Idiopathic Right Ventricular Outflow Tachycardia
Reproducibility of Ventricular Ectopy
Conduction Disturbances
First-Degree Atrioventricular Block
Second-Degree Atrioventricular Block
Fascicular Block
Left Anterior Division Block
Left Posterior Hemiblock
Congenital Long QT Syndrome
Rate-Related Bundle Branch Block
Right Bundle Branch Block
Left Bundle Branch Block
Third-Degree Atrioventricular Block
Accelerated Conduction (WPW Syndrome)

INTRODUCTION

Alterations in cardiac rhythm occur frequently with exercise and are considerably important in understanding a patient's function and in providing predictive information as to mortality and morbidity. Arrhythmias during exertion result from sympathetically enhanced phase IV repolarization of ectopic foci, so that if the rate of the ectopic focus is faster than the normal pacer tissue in the sinus node, the focus assumes predominance and sets the rhythm. Alterations in recovery time of cardiac tissues caused by ischemia, and probably battery effects associated with ischemic tissue adjacent to normally perfused myocardium, are important. After-potentials (low amplitude oscillations) seen in patients with large infarcts are triggered by catecholamines and enhanced by an influx of calcium. The abrupt withdrawal of much of the parasympathetic tone, which in most cases protects against arrhythmias, probably also plays an important role. The prevalence increases steadily with age[1] and has been reported to be 100% in a study of older subjects.[2] Busby also reports an age-related increase in normal individuals.[3]

Subendocardial ischemia is less arrhythmogenic than transmural ischemia, so we should be more concerned with arrhythmias combined with ST elevation than with those associated with ST depression. The imbalance between oxygen supply and demand induced in exercising patients with coronary artery disease (CAD) may be augmented during the recovery period. Peripheral dilatation induced by exercise, combined with a reduced venous return caused by abrupt cessation of muscular activity, may cause cardiac output and coronary flow to fall at a time when myocardial oxygen demand is still high, owing to tachycardia. These changes, in combination with elevated catecholamines, may explain the increase in arrhythmias commonly seen during recovery.

Although exercise testing is most frequently used to diagnose or evaluate ischemia, in some centers it is prescribed to detect arrhythmias and to evaluate the response to drug regimens. Young and colleagues[4] report the use of symptom-limited exercise testing specifically aimed at evaluating arrhythmias in 263 patients. Seventy-four percent had a history of ventricular tachycardia that compromised them hemodynamically or of ventricular fibrillation. These patients underwent 1377 maximum treadmill tests; complications occurred in 9.1%, and the remainder had 1345 tests without problems (97.7%). No death, myocardial infarction, or lasting morbid event occurred. The authors state that exercise testing can be conducted safely in patients with malignant arrhythmias.

SICK SINUS SYNDROME (CHRONOTROPIC INCOMPETENCE)

There exists a heterogeneous group of subjects who often have inappropriately low resting heart rates. Some are symptomatic and others may be unaware of this abnormality. Many have been diagnosed as having sick sinus syndrome. Some appear to have a high vagal tone; some have intrinsic disease of the nodal tissue, possibly due to ischemia or degenerative changes; and some have low resting heart rates due to causes not yet elucidated. Some patients with exercise-induced sinus bradycardia may also have syncope associated with a profound drop in blood pressure. This may be due to the Bezold-Jarisch reflex. It appears that hypersensitive mechanicoreceptors in the left ventricle activate nonmyelinated vagal afferents (C fibers), resulting in a significant increase in vagal tone.

When a slow resting pulse fails to accelerate normally with exercise, we have labeled it "chronotropic incompetence"; however, there is little doubt that our understanding of these syndromes is incomplete. A slower-than-normal acceleration of the heart rate during exercise would be a protective mechanism in ischemia, preserving a longer diastolic time to perfuse the myocardium.

We have found that the reduced heart rate response to exercise identifies a cohort of patients with poor ventricular function many of whom may have severe coronary narrowing who are subject to an increased prevalence of future coronary events.[5,6] The predictive power of this response is presented in Chapter 14.

Abbott and colleagues[7] performed bicycle ergometry on 16 patients with electrophysiologically confirmed sinus node dysfunction, who had a blunted heart rate response to exercise. Atropine increased their chronotropic response to normal at lower workloads, but with peak exercise their heart rates were still below predicted rates, suggesting that vagotonia was not the only mechanism involved. These patients probably suffer from a number of autonomic aberrations, and much is needed to improve our understanding of the complex factors controlling heart rate in patients with cardiac dysfunction.

A number of more recent papers by Lauer and colleagues confirms the importance of heart rate response to exercise.[8,9] A more complete discussion of the possible mechanisms has been published.[10]

SHORT PR INTERVAL

As early as 1965 Ostrand called attention to the syndrome of short PR interval without accelerated conduction and it's association with ST depression in normal individuals.[11] This is recently confirmed by Myrianthiefs of Cyprus.[12] When patients who have a low probability of coronary disease have modest ST depression at rest, a short PR interval should be looked for. If found it may be evidence to support the expectation that there is no ischemia. This may be due to the exaggerated influence of atrial repolarization.

SUPRAVENTRICULAR ARRHYTHMIAS

Although sinus arrhythmias tend to be reduced by the vagal withdrawal accompanying the onset of exercise, this and wandering pacemakers tend to recur early during the recovery period and have no special significance. The loss of the atrial transport mechanisms, however, results in a loss in stroke volume of from 5% to 30%, depending on the ventricular compliance and the heart rate. As early as 1912, Sir Thomas Lewis[13] demonstrated a drop in cardiac output and aortic pressure at the onset of atrial fibrillation, and reports by Kaplan and colleagues[14] and Killip and Baer[15] substantiate the belief that atrial contraction is important to function. Thus, the sinus node not only determines the chronotropic response to increased metabolic load, but also the appropriately timed atrial boost to ventricular filling is critical for optimal function at high workloads.

The incidence of any supraventricular arrhythmia during exercise testing varies from 4% to 18%, according to how the series was selected.[16] McHenry[17] reported 5% in normal volunteers and 40% in those with CAD. The incidence also increases with age.

Atrial Extrasystoles

Atrial premature beats often occur at lower workloads and have little clinical significance. As exercise increases, they usually subside and may then return during recovery. Supraventricular extrasystoles, however, may be an aid in the identification of ischemia. When the atrial extrasystole has ST depression greater than the preceding sinus beat, it has been shown to be a marker for ischemia. Michaelides and associates[18] reported a sensitivity of 74% and a specificity of 84% for this little-recognized finding. The same authors have also reported that the R wave in supraventricular beats in ischemic patients is taller than that in the normally conducted beats. In normals, the premature R wave is shorter than in the previous beat. An increased R wave or no change in premature supraventricular beats has a sensitivity of 79% and a specificity of 90% in those who had exercise-induced premature supraventricular contractions.[19] When some baseline ST depression is present and the premature atrial contraction shows less deviation than the sinus beat, then ischemia is rare. When a nodal premature beat is followed by a long pause and the following sinus beat shows accentuated ST depression, ischemia is also likely (Figs. 13–1 and 13–2).

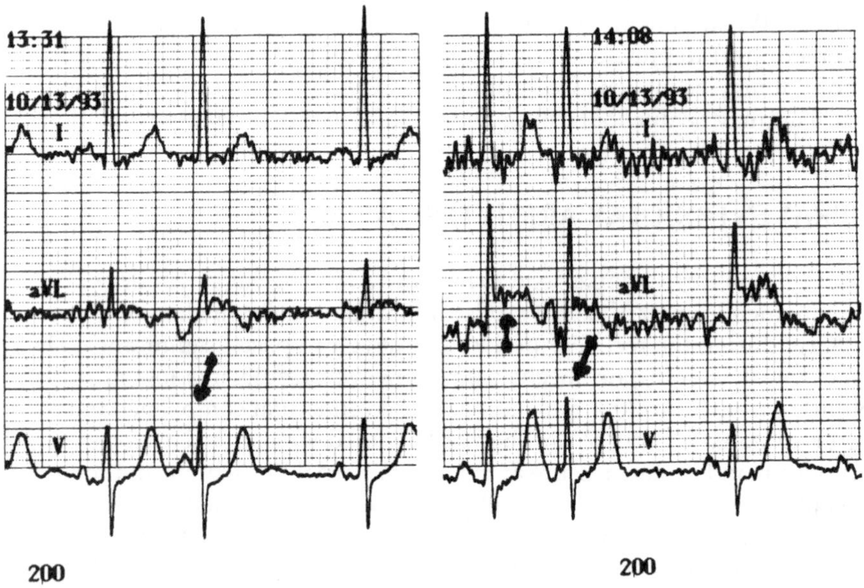

FIGURE 13–1. Panel on left illustrates atrial premature beat with R wave equal to previous sinus beat. Right panel is during exercise-induced ischemia. The R wave of the atrial premature beat is taller (see arrows).

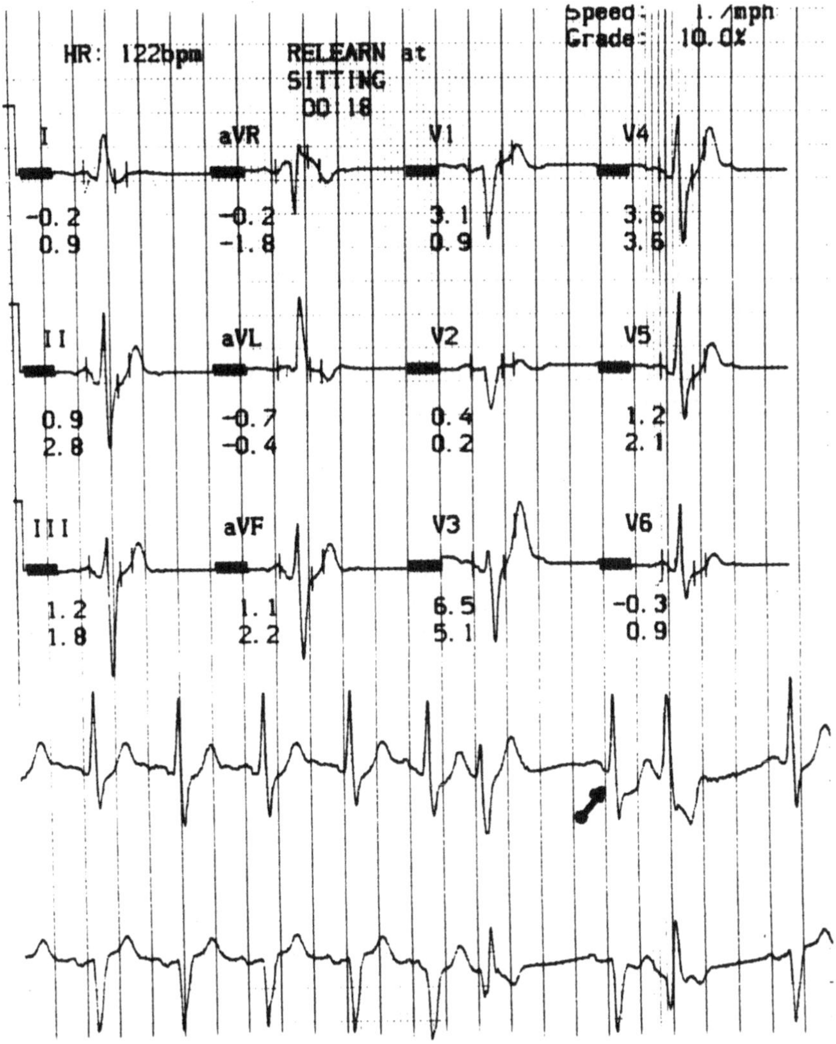

FIGURE 13–2. When ischemia is present, atrial premature beats have ST-segment depression not seen in the normally conducted beats.

Atrial Fibrillation or Flutter

Transient atrial fibrillation or flutter is seen frequently and can be associated with CAD, rheumatic heart disease, thyrotoxicosis, or myocarditis. It is also seen in people of all ages who have no other apparent abnormalities. Although no specific diagnosis can be made when this condition develops, it is an indication of malfunction; note the cardiac output with rapid rates of atrial fibrillation or flutter is far below that of a subject with sinus rhythm who has a similar ventricular response. Upon testing a subject with atrial fibrillation or flutter, the ventricular response tends to accelerate very rapidly, probably due to inadequate left-ventricular filling resulting in a decreased stroke volume. The ST-segment changes associated with ischemia are similar to those observed with a sinus rhythm and may be seen in rheumatic heart disease and other cardiac abnormalities. In these cases, the ST-segment depression may indicate left-ventricular dysfunction due to primary muscle change rather than to coexisting CAD. In addition, the very short diastolic intervals may produce subendocardial ischemia because of the inadequate perfusion time in the face of an otherwise-normal ventricular function. When atrial fibrillation or flutter is initiated by exercise, it does not necessarily implicate CAD as the underlying cause, although this is often the primary factor in older subjects. It may also be a tip-off that sustained atrial fibrillation will occur later (Figs. 13–3 and 13–4).

Paroxysmal Atrial Tachycardia

Two- or three-beat bursts of atrial or junctional tachycardia are occasionally seen with exercise, but sustained paroxysmal atrial tachycardia (PAT) is relatively rare. Graboys and Wright[20] reported 29 patients with sustained PAT in 3000 stress tests from a cohort of 207 patients referred for

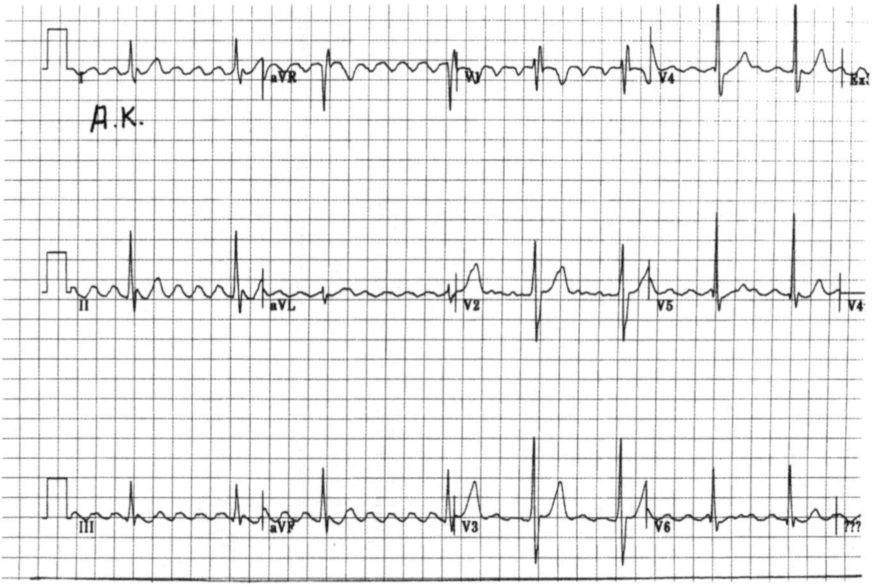

FIGURE 13–3. The resting tracing of a 42-year-old man who came to the emergency department with chest pain and palpitations. Note the flutter waves.

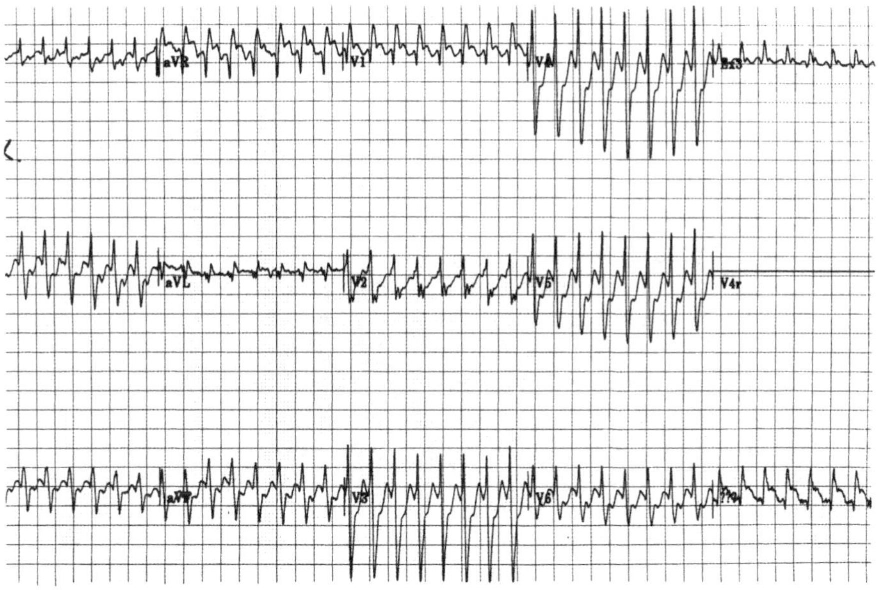

FIGURE 13–4. This tracing of the same patient illustrated in Figure 13–3 after 4 minutes of exercise, which caused shortness of breath and weakness. Note that the flutter resulted in a one to one conduction, causing a very fast heart rate with severe ST depression. A subsequent angiogram revealed normal coronary arteries.

evaluation of atrial arrhythmias. Gough[21] reported on the results of 880 stress tests, 315 of which were believed to be of normal subjects. Eleven patients had atrial tachycardia, nine had junctional tachycardia, and two had atrial fibrillation in short bursts. All but one spontaneously terminated within 90 seconds. Mauer and associates[22] from the Baltimore Gerontology Research Center reported the 7-year follow-up data on 85 subjects (6% of their total population). These normal individuals with exercise-induced supraventricular tachycardia failed to have any difference in their cardiovascular mortality but had a higher incidence of subsequent supraventricular tachycardia.

Even in persons prone to PAT, this rhythm is rarely initiated by exercise. In one of our patients, an intermittent supraventricular tachycardia was consistently terminated by exercise. The exact cause of this is obscure, but possibly the reentry pathway responsible for the tachycardia had become refractory during the exercise period. When PAT does appear during a stress test, ST-segment depression is commonly seen and is occasionally but not invariably associated with ischemia, but I believe it is prudent to terminate exercise.

VENTRICULAR ARRHYTHMIAS

Resting

Considerable disagreement exists regarding the significance of resting ventricular ectopic beats. Fisher and Tyroler[23] studied 1212 white male factory workers and concluded that although there was an increase in incidence of premature ventricular contractions (PVCs) of 2% to 15% with age, they could not statistically predict the incidence of sudden death or myocardial infarction. When Goldschlager and associates[24] compared the coronary angiograms of patients exhibiting premature contractions with the angiograms of those who did not, they found a much more severe degree of disease associated with the arrhythmia. Rodstein and coworkers[25] studied 712 insured persons with extrasystoles for an average period of 18 years. No change in mortality was observed, even when those older than and younger than aged 40 were compared. However, when exercise produced an increase in the number of arrhythmias in either age group, the incidence of mortality increased. A number of other studies claim that sudden death in subjects with resting ventricular arrhythmias is increased two- to threefold.[26] Alexander and colleagues[27] from the Lahey Clinic reported follow-up studies on 539 patients with PVCs at rest. They found that in patients with CAD there was a small but statistically significant increase in mortality when PVCs were recorded.

Buckingham and associates[28] have demonstrated that frequent PVCs detected in Holter monitor recordings in normal subjects are usually benign, and their results are now generally accepted by most workers. Frequent multiform PVCs only constitute a risk in those with poor ventricular function. On the other hand, if these PVCs occur in subjects with significant ventricular dysfunction, they are often harbingers of trouble. As it turns out, the same thing can be said for PVCs recorded during exercise testing.[29]

Exercise-Induced Ventricular Arrhythmias

Ventricular arrhythmias are usually produced by excess catecholamines and vagal withdrawal, as described in the beginning of this chapter. Occasionally, reentry and triggered activity also play a role.

In clinically normal subjects, maximum stress testing occasionally produces ventricular arrhythmias in 36% to 42%, usually at high workloads. In CAD patients, the prevalence is reported to be about 50% to 60%. In general, CAD patients manifest arrhythmias at a lower heart rate, which are somewhat more reproducible than those seen in clinically normal subjects. Sheps and coworkers[30] have reported that when stress tests are done consecutively on the same day, the second test produced significantly fewer PVCs.

In actively employed normal policemen[31] and air crewmen,[32] exercise-induced PVCs have been studied and were found to have no influence on subsequent morbidity and mortality. These data are generally believed to apply to all asymptomatic patients.

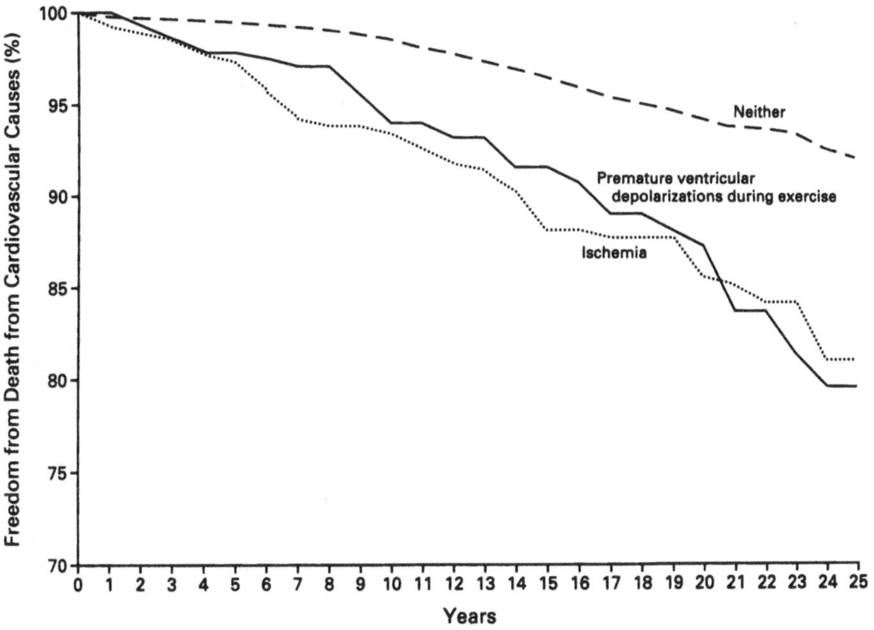

FIGURE 13–5. A life table illustrating survival of over a 23-year period of 6,101 asymptomatic men. The data shows that those who had PVCs during exercise had a mortality similar to those who had ST depression depicting ischemia. Reproduced with permission.[33]

A recent report from France on a large cohort (N=6101), of asymptomatic men suggests that exercise induced PVC's may have more predictive significance than previously reported.[33] The variation from some of the previous studies may be due to the long follow-up of 23 years (Fig. 13–5).

VENTRICULAR ECTOPY IN PATIENTS WITH CORONARY ARTERY DISEASE

PVCs are more common (10% to 40%) in CAD patients than in those without CAD.[34] Udall and I[29] have reported follow-up data on 1327 patients who had PVCs either before, during, or after exercise testing who were referred to our hospital mostly for chest pain syndromes. In this population, we found that the PVCs were associated with a moderate increase in morbidity and mortality compared with the normal population, even when these patients failed to have ischemic ST depression. However, when the CAD group developed ST depression, the mortality and number of coronary events almost doubled. Also, "ominous" PVCs increased the risk even more to about twice that of the others. Ominous PVCs were defined as multifocal, multiform, repetitive, and also ventricular tachycardia. Sami and associates[35] reported the follow-up of 1400 CAD patients enrolled in the CASS study. The mortality rate was 29% in 130 patients with ventricular arrhythmias compared with 25% in those without. Follow-up data on PVCs after myocardial infarction have also shown that when associated with mild disease and good left-ventricular function, they are of lesser clinical significance. However, when PVCs are recorded in patients with a low ejection fraction, they indicate a more grave prognosis (Fig. 13–6).[34]

A report from Durham, North Carolina, by Califf and colleagues[36] on 1293 stress tests in patients undergoing coronary angiography showed that their survival data are similar to ours. The investigators also found that those with greater ischemia (ie, three-vessel disease) had a higher incidence of more serious ventricular arrhythmias. McHenry and colleagues[37] reported that 27% of exercise-induced ventricular arrhythmias occurred in CAD patients compared with 7% in those with normal coronary arteries. It is interesting that Califf and colleagues[36] found a much higher incidence of ventricular arrhythmias among those on digitalis, thus confirming a previous report by Gough and McConnell,[38] who reported that 50% of the six patients taking digitalis in their series developed ventricular tachycardia.

Marieb and associates[39] reported on 383 subjects who had exercise thallium and angiography, 162 of whom had exercise-induced arrhythmias.

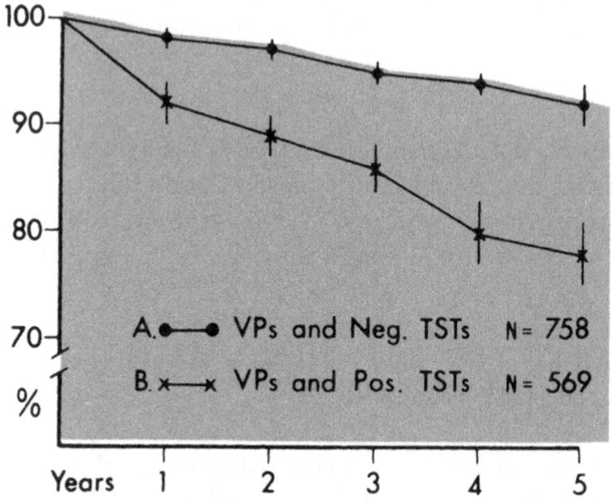

Subjects Analyzed Each Year

		0	1	2	3	4	5
A)	Sample #	758	333	250	193	137	97
B)	Sample #	569	267	178	130	100	64

FIGURE 13–6. Life table depicting the prevalence of coronary events for patients with ventricular premature beats and normal ST segments *(A)* and the same rhythm in patients with ST depression. *(B)* Patients in whom both abnormalities are present have more than a twofold greater prevalence of coronary events (angina, myocardial infarction, and death).

They found that ischemia was more likely to be found in those with ventricular arrhythmias than in those without and that the arrhythmias were useful in the prediction of subsequent cardiac events. Exercise-induced ventricular tachycardia will be discussed later.

Abolition of Arrhythmias by Exercise

The induction of arrhythmias by exercise is well recognized, but the abolition of ectopic activity is less commonly appreciated. The mechanisms responsible for this include rapid heart rate, which increases the relative time during the refractory period, providing a measure of overdrive suppression, and decreased automaticity of the Purkinje system, associated with rapid stimulation.

It is common to see young, apparently healthy subjects who have PVCs at rest but not during exercise. These persons have no evidence of cardiac abnormalities other than PVCs at rest. Our policy was to consider this type of arrhythmia benign, as proposed by Bourne[40] in 1977. This seemed so logical that we were surprised when our own study indicated that patients referred for stress testing in our laboratory whose PVCs were suppressed by exercise had a rate of cardiac events similar to that of those whose PVCs were initiated by exercise. Helfant and colleagues[41] have also reported a significant incidence of CAD in a small group (N=22) of subjects with PVCs that were decreased by exercise. McHenry and associates[37] reported exercise suppression of ventricular arrhythmias in 42% of these CAD patients.

TAKE-HOME MESSAGE

In CAD patients, many PVCs are abolished by exercise, just as they are in normals; therefore, this finding does not ensure that the patient is free of disease.

PVCs During Recovery

As the heart rate rapidly slows during recovery from exercise, PVCs commonly occur and usually have no clinical significance in our experience. As previously mentioned, this may be a time when metabolic adjustments in the heart are somewhat inappropriate, and therefore, occasionally serious disturbances in rhythm may be initiated. A recent report, however, suggests that the danger from arrhythmias during the cool-down may be considerable. Dimsdale[42] found that epinephrine and norepinephrine can shoot up to 10 times normal. The hormonal fluctuations can be minimized by a gradual cool-down. The drop in blood pressure during recovery appears to trigger the response. It is important to understand that even young subjects without established heart disease occasionally have ventricular tachycardia or even ventricular fibrillation after exercise. If this is to happen, it is better to happen while in the stress laboratory than while jogging in the park (see Fig. 13–7).

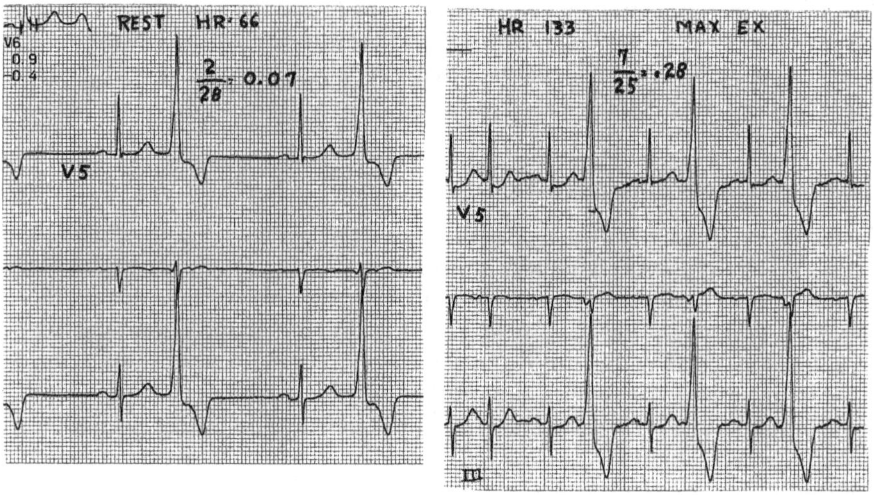

FIGURE 13–7. An 82-year-old man with infrequent angina had PVCs before and during an exercise test. The magnitude of the ST depression of the PVC is corrected for R-wave amplitude. Note the increase in the magnitude of the ST with exercise. Subsequent angiogram revealed high grade LAD narrowing.

ST Segments in Exercise-Induced PVCs

Over the years it has been believed that repolarization in ventricular ectopic beats had no diagnostic significance. Recently we have studied the magnitude of the ST depression in ventricular ectopic beats near peak exercise and found it to be of significant diagnostic value. Because most patients don't have PVCs during exercise, testing limits its value somewhat. The specificity however, of 90% suggests it may be of considerable help in patients with ventricular arrhythmias. ST depression of greater than 10 percent of the R wave amplitude is predictive of an ischemia response.[43]

> **TAKE-HOME MESSAGE**
> Look for increasing ST depression in PVCs occurring during or after exercise.

Ventricular Tachycardia

Only a few years ago ventricular tachycardia (VT) was defined as three consecutive PVCs. Now the term is usually reserved for at least four or more beats and modified by the term "nonsustained." Short runs of nonsustained VT may not have serious implications, especially in a patient with a normal heart. Yang and colleagues[44] reported on 55 patients and defined exercise-induced VT as three or more beats and sustained VT as five beats. The mean follow-up was 26 months with a mortality rate of 3.6 or about 18% per year for those with VT and 2.5% per year for those without VT. In my experience, however, nonsustained VT and multiform PVCs in CAD patients are more likely to be associated with more serious implications than in patients with no ectopy.

EXERCISE-INDUCED SUSTAINED VT

Sustained VT on the treadmill is relatively rare in most exercise laboratories, but when testing a group of patients with VT or ventricular fibrillation (VF) as their primary complaint, between 30% and 60% were found to develop VT.[45] Although there are some reports to the contrary, most data suggest that sustained VT or long runs of VT, even though nonsustained, portray serious underlying disease. Because VT often deteriorated into VF, it is obviously a cause for immediate termination of exercise. If the patient converts to sinus rhythm spontaneously very quickly, there is less cause for alarm; however, this rhythm still must be taken very seriously. Either CAD with ischemia or some type of cardiomyopathy should be suspected when VF occurs. Ventricular tachycardia caused by ischemia almost never has a left bundle branch block (LBBB) pattern. In the absence of overt cardiac pathology, after a thorough workup, most VT can be controlled by beta blockers. This was the case in the basketball player Hank Gathers, who unfortunately terminated his treatment with tragic results.

I believe that most adult men with VT associated with exercise have significant CAD, although occasionally they may have some other type of left-ventricular dysfunction. This rhythm is occasionally seen in children and young adults as a relatively benign process. Several subjects under our supervision with severe VT have had either myocardiopathies or very minimal coronary atheroma. In our follow-up study, there was a 12% death rate over a 5-year period in this group, and when the occurrence of VT was analyzed alone, the 5-year mortality rate was 37%. Therefore, we must conclude that the more irritable the ventricle, the more severe the implications.

EXERCISE TESTING TO EVALUATE SPONTANEOUS VT

Exercise testing is an important part of the workup in patients with sudden death or sustained VT. About 30% will develop VT if maximally stressed. Those who have spontaneous VT are less likely to have a ventricular arrhythmia with exercise than those who do not.[46] Although ischemia would seem to be the most likely initiating factor for an exercise-induced VT, it has been reported that measurable ischemia (ST-segment depression) is responsible for the arrhythmia in only about 10% or less.[47] It is also reported that exercise-induced VT correlates poorly with the findings in the electrophysiology laboratory. However, there is a small subset of patients who have VT only during exercise. Some of these patients may be discovered in your stress laboratory, and you must be prepared to treat them effectively.

There are times when patients develop left bundle branch block during testing and at first glance it may be very difficult to differentiate this rhythm from ventricular tachycardia. After exercise is discontinued, a relatively stable blood pressure and a comparison of the heart rate during the arrhythmia with that just prior to its inception will usually help make the correct diagnosis.

ARRHYTHROGENIC RIGHT VENTRICULAR DYSPLASIA

Patients with this abnormality often have VT, at times originated by exercise. The VT always manifests a LBBB pattern and prolongation of the QRS in the right precordial lead is common. Some patients with this syndrome have ST elevation in V2 and V3 during exercise and they often have a family history of sudden death.[48]

IDIOPATHIC RIGHT VENTRICULAR OUTFLOW TACHYCARDIA

This VT is more likely to be nonsustained and is very commonly induced by exercise. These patients are also likely to have many PVC's and coupled PVC's during exercise. They have normal LV function and are more likely to maintain a reasonable blood pressure during VT. The morphology is also a left bundle. An excellent discussion of right ventricular tachycardia has recently been published by Pinski.[49]

Reproducibility of Ventricular Ectopy

It has been experimentally shown that PVCs are frequently seen at the inception of acute ischemia. Thus, exercise-induced PVCs or VT may be an "ischemic equivalent," and good reproducibility would be expected. Unfortunately, this is not the case. Faris and colleagues[50] found that approximately a 50% reproducibility in clinically normal subjects after a 3-year interval was not too surprising. However, Sheps and associates[30] repeated the exercise test after 45 minutes and found that the second test resulted in a significant decrease in irritability. Jelinek and Lown[51] reported a reproducibility of 30% of PVCs and 50% for VT. Thus, when using a stress test to evaluate the efficacy of an antiarrhythmic agent, the degree of unreliability must be kept in mind. An even lower rate of reproducibility in Holter monitoring (10%) was reported by Jelinek and Lown.[51] Ryan and associates[52] and Glasser and coworkers[53] have reported, however, that for the detection of ventricular arrhythmias, Holter monitoring generally outperformed the exercise test. This is probably owing to the fact that many events in daily living besides exercise cause ventricular irritability. These include changes in pH and alterations in vagal and sympathetic tone either with or without the stimulus of emotional factors.

CONDUCTION DISTURBANCES

Exercise initiates a complex set of events that impinge on the conduction system. There is an increase in sympathetic drive and a withdrawal of vagal tone. Sympathetic enhancement of conduction is mediated somewhat by the increased sinus firing rate causing an increased number of impulses arriving at the atrioventricular (AV) node. The fatigue of the conduction tissue as a result of the increased traffic, and a relatively greater segment of the conduction time being occupied by the refractory period, may mitigate the effect of the excess sympathetic influence. In CAD patients, ischemia may also alter the conduction process, depending on its severity and location. In normals at maximum exercise, the PQ interval shortens to about 110 msec. Barrow and Ouer[54] reported that immediately after exercise, the PR interval is either decreased to a greater extent than would be predicted from the heart rate or is independent of the heart rate. Atrial pacing at increased heart rates almost always prolongs the PQ interval, probably because vagal tone is still intact and there is very little increase in sympathetic drive.

First-Degree Atrioventricular Block

First-degree AV block at rest commonly disappears with exercise owing to the vagal withdrawal. The same effect can be induced with atropine.[44] The development of a prolonged PQ segment after exercise has been reported in a patient with triple-vessel disease by Glasser and Clark,[55] who state that they have seen three patients with AV block after exercise in 2000 treadmill examinations. Sandberg[45] describes this phenomenon in two patients who have had myocarditis. This rare finding probably has little clinical significance.

Second-Degree Atrioventricular Block

Lepeschkin and colleagues[56] report a case of type II second-degree AV block after norepinephrine effusion. The absence of this type of abnormality in exercise testing is probably due to the fact that we rarely exercise a patient with a known infectious disease or active rheumatic fever. Bakst's group[57] reports a 74-year-old woman with CAD and a first- and second-degree AV block at rest. Both exercise testing and atropine produced a second-degree type II block. No change in PR interval occurred with either of these maneuvers when the sinus rate exceeded 68 beats per minute. Cases have also been reported by Moulopoulos and Anthopoulos[58] and Goodfriend and Barold.[59] The latter did His' bundle studies and reported the lesions to be above the His' spike and below the AV node. Gilchrist[60] in 1958 pointed out that type I AV block improves with exercise, whereas type II AV block deteriorates. This effect has also been emphasized by Rozanski's group,[61] who state, "an exercise-induced increase in sympathetic drive will enhance conduction through the AV node, but will have no effect on tissue below this level." As previously mentioned, first-degree AV block may be prolonged with atrial pacing at high heart rates until it becomes a second-degree block. Although second-degree AV block probably should be an indication for discontinuing exercise, it is not likely to lead to serious trouble.

Fascicular Block

Left Anterior Division Block

To my knowledge, there are no data on the risk of left anterior division hemiblock with exercise. Oliveros and associates[62] have reported two cases in which exercise-induced left anterior hemiblock was associated with a high-grade paroxysmal left anterior descending coronary lesion. Both patients also had typical ST-segment depression when normal conduction returned during recovery. During the period when hemiblock was evident, however, the ST changes tended to be masked in the frontal plane and to some degree in the precordial leads. Although Oliveros and associates[62] failed to comment on this in their paper, Gergueira-Gomes and colleagues,[63] in a general discussion of hemiblock, emphasized this point. They believe the changes were due to transient ischemia of the septum, because in one case following successful bypass surgery, conduction reverted to normal. In spite of the tendency of the axis shift to mask ischemia, the incidence of a positive test tends to increase when the presence of left anterior hemiblock is established. Miller and coworkers[64] described abnormal exercise test results in 14 of 20 subjects with left-axis deviation who were thought otherwise to be normal. Nine of these subjects had left anterior hemiblock using the criteria of more than a 35° axis. A matched control group with normal axis had an incidence of 40% positive tests for ischemia. This high incidence is rather surprising and makes me suspect that their control patients were a very select group. Mean age of the control group was 50.1, and from the experience in our laboratory, an abnormal response in this age group would be expected to be between 15% and 20%.

Figure 13–8 depicts the tracing of a 66-year-old man who had never experienced any symptoms of CAD. The resting ECG clearly demonstrated left anterior division block. As exercise progressed, temporary alterations in the axis resulted, presumably due to a change in the degree of block from beat to beat. In addition, the R wave in CM_5 diminished and returned toward that recorded at rest and during recovery. The patient experienced no symptoms during the test except for the usual fatigue and dyspnea. The ST-segment elevation in V_1 at rest, which was accentuated by exercise, might have been due to a dyskinetic area or an ischemic area in the septum (Fig. 13–9). ST-segment elevation at rest in V_2 and V_3 accentuated by exercise is usually due to residual anterior wall ischemia in an area of previous infarction.[64]

Left Posterior Hemiblock

Bobba and associates[65] reported four cases in which they proposed that the left posterior hemiblock was initiated by exercise. In their patients, the axis shifted inferiorly and to the right from 0° to approximately 110°. ST-segment depression developed in the classic V_4 and V_5 positions so that the recognition of ischemic changes was similar to that for the patient with a normal axis. The investigators described 4 such cases in 100 subjects, indicating that it

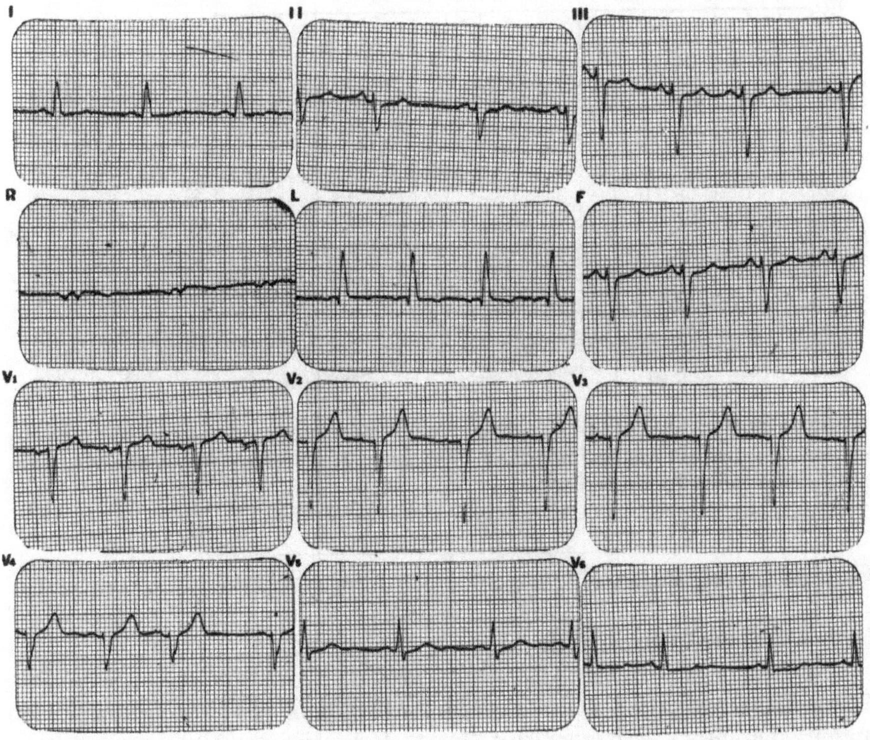

FIGURE 13–8. A resting 12-lead tracing of a 66-year-old asymptomatic man with a left anterior division hemiblock.

may not be unusual. No recent reports describing the prevalence of this finding have been discovered.

Congenital Long QT Syndrome

There is a rare group of young patients who suddenly pass out due to a spontaneous ventricular tachycardia and often have family members who have died suddenly. The long QT syndrome (LQTS) is an inherited disease whereby patients have a long QT interval due to genes encoding the cardiac ion channels that produce repolarizing current of the action potential. An abnormality in the inward and outward transmembrane potential can trigger polymorphic ventricular tachycardia.

At times these patients have a borderline QT interval at rest but exercise will usually resolve at a marked prolongation.[66] Thus, one of the ways to diagnose these patients, besides looking at their genotype, especially on chromosome 7, is to do a standard exercise test recognizing that there is some risk of initiating ventricular tachycardia (See Figure 13–10).[67]

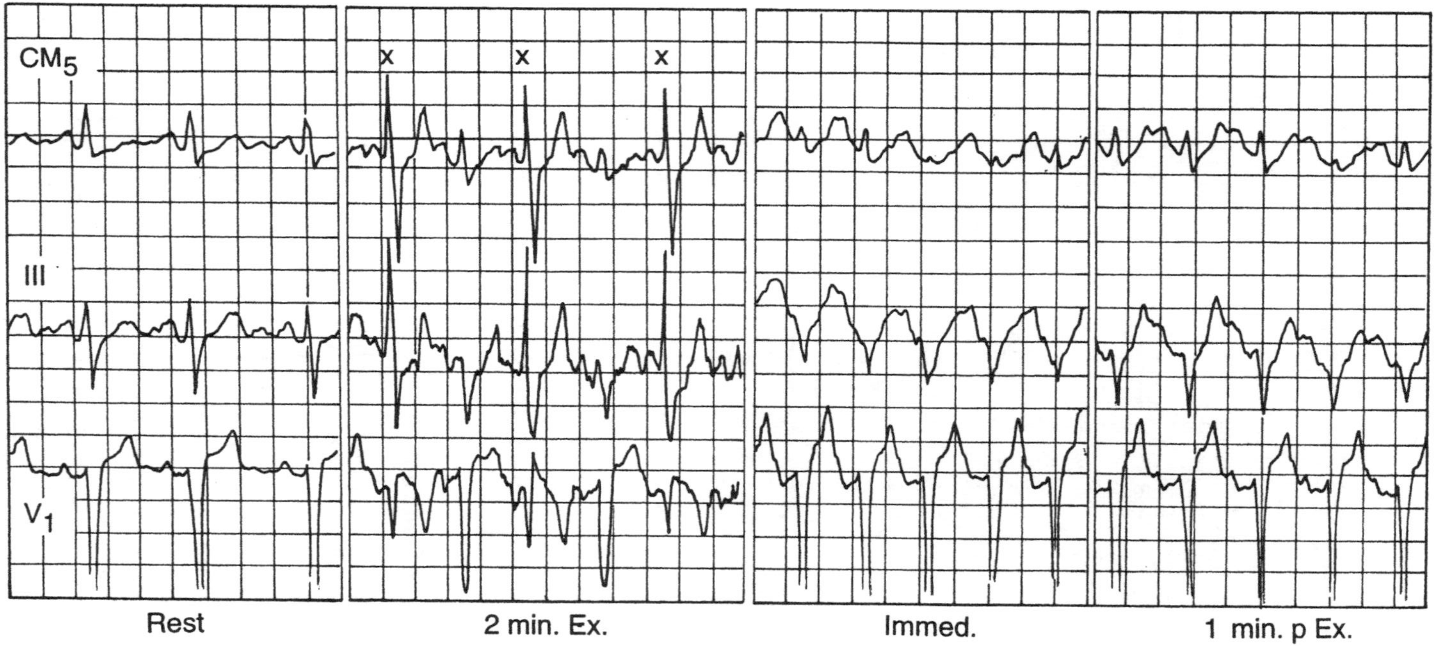

FIGURE 13–9. The exercise tracing of the man in Figure 13–5. With exercise, he developed intermittent alterations in axis deviation and ST-segment elevation in V_1 with exercise.

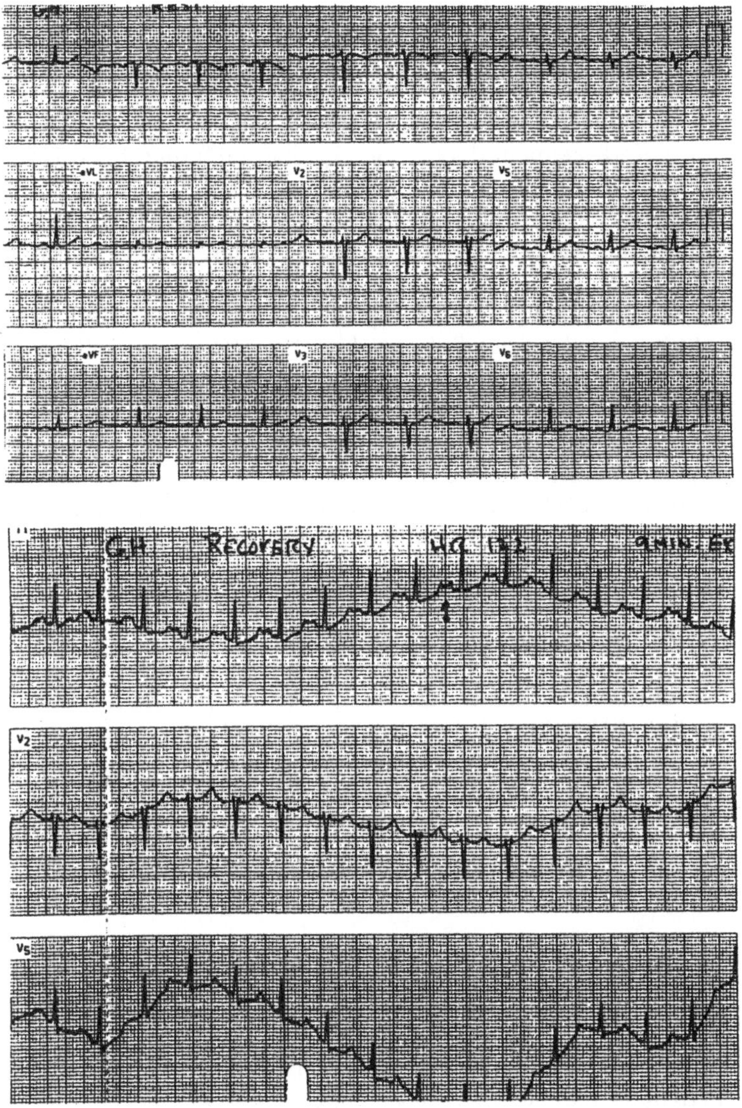

FIGURE 13–10. (A) Resting ECG of a 40 year old male with a strong family history of LQTS. QTc is borderline at 447 milliseconds. Two older brothers died in childhood suddenly and his mother experienced syncope as a child multiple times although she died of cancer at the age of 66. One month prior to this study, the patient and his wife celebrated the birth of a daughter whose QTc ws measured at 472 milliseconds. (B) Treadmill exercise ECG of the same patient after 9 minutes of exercise on the Bruce protocol. QTc is markedly prolonged at 500 milliseconds. Chronotropic incompetence is also evident—a maximum heart rate of 122 beats per minute was achieved (68% of predicted). The QTc actually prolonged further to 519 milliseconds 2 minutes into recovery. The patient was put on prophylactic beta-blockers.

Rate-Related Bundle Branch Block

Sandberg[45] studied nine cases of bundle branch block initiated by exercise, two of which were right bundle branch block (RBBB). In the young subjects (aged 30 to 40), the onset of the block appeared only at high workloads and in the absence of ST-segment depression. Sandberg felt that this was not associated with CAD and produced little change in function. He also found that bundle branch block could be caused by means other than exercise, such as the administration of amyl nitrate or atropine. There did not appear to be an exact heart rate or RR interval at which the patient would shift to a block pattern, but there was definitely a range after which this would invariably occur. The term *rate-related bundle branch block* has often implied the absence of significant coronary or myocardial pathology. Like so many findings in medicine, it cannot be judged without taking the total clinical picture into consideration. Evidence now suggests that in patients in the coronary age group, this process is often due to ischemia.[65] It was Sandberg's belief that in older subjects with CAD, the block would occur at slower heart rates.[45] Wayne and colleagues[68] however, found that 14 to 16 patients with "rate-related bundle branch blocks" had evidence strongly suggestive of CAD. Their patients' average age was 59. Eleven had left bundle branch block (LBBB) and five had RBBB.

Whenever a block pattern spontaneously occurs during exercise or with hyperventilation, one should consider the possibility of Wolff-Parkinson-White (WPW) syndrome. It is very important to recognize WPW syndrome because the ST-segment depression in this condition does not mean ischemic heart disease and the short PQ wave and delta wave are easy to overlook. Kattus[69] described a patient with variable RBBB who had ischemia in the normally conducted complexes, but not in those with the block pattern.

Right Bundle Branch Block

The reliability of exercise-induced ST-segment depression as a predictor of ischemia in patients with RBBB has been debated.[70] Most investigators argue that although the wide S wave makes the identification of the J-point somewhat more difficult, changes in the lateral precordial leads should be reliable.[70,71] Possibly the sensitivity is less satisfactory with this abnormality. Tanaka and coworkers[71] make the point that the ST depression must be manifested in the lateral precordial or similar leads to have significance. Several of their patients with normal coronary arteries had ST depression in V_1 to V_3. Kattus[69] also has made this point. In our laboratory, we have seen many patients with RBBB develop ST-segment depression with exercise. The 51-year-old man whose ECG is depicted in Figure 13–11 exhibits this finding. He had suffered two previous myocardial infarctions and exhibited ST-segment de-

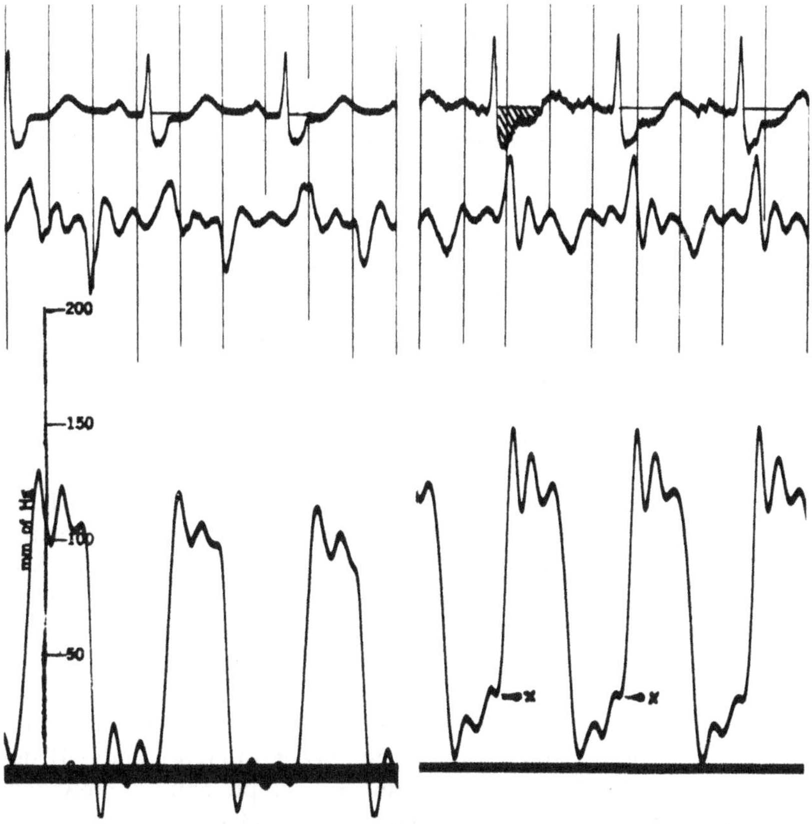

FIGURE 13–11. Resting and exercise left-ventricular pressures in a 51-year-old-man with advanced three-vessel disease by angiography. Note the increase in the LVEDP associated with ST-segment depression in a subject with RBBB. The wide S wave encroaches on the ST segment.

pression and experienced anginal pain immediately after exercise and during cardiac catheterization. Elevation of left-ventricular end-diastolic pressure (LVEDP) can be seen to correlate with the ST-segment depression.[72] Although the QRS is wide in RBBB, the total QT interval is not significantly prolonged. Therefore, the duration of the ST-segment depression is relatively shorter in RBBB because the wide S wave in CM_5 or in the lateral precordial lead encroaches on the ST segment.

Even so, RBBB, in contradistinction to LBBB, may (but usually does not) mask ischemic changes, at least in CM_5 or V_5.[73] ST depression in V_2 and V_3 is often seen in patients with RBBB without ischemia, probably because of repolarization changes secondary to the wide R prime often present in these leads (see Figure 13–11).

TAKE HOME MESSAGE

ST depression in leads V^2 and V^3 in patients with right bundle branch block *is not* ischemia. ST depression in V^5 and V^6 *is* ischemia.

Left Bundle Branch Block

In general, LBBB tends to be associated with decreased left-ventricular function and a poor prognosis. In patients who have LBBB alternating with normal conduction, the function of the ventricle during the beats associated with the block have been demonstrated to be less effective in subjects with reduced left-ventricular function. This has been shown, at least in congestive heart failure patients, to be due to dysynergy between the septum and the left ventricular free wall and an increase in mitral insufficiency.[74] This may be due to degenerative changes in the conduction system and not associated with CAD per se. It can also be due to myocarditis, severe left-ventricular hypertrophy, or myocardiopathy. Under such circumstances, the ECG changes associated with stress are difficult to evaluate with certainty. In asymptomatic symptomatic subjects, the stroke output and other measurements of left-ventricular function may at times be near-normal[75] (Fig. 13–12).

Cooksey and colleagues[76] report that if an ST depression of 1.5 mm more than at rest occurred with exercise, CAD should be suspected. Whinnery and Froelicher[73] on the other hand, found no significant difference in the ST depression of those with CAD when analyzing 31 asymptomatic air crewmen. Orzan and associates[77] studied 30 patients with CAD and 27 without and also found the ST-depression change with exercise to be of little value in identification. In their discussion, they commented that anginal pain was rarely associated with significant ST change and suggested that in LBBB the ST depression is probably not a manifestation of ischemia. Discussions of the possible electrophysiological reasons for these findings can be found in the work of Walston and colleagues[78] and Abildskov.[79] Gibbons[80] and the ACC Guidelines Committee have stated that ST depression has no diagnostic value in patients with LBBB.

In lead V_5, a fair number of patients with LBBB have a positive rather than a negative T wave. In these patients, the ST segments become more and more depressed during progressive exercise. This may be a reflection of decreased left-ventricular function, a higher filling pressure, or merely a secondary repolarization abnormality. This phenomenon often occurs in patients with hypertensive or idiopathic cardiomyopathies and may even occur when the disease is localized in the bundle itself. It is now well established that it is possible to recognize an acute myocardial infarction with left bundle branch block[81] and I believe it should be possible to identify criteria that correlate with ischemia. Although there is no consensus, we found that a significant decrease in ST segments in lead 2 has the sensitivity of 75% and specificity of 86%. Confirmations of our findings have not yet been published however.[82]

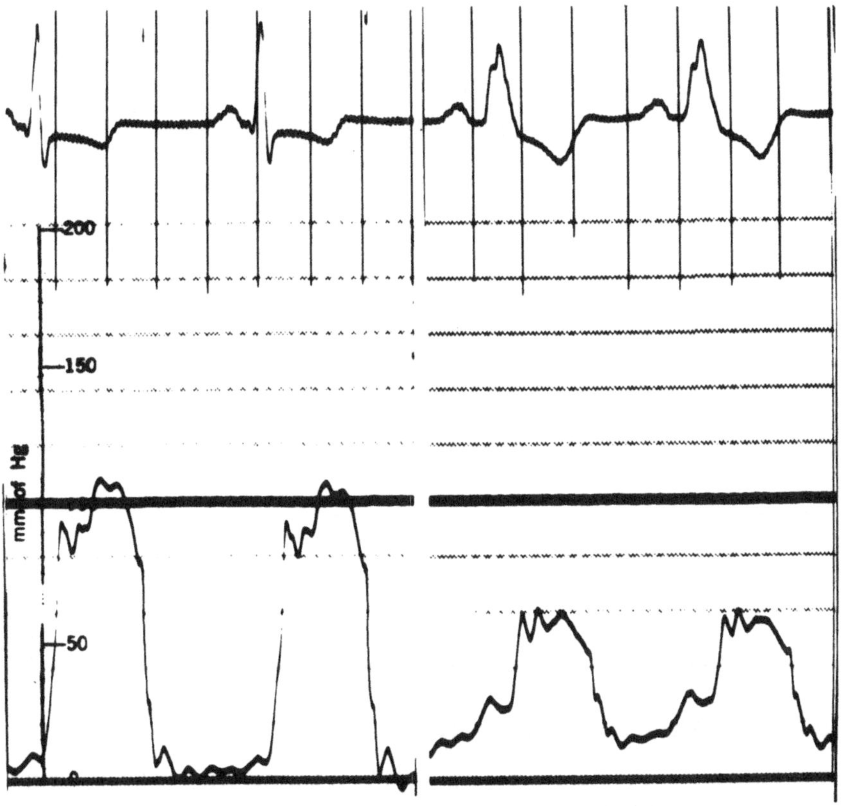

FIGURE 13–12. Left-ventricular tracings taken during catheterization in a 56-year-old-man. LBBB suddenly developed after the catheter was placed in the left ventricle. The decrease in left-ventricular systolic pressure and the increase in the LVEDP in the tracing on the right indicated a severe decrease in function.

There are times when patients with LBBB develop ST-segment depression that is clearly due to ischemia, either in the presence or absence of exercise.[4] A number of patients with normal ventricular conduction at rest develop LBBB during stress testing. They may or may not have CAD. Figure 13–13 illustrates the ECG of a patient who had LBBB not only with a stress test, but also after administration of atropine. The coronary angiograms of this patient were perfectly normal, although there was mild evidence of left-ventricular dysfunction as indicated by LVEDP elevations after angiography. The report of Wayne and colleagues,[68] previously mentioned, supports the growing trend to suspect ischemia in these patients. Bellet and associates[83] reported on a patient with LBBB at rest who maintained a normal pattern during exercise and reverted to LBBB during recovery. They claim that the patient had clear-cut hypertensive arteriosclerotic heart disease with congestive failure. I have seen one patient with LBBB, who was shown to have normal coronary arteries and good left-ventricular function, consistently convert to a normal pattern

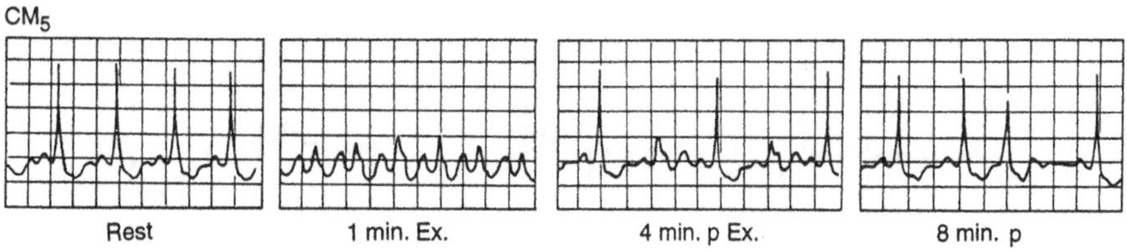

FIGURE 13–13. Exercise tracing of a 44-year-old woman who developed LBBB with exercise. Subsequent coronary angiography revealed normal vessels and left-ventricular function.

with exercise. A report by Lee and colleagues[84] suggests that R-wave changes may be useful in identifying CAD in patients with LBBB. Confirmation of their data needs to be published, however. The concept that patients who convert to LBBB at low heart rates are more likely to have CAD than those who convert at high heart rates has not been confirmed in our experience.

TAKE HOME MESSAGE

There is a consensus as stated in the ACC/AHA guidelines, that one cannot diagnose exercise-induced ischemia in patients with left bundle branch block from the EKG. I suspect this is an error.

Third-Degree Atrioventricular Block

In older patients with known or suspected CAD, third-degree heart block at rest should be a relative contraindication to stress testing. His' bundle electrograms demonstrate that the block may be proximal to, within, or distal to the His' spike. Congenital block is usually proximal to the His' bundle, and even in acquired block this location may have a lesser risk to the patient during exercise. No data to support this contention are available in acquired disease, however. It is well known that when patients with CAD develop complete AV block, the prognosis is poor. Whether or not this is the case in pre-His' bundle blocks is not known. On the other hand, if it is a congenital block or is present in vigorous younger patients with no other evidence of heart disease, testing may be done (Fig. 13–14). If patients develop complete AV block during exercise testing, exercise should be terminated immediately.

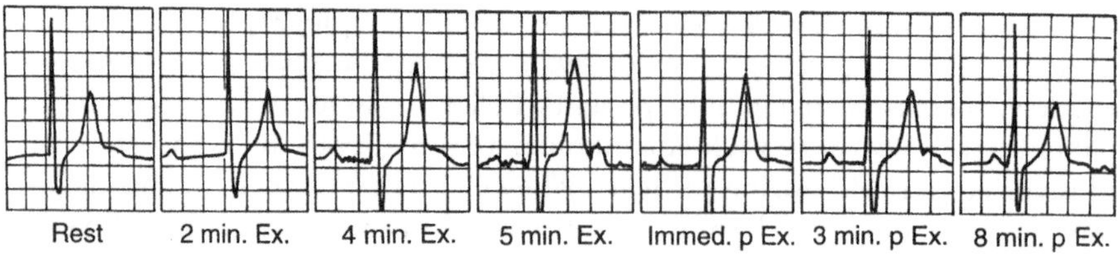

FIGURE 13–14. Tracings from a 23-year-old man with congenital heart block. The T-wave amplitude increases as exercise progresses.

ACCELERATED CONDUCTION (WPW SYNDROME)

It is now well established that patients with WPW syndrome have ST-segment depression when the accelerated conduction pathway intervenes. When accelerated conduction occurs intermittently, the changes in the ST-segment depression can be seen associated with each delta wave. A few isolated reports of coronary angiographic data on such patients have demonstrated normal coronary arteries.[85] Sandberg[45] reported 35 instances of patients with preexcitation syndrome who underwent exercise tests. He found that exercise may bring on the delta wave and preexcitation, may cause disappearance of the syndrome with a return during recovery, or may not affect the presence or absence of the syndrome at all. In two of Sandberg's patients, both in their 50s, this phenomenon was initiated by exercise. He suggested that these patients had acquired WPW syndrome because of CAD or some other myocardial dysfunction. In our laboratory, we occasionally see WPW syndrome initiated by exercise. Several of our patients underwent coronary angiography and had a normal coronary tree. Gazes[85] reported that 20 of 23 patients with WPW syndrome had ST-segment depression of 1.0 mm or more after exercise. We have also seen it initiated by hyperventilation.

The tracings in Figure 13–15 depict the stress test of a 46-year-old man with resting accelerated conduction who had ST-segment depression during exercise, even though the abnormal conduction pathways could not be recognized when the heart rate became rapid.

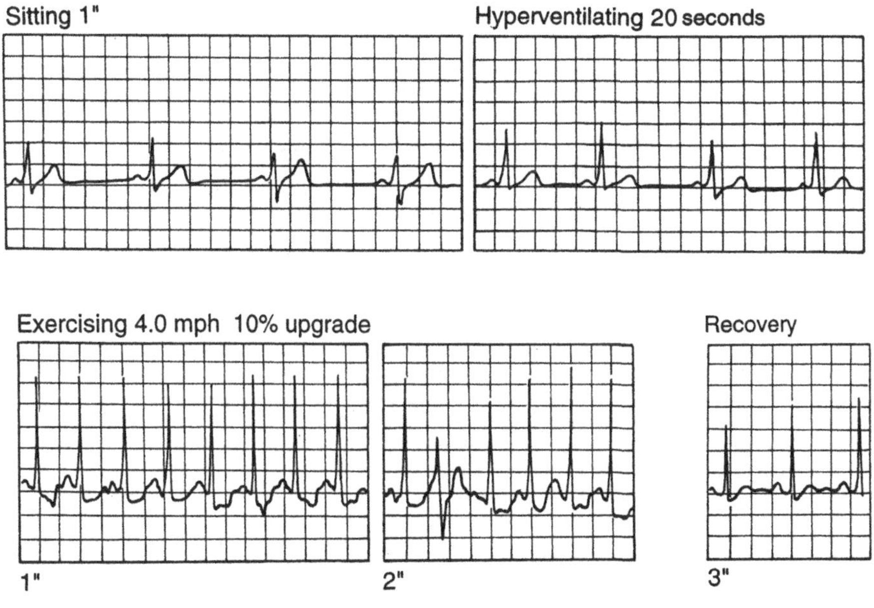

FIGURE 13–15. Exercise tracings of a 46-year-old man with normal coronary arteries manifesting ST-segment depression with exercise, and accelerated conduction at rest.

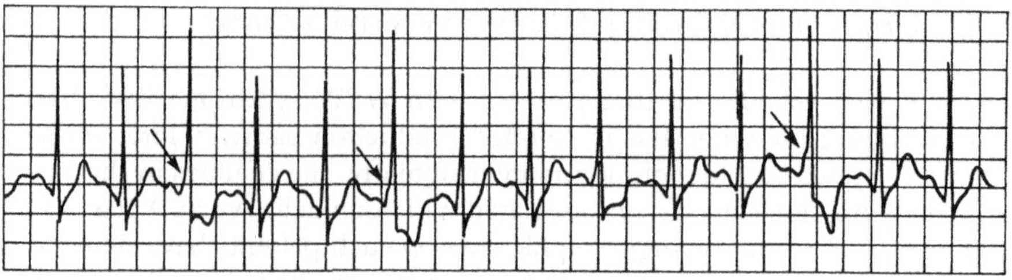

FIGURE 13–16. Tracing of a 52-year-old man illustrating transient WPW syndrome and ST-segment depression associated with each complex that exhibits a delta wave.

The preexcitation syndrome may be initiated in young patients whenever they exercise sufficiently; it is almost invariably associated with ST-segment depression. The exercise performance and aerobic capacity for Sandberg's patients were perfectly normal, suggesting that there were probably only minimal coronary abnormalities within the group. We have never seen a patient with WPW syndrome develop supraventricular tachycardia on the treadmill even though those with the disease have a history of attacks at unexpected times. Patients with accelerated conduction initiated by exercise should be considered to be free of CAD unless they have angina or other significant risk factors. (Fig. 13–16).

SUMMARY

Exercise-induced arrhythmias and conduction disturbances are abnormal in most cases. As with other findings during stress testing, however, they must be viewed in light of other clinical findings in each patient. In most patients who come to stress testing, these arrhythmias are potential causes for concern, but in special cases such as endurance athletes, especially young ones, certain of the arrhythmias have no clinical significance, even though concern may be engendered in both the examining physician and the patient (see Chapter 20).

REFERENCES

1. Bigger, JT Jr, et al: Ventricular arrhythmias in ischemic heart disease: Mechanism, prevalence, significance and management. Prog Cardiovasc Dis 19:255, 1977.
2. Faris, JV, et al: Prevalence and reproducibility of exercise-induced ventricular arrhythmias during maximal exercise testing in normal men. Am J Cardiol 37:617, 1976.
3. Busby, MJ, et al: Prevalence and long-term significance of exercise-induced frequent or repetitive ventricular ectopic beats in apparently healthy volunteers. ACC 14(7):1659, 1989.
4. Young, DZ, et al: Safety of maximal exercise testing in patients at high risk for ventricular arrhythmia. Circulation 70:184, 1984.
5. Ellestad, MH and Wan, MKC: Predictive implications of stress testing: follow-up of 2700 subjects after maximum treadmill stress testing. Circulation 51:363, 1975.

6. Chib, CF, et al: Chronotropic incompetence in exercise testing. Clin Cardiol 2:12, 1979.
7. Abbott, JA, et al: Graded exercises testing in patients with sinus node dysfunction. Am J Med 62:330, 1977.
8. Brener, SJ, et al: Chronotropic response to exercise predicts angiographic severity in patients with suspected or stable coronary artery disease. Am J Cardiol 76: 1228, 1995.
9. Lauer, MS, et al: Impaired heart rate response to graded exercise: prognostic implications of chronotropic incompetence in the Framingham Heart Study. Circulation 93:1520, 1996.
10. Ellestad, MH. Chronotropic incompetence: the implications of heart rate response to exercise (compensatory parasympathetic hyperactivity?) Circulation 93:1485, 1996.
11. Astrand, I. Exercise electrocardiograms recorded twice during an 8 year period. Acta Med. Scand 178:27, 1965.
12. Myrianthiefs, MM, et al: False positive ST-segment depression during exercise in subjects with short PR segment and angiographically normal coronaries. J of Electrocard 31(13):203, 1998.
13. Lewis, T: Fibrillation of the auricles: Its effects upon the circulation. J Exp Med 16:395, 1912.
14. Kaplan, MA, et al: Metabolic and homodynamic responses to exercise during atrial fibrillation and sinus rhythm. Am J Cardiol 22:543, 1968.
15. Killip, T and Baer, RA: Hemodynamic effects after reversion from atrial fibrillation to sinus rhythm by precordial shock. J. Clin Invest 45:658, 1966.
16. Jelinek, MV and Lown, B: Exercise testing for exposure of cardiac arrhythmia. Prog Cardiovasc Dis 16:497, 1974.
17. McHenry, PL: Clinical role of exercise testing for detection, evaluation, and treatment of ventricular arrhythmias. In Zipes, D and Jalife, RB (eds): Cardiac Electrophysiology: From the Cell to Bedside. WB Saunders, Philadelphia, p 832, 1990.
18. Michaelides, AP, et al: Significance of ST segment depression in exercise-induced supraventricular extrasystoles. Am Heart J 117:1035, 1989.
19. Michaelides, AP, et al: Significance of R wave changes in exercise-induced supraventricular extrasystoles. J Electrocardiol 26:197, 1993.
20. Graboys, TB and Wright, RF: Provocation of supraventricular tachycardia during exercise stress testing. Cardiovasc Rev Rep 1 (1):57, 1980.
21. Gough, AS: Exercise testing for detecting changes in cardiac rhythm and conduction. Am J Cardiol 30:741, 1972.
22. Mauer, MS, et al: Exercise induced supraventricular tachycardia in apparently healthy volunteers {abstract}. J Am Coll Cardiol 19:35A, 1992.
23. Fisher, FD and Tyroler, HA: Relationship between ventricular premature contractions in routine electrocardiograms and subsequent death from coronary heart disease. Circulation 47:712, 1963.
24. Goldschlager, N, et al: Treadmill stress tests as indicators of presence and severity of coronary artery disease. Ann Intern Med 85:277, 1976.
25. Rodstein, M, et al: A mortality study of the significance of extrasystoles in an insured population. Trans Assoc Life Ins Med Dir Am 54:91, 1971.
26. Lown, B and Wolf, M: Approaches to sudden death from coronary heart disease. Circulation 44:130, 1971.
27. Alexander, S, et al: Resting PVCs and their influence on mortality. Am Cardiol Conference, February 1973.
28. Buckingham, TA, et al: The clinical significance of ventricular arrhythmias in apparently healthy subjects. Pract Cardiol 9(8): 37, 1983.
29. Udall, JA and Ellestad, MH: Predictive implications of ventricular premature contractions associated with treadmill stress testing: A follow-up of 6,500 patients after maximum treadmill stress testing. Circulation 56:985, 1977.
30. Sheps, DC, et al: Decreased frequency of exercise induced ventricular ectopic activity in the second of two consecutive treadmill tests. Circulation 55:892, 1977.
31. McHenry, PL, et al: Exercise induced arrhythmia: Recognition, classification, and clinical significance. Cardiovasc Clin 6:245, 1974.
32. Froelicher, VF, et al: Epidemiologic study of asymptomatic men screened by maximal treadmill testing for latent coronary artery disease. Am J Cardiol 34:770, 1974.
33. Jouven, X, et al: Long-term outcome in asymptomatic men with exercise-induced premature ventricular depolarizations. N Engl J Med 343:826, 2000.
34. Weiner, DA, et al: Ventricular arrhythmias during exercise testing: Mechanisms, response to coronary bypass surgery and prognostic significance. Am J Cardiol 53:1553, 1984.

35. Sami, M, et al: Significance of exercise induced ventricular arrhythmias in stable coronary disease. Am J Cardiol 54:1182, 1984.
36. Califf, RM, et al: Prognostic value of ventricular arrhythmias associated with treadmill exercise testing patients studied with cardiac catheterization for suspected ischemic heart disease. J Am Coll Cardiol (6):1060, 1983.
37. McHenry, PL, et al: Comparative studies of exercise-induced ventricular arrhythmias in normal subjects and in patients with documented coronary artery disease. Am J Cardiol 37:609, 1976.
38. Gough, AS and McConnell, D: Analysis of transient arrhythmias and conduction disturbances occurring during submaximal treadmill exercise testing. Prog Cardiovasc Dis XIII(3):293, 1970.
39. Marieb, MA, et al: Clinical relevance of exercise-induced ventricular arrhythmias in suspected coronary disease. Am J Cardiol 66:172, 1990.
40. Bourne, G: An attempt at the clinical classification of premature ventricular beats. QJ Med 20:219, 1977.
41. Helfant, RH, et al: Exercise related ventricular premature complexes in coronary heart disease. Ann Intern Med 80:589, 1974.
42. Dimsdale, J: Etiology of post exercise sudden death. Discover 514:10, 1994.
43. Rasouli, ML and Ellestad, MH. Usefulness of ST depression in ventricular premature complexes to predict myocardial ischemia. Am J Cardiol 87:891, 2001.
44. Yang, JC, et al: Ventricular tachycardia during routine treadmill testing. Arch Intern Med 151:349, 1991.
45. Sandberg, L: Studies in electrocardiogram changes during exercise tests. Acta Med Scand (suppl)169:365, 1969.
46. Graboys, TB, et al: Long term survival of patients with malignant ventricular arrhythmias. Am J Cardiol 50:437, 1982.
47. Castle, LW, et al: Ventricular fibrillation and coronary atherosclerosis with normal maximal exercise test: Report of a case. Cleve Clin Q 39:163, 1973.
48. Towbin, JA, et al: Genetics of Brugada, long QT, and arrhythmogenic right ventricular dysplasia syndromes. J Electrocaridogr 33(suppl): 11, 2000.
49. Pinski, SL. The right ventricular tachycardias. J Electrocardiol, 33:103, 2000.
50. Faris, JV, et al: Prevalence and reproducibility of exercise-induced ventricular arrhythmias during maximal exercise testing in normal men. Am J Cardiol 37:617, 1976.
51. Jelinek, MV and Lown, B: Exercise stress testing for exposure of cardiac arrhythmia. Prog Cardiovasc Dis 16:497, 1974.
52. Ryan, M, et al: Comparison of ventricular ectopic activity during 24 hour monitoring and exercise testing in patients with coronary heart disease [abstract]. N Engl J Med 292:224, 1975.
53. Glasser, SP, et al: The occurrence of frequent complex arrhythmias detected by ambulatory monitoring in a healthy elderly population. Chest 75:565, 1979.
54. Barrow, WH and Ouer, RA: Electrocardiographic changes with exercise: Their relation to age and other factors. Arch Intern Med 71:547, 1943.
55. Glasser, SP and Clark, PI: The Clinical Approach to Exercise Testing. Harper & Row, New York, p 158, 1980.
56. Lepeschkin, E, et al: Effect of nifedipine and norepinephrine on the electrocardiograms of 100 normal subjects. Am J Cardiol 5:594, 1960.
57. Bakst, A, et al: Significance of exercise-induced second degree atrioventricular block. Br Heart J 37:984, 1975.
58. Moulopoulos, SD and Anthopoulos, LP: Reversible atrio-ventricular conduction changes during exercise. Acta Cardiol (Brux) 23:352, 1968.
59. Goodfriend, MA, and Barold, SS: Tachycardia-dependent and bradycardia-dependent Mobitz type II atrioventricular block within the bundle of HIS. Am J Cardiol 33:908, 1974.
60. Gilchrist, AR: Clinical aspects of high-grade heart block. Scott Med J 3:53, 1958.
61. Rozanski, JJ, et al: Paroxysmal second degree atrioventricular block induced by exercise. Heart Lung 9(5):887, 1980.
62. Oliveros, RS, et al: Intermittent left anterior hemiblock during treadmill exercise test. Chest 72:492, 1977.
63. Gergueira-Gomes, M, et al: Repolarization changes in left anterior hemi block. Adv Cardiol 14:148, 1975.

64. Miller, AB, et al: Left axis deviation: Diagnostic contribution of exercise stress testing. Chest 63:159, 1973.
65. Bobba, P, et al: Transient left posterior hemiblock: Report of four cases induced by exercise test. Circulation 44:931, 1972.
66. Arab, D, et al: usefulness of the QTc interval in predicting myocardial ischemia in patients undergoing exercise stress testing. Am J Cardiol 85:764, 2000.
67. Vincent, GM, et al: The inherited long QT syndrome: From ion channel to bedside. Cardiology in Review 7:44, 1999.
68. Wayne, VS, et al: Exercise induced bundle branch block. Am J Cardiol 52:283, 1983.
69. Kattus, AA: Exercise electrocardiography. Recognition of the ischemic response: False positive and negative patterns. Am J Cardiol 33:726, 1974.
70. Johnson, S, et al: The diagnostic accuracy of exercise ECG testing in the presence of complete RBBB [abstract]. Circulation 51,52(111):48, 1975.
71. Tanaka, T, et al: Diagnostic value of exercise-induced ST segment depression in patients with RBBB. Am J Cardiol 41:670,1978.
72. Johnson, S, et al: The diagnostic accuracy of exercise ECG testing in the presence of complete RBBB [abstract]. Circulation 51,52(111):48, 1975.
73. Whinnery, JE and Froelicher, V: Acquired BBB and its response to exercise testing in asymptomatic air crewmen: A review with case reports. Aviat Space Environ Med 43:1217, 1976.
74. Stellbrink, C, et al: Impact of cardiac resynchronization therapy using hemodynamically optimized pacing on left ventricular remodeling in patients with congestive heart failure and ventricular conduction disturbances. JACC 38(7):1957, 2001.
75. Goodfriend, MA, and Barold, SS: Tachycardia-dependent and bradycardia-dependent Mobitz type II atrioventricular block within the bundle of HIS. Am J Cardiol 33:908, 1974.
76. Cooksey, JD, et al: The diagnostic contribution of exercise testing in left bundle branch block. Am Heart J 88:482, 1974.
77. Orzan, F, et al: Is the treadmill exercise test useful for evaluating coronary artery disease in patients with complete LBBB? Am J Cardiol 42:36, 1978.
78. Walston, AL, et al: Relationship between ventricular depolarization and the QRS in right and left BBB. J Electrocardiol 1:55, 1968.
79. Abildskov, JA: Effects of activation sequence on the local recovery of ventricular excitability in the dog. Circ Res 38:240, 1976.
80. Gibbons, RJ, et al: ACC/AHA guidelines for exercise testing: A report of the American College of Cardiology/American Heart Association task force on practice guidelines (committee on exercise testing). ACC/AHA, 1997.
81. Sgarbossa, EB, et al: Electrocardiographic diagnosis of evolving acute myocardial infarction in the presence of left bundle branch block. N Engl J Med 334:48;1996.
82. Ibrahim, NS, et al: Detecting exercise-induced ischemia in left bundle branch block using the electrocardiogram. Am J Cardiol 82:832, 1998.
83. Bellet, S, et al: Radioelectrocardiographic changes during strenuous exercise in normal subjects. Circulation 25:686, 1962.
84. Lee, G, et al: Accuracy of left precordial R wave analysis during exercise testing in reliably detecting coronary disease in LBBB patients. Am J Cardiol 52:876, 1983.
85. Gazes, PC: False positive exercise test in the presence of Wolff-Parkinson-White syndrome. Am Heart J 78:13, 1969.

14
Predictive Implications

Bayes' Theorem
Sensitivity and Specificity
Sensitivity
Specificity
Predictive Value and Relative Risk
Disease Prevalence
Effect of Prevalence on Exercise-Induced ST Depression
Critique of Bayes' Theorem
Population Groups
Limited Challenge
Correlation of ST Depression with Coronary Angiography
False-Positive Tests
False-Negative Tests
Long-Term Follow-up Studies
Master's Test
Memorial Medical Center Follow-Up Study—1975
Duke Study—1978
Heart Watch—1980
CASS Study—1982
Cooper Clinic Study—2000
VA Study
Time of Onset of ST-Segment Depression
Magnitude of ST-Segment Depression
Time of Recovery from ST-Segment Depression
Poor Chronotropic Response
Delta Heart Rate
Heart Rate Recovery
Anginal Pain
Exercise Duration
Effect of Age
Effect of Previous Myocardial Infarction
Exercise Test Scores
Multivariate Analysis
The Duke Score
Froelicher Score
Morise Score
Comments About Manipulation of Data to Produce Scores

Prediction of disease is one of the primary functions of stress testing. We would like to be able to predict in each patient:

1. The anatomical condition of the coronary arteries
2. The functional status of the heart
3. The ultimate outcome of the patient as influenced by the above two parameters

It is commonly but erroneously assumed that items 2 and 3 are easy to determine when we know item 1. So many factors influence the outcome of any given patient with clinically significant coronary artery disease (CAD) that knowing the anatomical condition of the coronary arteries as assessed by the angiogram may give very little information about items 2 and 3, especially if we are only examining the coronary angiogram. We should not be too surprised when a patient with a normal maximum exercise test suddenly has an infarction or ventricular fibrillation a few weeks later. Although this occurs infrequently, the dynamic nature of coronary atheroma certainly can result in sudden reductions in perfusion with all the attendant dramatic sequelae. In this chapter, I present some of the concepts necessary to understand how information derived from stress testing can be used to predict the patient's outcome.

One of the difficulties in interpreting a diagnostic report stems from the fact that many of us are not used to being precise in our statements. We know that very few tests are 100% reliable, but we rarely stop to consider just how reliable our tests are. Unfortunately, limited data prevent us from deriving a high degree of certainty from stress testing in its present form. Most of us combine so many different variables in arriving at the final conclusion that it should be called a "consultation" rather than a "test." However, if we limit our discussion to ST-segment depression, about which there is a great deal of information, we can illustrate some important principles. There is a tendency by most doctors to ignore a good deal of the information available in the literature.

BAYES' THEOREM

Bayes' theorem is a mathematical rule that relates the interpretation of present observation to past experience (Fig. 14–1). It relates the probability of disease (pretest probability) in the patient before the test is performed to the probability of disease after the test (post-test probability).[1] This is best understood by considering Figure 14–2. If the pretest probability of disease in question is 10% and the information content (power of the test to increase information) is known to be 50%, for example, then we can calculate the post-test uncertainty or, conversely, the probability.

In Figure 14–2, the information content of the test is 50%, leaving us with a post-test probability of 60% or a remaining uncertainty of 40%. The information content varies with the nature of the test and the prevalence of disease in the population under study, which also determines the pretest probability.[2] Therefore, the information content of a test varies to some degree according to the individual being tested. This concept may be difficult for some clinicians because we think in terms of individual patients and consider the test's value to be intrinsic to the test. If we use Bayes' theorem, we consider the test in the context of the population to which the patient belongs. By collating data from large population studies, Diamond and Forrester[3] estimated the information gained by the discovery that 1 mm of ST-segment depression varies according to the type of chest pain because of the difference in the pretest probability. Thus, the information gained or diagnostic

PAST EXPERIENCE + PRESENT OBSERVATIONS = FUTURE INTERPRETATION

FIGURE 14–1. Bayes' theorem.

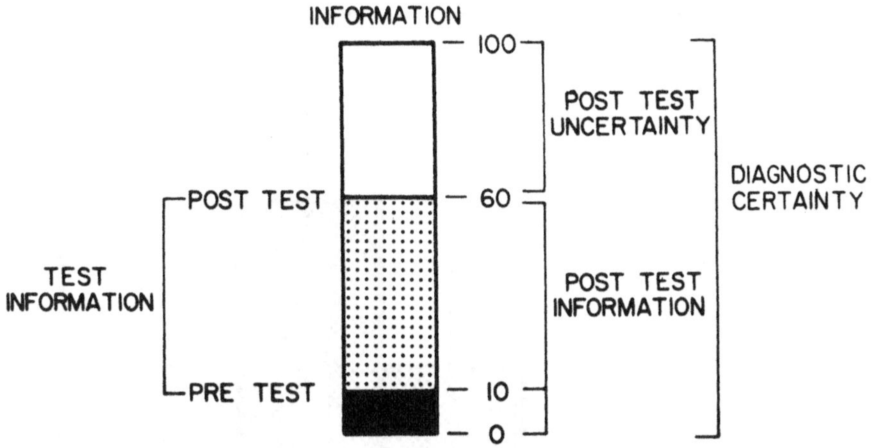

FIGURE 14–2. The total information about the patient's diagnosis is depicted by the bar. It is divided into pretest *(black)*, which is the probability of disease as estimated from clinical data; the test information *(stippled)*, which represents the increase in information supplied by the diagnostic test; and the uncertainty after the test is finished, which is the diagnostic difference between the post-test probability or post-test information content and 100%. (From Diamond et al,[2] by permission of the American Heart Association, Inc.)

use is five times more in a subject with atypical angina than in a subject without symptoms and two and one-half times that of someone with typical angina (Fig. 14–3).

The diagnostic use of the stress test is highest when applied to a population in which the diagnosis is most uncertain. ST depression in patients with typical angina adds little because this group already has a high likelihood of CAD.

For the purpose of this discussion, we will assume that the prevalence of disease is accurate in each of the pain categories described by Diamond and Forrester. We know, of course, that the prevalence of disease in each of these categories would also be influenced by sex, age, cholesterol, family history, smoking habits, and other determinants.[4]

SENSITIVITY AND SPECIFICITY

We have accepted the coronary angiogram as the gold standard in determining the presence of CAD. Most of the literature assumes that a coronary artery obstruction of 70% or greater is significant and one that is less than 70% is not significant. Although this is highly arbitrary and is probably only partly true, we will accept it for now in order to explain the principle. A group of patients studied by angiography and exercise testing can be categorized by means of the contingency table (Table 14–1).

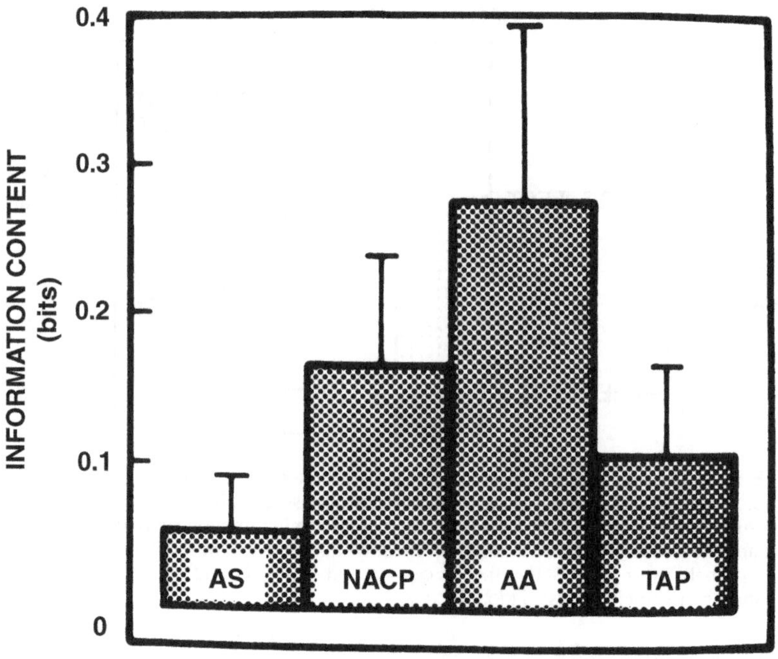

FIGURE 14–3. The pretest information content (equivalent to the black part of the bar in Fig. 14–2) according to the patient's symptoms. AS = asymptomatic; NACP = nonanginal chest pain; AA = atypical angina; TAP = typical anginal pain. Atypical angina is a very reliable symptom and thus starts with the largest pretest probability. (From Diamond, et al,[2] with permission.)

Sensitivity

Sensitivity is the measure of reliability in identifying the presence of disease or the percentage of patients with an abnormal stress test* out of all those studied with significant CAD.

$$\text{Sensitivity} = \frac{\text{Patients with abnormal stress tests and abnormal angiograms}}{\text{All patients with abnormal angiograms}} \times 100$$

True-positives = Patients with both abnormal stress tests and abnormal angiograms

False-positives = Patients with abnormal stress tests and normal angiograms

*Abnormal angiograms are used in this example for illustration purposes. Coronary artery abnrmalities are only one cause of abnormal stress tests.

Table 14–1. **2 × 2 Contingency Table**

Test Result	*Disease*	
	Present	**Absent**
Positive	True-positives	False-positives
Negative	False-negatives	True-negatives

Sensitivity is not only a function of the prevalence of disease in the population under study. It can be enhanced by increasing the stress applied, by using more leads, and by liberalizing the criteria for anabnormal test. If this is done, for example, by accepting 0.5 mm of ST depression rather than 1.0 mm, we will identify more of those with disease; however, more false-positives will be identified. False-negative tests will be increased by reducing the stress applied, increasing the amount of ST depression required for a positive test, and balancing ST vectors, inadequate critical mass of ischemic muscle, and so forth.

Specificity

Specificity is the measure of reliability in identifying by stress test the absence of disease or the percentage of those with a normal stress test out of all studied with normal angiograms.

$$\text{Specificity} = \frac{\text{Patients with normal stress tests and normal angiograms}}{\text{All patients with normal angiograms}} \times 100$$

True-negatives = Patients with normal stress tests who have normal angiograms

False-negatives = Patients with a normal stress test who have abnormal angiograms

As specificity increases, the false-positives decrease. The false-positive, or subject who has ST depression and normal coronary arteries, creates the biggest problem for clinicians. The term "specificity" in this sense has a slightly different meaning than is commonly understood. In common parlance, specificity refers to the reliability or predictive power of a test. We term this the *correct classification rate.*

PREDICTIVE VALUE AND RELATIVE RISK

The data to be presented in this chapter describing sensitivity and specificity of stress Testing are of necessity usually based on patients being admitted for coronary angiography. This results in a cohort of patients with a high prevalence of disease. Let us examine how this affects the results.

$$\text{Predictive value} = \frac{\text{True-positives}}{\text{True-positives} + \text{false-positives}}$$

The predictive value of a positive or an abnormal test is defined as the true-positives over true-positives plus false-positives. The predictive value is the percentage of those identified correctly. It can be for a positive or for a negative test. The predictive value of a positive test does not tell how many abnormal patients have been diagnosed as normal, however. Bayes' theorem states that the predictive value of a test is directly related to the prevalence of disease in the population being studied[1] (Table 14–2).

If we examine a population with a 1% prevalence of disease with a test that has a 60% sensitivity and a 90% specificity (values not far removed from those reported for ST-segment depression), the result will be as shown in Table 14–3. If we select another population to study with the prevalence of disease at 10%, the predictive value will increase to 40% (Table 14–4).

Table 14–2. **Relation of Prevalence of a Disease and Predictive Value of a Test***

Actual Disease Prevalence (%)	Predictive Value of a Positive Test (%)	Predictive Value of a Negative Test (%)
1	16.1	99.9
2	27.9	99.9
5	50.0	99.7
10	67.9	99.4
20	82.6	98.7
50	95.0	95.0
75	98.3	83.7
100	100.0	–

*Sensitivity and specificity rates each equal 95%.
From Vecchio, TH: Predictive value of a single diagnostic test in unselected populations. N Engl J Med 274:1171, 1966, with permission.

Table 14–3. **Performance of a Test with a 60% Sensitivity and a 90% Specificity in a Population with a 1% Prevalence of Disease**

Subjects	No. with Abnormal Test			No. with Normal Test	
100 diseased	60	(TP)	(Sensitivity)	40	(FN)
9900 nondiseased	990	(FP)	(Specificity)	8910	(TN)
Total	1050			8950	

$$\text{Predictive value of an abnormal test} = \frac{TP}{TP + FP} = \frac{60}{1050} = 5.7\%$$

False-positive rate = 100 − 5.7 = 94.3%.
TP = true-positives; FP = false-positives; FN = false-negatives; TN = true-negatives.

Table 14–4. **Performance of a Test with a 60% Sensitivity and a 90% Specificity in a Population with a 10% Prevalence of Disease**

Subjects	No. with Abnormal Test			No. with Normal Test	
1000 diseased	600	(TP)		400	(FN)
			(Sensitivity)		
9000 nondiseased	900	(FP)		8100	(TN)
			(Specificity)		
Total	1500			8500	

Predictive value of an abnormal test $= \frac{TP}{TP + FP} = \frac{600}{1500} = 40\%$

False-positive rate = 100 − 40 = 60%

It can be seen from the previous numbers that the inherent accuracy of the test as previously stated is defined by the sensitivity and specificity and that the results when applied to the individual depend on the prevalence of disease in the population to which the individual belongs.

Obviously, two of the most important factors in the analysis of patients undergoing stress testing are (1) pretest prevalence of disease and (2) sensitivity and specificity of the test.

DISEASE PREVALENCE

There are a number of ways to estimate disease prevalence, and there is considerable disagreement in this area. Diamond and Forrester[3] believe that patients should be categorized according to their pain pattern (Fig. 14–4). This is then modified by age, sex, and other factors. The researchers have published tables that provide information gleaned from a review of the literature. These tables or their computer program (Cadenza) can be used to eval-

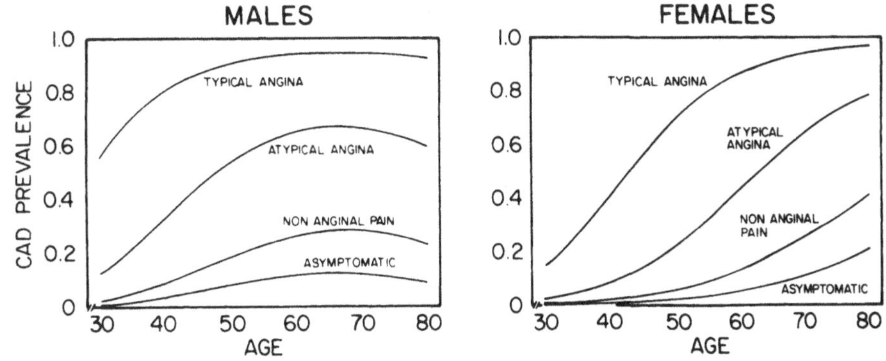

FIGURE 14–4. Prevalence of CAD according to age, sex, and symptom classification. (From Diamond and Forrester,[3] with permission.)

uate the probability of disease.[3] Both pretest and post-test probability will be calculated after a stress test or a series of noninvasive tests including cardiokymography, coronary calcification by fluoroscopy, and thallium scintigraphy.

Hossack and colleagues[5] believe one can do as well with the conventional risk factors combined with exercise risk factors obtained during treadmill stress testing. The Framingham risk factor tables are well known and have been used by the Seattle Group in their Heart Watch study for a number of years. The use of symptoms for disease prevalence presumes that the patient will tell you about pain. Many subjects withhold or modify information for various reasons; commercial airline pilots are a typical example.

EFFECT OF PREVALENCE ON EXERCISE-INDUCED ST DEPRESSION

To proceed with the application of Bayes' theorem, the probability of significant CAD is presented from Diamond's calculations based on the pretest probability. Figure 14–5 illustrates the degree of diagnostic uncertainty according to the magnitude of ST-segment depression and the pretest probability.

The data suggest that even if the pretest probability was only 20%, exercise-induced ST depression of greater than 2.5 mm gives a probability of disease in the range of 90%, whereas slightly less than 2 mm of ST depression results in a probability of about 50%. This information can be used after the exercise test and in other tests such as a nuclear scintigram. For example, if the post-test probability is 70% after a stress test and the information content of a nuclear test is 25%, an abnormal nuclear scintigram will give a probability of 95%, however, a normal nuclear test following the abnormal stress test will reduce the probability to 55%.

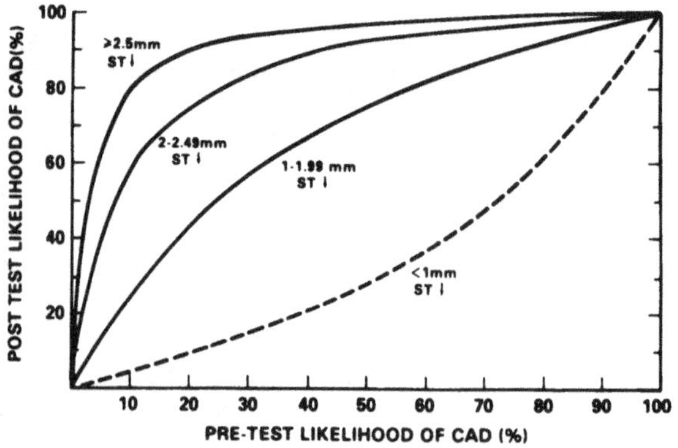

FIGURE 14–5. Family of ST-segment depression curves and the likelihood of CAD. (From Epstein,[6] with permission.)

CRITIQUE OF BAYES' THEOREM

The numbers presented here provide a highly simplified approach to a complex problem. Although the concept is valid, when we apply it to our patients we must remember that important elements in the calculations are not actually known with certainty.

The sensitivity and specificity of stress testing in the day-to-day management of particular patients are uncertain. Most of the data available to us come from cardiac centers where the referral pattern may influence the prevalence of disease in the study.[7] Sensitivity and specificity from such centers are known to vary. How then do we relate these data to our individual patients? In clinical practice, most of us instinctively use a number of variables to determine the presence of disease. In some laboratories, a computer-generated probability based on a multivariate analysis of a number of variables is used. However, we have no information that indicates how well this approach would work in an outpatient-oriented clinic, a private practice of cardiology, or an internal medical office.

POPULATION GROUPS

In a cardiology practice in an area where prevalence of CAD is very high (especially if the physician is a recognized expert in this field), there would be a larger percentage of patients with CAD than in the office of a general internist, in an industrial clinic, or in a military installation. An example of this concept is illustrated in Table 14–5, in which two groups of subjects were studied in relationship to the prevalence of exercise-induced ST depression (positive stress tests).

Those referred for evaluation in the Memorial Hospital Cardiology Laboratory, as expected, resulted in two to four times more positive tests than those studied in an asymptomatic group solicited by the Long Beach Heart Association.[8] Actually, most physicians do stress tests on subjects who, by their age and sex, are in a population with a higher prevalence of CAD.

Table 14–5. **Percent of Positive Stress Tests According to Age and Sex in Two Studies**

Age	MHLB* Female	LBHA† Female	MHLB Male	LBHA Male
21–30	0	0	2.5	1.2
31–40	10.1	2.1	11.7	4.3
41–50	19.9	2.0	29.5	11.4
51–60	29.1	7.4	48.0	26.9
Over 60	43.3	12.1	58.2	29.3
Mean	23.3	4.6	34.3	13.5

*Memorial Hospital Cardiology Laboratory.
†Long Beach Heart Association.
From Ellestad, Allen, and Stuart, with permission.[46]

Using Table 14–5, it would be fair to estimate a disease prevalence of approximately 19% (26.9 + 11.4 = 19) ÷ 2 in men between ages 40 and 60. In this population, there would be a significant number of false-positives and false-negatives. If we were to agree that about 20% were false-positives, we might calculate the predictive value if we analyzed 500 men as follows:

	No. with abnormal test	No. with normal test
100 diseased	70 (TP) (Sensitivity = 70%)	30 FN
400 nondiseased	80 (FP) (Specificity = 80%)	320 TN
	Total 150	350

$$\text{Predicted value of abnormal test} = \frac{TP}{TP + FP} = \frac{70}{150} = 46\%$$

where TP = true-positive; TN = true-negative; FP = false-positive; and FN = false-negative.

Thus, almost 50% of this group of men would be correctly identified by ST segments and age alone. It would be prudent to evaluate the abnormal responders by considering risk factors and other exercise variables (see Chapter 19).

LIMITED CHALLENGE

When evaluating patients to determine the accuracy of the test some investigators have compared patients with a high probability of disease, i.e. patients with chest pain, with a group who obviously have a low probability, such as normal volunteers. This has been termed "limited challenge" because it exaggerates the tendency for normal patients to have a negative test and thus increase the specificity. The best way to know the usefulness of the test is to compare only patients who are suspected of ischemia, usually because they present with chest pain.

The final caveat has to do with the difficulties with angiographic estimates of coronary narrowing and their effect on coronary flow during metabolically induced hyperemia.[9] When we consider that all our data, using angiographically estimated percentage of narrowing, are subject to considerable question (see Chapter 4), it may take a few years before the reliability of any test in estimating coronary ischemia can be based on more certain criteria. For a more detailed critique of this subject, I suggest that the serious reader review Feinstein's[10] essay, "The Haze of Bayes, the Aerial Palaces of Decision Analysis, and the Computerized Ouija Board."

CORRELATION OF ST DEPRESSION WITH CORONARY ANGIOGRAPHY

Published reports correlating the association of exercise-induced ST depression with coronary angiography offer some insight into the reliability of this method in a population being referred to a cardiac center.[11,12] A few of these studies are illustrated in Table 14–6. The investigators considered 1 mm of horizontal or downsloping ST depression to denote a positive test and used 50% to 75% cross-sectional narrowing as a significant coronary lesion. In spite of the fact that coronary stenosis is often misjudged on angiography and other factors such as embolism and coronary spasm often cause ischemia, the results are similar. It is evident that the similar results are due in part to the similar prevalence of CAD in the groups studied. Other factors would be the lead systems used, criteria for performing and terminating the test, and the mix of single- versus three-vessel disease in the population.

Some time ago, Weiner and associates[16] attracted a good deal of attention in the press when they reported that stress testing has very little diagnostic value. They found that a positive stress test—one resulting in horizontal or downsloping ST segments—increased the post-test risk of CAD by only 6% to 20%, and a negative test decreased the post-test risk by only 2% to 28%. They really presented nothing new but emphasized that in the subjects with typical angina, depressed ST segments added little to the diagnosis. What they failed to say was that ST depression added a great deal to the prognosis. The reasons for their findings are understandable from our discussion of prevalence and Bayes' theorem.

Claims are being made that computer evaluation of ST segments can give a better discrimination between diseased and normal patients of this type of population. Simoons and Hugenholtz[17] report that by using measurements of ST segments at 20 and 80 msec after the QRS in the X lead, they found a sensitivity of 85% and a specificity of 91%. The specificity is similar to that of other investigators, but the sensitivity is somewhat better. The major improvement reported is in the sensitivity, or the ability to correctly iden-

Table 14–6. **Sensitivity and Specificity of Stress Testing Reported by Various Investigators**

			Sensitivity			
Study	**N**	**Specificity**	**1 Vessel**	**2 Vessels**	**3 Vessels**	**Total**
Kassebaum et al,[13]	68	97%	25%	38%	85%	53%
Martin et al,[14]	100	89%	35%	67%	86%	62%
McHenry et al,[12]	166	95%	61%	91%	100%	81%
Helfant et al,[15]	63	83%	60%	83%	91%	79%
Bartel et al,[19]	609	94%	39%	62%	73%	63%
Goldschlager et al,[35]	410	93%	40%	63%	79%	64%

tify diseased patients. Simoons[18] also found that correcting for heart rate enhanced the results.

Bartel and colleagues[19] report a specificity of 88% to 97%, but a sensitivity of 53% to 73%. One can see that the false- negatives remain a prominent shortcoming when using ST segments alone.

We found that between 70% and 80% of those with high-grade and two- and three-vessel disease have an abnormal ST-segment response to exercise (Fig. 14–6). On the other hand, the reliability of the ST segment decreases in single-vessel disease in our study[20] and studies by others. Most reports suggest that single-vessel disease can be detected in about 50% to 60% of men with an obstruction of 70% or more. We must then accept at least a 40% false-negative response using the ST segment alone as an identifier. Bruschke and associates[21] and later McNeer and colleagues[22] demonstrated that the single-vessel disease patients have a relatively good long-term outlook, however. Chaitman and coworkers,[23] who originally suggested the subgrouping according to symptoms discussed under the Bayes' theorem, used a 14–lead system and reported that the predictive value of a positive test was 100% in men with typical angina, 85% in men with probable angina, and only 45% in

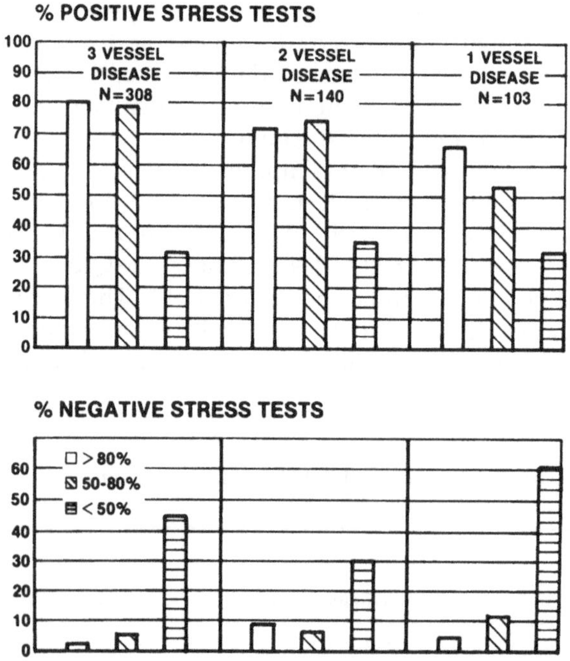

FIGURE 14–6. The bar graph illustrates the percentage of those having a positive test according to the number and severity of coronary artery narrowing. Patients with lesions of less than 50% have positive test results only about 30% of the time, even if low-grade plaques are in all three vessels. The percentages in the bar graphs do not add up to 100% because those with equivocal tests were not included. This constitutes a sizable number of subjects in each group.

men with atypical chest pain. The predictive value of a negative test was 83% in men with nonspecific chest pain, 70% in men with probable angina, and 55% in men with typical angina. When men with probable or typical angina and a limited work time of less than 360 seconds on the Bruce protocol had a positive test, the predictive value of multivessel disease was 92%. It is important to mention that a good exercise tolerance does not rule out severe disease. Chaitman and coworkers[23] found that 47% of their patients reaching Bruce stage IV of the Bruce protocol had significant disease.

From the data available, the following statements regarding average correlations between catheterization data and maximum stress testing seem to be appropriate if ST segments are taken as the only marker for coronary ischemia in a cohort referred for angiography, mostly for chest pain.

1. Men with single-vessel disease and significant coronary narrowing of 70% of luminal diameter have about 50% to 60% chance of having ST depression.
2. Men with two-vessel disease have a 65% chance of having ST depression.
3. Men with three-vessel disease have a 78% chance of having ST depression.
4. Men with left main coronary artery disease have an 85% chance of having ST depression.
5. Men admitted for evaluation of chest pain who are older than aged 45 with 1.0 mm of ST-segment depression have a 90% chance of having CAD or 2.0 evidence of significant left-ventricular dysfunction.
6. Men in the latter category with 1.5 mm of ST depression have a 94% to 95% chance of having CAD or evidence of significant left-ventricular dysfunction.
7. Men older than aged 45 with 2.0 mm or more ST-segment depression have a 98% chance of having CAD or evidence of significant left-ventricular dysfunction.

When evaluating subjects with lesser degrees of coronary narrowing, the number of false-negative tests increases. If the location of the lesion is proximal in a large artery the probability of ST depression increases.

Some might be critical that the above data are given for men only. This is because similar information in women is more difficult to come by (see Chapter 15.)

FALSE-POSITIVE TESTS

Because ST depression has been equated with CAD, patients with this finding who have less than a critical coronary narrowing have been called false-positives. Upon careful scrutiny of these patients, however, most are found to have some process or condition that could explain the repolarization ab-

Table 14–7. **Summary of Cardiac Catheterization Data**

	Stress Test (%)	
	True Positive	**False Positive**
Contraction patterns in ventriculogram		
Normal	46	73
Akinesia	33	9
Hypokinesia	5	18
Dyskinesia	16	1
LVEDP >12 mm Hg		
At rest	41	35
After exercise	64	57
Other findings		
Mild mitral insufficiency	6	3
Papillary muscle dysfunction	3	0
Mild aortic insufficiency	4	6
Mild cardiomyopathy	1	22
Infarction	31	9
Left-ventricular hypertrophy	6	8
Bundle branch block	3	5
IHSS	0	2
Hypertension	9	20
Hyperdynamic heart	1	14

LVEDP = left-ventricular end-diastolic pressure; IHSS = idiopathic hypertrophic subaortic stenosis.

normality[24] (Table 14–7). In a study of 95 patients with ST-segment depression and normal coronary arteries, we found only 13% without some possible explanation. Erikssen and Myhre[25] followed up 36 men for 7 years with normal coronary arteries and ST depression. The incidence of cardiac events after 7 years was the same in this group as in those who were found to have significant CAD. Moreover, none was believed upon entry to have any of the conditions listed in Table 14–7. The investigators believe that many of these patients represent early myocardiopathies and that the ST changes were due to abnormalities in the vasodilator reserve. It is now known that coronary atheroma that do not appear to be flow limiting may cause decreased perfusion and thus ischemia. Thus, the term false-positive ST depression should be abandoned and replaced with abnormal ST depression of unknown cause.

FALSE-NEGATIVE TESTS

When patients are found to have significant coronary narrowing and fail to have exercise-induced ST depression, they have been labeled false-negative. We can understand this when the obstructed artery subtends an area of scar, suggesting that there is no ischemic muscle to produce the characteristic ECG changes. Indeed, the prevalence of an ischemic ST response is reduced in subjects with a previous infarction, especially if it is a large anterior wall scar.[26] Harder to understand is the patient who has no known previous infarction but has classic angina on exercising with no detectable ST change. This has been observed even in patients with left main coronary artery disease.[27] In one series, this phenomenon occurred in 22% of those with left main coronary artery stenosis. It might be postulated that if we had enough leads this would never occur, but even with precordial maps false-negatives occur in about 10% of those tested. Weiner and colleagues[28] analyzed the false-negative tests from the CASS study and reported that they were as common in patients with multivessel disease as in those with single-vessel disease. They found that even in patients with three-vessel disease, the absence of ST depression (horizontal or downsloping) predicted a very low probability of a coronary event in 4 years. Weiner and colleagues[28] also claim that the achieved heart rate response had no effect on the likelihood of a false-negative, although this would be at odds with reports from other workers.[14,17,20] The results must be viewed with the knowledge that they excluded upsloping ST depression and therefore increased the number of false negative findings considerably.

In some patients, the magnitude of ischemia is probably inadequate to produce a significant current of injury; in others, the ischemia may be in both the anterior and posterior wall so that the ST changes cancel each other out. Because ST depression is due to subendocardial ischemia with the attendant potassium shift, factors that would alter this process may come into play (see Chapter 3). Probably the most common factor, in patients with severe three-vessel disease, is patchy scarring of the subendocardium, often unrecognized in the resting ECG. Low voltage can also be a factor.

Hakki and colleagues[29] report that when evidence of infarction on the ECG is taken into consideration, false-negatives should constitute only about 10% of a population referred for angiography (less than 50% of that found by Weiner and associates[28]) and 75% of these would be identified by nuclear scintigraphy. A few more can be identified by analysis of multiple variables such as heart rate response, septal Q-wave changes, prolongation in P-wave duration, intraventricular conduction abnormalities, and the presence of anginal pain.

By combining a number of noninvasive parameters, most significant (but not all) coronary narrowing might eventually be detectable by stress testing.

LONG-TERM FOLLOW-UP STUDIES

A knowledge of the capacity of stress test findings to predict subsequent coronary events is important in making clinical judgments in managing individual patients. Events are influenced by myocardial function and many other factors besides the coronary anatomy.

Master's Test

The first large actuarial study of survival following a stress test was that of Robb and coworkers[30] in 1957, later expanded in 1967. They reported that the incidence of mortality was 56.8 per 1000 patient-years of observation when an abnormal test was present in patients with CAD and that this was more than five times higher than in those with a normal test with an incidence of mortality of 11.5 per 1000. When evaluating sudden death, the mortality of those with abnormal tests increased to six times that of the normal. When they reviewed the data on 2224 patients in 1967, the maximum period of observation was 15 years with an average of 5 years. At this time, they reported an incidence of 25 per 1000 patient-years of observation in the subjects with abnormal tests. The mortality ratio was 1.2 for normal responders, 0.9 for those with J-point depression, and 4.3 for those with an abnormal test. In 1972, Robb[31] again reviewed the data, and those subjects with more than 2.0-mm ST depression had an average mortality rate of approximately 8% per year for 8 years. Those subjects whose tests were read as abnormal, including all those with 0.5-mm ST segment depression or more, had an average mortality of about 3% per year with the standard insurance risk being about 2%. His data suggest that some of Robb's abnormal responders (those with 0.5-mm ST depression) probably had normal hearts but abnormal-appearing ST segments due to abnormalities not associated with CAD. However, our 6-year study of 658 abnormal responders to a treadmill test showed a mortality rate of 20% or 3.3% per year.[20]

In 1962, Mattingly[32] reviewed data compiled over a 10-year period on 1920 military personnel. He reported 56 coronary episodes in 145 abnormal responders (with 0.5-mm or more ST-segment depression), which is about 3.8% per year. The subjects with abnormal tests had approximately 10 times more coronary events than did those with normal tests.

The significant differences reported between the abnormal and normal responders to the Master's test indicate that stress testing was of definite value in predicting death as a result of CAD. The data to follow extend this concept to the maximum treadmill stress test.

The predictive capacity reported in several of the earlier follow-up studies is summarized in Table 14–8. The sensitivity and specificity in these studies are surprisingly similar to those reported in the angiographic studies.

When ST-segment depression occurs in subjects who have yet to have a clinical manifestation of coronary narrowing, even though they may have high-grade stenosis, they would be termed "false-positive."

Memorial Medical Center Follow-Up Study—1975

We obtained follow-up data on about 6000 patients previously referred for maximum treadmill tests.[20] Most subjects were referred for evaluation of pain syndromes, with 17% being referred for a routine screening test. The

Table 14–8. **Risk Ratio, Sensitivity, Specificity, and Predictive Value of Stress Testing Calculated from Follow-up Data of Various Investigators**

Study	Risk Ratio	Sensitivity	Specificity	Predictive Value
Bruce	13.6×	60%	91%	13.6%
Aranow	13.6×	67%	92%	46%
Froelicher	14.3×	61%	92%	20%
Cumming	10×	58%	90%	25%
Ellestad	6.3×	75%	86%	75%

When using follow-up data, note that if CAD is present but not yet symptomatic, the result will be false-negative findings, which will reduce the sensitivity.

events recorded as significant in follow-up were (1) progression of angina, (2) myocardial infarction (MI), and (3) death due to heart disease.

Subjects were diagnosed as abnormal if they had ST-segment depression of 1.5 mm or more 0.08 second from the J point. Flat, upsloping, or downsloping ST segments were included. Subjects diagnosed as equivocal included those with ST-segment depression of 0.5 to 1.4 mm, multifocal or frequent premature ventricular contractions with exercise, and poor chronotropic response falling more than 1 standard deviation below the mean heart rate response for age and sex.

The prevalence of any coronary event by year is depicted in Figure 14–7 for normal, equivocal, and abnormal responders. The prevalence of coronary events in the abnormal responders is almost 10% per year. Those with equiv-

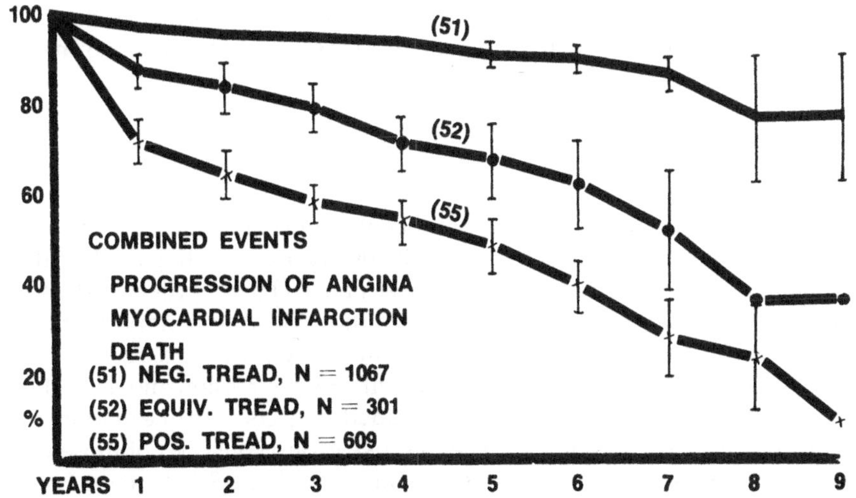

FIGURE 14–7. Survival without all coronary events in the negative responders (51), in equivocal responders (those with ST-segment depression from 0.5–1.4 mm) (52), and in classically positive responders (ST-segment depression of 1.5 or more mm) (55).

ocal results fall so far below those with a normal pattern that there must be a large number of subjects with CAD in this group. The prevalence of coronary events over a 4-year period in those diagnosed as positive is 46% compared with 77% in the normal responders, almost a seven fold difference. The 25% prevalence of coronary events in subjects with equivocal results resulted in our revision of the criterion for an abnormal stress test to 1.0-mm ST-segment depression at 0.08 second from the J point.

After 8 years, 76% of the abnormal responders had some coronary event; this amounts to 9.5% per year. The prevalence of MI over a 4-year period is 15% in positive responders in contrast to 1% in negative responders. The prevalence of 5% in those with equivocal results (five times that of normal subjects) also suggests that some of these tests should have been read as abnormal. The data compiled for an 8-year period are similar, showing infarctions in 27% of those with abnormal tests, resulting in an average of about 3.5% per year. It is interesting how closely this fits Mattingly's data[32] from the double Master's test in which the prevalence of death is similar to that for MI, averaging about 3.3% per year. Some of the data from the early studies are omitted here but can be found in the 4th edition or in the published papers.[33]

Duke Study—1978

The excellent registry at Duke has made it possible to publish follow-up data in subjects who have had not only exercise tests but also angiograms[22] (Fig. 14–8). The mortality rate in their patients with ST depression is about 6% per year—about double our findings—undoubtedly due to patient selection. Also, the 3% annual mortality rate compared with our normals reflects the same bias. I suspect that a high percentage of their subjects with a normal ST response may have a single-vessel disease.

Heart Watch—1980

Although the early reports from the excellent multicenter study by Bruce and colleagues[33] began to appear in the late 1970s, we are reporting on their data on patients (656 men) with atypical chest pain.[5] (Their earlier work is reported in Chapter 19.) Because it had been recognized how important multiple variables can be, the investigators categorized the subjects into three groups. The high-risk group were those with ST depression and a short exercise time. The moderate-risk group included subjects with one or more risk factors but no exercise findings. The low-risk group consisted of those with no risk factors and normal exercise tolerance without ST changes. Figure 14–9 illustrates the importance of ST depression, especially when combined with a short exercise time, the coronary event rate being about seven times more likely than in those without these findings.

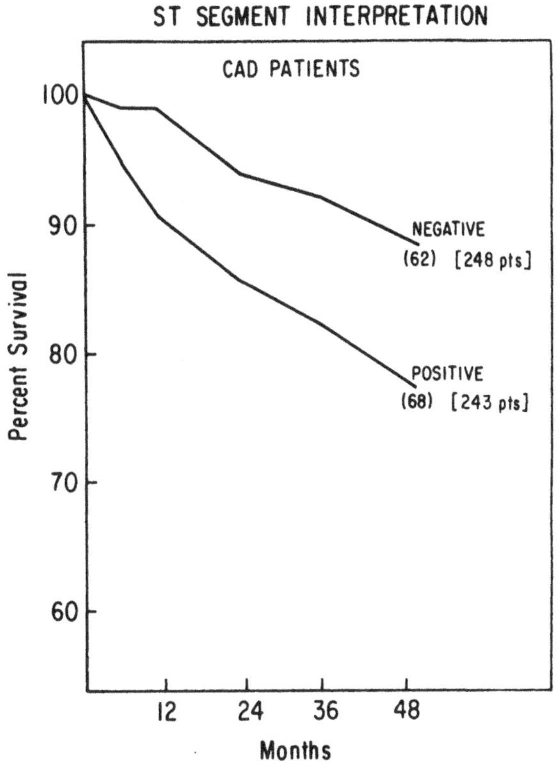

FIGURE 14–8. In patients with angiographically demonstrated CAD, the mortality is greater in those with ischemic ST segments. (From McNeer et al,[22] with permission.)

CASS Study—1982

The CASS multicenter study based on 4083 patients deals with a different population but provides us with similar evidence that exercise ST-segment depression is a good discriminator of events.[35] Patients in this study were stratified according to various risk factors and in essence confirmed the previously cited studies. The researchers found that a short exercise time and ST depression of greater than 2 mm identified a cohort with a high risk of developing coronary events. Those who had 1 mm of ST depression and could not exceed Bruce stage I had an annual mortality rate of more than 5%. The predictive importance of short exercise duration reported by our group in 1975[20] has now been confirmed by subsequent studies.[33,34]

Cooper Clinic Study—2000

A large long term–follow up study of clinically normal men from the Cooper Clinic correlated risk factors and ST depression (Fig. 14–10).[35] It

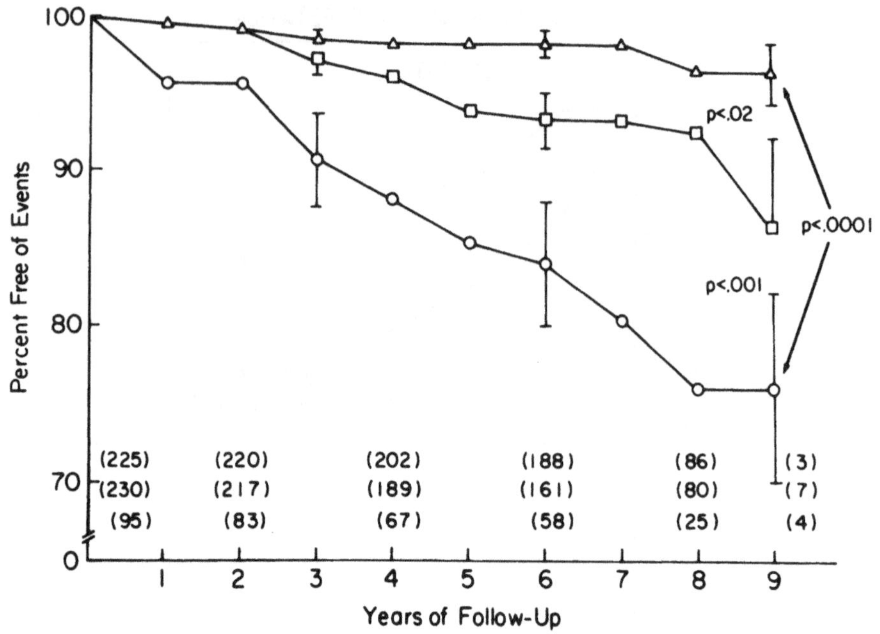

FIGURE 14–9. A life table depicting the effect of ST depression in coronary events in men with atypical chest pain.
Δ Low risk = no risk factors, no ST depression, and excellent exercise tolerance.
□ Medium risk = one or more risk factors but no abnormal exercise findings.
O High risk = either exercise-induced ST depression or exercise capacity more than 30% below predicted for age and sex. (From Hossack et al,[5] with permission.)

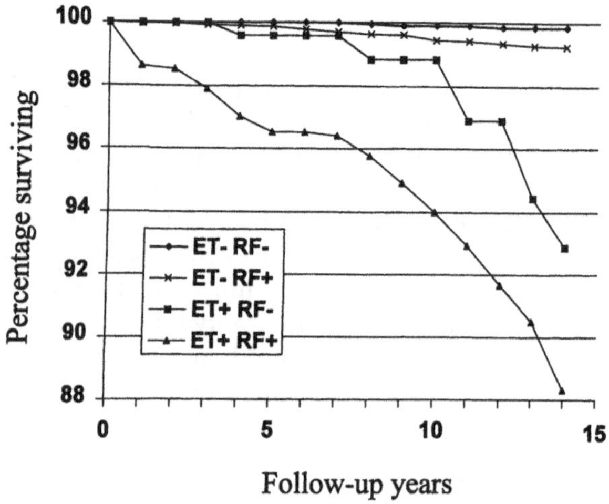

FIGURE 14–10. Life table of a coronary heart disease survival as related to the exercise test and the conventional risk factors in 25,927 men followed for 8.4 years. With permission of publisher.[35]

can be seen that exercise induced ST depression is a good predictor of survival in their study.

VA Study

Froelicher's group recently reported on 6,000 men, mostly tested for chest pain and found that ST depression resulted in a risk ratio of 1.8 and that >6 pvc's per minute resulted in a similar risk, and that a treadmill score can stratify risk. The important predictors were age >65, low exercise capacity and LVH.

TIME OF ONSET OF ST-SEGMENT DEPRESSION

A logical conclusion would be that ischemia reflected by ST-segment depression resulting from very mild exercise is more severe than that occurring at a workload near peak capacity. We analyzed the follow-up events in those who had ST depression of 2.0 mm or more manifested at the various work levels of our protocol, that is, 3, 5, and 7 minutes.

Figure 14–11 clearly supports the concept that the workload at which the ischemic changes are determined is of prime importance in the evaluation of the severity of the disease. The incidence of coronary events in a subject with a 2.0-mm ST-segment depression at 3 minutes of our protocol (walking at 1.7 mph on a 108 incline) is four times that of a subject requiring 4 mph to initiate ST-segment changes (seventh minute of our protocol). The prevalence of anginal pain associated with ischemia at high levels of exercise is also decreased.

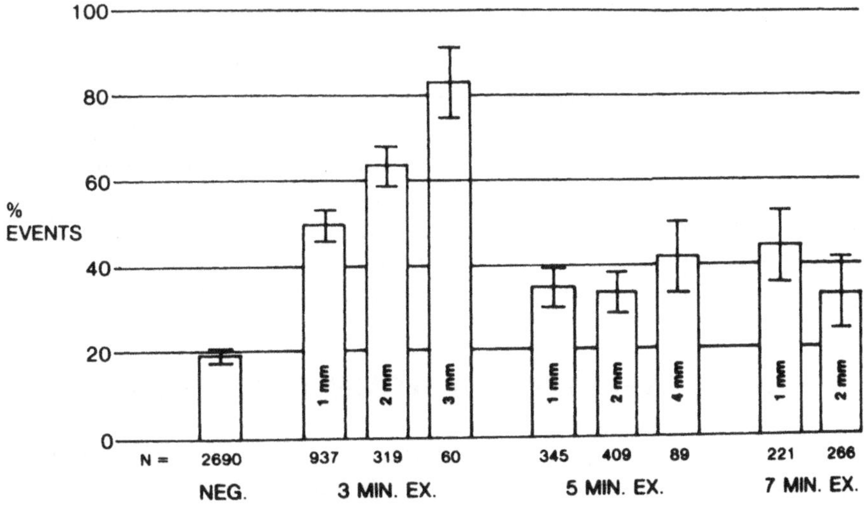

FIGURE 14–11. The incidence of subsequent coronary events (progression of angina, MI, and death) increases with the magnitude of the ST-segment depression only when analyzed at a light workload (3 minutes of exercise = 4 METS; time span = 6 years).

When the onset of 1 mm of ST depression is used as an indicator, the difference at various workloads is also significant, although not so marked. Goldschlager and colleagues,[37] McNeer and associates,[22] and Weiner and coworkers[34] have confirmed our life table studies by demonstrating a higher proportion of multivessel disease in those with onset of ischemia at low workloads. Schneider and colleagues[38] report that the onset of ST depression in Bruce stage I or II predicts a 30% incidence of left main coronary artery stenosis.

MAGNITUDE OF ST-SEGMENT DEPRESSION

The original work of Robb and associates[30] indicates that the deeper the ST-segment depression, the more serious the disease. This seems valid when considering the progression of ST-segment depression during exercise. In 1975, we reported that there appeared to be no predictive value in the magnitude of ST depression measured immediately after exercise. [20] In a subsequent study, however, it appeared that when analyzed at low workloads, those subjects with deep ST depression definitely have a more serious prognosis[8] (see Fig. 14–11). In a study in our laboratory, Hustead and I[39] found that the sum of the ST depression in all leads at maximum exercise failed to predict the number of diseased vessels or the size of the nuclear deficit. This has also been confirmed by Bogaty and associates.[40]

The debate over the importance of the magnitude of STdepression has continued. Podrid and colleagues[41] reported "profound ST segment depression" or a "strongly positive test" did not have a serious prognosis in 212 men followed up for 20 to 59 months. Careful analysis of their report reveals that four of their patients (26%) who had early-onset ST surgery and that four others who were treated medically died. The event rate of 17% translated to approximately 4% per year. Deganis and coworkers[42] from Quebec Heart Institute reported similar data confirming that early-onset ST depression reflects a serious prognosis, but when combined with a good exercise tolerance, deep ST depression must be suspected as being noncoronary or at least associated with less severe disease. Animal studies suggest that the magnitude of ST depression in a single lead may reflect the severity of ischemia in some segment of the myocardium but not the amount of muscle that is ischemic.[43]

TIME OF RECOVERY FROM ST-SEGMENT DEPRESSION

It had been our opinion that the longer it takes a patient to recover from ST-segment depression, the more serious the degree of ischemia and therefore the more serious the prognosis. However, we were unable to demonstrate this with follow-up data. This was surprising and may be due to the fact that in those with more severe disease, exercise is terminated sooner; therefore, their recovery was more rapid than those who had less severe disease and exercised longer before being forced to terminate exertion.

Goldschlager and associates[37] reported that the severity of coronary narrowing correlates with the duration of the ischemic response after exercise is terminated. It is of interest that their protocol calls for the termination of exercise after clear-cut ST-segment depression is established. Thus, on the average, their ischemic patients were exposed to less exercise after onset of significant abnormalities. With the evidence available, the time necessary for resolution of ST-segment depression should correlate with the severity of ischemia and in most cases the severity of coronary narrowing, but it is dependent on the indications for termination of exercise. When patients are given nitroglycerin prior to the exercise test, it has been shown that the ST depression recovers more quickly, suggesting that the magnitude of ischemia is a factor in the recovery time.[38,44]

POOR CHRONOTROPIC RESPONSE

When the heart rate response to exercise falls considerably below the average rate for age and sex, the incidence of a future MI and all coronary events is slightly greater than in those with ischemic ST-segment depression and a normal heart rate response. Figure 14–12 demonstrates the prevalence of any

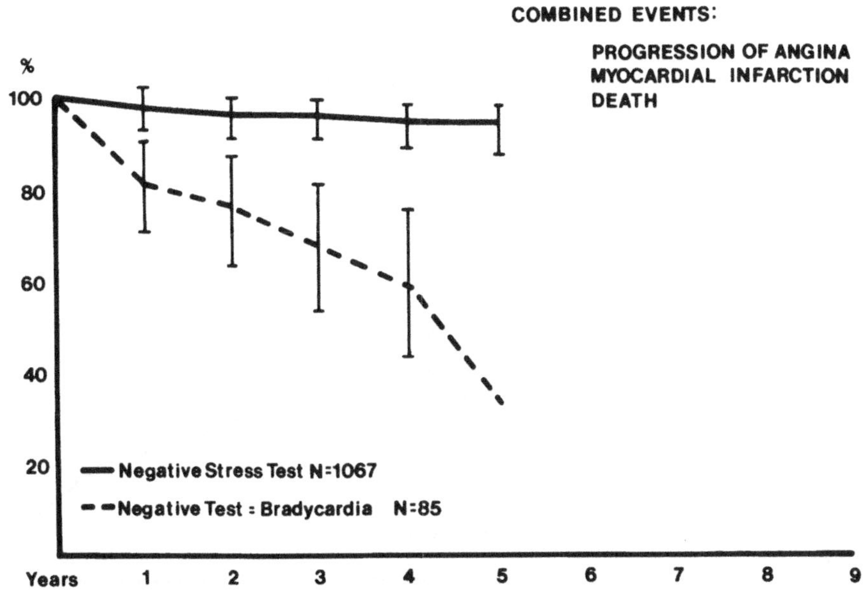

FIGURE 14–12. Those with chronotrophic incompetence (pulse below the 95% confidence limits for age and sex) and normal ST segments have a high incidence of combined events (similar to those with ST-segment depression).

coronary event in subjects with normal ST segments and a slow heart rate compared with all subjects whose tests were diagnosed as normal. A poor heart rate response appears to have the same long-term significance, even in the absence of ischemic ST segments, as an early classic ischemic response. Approximately 15% per year of those with slow pulse had some coronary event. Figure 14–13 compares those with ST-segment depression and bradycardia with all abnormal responders.

Our study group was characterized by a consistently low heart rate response to each workload, but even those who have an appropriate response to a given workload but failed to achieve their predicted maximum heart rate have an increased incidence of events. Figure 14–14 illustrates that there is almost a twofold increase in events when achieved heart rate is significantly reduced. The data of McNeer and colleagues[22] confirm this, even when the population is limited to those with significant CAD. More recently, Hammond and associates[45] studied this in patients with radionuclide imaging and found a high percentage of angina or myocardial scarring, and Lauer has confirmed the importance of this finding in several large population groups (Fig. 14–15).[46]

DELTA HEART RATE

Erriksen's group in Oslo reported that the difference between heart rate at rest and heart rate at maximum exercise is a good predictor of survival.[47]

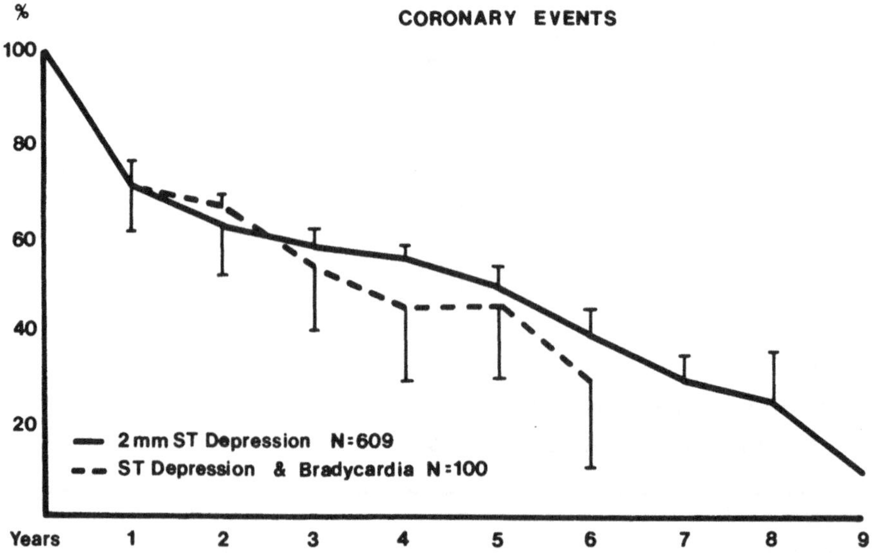

FIGURE 14–13. Those with ST-segment depression and chronotrophic incompetence have a high incidence of coronary events (50% in 5 years). Bradycardia-chronotrophic incompetance.

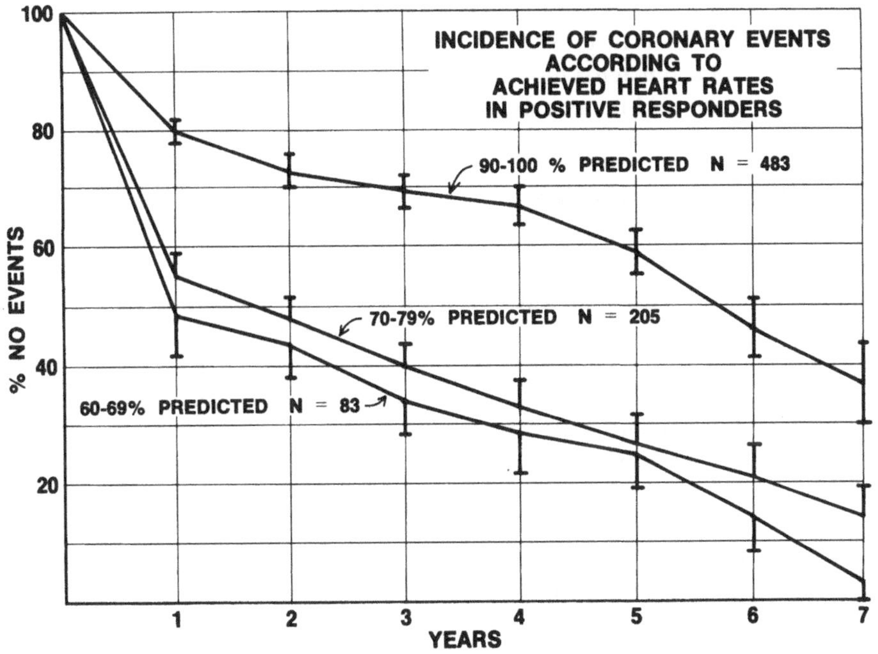

FIGURE 14–14. When all patients with abnormal ST segments are stratified according to achieved heart rate, it is evident that those stopping at lower heart rates have a higher prevalence of events and presumably more severe CAD.

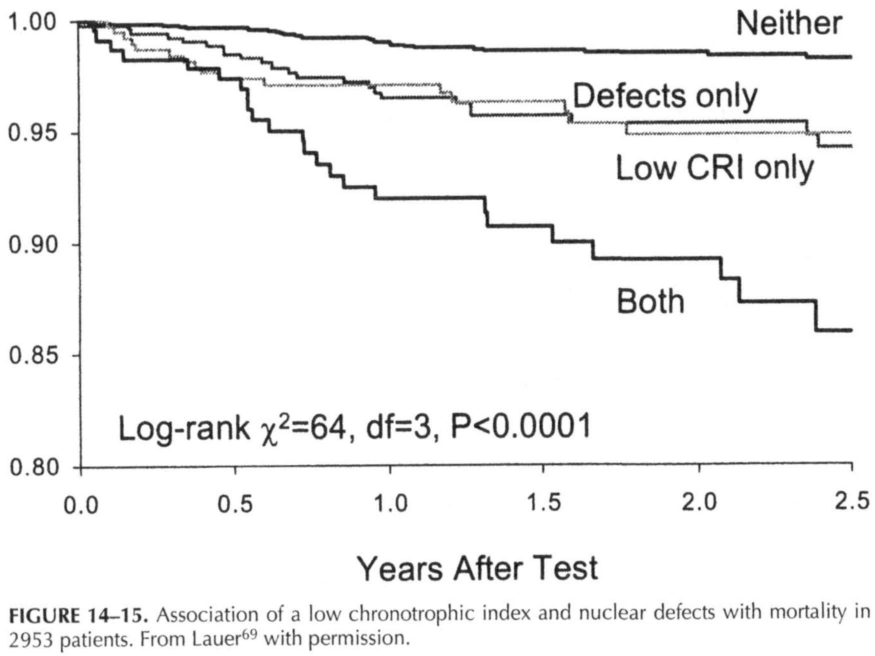

FIGURE 14–15. Association of a low chronotrophic index and nuclear defects with mortality in 2953 patients. From Lauer[69] with permission.

There have been a number of reports that resting heart rate is correlated with cardiovascular mortality,[47,48,49] so that when a patient has a slow resting heart rate and can reach a high rate during exercise testing, it should follow that he or she would have an improved survival.

HEART RATE RECOVERY

It appears that when the heart rate returns to normal rapidly during recovery, ischemia is less likely because when the recovery heart rate remains high it is predictive of a poor prognosis.[53] It is of interest that in 1929 Arthur Master published a paper on exercise testing to evaluate cardiac function and reported that the failure of the heart rate to recover rapidly indicated coronary disease.[59] More recently Lauer rediscovered this fact and has demonstrated its predictive capacity in several papers, which have been confirmed by others.

In patients who stop exercise abruptly Lauer[69] reports that those who fail decrease their heart rate more than 18 beats one minute after termination are significantly more at risk for a cardiac event.

These changes are undoubtedly related to changes in sympathetic and vagal balance. A brief discussion of this concept has recently been published.[57]

ANGINAL PAIN

Although our experience is that anginal pain occurs in less than 50% of those manifesting ST-segment depression,[50] Cole and I,[51] showed that this symptom gives added significance to the presence of the ischemic ST segment. Subjects with pain associated with ischemic ST segments have twice the number of subsequent coronary events as those with ST changes and no pain. This difference was also present when analyzing for any of the events (MI, increased angina, and coronary death) individually (Fig. 14–16). The difference was even more striking when the analysis was restricted to men between ages 41 and 50. In this relatively young group, pain was associated with a threefold increase in events. It was also demonstrated that pain manifested early in the test, at low workloads, also was a marker for a higher incidence of future events.

Weiner and colleagues[52] from Boston City Hospital have reviewed the importance of chest pain during testing and report that classic angina during testing, even in the absence of ST depression, has a 90% predictive accuracy. Other authors have found a similar reliability.[53]

There is a high correlation between those unable to attain high heart rates and those with early onset of ischemia and pain. Thus, these various indicators are probably all telling us the same thing, although not always appearing

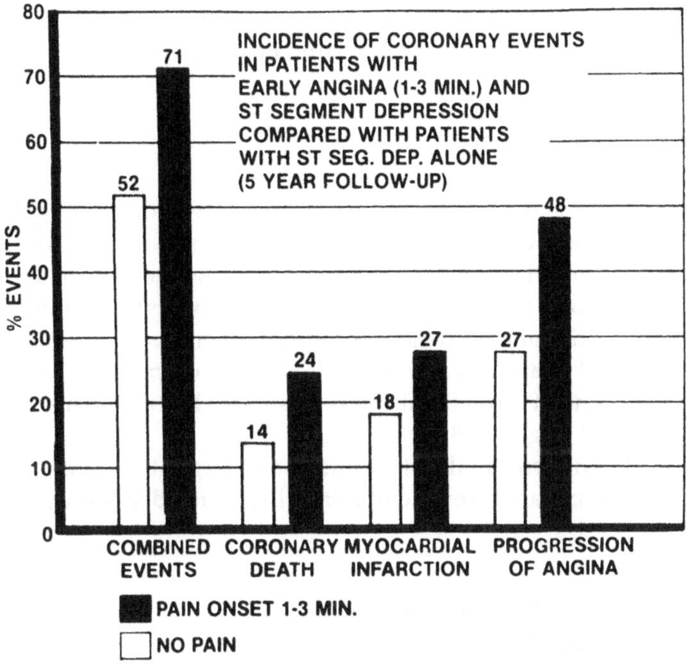

FIGURE 14–16. When pain manifested early in the test was analyzed, it identified a group with a higher incidence of events. (From Cole and Ellestad,[47] with permission.)

together. They indicate that there is a larger area of ischemic heart muscle during exercise and that ventricular function is seriously compromised.

Hayet and Kellerman[54] from Tel Aviv have used the heart rate and angina threshold as predictor of a subsequent coronary event. In a 5-year follow-up study, their group found an increased prevalence of bypass surgery, infarction, and cardiac death compared with those who developed pain at a heart rate greater than 120 beats per minute. In contrast to the above data, more recent reports claim that silent ischemia is equally as serious as that which produces pain.[55] Although there is little doubt that many patients who do not complain of angina get in severe trouble, I have yet to be convinced that anginal pain often does not alert us to a more severe process.

EXERCISE DURATION

One of the most consistent findings in large-scale studies is the favorable prognosis seen in patients who have a prolonged exercise duration on the treadmill. This was demonstrated in the CASS study,[28] the Framingham data,[48] and in Bruce's Heart Watch Group and recently in a large study from the Veterans Administration.[36] The reverse is also true. A short exercise time has a poor prognosis, as does a high resting heart rate.[47,57]

EFFECT OF AGE

There has been some divergence in our studies when considering the influence of age on those with an abnormal ST response. In our earlier life table analysis, it appeared that age had no effect on subsequent coronary events. In another study[8] on a much larger sample (2667 subjects), we found that age seemed to have a definite influence on coronaryevents when 1 mm of ST depression was used as an indicator (Fig. 14–17). When 2 mm of ST depression at a prescribed time of onset (5 minutes) was used, less difference in the age groups was found (Fig. 14–18).

The number of abnormal test results in any large study will increase as age increases. If one analyzes the abnormal tests for death only and com-

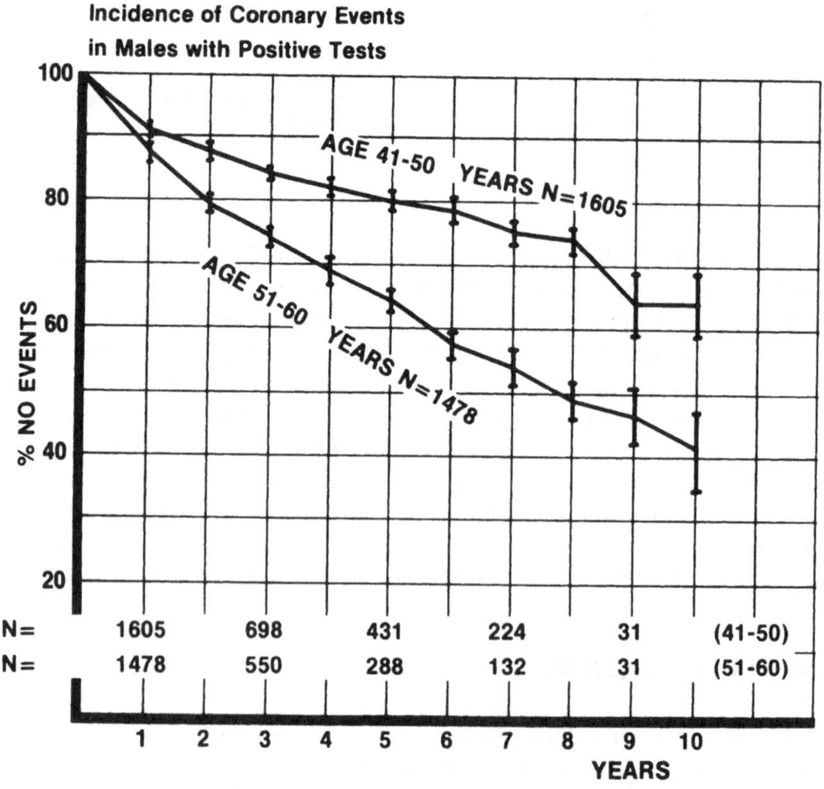

FIGURE 14–17. When the coronary events are stratified according to age and 1 mm of ST depression, it appears that the older subjects (aged 51–60) are at higher risk.

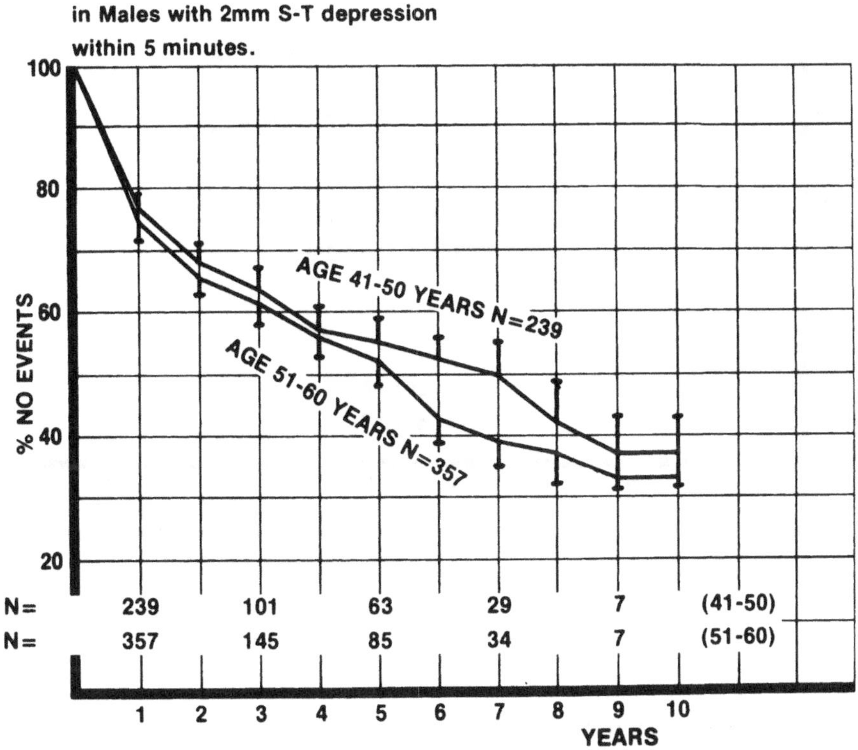

FIGURE 14–18. When an abnormal test is characterized by 2 mm of ST depression, age then loses some of its impact on the ultimate outcome. It appears that in those with more severe degrees of ischemia, age has less effect on the long-term outcome.

pares age group 41 to 50 with age group older than 50, there is no difference (Fig. 14–19).

The slight trend for the younger groups to manifest a greater mortality at 7 years is not statistically significant. If the negative responders are divided into age groups and analyzed for death alone, the older subjects tend to have an increased prevalence, as would be expected. The same trend for MI was also found.

EFFECT OF PREVIOUS MYOCARDIAL INFARCTION

Early stress testing after an MI was reviewed in Chapter 10. The data here deal with the effect of a stable scar on the predictive value of exercise testing. Bruce[55] has shown that when ST depression is used as a marker for CAD, the prevalence of abnormal stress tests is decreased if there is evidence of a previous MI. Even though a previous MI decreases the sensitivity of the test, pa-

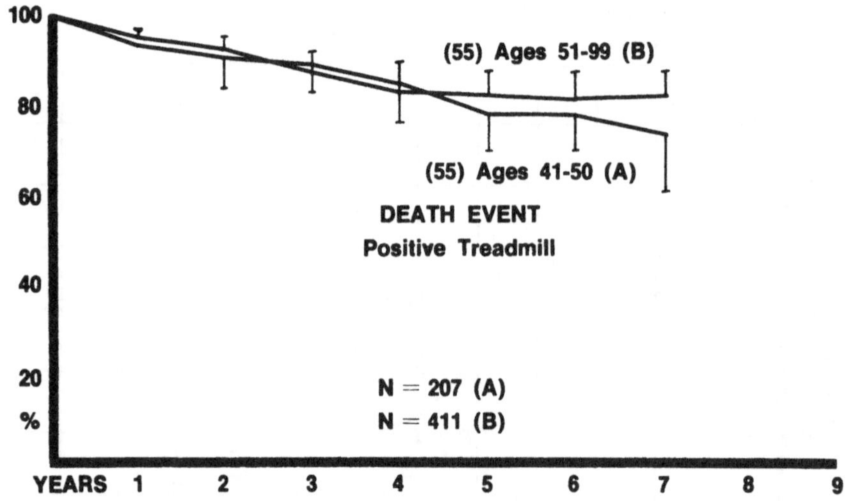

FIGURE 14–19. The incidence of death in the two age groups is similar, as well as the incidence of the events depicted in Figure 14–25.

tients who had suffered this complication have a more serious prognosis than those who had not, averaging 7.5% per year.

Figure 14–20 shows that even a negative stress test in a subject with a previous MI is no protection against the appearance of a coronary event. Those who have ST depression after sustaining an MI have an 81% probability of having some coronary event within 5 years. However, those who have not had an MI have a 34% chance of a coronary event—less than half the probability of the MI group. It can be seen from the standard deviations that the difference is highly significant between these groups.

To fully evaluate postinfarction testing, localization of the scar must be considered. Castellanet and colleagues[26] have studied the effect of various infarction patterns on the reliability of the ST segment to identify ischemia in noninfarcted areas of the heart. They have shown that in those with inferior infarction, the sensitivity of the stress test is 84%. When a large anterior wall scar is present, it may mask ischemia in other areas and reduce the sensitivity to 33%. Reliability of the test in patients with anterior infarction is inversely related to the magnitude of the scar. Their work has been confirmed by Myers and associates[57] and Weiner and coworkers.[58] Thus, one is on fairly safe ground when coming to a clinical decision based on the stress test when the infarction is inferior, but when the test appears normal following a large anterior infarction, other areas of muscle may be ischemic without influencing the ST segment.

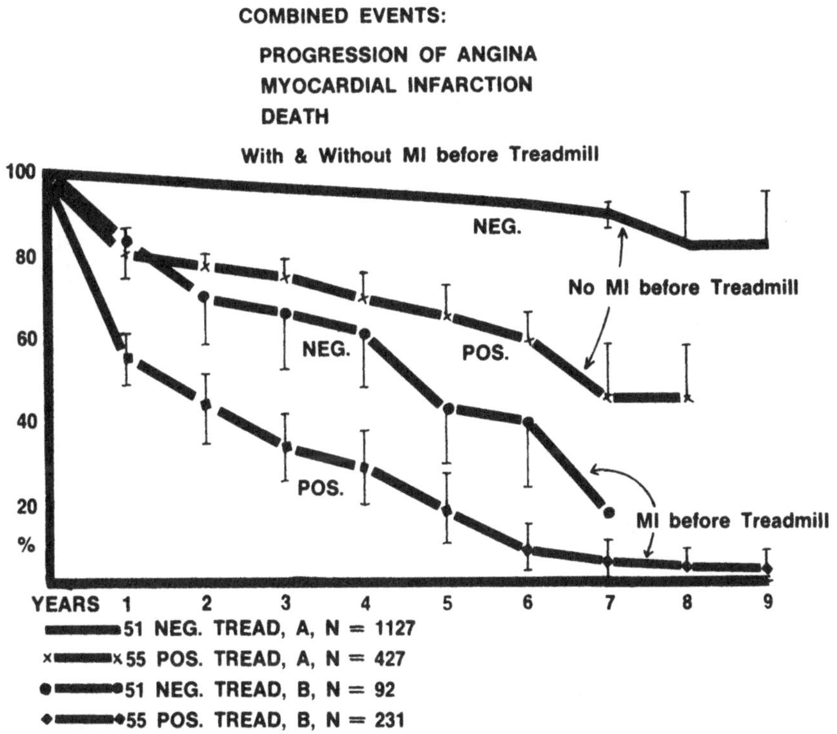

FIGURE 14–20. Those with a previous infarction *(B)* have a much higher risk of coronary event than those without *(A)*, even if they have a negative stress test.

EXERCISE TEST SCORES

The use of exercise data to predict probability of coronary artery disease or the probability of subsequent coronary events has been a goal of investigators since the Masters Step Test was proposed.[59] Although the final score is yet to be designed, a few of the most accurate will be presented for review. These include: (1) multivariate analysis, (2) Duke Score, (3) Froelicher Score, and (4) Morise Score.

Multivariate Analysis

In 1980 we examined a group of patients who had treadmill tests and coronary angiograms to determine which variables were predictive of significant disease.[60,61] Using multivariate analysis we found that durations of exercise, infarct by EKG, and ST depression were the significant predictors in males. Five variables in women were significant, including previous infarction, angina during the test, ST changes and age. The sensitivity and specificity for men were 84% and 80% and for females 85% and 86%, respectively. Since than numerous papers by Diamond, Detrano and others have validated this approach, with similar results.[62,63]

The Duke Score

The excellent registry at Duke University was used by Mark[64] to construct a simple score to categorize patients into high, medium and low risk that can be calculated easily without a computer. They used exercise time, magnitude of ST depression, and presence of angina. This has become quie popular and has been validated by subsequent reports.

A Duke Score of 11 predicts a 5-year survival of 72% labeled a high risk, a score of −10 to +4 is a moderate risk and predicts a 5-year survival of 91% and a score of +5 or more predicts a survival of 97% and is labeled a low risk. Predictive data of this type do not take into consideration our current modes of therapy. There are data to suggest that the predictive value does not apply to older patients.

Froelicher Score

Froelicher and others working in the VA system have proposed a series of scores[65] to help characterize the clinical importance of coronary disease from clinical risk factors and exercise results. Because the data were collected largely from VA hospitals on men only, it is not known how applicable these are to general populations. The score was validated by comparing the results of coronary angiograms using a coronary lesion with a narrowing greater than 50% as evidence of clinically important coronary artery disease. Froelicher claims a 90% correct diagnosis for this method but he achieves this by assuming all those in the intermediate group would go to angiography and have an angiogram and, therefore, be 100% correct. The clinical variables scored include age, sex, character of the angina, estrogen status, and standard risk factors, including diabetes, hypertension, smoking, family history, hyperlipidemia, and obesity. Patients are stratified into low probability, intermediate and high probability. Patients are stratified into low probability, 0–28 points (prevalence of coronary artery disease = 16%, intermediate probability, 9–15 points (prevalence of coronary artery disease = 44%) and high probability, 16–24 points (prevalence of coronary artery disease = 69%). The most recent itteration of his score was compared to a diagnosis made by expert cardiologists and was similar in accuracy, but it performed better than most other physician groups.[66]

Morise Score

This score,[67] which is similar to that of Froelicher's but was derived from a population seen at West Virginia University School of Medicine, includes the data from women using the same risk factors but including the nature of anginal symptoms as proposed by Berman.[68] He believes that this score would be useful in non-VA populations as well as Froelicher's Score.

COMMENTS ABOUT MANIPULATION OF DATA TO PRODUCE SCORES

1. They are based on a tarnished gold standard. Recent work has documented that examining the angiogram and using 50% stenosis as a marker for clinical ischemia leads to many incorrect conclusions (see page 7).
2. Work up bias. Patients who are sent for angiograms have a high prevalence of coronary artery disease; therefore the sensitivity of the test is arbitrarily high.
3. If the population tested are from individuals who are clinically normal and do not have angiograms, the specificity is arbitrarily high.
4. The indication for terminating exercise affects the results. When published age predicted target heart rates are used many subjects may have exercise terminated prematurely and thus have inadequate stress to the degree that it will fail to produce ischemia.
5. Restricted EKG criteria for ischemia. Most scores only use 1 mm of horizontal or downsloping ST depression in this calculation. If one reviews Chapter 12 he/she will immediately see that sensitivity is falsely low with this restriction because there are other ECG markers of ischemia.
6. Predictors of mortality, such as maximum achieved workload, recovery heart rate, chronotropic incompetence, recovery blood pressure, and ST depression are almost all based on "all cause" mortality data, although most people in these studies probably die of cardiac causes, a significant percent have other reasons to die, which are obviously not related to exercise-testing variables. For this reason I believe we have to look upon exercise-based scores as being very useful for evaluating population studies but only marginally useful in treating individual patients.

CONCLUSIONS

The predictive power of the normal as well as the abnormal maximum stress test can provide us with a very useful tool in the clinical management of CAD patients. The early studies of the Master's test suggested this, but validation with the maximum test was needed to confirm it.

The fact that all abnormal responders to stress tests are not the same needs reemphasis. Marked differences exist between those with early onset

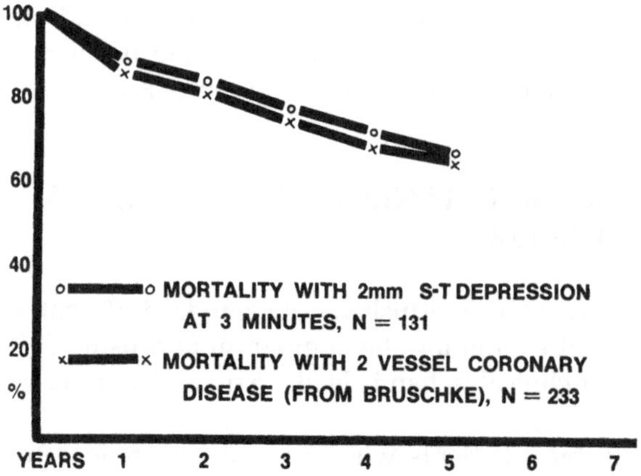

FIGURE 14–21. The mortality predicted by two-vessel CAD and by 2 mm of ST segment depression on the third minute of our protocol is the same. (Coronary angiogram mortality data from Bruschke et al,[21] with permission.)

of ischemia and those with changes near peak cardiac output. Among those with early-onset ischemia are patients who have lesions in the left main coronary and proximal branches of the circumflex and left anterior descending arteries. When the blood pressure and heart rate responses, ST configuration, R-wave changes, and other variables are considered, we can often come to a useful clinical diagnosis.

Coronary angiography has long been believed to be the ultimate test for helping to predict the future of subjects with CAD. As new information identifies the limits of angiography in defining flow, there is no doubt that some type of dynamic evaluation will be considered superior.[55] If our preliminary data are confirmed, stress testing may be considered as reliable. In a recent editorial Lauer proposes that exercise capacity, chronotropic response, and heart rate recovery are equal to exercise Echo or exercise nuclear studies in predicting death.[46,69] When comparing the life table figures of Bruschke and associates[21] with our subjects having early onset of ischemia, the curves are statistically equivalent (Fig. 14–21). The usefulness of the maximum stress test in predicting future events seems well established. Apparently, subsequent experiences can only result in further refinements in enhancing the usefulness of a test that has gained wide acceptance.

REFERENCES

1. Diamond, GA: Bayes' theorem: A practical aid to clinical judgment for diagnosis of coronary artery disease. Pract Cardiol 10(6):47–77, 1984.
2. Diamond, GA, et al: Application of information theory to clinical diagnostic testing. Circulation 63(4):915–921, 1981.

3. Diamond, GA and Forrester, JS: Analysis of probability as an aid in the clinical diagnosis of coronary artery disease. N Engl J Med 1350–1358, 1979.
4. Coronary Risk Handbook: New York Heart Association, 1973.
5. Hossack, KF, et al: Prognostic value of risk factors and exercise testing in men with atypical chest pain. Int J Cardiol 3:37–50, 1983.
6. Epstein, SE: Implications of probability analysis on the strategy used for non-invasive detection of coronary artery disease. Am J Cardiol 46:491–499, 1980.
7. Detrano, R, Gianrossi, R, and Mulvihill, D: Exercise-induced ST segment depression in the diagnosis of multivessel coronary disease. Am J Cardiol 14:1501–1508, 1989.
8. Ellestad, MH and Halliday, WK: Stress testing in the prognosis and management of ischemic heart disease. Angiology 28:149, 1977.
9. Marcus, ML: The Coronary Circulation in Health and Disease. McGraw-Hill, New York, 1983.
10. Feinstein, AR: The haze of Bayes, the aerial palaces of decision analysis, and the computerized Ouija board. Clin Pharmacol Ther 21:482–495, 1979.
11. Chaitman, BR, et al: Improved efficiency of treadmill exercise testing using a multiple lead ECG system and basic hemodynamic response. Circulation 57:71, 1978.
12. McHenry, PL, Phillips, JF, and Knobebel, SB: Correlation of computer quantitated treadmill exercise ECG with arteriographic location of coronary artery disease. Am J Cardiol 30:747, 1972.
13. Kassebaum, DG, Sutherland, KI, and Judkins, MP: A comparison of hypoxemia and exercise electrocardiography in coronary disease. Am Heart J 7:371, 1932.
14. Martin, CM and McConahay, DR: Maximal treadmill exercise electrocardiography: Correlations with coronary arteriography and cardiac hemodynamics. Circulation 46:956, 1972.
15. Helfant, RH, et al: Exercise related ventricular premature complexes in coronary heart disease. Ann Intern Med 80:589, 1974.
16. Weiner, DA, et al: Correlations among history of angina, ST segment response and prevalence of coronary artery disease in the Coronary Artery Surgery Study. N Engl J Med 301:230, 1979.
17. Simoons, ML and Hugenholtz, PG: Estimation of probability of exercise-induced ischemia by quantitative ECG analysis. Am J Cardiol 56:522, 1977.
18. Simoons, ML: Optimal measurements for detection of coronary artery disease by exercise ECG. Comput Biomed Res 10:483, 1977.
19. Bartel, AG, et al: Graded exercise stress tests in angiographically documented coronary artery disease. Circulation 49:348, 1974.
20. Ellestad, MH and Wan, MKC: Predictive implications of stress testing: Follow-up of 1700 subjects after maximum treadmill stress testing. Circulation 51:363, 1975.
21. Bruschke, AVG, Proudfoot, WL, and Sones, FM Jr: Progress study of 590 consecutive nonsurgical cases of coronary disease followed 5–9 years: Arteriographic correlations. Circulation 42:1154, 1973.
22. McNeer, JF, et al: The role of the exercise test in the evaluation of patients for ischemic heart disease. Circulation 57:64, 1978.
23. Chaitman, BR, et al: The importance of clinical subsets in interpreting maximal treadmill exercise test results: The role of multiple lead ECG systems. Circulation 59:560, 1979.
24. Ellestad, MH, et al: The false positive stress test multivariate analysis of 215 subjects with hemodynamic, angiographic and clinical data. Am J Cardiol 40:681–685, 1977.
25. Erikssen, J and Myhre, E: False positive exercise ECG: A misnomer? Int J Cardiol 6:263–268, 1984.
26. Castellanet, M, Greenberg, PS, and Ellestad, MH: Comparison of ST segment changes on exercise testing of angiographic findings in patients with prior myocardial infarction. Am J Cardiol 42:24–35, 1978.
27. Stone, PH, Lafollette, LE, and Cohn, K: Patterns of exercise treadmill test performance in patients with left main coronary artery disease: Detection dependent on left coronary dominance or coexistent dominant right coronary disease. Am Heart J 104(1):13–19, 1982.
28. Weiner, DA, et al: Assessment of the negative exercise test in 4,373 patients from the coronary artery surgery study (CASS). J Cardiac Rehabil 2(71):562–568, 1982.
29. Hakki, AH, et al: Implications of normal exercise electrocardiographic results in patients with angiographically documented coronary artery disease: Correlation with left ventricular function and myocardial perfusion. Am J Med 75:439–444, 1983.

30. Robb, GP, Marks, HH, and Mattingly, TW: The value of the double standard 2 step exercise test in detecting coronary disease in a follow-up study of 1,000 military personnel. Research Report AMSG-21-54, Army Medical Service Graduate School, Walter Reed Army Medical Center, Washington, DC, September 1957.
31. Robb, GP: Metropolitan Life Statistical Bulletin. 53, 1972.
32. Mattingly, TW: The postexercise electrocardiogram: Its value in the diagnosis and prognosis of coronary arterial disease. Am J Cardiol 9:395, 1962.
33. Bruce, RA, DeRouen, TA, and Hossack, KF: Value of maximal exercise tests in risk assessment of primary coronary heart disease events in healthy men: Five years' experience of the Seattle Heart Watch Study. Am J Cardiol 46:371–378, 1980.
34. Weiner, DA, et al: Prognostic importance of a clinical profile and exercise test in medically treated patients with coronary artery disease. J Am Coll Cardiol 3(3):772–779, 1984.
35. Gibbons, LW, et al: Maximal exercise test as a predictor of risk for mortality from coronary heart disease in asymptomatic men. Am J Cardiol 86:53, 2000.
36. Myers, J, et al: Exercise capacity and mortality among men preferred for exercise testing. New Engl J of Med 346 (11):793, 2002.
37. Goldschlager, H, et al: Treadmill stress tests as indicators of presence and severity of coronary artery disease. Ann Intern Med 85:277, 1976.
38. Schneider, RM, et al: Early positive exercise test: Implications for prognosis. Prim Cardiol: 49, 1983.
39. Hustead, R and Ellestad, MH: Failure of the magnitude of ST segment depression to predict the severity of ischemia. Circulation 88(4)I:109, 1993.
40. Bogaty, P, et al: Does more ST segment depression on the 12-lead exercise electrocardiogram signify more severe ischemic heart disease? (Abstract) Circulation 88(suppl 2):1, 1993.
41. Podrid, PJ, et al: Prognosis of medically treated patients with coronary artery disease with profound ST segment depression during exercise testing. N Engl J Med305(19):1111, 1981.
42. Deganis, GR, et al: Survival of patients with a strongly positive exercise ECG. Circulation 65:452, 1982.
43. Mirvis, DM, et al: Regional blood flow correlates of ST segment depression in tachycardia-induced myocardial ischemia. Circulation 73:365, 1986.
44. Pupita, G, et al: Reproducibility and relation to the degree of myocardial ischemia of postexercise electrocardiographic changes in stable angina pectoris. Am J Cardiol 68:1397, 1991.
45. Hammond, HK, et al: Radionuclide imaging correlatives of heart rate impairment during maximal exercise testing. J Am Coll Cardiol 2(5):826, 1983.
46. Lauer, MS: Chronotropic Incompetence and Heart Rate Recovery. Exercise Testing: New Concepts for the New Century, Kluwer, 2001.
47. Sandvik, L, et al: Hert rate increase and maximal hert rate during exercise as predictors of Cardiovascular mortality: A 16-year follow-up study of 1960 healthy men. Coron Artery Dis. 5:667, 1995.
48. Kannel, WB, et al: Heart rate and cardiovascular mortality: The Framingham study. Am Heart J 113:1489, 1987.
49. Dyer, AR, et al: Heart rate as a prognostic factor for coronary heart disease and mortality. Am J Epidemiol 736, 1980.
50. Ellestad, MH, et al: Diagnostic and prognostic information derived from stress testing. In Wenger, NK (ed): Exercise and the Heart. FA Davis, Philadelphia, 1978.
51. Cole, J and Ellestad, MH: Significance of chest pain during treadmill exercise. Am J Cardiol 41:227, 1978.
52. Weiner, DA, et al: The predictive value of anginal chest pain as an indicator of coronary disease during exercise testing. Am Heart J 96(4):458, 1978.
53. Jelinek, VM, et al: The significance of chest pain occurring with the Master Two Step Test. Aust NZ J Med 6:22, 1976.
54. Hayet, M and Kellerman, JJ: The angina pectoris, heart rate threshold as a prognostic sign. Cardiology 68(suppl 2):78, 1981.
55. Bruce, RA: Exercise testing of patients with coronary heart disease. Ann Clin Res 3:323, 1971.
56. Abbott, RD, et al: Cardiovascular risk factors and graded treadmill exercise endurance in healthy adults. Am J Cardiol 63:342, 1989.
57. Myers, J, et al: Exercise capacity and mortality among men referred for exercise testing. N Engl J Med 346:793, 2002.
58. Weiner, DA, et al: Exercise induced ST changes, post-infarction: Predictive value for multivessel disease [abstract]. Circulation 111 (suppl 55 & 56)111, 1977.

59. Master, AM and Oppenheimer, ET: A simple exercise tolerance test for circulatory efficiency with standard tables for normal individuals. Am J Med Sci 177:223, 1929.
60. Greenberg, PS, et al: Use of the multivariate approach to enhance the diagnostic accuracy of the treadmill stress test. J Electrocardiol 13 (3):227, 1980.
61. Greenberg, PS, et al: Comparison of the multivariate analysis and CADENZA systems for determination of the probability of coronary artery disease. Am J Cardiol 53:493, 1984.
62. Diamond, GA, et al: Computer assisted diagnosis in the noninvasive evaluation of patients with suspected coronary artery disease. J Am Coll Cardiol. 1:444, 1983.
63. Detrano, R, et al. Factors affecting sensitivity and specificity of a diagnostic test: The exercise thallium scintingram. Am J Med 84:699, 1988.
64. Shaw, LJ, et al: Use of prognostic treadmill score in identifying diagnostic coronary disease subgroups. Circulation Oct 20;98 (16):1622, 1998.
65. Do, D, et al: A consensus approach to diagnosing coronary Artery disease based on clinical and exercise test data*: Chest 111(6):1742, 1997.
66. Lipinski, M, et al: Comparison of treadmill scores with physician estimates of diagnosis and prognosis in patients with coronary artery disease. Am Heart J 143:650, 2002.
67. Morise, AP, et al: Development and validation of a clinical score to estimate the probability of coronary artery disease in men and women presenting with suspected coronary disease. Am J Med 102:350, 1997.
68. Berman, JL, et al: Value of a multivariate approach for interpreting treadmill exercise tests in coronary heart disease [abstract]. Am J Cardiol 41:375, 1978.
69. Lauer, M: The "exercise" part of exercise echocardiography. JACC 39(8); 1353, 2002.

15
Stress Testing in Women

Prevalence of Coronary Artery Disease in Women Versus Men
Sensitivity and Specificity of ST Changes
Findings According to Symptoms
Typical Angina
Probable Angina
Mechanisms
Strategy to Separate True-Positive From False-Positive Patients

Since the early days of exercise stress testing, ST-segment depression has been the focus of interest as a marker for ischemia. The increased tendency for a false-positive ST response was first noted in women by Scherlis and associates[1] as early as 1950 and confirmed by Lepeschkin and Surawicz[2] in 1958 and Astrand[3] in 1965. Because the trends in coronary artery disease (CAD) in women seem to parallel those of lung cancer, another disease often induced by smoking, we expect to be treating more women with this problem than ever before. Is there a way to deal with ST changes in women? What is the cause? Is ST depression in women with normal coronary arteries truly a false-positive? Is it due to ischemia?

This chapter reviews information available bearing on these perplexing problems, suggests some partial answers, and offers guidelines that we have found useful.

PREVALENCE OF CORONARY ARTERY DISEASE IN WOMEN VERSUS MEN

Exact information on prevalence of CAD in women is difficult to acquire because we are dependent on symptoms to lead us to the diagnosis, especially in younger subjects. Data on mortality, however, suggest that women lag behind men by about 10 years, and the age-adjusted mortality in men is about 2.5 times that of women[4,5] (Fig. 15–1). At younger ages, however, CAD in men exceeds that found in women by 5 to 1. It has been found that risk factors of smoking and use of oral contraceptives are almost always present when CAD is found in premenopausal nondiabetic women.[6] On the other hand, Engel and colleagues[6] found family history to be the most important risk factor in these patients. It is paradoxical that exercise-induced ST de-

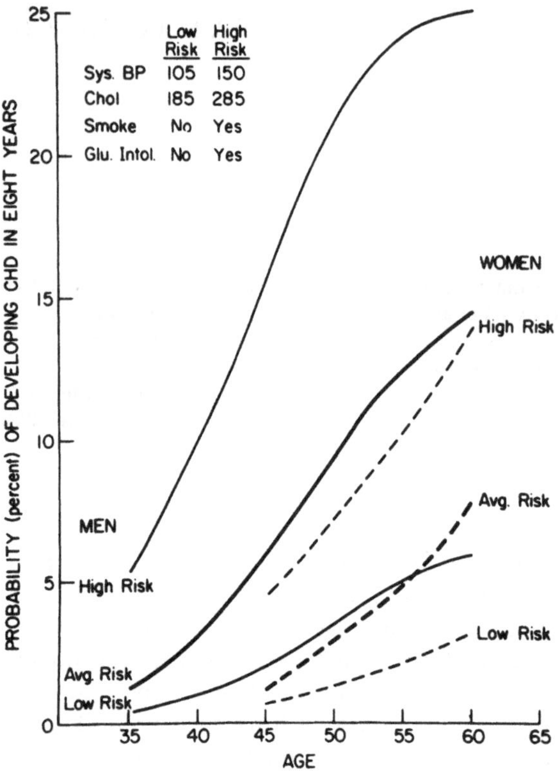

FIGURE 15–1. Probability of women developing CAD in 8 years according to age, sex, and risk. Men ——; Women ------ (From the Framingham Heart Study, with permission.)[4]

pression in normal women younger than age 45 has been found to be much more common than in men (almost four times)—by both Wu's group[7] in Milan and Profant and associates[8] in Seattle. Because CAD is known to be less prevalent in women than in men, these changes must be presumed to be due to some process independent of coronary atherosclerosis. As the women in the study of Wu and associates aged, however, the prevalence of ST depression fell.[7] In women older than age 45, during the years we know they are more susceptible to CAD, the prevalence of ST depression was exceeded by the men in their study (Fig. 15–2). Our experience with a group of normal volunteers did not reflect this trend, however (see Table 14–5).

SENSITIVITY AND SPECIFICITY OF ST CHANGES

As in all studies, we must remember that the population under scrutiny determines the findings. Most reported series analyzing ST depression in

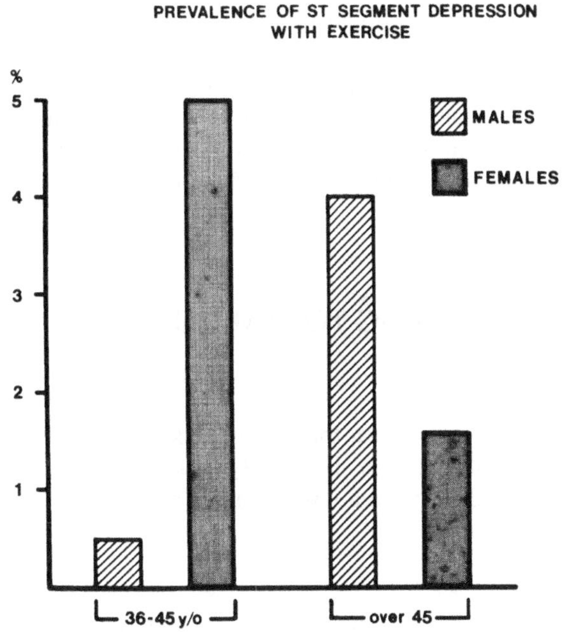

FIGURE 15–2. Prevalence of exercise-induced ST depression in normal subjects according to age. The young women with a low prevalence of CAD and a high estrogen level show a higher prevalence than men. This ratio reverses in patients older than aged 45. (Drawn from data in Wu[7].)

women are from cardiac centers where women with chest pain syndromes are sent for angiography. Thus, the symptoms and signs determine the sampling. When women with chest discomfort, for whatever cause, come to undergo angiography, they are likely to have been screened with an exercise test. If the test is normal, few are sent for angiography. Thus, the sampling favors those with ST depression. This is also true for men. Of the various studies comparing men and women, Sketch and associates[9] in Nebraska found that 8% of men and 67% of women had false-positive ST changes. Linhart and coworkers,[10] on the other hand, found that only 22% of their female subjects had false-positive ST depression and only 5% when they excluded those with abnormal resting ECGs and those on drugs. It is unlikely that women in Omaha were much different from those in Philadelphia. Koppes and colleagues[11] report false-positive rates of 24% to 35% in four studies they reviewed, and Amsterdam and associates[12] reviewed 96 men and 65 women with normal coronary angiograms and reported the false-positive rate of 15% in women compared with 11% in men. Weiner and coworkers[13] studied 3153 patients in the CASS study and reported a false-positive rate of 3% in men and 14% in women. The false-negative rate was 38% and 22%, respectively. The investigators then matched men and women for age, previous infarction, and coronary anatomy and found the false-positive and false-negative rates to be almost identical. When Guiteras and associates[14] and Chaitman and colleagues[15] at the Montreal Heart Institute evaluated 112 women according to symptoms, as well as different lead systems, the overall sensitivity was 79% and the specificity 66% using 14 leads. This is considerably lower than that reported in most studies of men. In a study by Guiteras,[15] the specificity in men was 82%. Similar results were obtained using only CC_5 or CM_5.

FINDINGS ACCORDING TO SYMPTOMS

Typical Angina

In women with typical angina, the pretest risk in the CASS study was 0.75 and postexercise test risk with abnormal ST depression was 0.83. These data were similar to the data of men with typical angina.

Probable Angina

In women with probable angina, the pretest risk was 0.36 and after ST depression with exercise, 0.5.[14] This group turns out to have a high false-positive rate and a low specificity. In those with nonspecific chest pain, the post-test likelihood was zero. The researchers in the CASS study found typical angina during testing and exercise ST elevation to be 100% reliable in detecting CAD, however. On the other hand, ST depression found only during exercise and not immediately afterward had a low specificity (89% false-positive).

Sketch and Aronow[16] categorized their data according to symptoms and constructed Figure 15–3. The sensitivity of their data varied more between sexes than did the specificity, thus their false-positive rate remained low in all groups. Some of the above data suggest that the false-positive tracings are due to prevalence alone. This presupposes that many known causes such as mitral prolapse, vasoregulatory asthenia, and drug effects are excluded. Certainly, some of these problems are more common in women than men.

The most encouraging progress in the analysis of women comes from work by Hung[17] from Montreal and Okin and Kligfield[18] from New York. The former investigators used logistic discriminant analysis of a number of exercise variables, and in 135 infarct-free women reported a sensitivity of 70% and a specificity of 93%. The three variables of significance were maximum heart rate, maximum workload and ST depression in lead X (the orthogonal lead most similar to lead V_5). Okin and Kligfield reported even better results using their ST/HR slope. They found a sensitivity of 97% and a specificity of 93%. Although their work using this approach seems physiologically sound, it has been challenged by Frolicher and colleagues[19] and others,[20] and the final verdict is still out.

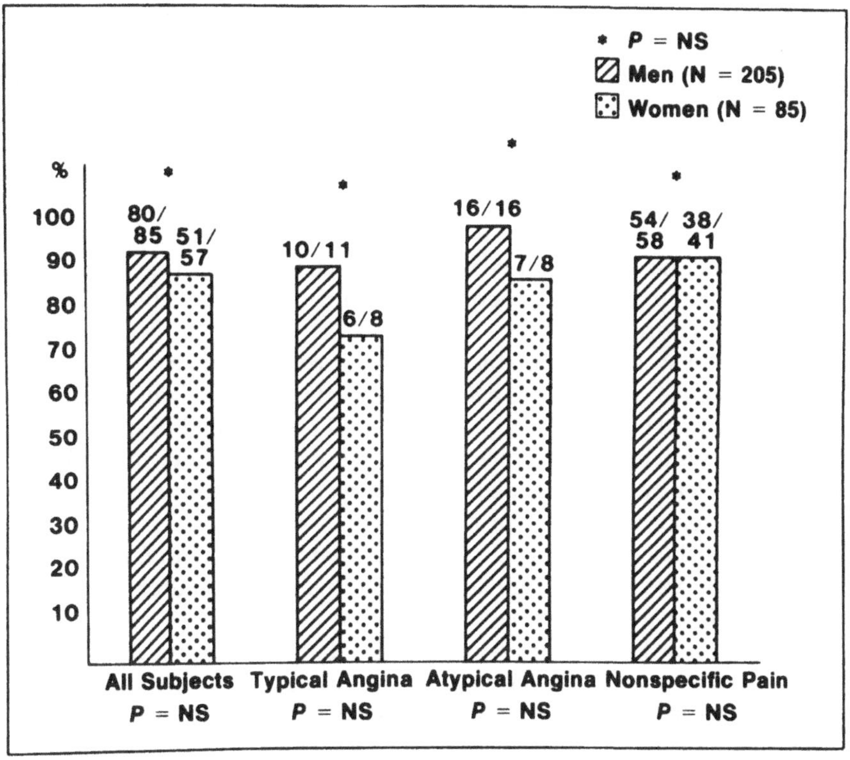

FIGURE 15–3. The specificity of an abnormal exercise test for men and women according to chest pain syndrome. These data differ from those of other workers in that there is a lower prevalence of false-positive responders among the women. This would be expected if most of the women were older. (From Sketch and Aronow,[16] with permission.)

MECHANISMS

Estrogens have been implicated as a cause of ST depression. Jaffe[21] has reported that oral estrogens increase the prevalence of ST depression and androgens decrease the effect. Estrogens have a similar chemical structure to that of digitalis, which is known to cause ST depression and has been believed to function as a coronary vasoconstrictor. This mechanism has been proposed as a likely explanation for some of the changes seen. Recent reports have cast doubt on these concepts, however. Glasser and Clarke[22] followed up 18 healthy young women, ages 18 through 35, and correlated exercise-induced ST changes with fluctuations in estrogen and progesterone. Seven had exercise-induced ST depression at some time in their cycle—some when estrogen levels were high and some when estrogens levels were low—but none had ST changes when progesterone levels were high. The conclusions of Glasser and Clark were that a proportion of these two hormones had some effect on ST depression, but they could offer no clear mechanism for their findings. Williams and associates[23] have recently reported that estrogen in atherosclerotic female monkeys caused inhibition of acetylcholine-induced constriction of the coronary tree by its effect on the vascular endothelium. This finding also casts doubt on the role of estrogen as a coronary vasoconstrictor. Dalal and Morise[24] have reported a reduced prevalence of abnormal exercise tests in postmenopausal women who take estrogens, suggesting that these hormones have a protective influence on the coronary tree. High doses of estrogens have also been reported to improve coronary blood flow in women with syndrome X.[25]

For years it seemed certain that estrogens protect women from coronary artery disease. This concept has been challenged recently,[26,27] although there is still a good deal of controversy. Also, several reports tend to strongly link the hormone with exercise induced ST depression.[26] Vaitkevicius and associates[28] have clearly demonstrated that hyperventilation-induced ST depression in postmenopausal women is related in some way to estrogens, and Marmor and colleagues[29] have documented that women with false-positive ST-segment depression during exercise lose this response after surgical removal of their ovaries. They have shown that not only does removing the estrogen eliminate the ST depression, but also that replacing it in two women who changed from an abnormal response to a normal response with surgery results in a return of ST depression with exercise. In my mind, this fulfills Koch's postulates.

Subclinical disturbances in muscle function that are associated with reduced left-ventricular compliance may be more common in women. These changes may be due to a nonspecific cardiomyopathy or the hypertrophy associated with hypertension.[30] Kasumi and coworkers[31] studied left-ventricular dynamics in women with ST depression compared with normal subjects and described higher vascular resistance and an increased oxygen demand, especially at the subendocardial level. They postulate that this is an important cause for false-positive changes.

Syndrome X patients, mostly women with angina relieved by nitroglycerin, who have normal coronary arteries may well have reduced coronary vasodilator reserve.[32] Abnormal lactate excretion has been shown in these patients with atrial pacing. Whether this phenomenon is hormonal, autonomic, or mechanical has yet to be elucidated. Higgenbotham[33] found that normal women do not show an increase in ejection fraction with exercise, as measured by radionuclide angiography, and also that they have a greater increase in diastolic volume. If we remember that asymptomatic women with exercise-induced ST depression have a higher mean pulmonary pressure with exercise than women without this change,[31] it can be assumed that there is a subset of women who, for reasons unknown, have an abnormal hemodynamic response to exercise. It may be that so-called normal women with exercise-induced ST depression have abnormal left-ventricular function and a limited vasodilator reserve. This process may be the first stage of what eventually becomes syndrome X.

I expect that in time some of the mechanisms will be better understood. Various maneuvers are now under study to help to identify them.

An excellent article by Morise discusses this issue in detail and I would urge the serious student to review it.[34]

STRATEGY TO SEPARATE TRUE-POSITIVE FROM FALSE-POSITIVE PATIENTS

When testing women the pretest likelihood cannot be ignored.

Careful attention to the history of pain, medications, physical signs, and other laboratory signs of disease will go a long way toward helping to distinguish the true disease process. Mitral prolapse is often associated with ST depression in young premenopausal women.

Rapid upsloping ST, increasing septal Q amplitude, and large P waves suggesting the possibility of a large Ta wave can also alert us to the probability of a false-positive.

Repeating the test with the patient in a fasting state, if the abnormal one was done soon after a meal, may help.[35]

The use of beta blockers has been shown to correct abnormal ST changes in the absence of CAD[33,36] (see Chapter 19). Okin and Kligfield[18] have reported that the ST/HR slope can improve the reliability when testing women.

If indicated, thallium stress testing[37] performed in high-quality laboratories may add data to confirm or negate the results suggested by ST-segment depression after the standard exercise test has been completed. The American Heart Association and the American College of Cardiology have published guidelines that state "currently there is insufficient data to justify stress imaging tests as the initial test in women". [38] However, we have found nuclear perfusion studies also to have a higher false-positive rate in women. I believe that the ST/HR slope holds the most promise for a highly accurate exercise test in women. It is hoped that the work of the Cornell group will be confirmed by others.[18]

Angiography is indicated in certain clinical situations even when normal coronary arteries are suspected. Clearing up uncertainty is important, especially since the risk of angiography is virtually zero in top-flight laboratories. We should remember that normal epicardial coronary arteries on angiography do not rule out myocardial ischemia. Therefore, labeling a patient with syndrome X as a neurotic is a disservice to the patient as well as to the physician.

CONCLUSIONS

It appears that even using careful clinical analysis and all the information available during stress testing, the reliability of the stress test in women is lower than that of men. In most cases, when the ST depression is suspected to be due to noncoronary causes, it can be confirmed with some certainty short of an angiogram.

It is important to remember that the prevalence of false-positive ST depression is high in younger women, who are unlikely to have CAD on the basis of age alone. As they age, the number of false-positive changes decreases, and ST depression becomes a more reliable marker for CAD. Even though there are more false-positive tests in women, a negative test provides a greater assurance that there is no disease than a negative test in men.

When dealing with women with pain and normal coronary arteries, reassurance, understanding, and careful follow-up are essential in providing a proper program to minimize disability.

REFERENCES

1. Scherlis, L, et al: Effects of single and double two step exercise tests upon the electrocardiogram of 200 normal persons. J Mt Sinai Hosp 7:242–253, 1950.
2. Lepeschkin, E and Surawicz, B: Characteristics of true positive and false positive results of electrocardiographic Masters two step tests. N Engl J Med 258:511–520, 1958.
3. Astrand, I: Electrocardiograms recorded twice within a 8 year interval in a group of 204 women and men. Acta Med Scand 178:27–39, 1965.
4. Levy, RI and Feinleib, M: Risk factors for coronary artery disease and their management. In Braunwald, E (ed): Heart Disease. WB Saunders, Philadelphia, 1984, p 1206.
5. World Health Organization: World Health Statistics Annual. Geneva, WHO 1980.
6. Engel, HJ, Page, HL Jr, and Campbell, WB: Coronary artery disease in young women. JAMA 230(11):1531–1534, 1974.
7. Wu, SC, et al: Sex differences in the prevalence of ischemic heart disease and in the response to a stress test in a working population. Eur Heart J 2:461–465, 1981.
8. Profant, GR, et al: Responses to maximum exercise in healthy middle-aged women. J Appl Physiol 33:595, 1972.
9. Sketch, MH, et al: Significant sex differences in the correlation of electrocardiographic exercise testing and coronary arteriograms. Am J Cardiol 36:169–173, 1975.
10. Linhart, JW, Laws, JG, and Satinsky JD: Maximum treadmill exercise electrocardiography in female patients. Circulation 50:1173–1178, 1974.
11. Koppes, G, et al: Treadmill exercise testing. Curr Probl Cardiol 8:1, 1977.
12. Amsterdam, EA, et al: Exercise stress testing in patients with angiographically normal coronary arteries: Similar frequency of false positive ischemic responses in males and females. Am J Cardiol 41:378, 1978.
13. Weiner, DA, et al: Correlations among history of angina, ST segment response and prevalence of coronary artery disease in the coronary artery surgery study (CASS). N Engl J Med 301:230, 1979.
14. Guiteras, P, et al: Diagnostic accuracy of exercise ECG lead systems in clinical subsets of women. Circulation 65(7):1465–1474, 1982.
15. Chaitman, BR, et al: Improved efficiency of treadmill exercise testing using a multiple lead ECG system and basic hemodynamic exercise response. Circulation 57:71, 1978.
16. Sketch, MH and Aronow, WS: Continuing education: Diagnostic and prognostic value of exercise testing. J Cardiac Rehab 3:495–508, 1983.
17. Hung, J, et al: Noninvasive diagnostic test choices for the evaluation of coronary artery disease in women. J Am Coll Cardiol 4:8–16, 1984.

18. Okin, PM and Kligfield, P: Identifying coronary artery disease in women by heart rate adjustment of ST segment depression. Am J Cardiol 69:297–302, 1992.
19. Froelicher, V, et al: Exercise-induced ST depression in the diagnosis of coronary disease: A meta-analysis. Circulation 80:87–97, 1989.
20. Bobbio, M and Detrano, R: A lesson from the controversy about HR adjustment of ST segment depression. Circulation: 84:1410–1413, 1991.
21. Jaffe, MD: Effect of testosterone cypionate on post exercise ST segment depression. Br Heart J 39:1217, 1977.
22. Glasser, SP and Clark, PI: Interpretation of exercise test results in women. Pract Cardiol 14(8):85–90, 1988.
23. Williams, JK, et al: Short-term administration of estrogen and vascular response of atherosclerotic coronary arteries. J Am Coll Cardiol 20:452–720, 1992.
24. Dalal, LN and Morise, AP: Exercise testing in women. Cardiology 25:57–60, 1992.
25. Steingart, RM, et al: Coronary disease in women: Underdiagnosed and undertreated. J Myocardl Ischemia 4:61, 1992.
26. Hulley, S, et al: Randomized trial of estrogen plus progestin for secondary prevention of coronary heart disease in post-menopausal women. JAMA 280 (7):605, 1998.
27. Grodstein, F, et al: Postmenopausal estrogen andprogestin use and the risk of cardiovascular disease. New Engl J Med 335:453, 1996.
28. Vaitkevicius, P, et al: Effect of estrogen replacement therapy on the ST segment response to postural and hyperventilation stimuli. Am J Cardiol 64:1076, 1989.
29. Marmor, A, et al: Effects of bilateral hystero-salpingo-oophorectomy, on exercise induced ST segment abnormalities in young women. Am J Cardiol 71:1118, 1993.
30. Ellestad, MH, et al: The false positive stress test multivariate analysis of 215 subjects with hemodynamic, angiographic and clinical data. Am J Cardiol 40:681, 1977.
31. Kasumi, F, et al: Elevated arterial pressure and post-exertional ST segment depression inmiddle aged women. Am Heart J 92(5):576, 1976.
32. Marcus, ML: The Coronary Circulation in Health and Disease. McGraw-Hill, New York, 1983.
33. Higgenbotham, MB, et al: Sex related differences in the normal cardiac response to upright exercise. Circulation 70:357, 1984.
34. Morise, AP. Exercise electrocardiography in women with suspected coronary disease. Exercise Testing: New Concepts for the New Century. Kluwer Academic Publishers, 2002.
35. McHenry, PI and Morris, SN: Exercise electrocardiography: Current state of the art. In Schlant, RC and Hurst, JW (eds): Advances in Electrocardiography. Grune & Stratton, New York, pp 265, 1976.
36. Marcomichelakis, J, et al: Exercise testing after beta-blockade: Improved specificity and predictive value in detecting coronary heart disease. Br Heart J 43:252, 1980.
37. Friedman, TD, et al: Exercise thallium-201 myocardial scintigraphy in women: Correlation with coronary arteriography. Am J Cardiol 49:1632, 1982.
38. Gibbons, RJ, et al: ACC/AHA guidelines for exercise testing: a report of the American College of Cardiology/American Heart Association Task Force on Practice Guidelines (Committee on Exercise Testing). J Am Coll Cardiol 30:260, 1997.

16 Exercise Testing in Congestive Heart Failure

Measurement of VO_2 Max in Normal Patients
Oxygen Transport
Caveats in the Use of VO_2 Max
VO_2 Max in Congestive Heart Failure Patients
Treadmill Protocol
6-Minute–Walk Test
Instrumentation
Heart Rate
Exercise Duration
Can Exercise Capacity Predict Events?

The use of exercise testing in congestive heart failure has become fairly common in the last few years and it seems appropriate to include a chapter reviewing the concepts and the practical applications now being applied. It has now become apparent that the usual indices of ventricular function such as ejection fraction, stroke volume or pulmonary wedge pressure do not correlate with the patient's capacity for exercise. Naughton was one of the first to use exercise testing to obtain an objective measurement of exercise capacity in heart failure, correlating it with total body oxygen consumption.[1] He reported that when a patient's maximum oxygen consumption was less than 20 milliliters per kilogram per minute they invariably had symptoms that limited their performance (Table 16–1).

Previously, patients with heart failure were classified according to the criteria of the New York Heart Association based on the amount of activity they could sustain without exercise symptoms.[2] These subjective categories were of limited use when attempting to evaluate therapy. The idea that the plateau in oxygen uptake occurring during progressive exercise was a function of the maximum capacity of the circulatory and respiratory systems was first proposed by Hill and Lipton over 75 years ago (Table 16–2).[3]

MEASUREMENT OF VO_2 MAX IN NORMAL PATIENTS

In order to understand the use of maximal oxygen consumption in congestive heart failure, a few comments about the response in normal individuals is in order. Experience has demonstrated that to obtain accurate measurements of VO_2 max exercise must involve at least 50% of the person's total

Table 16–1. **Grading the Severity of Chronic Cardiac Failure According to Aerobic Activity**

Class	Severity	Aerobic Capacity (mL/min/kg)*
A	None to little	>20
B	Mild to moderate	16–20
C	Moderate to severe	10–16
D	Severe	<10

*Measured as maximum oxygen uptake.

Table 16–2. **NYHA Functional Classification**

Class I	*Class III*
No limitation. Ordinary physical activity does not cause symptoms.	Marked limitation of physical activity. Less than ordinary activity leads to symptoms.
Class II	***Class IV***
Slight limitation of physical activity. Ordinary physical activity will result in symptoms.	Inability to carry on any activity without symptoms. Symptoms are present at rest.

muscle mass.[4] Thus, walking or running has become the standard, although bicycling, which results in values about 10% below treadmill performance, is occasionally used. During progressive exercise on a treadmill for every 100 ml/min/m_2 increment in oxygen uptake the heart normally provides approximately 600 ml/min/m_2 of cardiac output.[5]

Measuring oxygen uptake requires determining the volume of expired gas, the faction of oxygen and the faction of carbon dioxide, the expired gas temperature and the barometric pressure.

The amount of carbon dioxide produced divided by the oxygen that is consumed is the respiratory exchange ratio or respiratory quotient ($R = VO_2/VCO_2$). During submaximal steady state exercise the R value ranges from .6 to .8 and, when the subject is near exhaustion, it increases to 1.0. The point when R = 1.0 has been termed the anaerobic threshold. The increase in CO_2 results from an increase in lactic acid as an energy substrate as the supply of oxygen becomes inadequate to supply the increased energy demand. This is because the lactate is buffered by bicarbonate, leading to the production of carbonate acid, which converts to CO_2 and water. This nonmetabolic source of CO_2 raises the respiratory quotient to 1.0.[4] With maximum exertion oxygen consumption plateaus and, in normals, this is a very reproducible measurement. This can be increased by physical conditioning in normals by as much as 15% to 20% in active subjects and in sedentary people by as much as 40%.

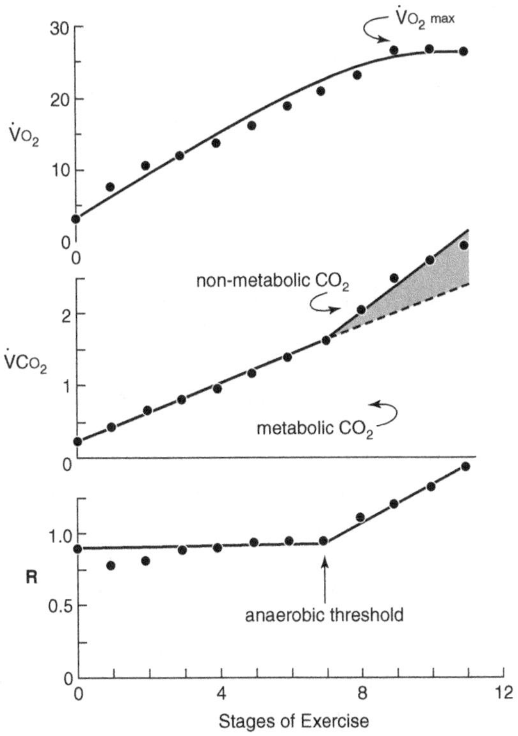

Figure 16–1. The response in CO_2 production, O_2 uptake is depicted during exercise. The respiratory gas exchange ratio (R) to progressive exercise and increasing O_2 uptake is shown. The metabolic and nonmetabolic components of VCO_2 response are indicated and the onset of anaerobic metabolism is identified as the anaerobic threshold, with permission of publisher.[4]

OXYGEN TRANSPORT

Oxygen delivery to the working muscle is also influenced by oxygen transport, or the amount carried by hemoglobin. Arterial oxygen transport (ml/min) = hemoglobin concentration × 1.35 × arterial oxygen saturation × cardiac output × 10. 1.35 is the oxygen-carrying capacity of 1 gm of hemoglobin. This factor is especially important where chronic anemia is present.[5]

Caveats in the Use of VO_2 Max

Measurements of VO_2 max and the respiratory equivalent are dependent not only on accurate measurements and sampling techniques, but on several physiological mechanisms that are difficult to predict. The utilization of lactic acid by the muscles is one of the most important and is dependent on the

AV O_2 difference, the glycogen stores, free fatty acid metabolism, obesity, blood flow in various muscle beds, insulin resistance and several more.

Age also has a significant effect on Vo_2 uptake and muscle metabolism, as well as blood flow. All of these effects make normal values for any subject difficult to characterize and attempts to establish normal ranges for population groups have resulted in wide variations.

Vo_2 MAX IN CONGESTIVE HEART FAILURE PATIENTS

Patients with poor ventricular function in congestive heart failure have a limited reaching a plateau or steady state. Because of this limitation "peak" oxygen uptake, which is almost the same or just slightly above the anaerobic threshold is used as an objective measurement of exercise capacity rather than when oxygen consumption reaches a plateau. This measurement varies as much as 20% to 30% in some patients while Vo_2 max in normal subjects is repeatable within 5%.[6] Thus, measurements of peak Vo_2 in congestive heart failure are helpful but do not always parallel changes in cardiac output, probably because cardiac output and increased muscular blood flow do not always appear simultaneously. The factors mentioned in the preceding paragraph are also important. Maximum Vo_2 however, has been demonstrated to be useful in not only measuring progress, or the lack thereof, but also in predicting mortality (Fig. 16–2).[7]

TREADMILL PROTOCOL

Because of the expectation that capacity is limited, a slow protocol is usually used. A modified Naughton Protocol with 2-minute stages is convenient and the most commonly used. We have found it to be very satisfactory. Patients on a treadmill stop because of either fatigue or dyspnea. If the exercise load is increased rapidly, breathlessness will usually cause termination, but if a slow protocol is used fatigue will be the reason to stop exercise. In general, the former situation will result in a higher maximum Vo_2, thus if the patient's clinical progress is being measured with maximum oxygen uptake, the same protocol should be used for each test (Table 16–3).[8]

6-MINUTE–WALK TEST

This simple protocol is quite popular and has been used to estimate exercise capacity and function in congestive heart failure patients in many therapeutic trials.[8] A 20 meter long enclosed corridor is marked off and the patient is

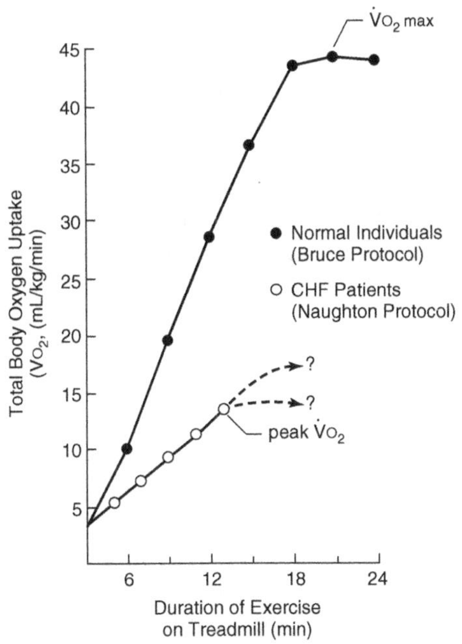

Figure 16–2. The relationship between oxygen consumption and duration of exercise in normal individuals who reach a plateau and in patients with congestive heart failure who, because of symptoms, do not reach a plateau, with permission of publisher.[7]

encouraged to walk back and forth for 6 minutes at his best rate possible. The distance covered is recorded and used as a measure of cardiac function. This test has been reported to be an excellent predictor of mortality and morbidity, however we have found it to be most useful in the more severe patients, i.e., N.Y. Heart Classification III and IV.

Table 16–3. **Naughton Protocol**

		Patient Data	
Stage	**Speed (MPH)**	**Grade**	**Duration (min)**
0 (Rest)	0	0.0	3.0
1	1.0	0.0	2.0
2	2.0	0.0	2.0
3	2.0	3.5	2.0
4	2.0	7.0	2.0
5	2.0	10.5	2.0
6	2.0	14.0	2.0
7	2.0	17.5	2.0
8	3.0	12.5	2.0
9	3.0	15.0	2.0
10	3.0	17.5	2.0

INSTRUMENTATION

There are a number of excellent systems that measure oxygen and CO_2 with electrodes and a flow meter in a mouthpiece and, combined with an excellent computer program, may calculate the necessary values on line during the exercise test. One can estimate the anaerobic threshold by the R-value or by the change in ventilatory volume that usually occurs as the lactic acid level increases. A detailed discussion of this technology can be found in an excellent text by Weber.[4]

HEART RATE

The heart rate response to isotonic exercise should be appropriate for the level of muscle work and Vo_2 consumption. There was a time when a slow heart rate during exercise was believed to identify excellent conditioning. Although this is to some extent true, an inappropriately reduced chronotropic response is now recognized as a predictor of poor prognosis.[10] Most patients with severe congestive heart failure are unable to reach their age predicted heart rate.[11] This is probably due to an adjustment in their autonomic control as the heart rate in these patients can be accelerated during exercise by intravenous atropine. There is a sub group of heart failure patients who have inappropriate sinus tachycardia. This compromises myocardial relaxation, ventricular filling and coronary perfusion, which is mostly a diastolic event. Patients with atrial fibrillation usually fall into this category. Reducing their heart rate with beta-blockers is usually beneficial in these patients (Fig. 16–3).

EXERCISE DURATION

Although in normals, an increase in exercise duration is usually believed to reflect a more efficient cardiovascular system, in congestive heart failure there may be exceptions to this dictum. At times an increase in exercise duration and an increase in peak Vo_2 consumption may not increase in parallel. Certain pharmacological interventions, such as vasodilators, may delay lactate accumulation during exercise due to improved circulation to skeletal muscles.[12] This has been reported with the inotropic milrinone.[13]

CAN EXERCISE CAPACITY PREDICT EVENTS?

A good deal of data have been accumulated to suggest that peak Vo_2 can predict survival.[14] Patients with a peak Vo_2 of less than 10 to 12 ccs per minute per kilogram have been identified to be in a group with a very poor one year

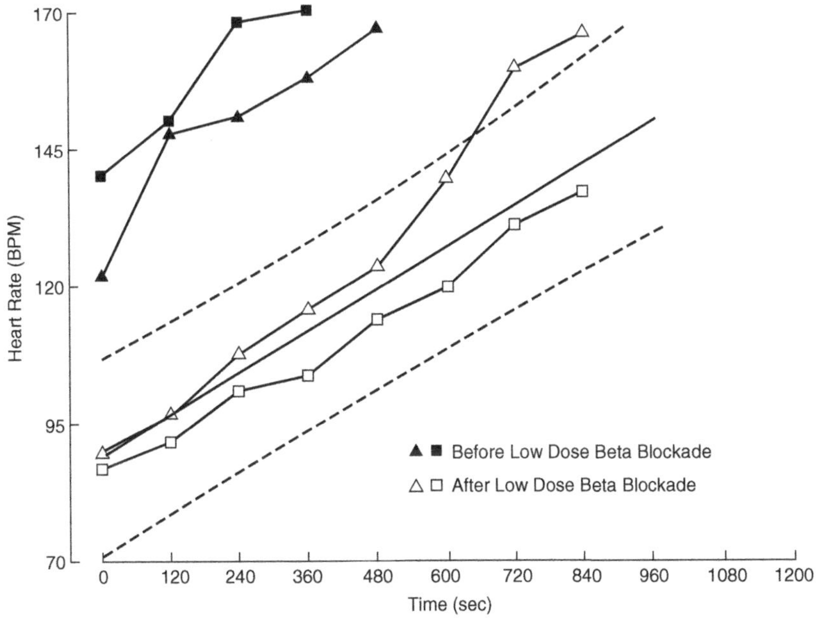

Figure 16–3. The heart rate response to treadmill exercise in congestive heart failure patients who had an inappropriate sinus tachycardia at rest and during exercise. Following low dose beta-blocker therapy, the heart rate response to exercise as normalized, with permission of publisher.[4]

survival and, in some programs,[15] this information is used to place them on the transplant list.

There have been interventions reported however, that improve survival without improving peak oxygen consumption. Exercise conditioning in congestive heart failure has been shown to improve peak VO_2 but there is no data at this time to be sure that it will reduce mortality. Beta-blockers improve survival and result in an increase in ejection fraction but do not appear to increase VO_2 max. It should be recognized that VO_2 max, exercise time, ejection fraction, and almost any other measure of cardiac performance in congestive heart failure are only a rough predictor of survival.[16] In today's world because of the rapid introduction of new medications and methods for treating heart failure, it is questionable how well these measurements will perform in patients on a full pharmacy of medication and who are applying meticulous control to their heart failure signs and symptoms.

REFERENCES

1. Patterson, JA, et al: Treadmill exercise in assessment of the functional capacity of patients with cardiac disease. *Am J Cardiol* 30:757, 1972.

2. Criteria Committee of the New York Heart Association, Kossmars, CE, Chairman: Diseases of the Heart and Blood Vessels: Nomenclature and Criteria for Diagnosis, 6th ed. Boston, 1964.
3. Hill, AV and Lupton, H: Muscular exercise, lactic acid, and supply and utilization of oxygen. *Q J Med* 16:135, 1923.
4. Weber, KT, et al: Oxygen utilization and ventilation during exercise in patients with chronic cardiac failure. *Circulation* 65:1213, 1982.
5. Weber, KT and Janicki, JS: Pathophysiologic responses to exercise in patients with chronic cardiac failure. *Heart Failure* May/June:139, 1985.
6. Miyagi, Y, et al: Relation of exercise capacity to resting arterial oxygen transport in left ventricular dysfunction. *Am J Cardiol* 63:457, 1989.
7. LeJemtel, TH, et al: Clinical response to long-term milrinone therapy in patients with severe congestive heart failure: 12-month experience, in Braunwald E, Sonnenblick EH, Chackrin LW, et al (eds): *Milrinone: Investigation of a New Inotropic Therapy for Congestive Heart Failure.* New York, Raven Press, p. 177, 1984.
8. Ellestad MH and Wan MKC: Predictive implications of stress testing: Follow-up of 1700 subjects after maximum treadmill testing. *Circulation* 51:363, 1975.
9. Lipkin, DP, et al: Six minute walking test for assessing exercise capacity in chronic heart failure. *Br Med J* 292:653, 1986.
10. Collucci, WS, et al: Impaired chronotropic response to exercise in patients with congestive heart failure. Role of postsynaptic β-adrenergic desensitization. *Circulation* 80:314, 1989.
11. Astrand, PO: Aerobic work capacity during maximal performance under various conditions. *Circ Res* 209(suppl):202, 1967.
12. Ziesche, S, et al: Hydralazine and isosorbide dinitrate combination improves exercise tolerance in heart failure. *Circulation* 87:VI-56-VI-64, 1993.
13. Alousi, AA, et al: Pharmacology of milrinone. In Braunwald, ,. et al (eds): *Milrinone: Investigation of New Inotropic Therapy for Congestive Heart Failure.* New York, Sterling Winthrop, p. 21, 1984.
14. van den Brock, SAJ, et al: Mode of death in patients with congestive heart failure: Comparison between possible candidates for heart transplantation and patients with less advanced disease. *J Heart Lung Transplant* 12:367, 1993.
15. Szlachcic, J, et al: Correlates and prognostic implications of exercise capacity in chronic congestive heart failure. *Am J Cardiol* 55:1037, 1985.
16. Wilson, JR, et al: Dissociation between peak exercise oxygen consumption and hemodynamic dysfunction in potential heart transplant candidates. *J Am Coll Cardiol* 26:429, 1995.

17
Chest Pain and Normal Coronary Arteries

Prevalence
Clinical Syndromes
Myocardial Infarction
Prinzmetal's Angina
Cardiomyopathy
Syndrome X (Microvascular Angina)
Esophageal Dysfunction
Other Mechanisms
Treadmill Findings
Therapy
Prognosis

A relieved 42-year-old woman, upon being told she had just sustained a myocardial infarction, exclaimed, "Thank God, now everyone will know the pain wasn't all in my mind." Between 10% and 30% of patients subjected to coronary angiograms have epicardial coronary arteries thought to be normal or have disease inadequate to explain their chest pain.[1] In an age when many people are obtaining relief of symptoms with coronary bypass surgery or angioplasty, the failure to demonstrate anatomical stenosis is frustrating to both physician and patient. The finding is even more perplexing when exercise-induced ST depression or relief of pain by nitroglycerin is also present. This chapter reviews present concepts pertinent to the understanding of this syndrome and the place of exercise testing in diagnosis and management.

PREVALENCE

The occurrence of chest pain with normal coronary arteries in any center or hospital depends a good deal on the referral patterns. In areas where only those with late, severe, typical angina are referred for study, this is seen infrequently. Centers in which the sensitivity and specificity of stress testing are reported to be very high must not be seeing many of these types of patients because a significant number (about 20%) have ST-segment depression with exercise.[2] After ergonovine testing became popular, many patients who had chest pain with normal coronary arteries were subjected to provocative testing, but those who failed to have classic epicardial coronary spasm and ST-segment elevation (most) were still left without a clear-cut diagnosis. Most cardiac centers report that about 10% to 12% of their patients referred for angiography fall into this category if those with well-understood mechanisms for their pain are excluded.[3–6] These known conditions responsible for false-positive ST depression include aortic stenosis, severe hypertensive left-ventricular hypertrophy, classic obstructive cardiomyopathy, mitral prolapse, and possibly certain drugs such as cocaine.

CLINICAL SYNDROMES

Myocardial Infarction

Although patients with this syndrome who have a myocardial infarction (MI) rarely have classic angina, they are included here because this subset may be important in understanding the syndrome of chest pain and normal arteries as a whole. Typically, patients are younger, often under age 35. The sex ratio is predominantly female. The most common risk factors for MI are smoking and oral contraceptives, at least in women.[7] The three possible mechanisms involved are coronary spasm, thrombosis, and coronary embolus. All the evidence implicating spasm is somewhat scant; Maseri and colleagues[8] reported a patient with spasm at the onset of an infarction who died 6 hours later. A fresh thrombus was found at necropsy in the area seen on angiography as being severe spasm. Engle and associates[9] have attributed infarcts during angiography to a spasm, and infarction has been reported following the withdrawal of nitrates.[10]

In women taking oral contraceptives, abnormalities in clotting have been demonstrated and blamed for infarction.[11] Postinfarction angiograms lend some credence to the concept that thrombosis, which later is lysed out, may be the villain. The rare case of coronary embolus, excluding that caused by bacterial colonies on the aortic valve, remains hard to explain. The natural history of this syndrome is yet to be fully described. It is now becoming fairly common to see anginal pain and MI in young people who use cocaine.

Prinzmetal's Angina

The syndrome of vasospastic angina should be suspected when patients with known coronary artery disease (CAD) have rest pain or when the early morning spontaneous attacks of angina, earlier described by Prinzmetal and coworkers,[12] recur repeatedly. These are usually relieved by nitroglycerin and may be initiated by ergonovine, hyperventilation, or the cold pressor test. When ST elevation accompanies pain and rhythm disturbances are seen, the provocative use of ergonovine is likely to be positive during the coronary angiogram. Because Prinzmetal's angina has been so well described, I will mention only that these subjects may have either ST elevation or depression during stress testing. Those with ST depression are more likely to have coexisting coronary atheroma. Most patients with pure spasm and normal coronary anatomy have a normal exercise test. Patients with Prinzmetal's angina are rare at our center.

Cardiomyopathy

In patients without overt cardiac enlargement caused by congestive or obstructive cardiomyopathy, it is common to find abnormalities in contraction or increased left-ventricular end-diastolic pressure (LVEDP), especially after contrast injection.[13] Goodin and colleagues[2] found that 46% had an increased LVEDP after contrast was injected. Erikssen and associates[14] from Oslo did coronary angiograms on 105 asymptomatic men who had ST depression on a treadmill and identified 36 with normal coronary arteries. After a 7-year follow-up, three were dead of heart failure, four had clear-cut cardiomyopathies, one had aortic incompetence and left-ventricular dilatation, and one had developed severe angina thought to be caused by CAD found on an abnormal multiple gated acquisition (MUGA) scan. Thus, 22% had developed significant myocardial disease and about 50% had an abnormal ejection fraction with exercise MUGA scan on follow-up. In asymptomatic men, ST depression and normal coronary arteries may identify a cohort with poor function and a poor long-term prognosis. Pasternac and associates[15] have shown that in hypertrophic and congestive cardiomyopathy, subendocardial ischemia occurs at rest and during exercise and that most patients develop chest pain and lactate excretion with atrial pacing. They implicate a reduced diastolic pressure time interval to systolic pressure time interval ratio and the compressive forces associated with the myocardial hypertrophy. We analyzed 100 false-positive stress test patients and found that 57% had an increased LVEDP[16]; Goodin and colleagues[2] found that 18% of their 60 patients with chest pain and normal coronary arteries had the same finding. Thus, a significant percentage of this population may have some type of poorly understood cardiomyopathy (see Chapter 4).

Syndrome X (Microvascular Angina)

The term syndrome X was first applied by Likoff and coworkers[17] in Philadelphia. They recognized that the mechanisms explaining the pain were unknown. Their belief, however, was that most of these patients had myocardial ischemia, because their classic pain was at times relieved by nitroglycerin, even though coronary atheroma could not be demonstrated. Only recently are we beginning to understand more about the underlying mechanisms responsible for this process. Following Marcus's[18] demonstration in the operating room that in some patients with normal coronary arteries blood flow was not increased appropriately during reactive hyperemia, Cannon and colleagues[1] at the National Heart, Lung, and Blood Institute have used coronary sinus flow measurements to demonstrate a reduced increase in coronary perfusion following atrial pacing. They also found a reduction in coronary sinus flow after ergonovine and the cold pressor tests, even though no epicardial narrowing was present. Cannon and colleagues initially labeled this condition "reduced vasodilator reserve" and believed the obstruction was in the arterioles, which explains many of the findings that were heretofore hard to understand. Subsequent studies in their laboratory have confirmed their original concepts, and they have now labeled the syndrome "microvascular angina."[19] They report an increase in left-ventricular filling pressure during pacing, less decrease in coronary resistance during dipyridamole infusion, and consistent chest pain during atrial pacing. They reported a lower sensitivity with exercise testing than with some of their invasive tests and also a lower sensitivity than in patients with CAD. They found that more than 60% were postmenopausal women.

Vrints and colleagues[20] in Belgium reported that these patients have impaired endothelin-dependent cholinergic coronary dilatation. Thus, it appears that, as in patients with coronary atheroma, endothelin is not causing dilatation with exercise, as it does normally, but is causing vasoconstriction instead. The active substance in endothelin, nitrous oxide, is an endogenous agent similar to the nitrates we have been using for years to relieve coronary artery spasm.[21]

This is supported by the positron emission tomography studies of Camici and coworkers[22] in Pisa, who reported reduced myocardial blood flow as measured by N-labeled ammonia. It is of interest that in the patients with the most reduction in flow, 86% had ST-segment depression with exercise. The investigators also reported that 16 (55%) of 29 patients studied who had normal flow also had ST depression, and they suggested that although the sensitivity is good, the specificity is rather poor. "There is evidence that some of these patients have endothelial dysfunction in their coronary arteries".[23] Panting from London, using MRI, has demonstrated that the subepicardium is hypo perfused during adenosine infusion, which is associated with intense chest pain.[24]

Patients with ST depression are likely to have an increase in lactate excretion, confirming that the ST depression is not a false-positive finding, but reflects ischemia. ST depression with exercise on atrial pacing was demonstrated in 72% in a series of cases reported by Bemiller and associates[25] but was found in only 36% in a series by Waxler and colleagues.[26] When Berland and coworkers[27] divided their patients into those with abnormal lactate excretion and those without, typical anginal pain and ST depression on exercise were more common in the former.

Esophageal Dysfunction

Esophageal dysfunction is so common and so difficult to distinguish from angina by symptoms alone that it warrants a brief discussion. Tibbling[28] from Sweden studied 217 patients diagnosed as having esophageal dysfunction by acid perfusion or by esophageal manometry and found that 60% to 70% had effort-related pain. Tibbling and Wranne[29] found that 50% of one group referred for exercise tests had esophageal dysfunction. In their data, however, more than 50% of their patients described their symptoms as heartburn, a term that should not be ignored by the physician. Kramer and Hollander[30] inflated esophageal balloons in patients with ischemic heart disease and 7 of 19 complained of pain identical with their angina, which was relieved immediately when the balloon was deflated. Most of the reports suggest that ischemic ST depression in patients with esophageal dysfunction is rare (2% to 5%), although nonspecific T-wave changes are common.

The reason for exercise-induced chest pain in esophageal dysfunction may be explained by the recent work of Harrison and colleagues,[31] who found gastroesophageal reflux (GER) in exercising patients who had eaten or who had previous acid loading. The GER was measured with a pH electrode in the esophagus above the gastroesophageal junction. Only 1 of 33 fasting patients had GER, however. It is of interest that smoking aggravates this response. Thus, when our patients with anginal pain have a negative coronary angiogram, esophageal disease must be suspected, but if they are tested in a fasting state, confusion is less likely to occur.

Other Mechanisms

We don't know at this time how many cases of syndrome X are caused by esophageal dysfunction. Myocardial bridging, musculoskeletal syndrome, esophageal spasm, and psychosomatic disorders all have been proposed.

Bass and colleagues[32] report that patients with chest pain have a high percentage of psychological syndromes such as sighing and gasping during rest and breathlessness after trivial exertion, during conversation, and with emotional tension. They believe that the angina is often a somatic expression of anxiety. The investigators also report that chronic hyperventilation in some of these subjects may cause peripheral and coronary vasoconstriction due to hypocapnia. Case[33] has adequately demonstrated marked myocardial hypoxia secondary to hypocapnia and alkalosis. Waxler and associates[26] also found that 40% of subjects with this syndrome had some type of anxiety neurosis. The presence of an abnormal hemoglobin dissociation curve reported by Eliot and Bratt[34] has not been confirmed by others. In recent years a metabolic syndrome, consisting of insulin resistance, truncal obesity and high glycerides, has at times been termed Syndrome X.[35] Most of these patients do not have angina however.

TREADMILL FINDINGS

Are there any tips that can help differentiate patients with chest pain and normal coronary arteries from those with anatomically significant CAD? We selected a group of false-positive patients and compared them with true-positive patients to try to answer this question.[16] We found that in men, false-positive patients were more likely to be younger, to be able to exercise longer, to have atypical chest pain, and to have hyperventilation-induced ST changes. This can be suspected when ST depression is associated with significant septal Q waves (see Chapter 12). In women, exercise time was not helpful, but the patients were younger, usually postmenopausal, had more atypical pain, and were more likely to have significant changes on hyperventilation; some had abnormal ECGs at rest (see Chapter 15).

If the angina is due to myocardial ischemia and induced by exercise, we must recognize that a number of patients will be clinically indistinguishable from those with epicardial coronary narrowing. Radice and coworkers[36] performed exercise tests after sublingual nitroglycerin on 23 patients with syndrome X and 19 with CAD. They found that the ischemic threshold was increased in CAD patients but not in those without epicardial coronary disease. They also found that some syndrome X patients had a lower exercise tolerance after nitroglycerin and suggested that these changes may be a tool to aid in the diagnosis of this syndrome. These patients, as long as they are with us, promise to keep stress testing from being 100% reliable in predicting anatomical CAD.

THERAPY

If our present perceptions are accurate and a significant number of patients with angina and normal coronary arteries have significant myocardial ischemia, then the use of nitrates, calcium blockers, and beta blockers seem appropriate. We have had modest success with imipramine in some, dipyridamole in others and a few with L-arginine. A significant proportion of our patients failed to be relieved by these agents, however, suggesting that there are mechanisms yet to be elucidated. When symptoms are atypical, a careful search for noncardiac causes of pain may be rewarding. Chest wall pain and esophageal pain can usually be recognized once one suspects that the heart may not be the culprit.

PROGNOSIS

Most studies indicate that patients with chest pain and normal coronary arteries have a good prognosis.[25,37] Goodin and coworkers[2] report that after a 2-year follow-up, 49% of 80 patients are improved or have no symptoms. MI and death were absent in this short follow-up. Bemiller and colleagues[25] report that after 4 years, 80% of their patients claimed that their angina was decreased and the other 19% reported it had remained stable. The investigators also reported one patient with sudden death, however, who was found to have normal coronary arteries at autopsy. Goodin and colleagues[2] report that 50% of their patients had marked improvement or a complete loss of pain in 2 years.

CONCLUSIONS

It is clear that patients with chest pain and normal coronary arteries are not all that they seem. At one end of the spectrum, there may be a few who have significant CAD that was missed on the angiogram. At the other end are patients with a neurosis or some type of noncardiac pain. In the middle, probably representing 40% to 50%, is a group with definite myocardial ischemia. Many of these patients will have ischemic ST depression on exercise and lactate excretion when challenged by atrial pacing. Some have lactate excretion and negative exercise tests and vice versa, however. Many of those with true ischemia probably have a reduced vasodilator reserve.

The syndrome described herein can be enormously disabling. Goodin and coworkers[2] reported that 78% of their patients had one or more hospitalizations for chest pain in the year prior to study. A complete cardiac study often relieves anxiety, allows for a more sensible approach to therapy, and minimizes subsequent hospitalizations. No longer should these patients be embarrassed by their pain syndromes and live in fear of imminent infarction and death.

The following conclusions can be made:

Typical angina and exercise ST depression are more likely to be associated with myocardial ischemia, even though the epicardial coronary arteries may be normal.

Atypical angina and negative exercise tests are more likely to be found in those in whom ischemia cannot be demonstrated.

REFERENCES

1. Cannon, RO, III, et al: Angina caused by reduced vasodilator reserve of the small coronary arteries. J Am Coll Cardiol 1(6):1359–1373, 1983.
2. Goodin, RR, et al: Exercise stress testing in patients with chest pain and normal coronary arteriography: With review of the literature. Cathet Cardiovasc Diagn 1:251–259, 1975.
3. Ockene, IS, et al: Unexplained chest pain in patients with normal coronary arteriograms. N Engl J Med 303:1249–1252, 1980.
4. Boden, WE: The anginal syndrome with normal coronary arteriograms. Cardiovasc Intervent Radiol 6:12–16, 1991.
5. Proudfoot WL, Shirey, EK, and Sones, FM: Selective cine coronary arteriography: Correlation with clinical findings in 1,000 patients. Circulation 33:901–910, 1966.
6. Kemp, HG, et al: The anginal syndrome associated with normal coronary arteriograms: Report of a six year experience. Am J Med 54:735–742, 1973.
7. Khandheria, B and Segal, BL: Myocardial infarction in patients with normal coronary arteries. Pract Cardiol 10(3):68–73, 1984.
8. Maseri, A, et al: Coronary vasospasms as a possible cause of myocardial infarction. N Engl J Med 299:1271–1277, 1978.

9. Engle, HJ, et al: Coronary artery spasm as the cause of myocardial infarction during coronary arteriography. Am Heart J 91(4):500–506, 1976.
10. Lange, RI, et al: Nonatheromatous ischemia heart disease following withdrawal from chronic industrial nitroglycerin exposure. Circulation 46:666, 1972.
11. Schuster, EH, et al: Multiple coronary thromboses in previously normal coronary arteries: A rare cause of acute MI. Am Heart J 99(4):506–509, 1980.
12. Prinzmetal, M, et al: Correlation between intracellular and surface electrograms in acute myocardial ischemia. J Electrocardiol 1:161–166, 1968.
13. Ohlmeier, H and Gleichmann, U: Abnormal left ventricular compliance as a cause of exercise-induced angina in patients without coronary-artery disease. Pract Cardiol 10(4):97–104, 1984.
14. Erikssen, J, et al: False suspicion of coronary heart disease: A 7 year follow-up study of 36 apparently healthy middle-aged men. Circulation 68(3):490–497, 1983.
15. Pasternac, A, et al: Pathophysiology of chest pain in patients with cardiomyopathies and normal coronary arteries. Circulation 65(4):778–789, 1982.
16. Ellestad, MH, et al: The false-positive stress test multivariate analysis of 215 subjects with hemodynamic, angiographic and clinical data. Am J Cardiol 40:681–685, 1977.
17. Likoff, W, Segal BL, and Kasparian, H: Paradox of normal coronary arteriograms in patients considered to have unmistakable coronary heart disease. N Engl J Med 276:1063–1066, 1966.
18. Marcus, ML: The Coronary Circulation in Health and Disease. McGraw-Hill, New York, 1983.
19. Cannon, RO and Epstein, SE: "Microvascular angina" as a cause of chest pain with angiographically normal coronary arteries. Am J Cardiol 61:1338–1343, 1988.
20. Vrints, CJ, Bult, H, and Hitter, E: Impaired endothelin-dependent cholinergic coronary vasodilatation in patients with angina and normal coronary arteries. J Am Coll Cardiol 19:21–31, 1992.
21. Cohen, R: Pathways controlling healthy and diseased arterial smooth muscle. Am J Cardiol 72:39C, 1993.
22. Camici, PG, et al: Coronary reserve and exercise ECG inpatients with chest pain and normal coronary arteriograms. Circulation 86:179, 1992.
23. Gokce, N, et al: Risk stratification for postoperative cardiovascular events via noninvasive assessment of endothelial function: A prospective study. Circulation 105:1567, 2002.
24. Panting, JR, et al: Abnormal subendocardial perfusion in cardiac syndrome x detected by cardiovascular magnetic resonance imaging. N Engl J Med 346:1948, 2002.
25. Bemiller, CR, et al: Long-term observations in patients with angina and normal coronary arteriograms. Circulation 47:36, 1973.
26. Waxler, EB, et al: The fate of women with normal coronary arteriograms and chest pain resembling angina pectoris. Am J Cardiol 28:25, 1971.
27. Berland, J, et al: Angina pectoris with angiographically normal coronary arteries: A clinical hemodynamic, and metabolic study. Clin Cardiol 7:485, 1984.
28. Tibbling, L: Angina-like chest pain in patients with oesophageal dysfunction. Acta Med Scand 644(Suppl):56, 1981.
29. Tibbling, L and Wranne, B: Esophageal dysfunction in male patients with angina-like pain. Acta Med Scand 200:391, 1976.
30. Kramer, P and Hollander, W: Comparison of experimental esophageal pain with clinical pain of angina pectoris and esophageal disease. Gastroenterology 29:719, 1955.
31. Harrison, MR, et al: Gastroesophageal reflux occurring during treadmill exercise testing. Prac Cardiol 16:43, 1985.
32. Bass, C, et al: Angina-like chest pain: Is it the somatic expression of anxiety? Mod Med September: 161, 1983.
33. Case, RB: The response of canine coronary vascular resistance to local alterations incoronary arterial pCO_2. Circ Res 39:558, 1976.
34. Elliot, RS and Bratt, G: The paradox of myocardial ischemia and necrosis in young women with normal coronary arteriogram. Am J Cardiol 23:633, 1969.
35. Arcaro, G, et al: Insulin causes endothelial dysfunction in humans: Sites and mechanisms. Circulation 105:576, 2002.
36. Radice, M, et al: Usefulness of changes in exercise tolerance induced by nitroglycerine in identifying patients with syndrome X. Am Heart J 127:531, 1994.
37. Selzer, A: Cardiac ischemic pain in patients with normal coronary arteriograms. Am J Med 63:651, 1977.

18
Blood Pressure Measurements During Exercise

Introduction
Reliability of Blood Pressure Recording
Problems with Auscultation
Correctable Sources of Error
Observer Bias
Automated Blood Pressure Measurement
Physiology
Normal Blood Pressure Response
Hypertensive Response
BP Response with Age
BP Response in Patients with Resting Hypertension
Effect of Left-Ventricular Hypertrophy on Myocardial Function During Exercise
Hypertensive Response in CAD Patients
Hypotensive Response
Late in Exercise
Early in Exercise
BP Response with Ischemia
Recovery Blood Pressure
Cardiomyopathies
The Effects of Medications

INTRODUCTION

Reliability of Blood Pressure Recording

The limitations of our ability to accurately measure BP were highlighted by the study done at The Johns Hopkins Hospital by Russell.[1] The investigators set up a sound film of the BP being recorded on a patient. Physicians listened to the sounds while they watched a manometer on the film and then recorded their estimation of the BP. When the true readings were compared with the physicians' ranges of responses, significant intra- and interobserver variability was present. The wide variations were more surprising because these experienced physicians knew that the accuracy of their technique was being tested and that they would be expected to take extra care in the measurements. How could the results be so inconsistent, especially when most of the common errors that lead to faulty BP readings were eliminated by the testing methodology? Eliminated were equipment and technique problems such as inaccurate aneroid manometers, inappropriate-sized air bladders and cuffs, heavy pressure on the stethoscope, too-rapid deflation rate, terminal digit bias, systolic recheck, and many others.

Problems with Auscultation

The audible sounds, called Korotkoff sounds, heard through an acoustical stethoscope, range from 18 to 26 Hz at systolic cuff pressures and 40 to 60 Hz at diastolic pressure.[2] For phases 1 and 4, most of the sound is lower than 20 Hz, whereas phases 2 and 3 are broadly distributed in the 5- to 50-Hz range. When we learned the manual technique, we listened for the clear tapping sound at phase 1, followed by the swishing sound at the phase 2 mid-pressure range. Amplification of the swishing sound occurs at phase 3, when the cuff pressure is low enough for the partially compressed artery to allow a sizable amount of blood to pass through. Phase 4 diastolic pressure is then characterized by abrupt muffling of sounds, with complete disappearance of sound at phase 5. There is still considerable disagreement as to whether phase 4 or phase 5 best identifies diastole.

These audible differences result from frequency and intensity changes occurring during the cuff deflation. The frequencies shift toward the low end of the frequency spectrum and progress from diastole to systole, reaching the lowest values at the true systolic point (Fig. 18–1). The human ear is a very sensitive organ; however, because of its intricacies, the ear is far more sensitive to some frequencies than others. The ear hears best between 200 and 4000 Hz. The lowest frequency at which the ideal human ear can appreciate a sound is about 16 Hz.[3]

Figure 18–1 is a graph of the auditory area of perception of a person with good hearing.[4–6] Represented is a range of frequencies and intensities of sound to which the ear is sensitive. The vertical axis represents the intensity in decibels (dB) that sound of a given frequency must have in order to be heard. It can be seen that the ear is most sensitive to frequencies between 2000 and 3000 Hz, where the threshold of hearing is defined as 0 dB. Human speech is in the range of 120 to 250 Hz.[7]

By comparison, the frequencies of systolic and diastolic sounds require respective intensities of about 80 and 30 dB, that is, intensities greater than normal conversational sound, to produce the same audible sensation. Thus, the ear is more sensitive to conversational sound than to the very low frequencies of Korotkoff sounds. Inspection of the curve will reveal that systolic frequencies lower than the 20-Hz range may approach intensities that many people will be able to detect. This is compounded by the fact that by age 50 most humans have a loss of at least 20 dBs, and this occurs a good deal earlier in people repeatedly exposed to very loud sounds such as rock music. Recording of accurate BP has long plagued those of us doing exercise testing.

Correctable Sources of Error

The American Heart Association task force on BP recording has emphasized three sources of error that can be minimized. These are observer bias, faulty equipment, and poor technique.

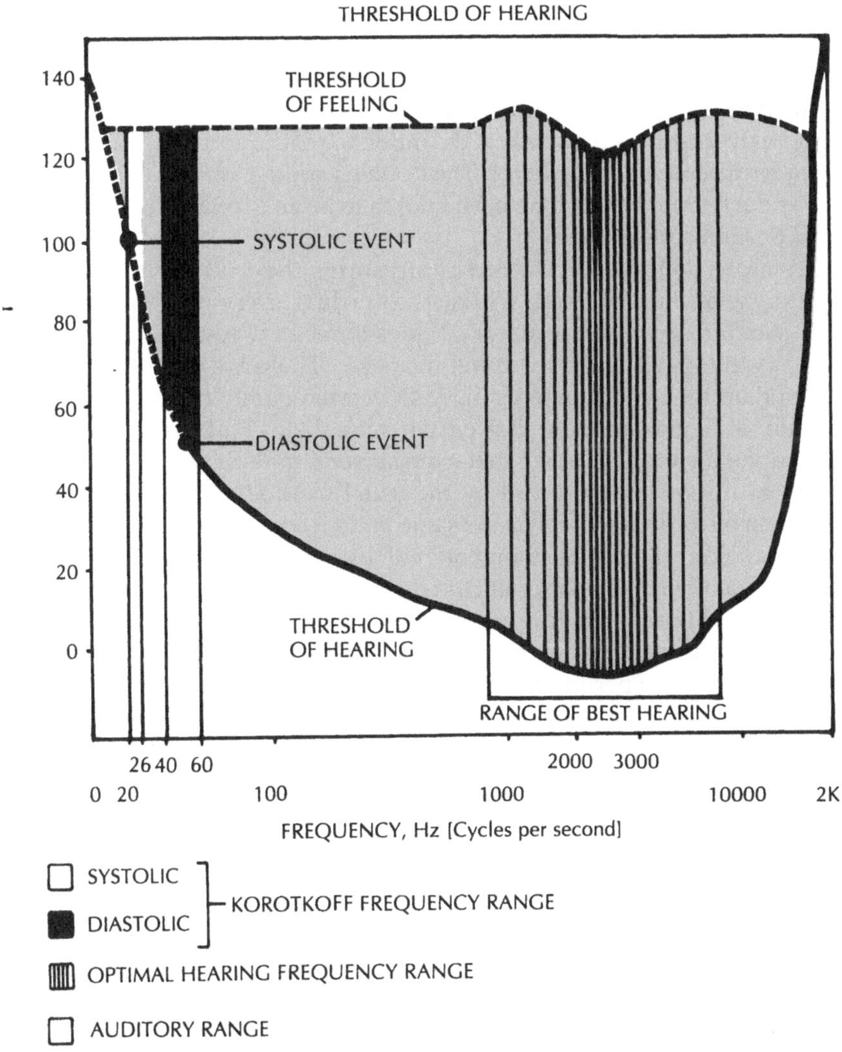

FIGURE 18–1. Auditory capacity of the human ear. The diagram shows that as the frequency decreases, the human ear loses the ability to detect sound. This is particularly important at the onset of the systolic component of the Korotkoff sound. (From Ellestad,[3] with permission.)

Observer Bias

Certain physicians or technicians habitually record pressure either higher or lower than the point at which they actually hear the sounds. Some prefer certain terminal digits, the most common being 0. Wilcox[8] reported that this type of observer error may be responsible for deviations as high as 45 mm Hg.

Observers often differ in their interpretation of Korotkoff's sounds. Some seem to hear the first sound later than others do; this may be due to a variation in reaction time. Others differ according to which sound they use to designate diastole. It is now accepted that diastole should be identified at the fifth sound; otherwise, Korotkoff sounds disappear altogether.

In spite of the inherent inadequacies, the importance of measuring BP cannot be overestimated in view of the influence of the aortic pressure on the oxygen requirements of the heart. The double product, or systolic BP multiplied by the heart rate, has long been known to be an excellent index of myocardial oxygen consumption.

A simple, noninvasive method of measuring the central aortic pressure has yet to be found. Although we use the brachial artery pressure recorded in the standard way, its accuracy is questionable at rest and diminishes rapidly as the speed of the treadmill increases. There are patients who, because of their well-coordinated gait, walk very smoothly or even jog with a minimum of jiggle; therefore, it is easy to take their BP at even 5 or 6 mph. Other patients vibrate so much that even at 3 or 4 mph their BP is extremely difficult or impossible to record by the usual method. Simultaneous pressures taken by two examiners on the same patient on opposite arms are fairly widespread (Fig. 18–2). Measurement of BP by catheter in the brachial artery and the aorta often reveals a significant increase, even at rest, as one proceeds distally. This difference during exercise may well be accentuated, especially in patients with inadequate cardiac outputs, because of their well-known tendency to develop peripheral vasoconstriction.

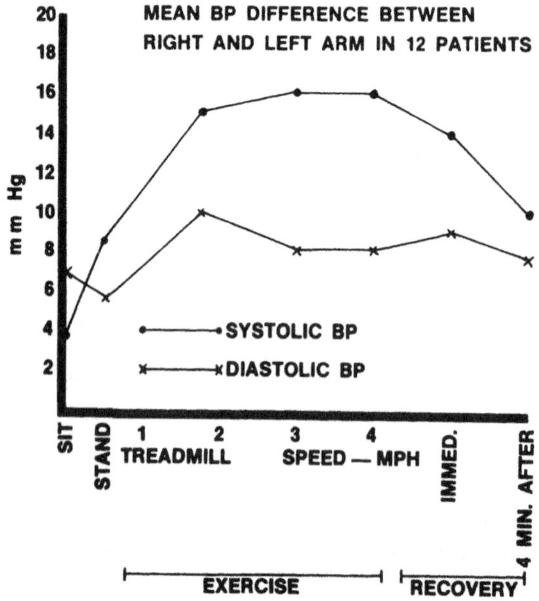

FIGURE 18–2. The difference between two simultaneously recorded blood pressures using aneroid manometers on the right and left arms is plotted. The difference between the two measures tends to increase during exercise and to decrease again as soon as exercise is terminated.

AUTOMATED BLOOD PRESSURE MEASUREMENT

Automated blood pressure measurement at rest has become a common practice in hospitals but this is not so easy during exercise. The measurement of blood pressure by automatic means for exercise testing has been studied by a number of equipment companies and we have tested several. By filtering Korotkoff sounds and blocking the sound pick-up, except at the appropriate time by triggering the sound circuit from the electrocardiogram, the accuracy of the mechanical devices has been improved somewhat. We are now using one made by Suntech Medical Instruments. When using a cuff of the appropriate size and the patient is not too obese, the systolic pressure appears to be reasonably accurate during rest and during walking. The accuracy decreases during exercise and the diastolic pressure at high workloads is usually over estimated. Our practice is to check these pressures by manometer to come up with a more accurate estimate.

According to the vendors, the system exceeds that obtained by the conventional method. If this accuracy is confirmed by careful experimental work, it will be a major advance but I have yet to see convincing evidence of this.

In spite of the inherent inadequacies, BP should be recorded frequently before, during, and after the stress test. We do this at minute intervals as long as possible as the rate of exercise increases and continue during at least 6 minutes of recovery.

PHYSIOLOGY

Many complex factors are involved in the control of BP response with exercise. An understanding of these various factors and how they interact with each other is necessary to draw conclusions concerning BP response and the patient's condition, based on BP changes with exercise and the degree of underlying myocardial impairment.

Normal Blood Pressure Response

The interaction between the peripheral vasculature and the heart during exercise is modulated through the central nervous system via the sympathetic nervous system as well as locally by factors that are responsible for autoregulation on an arteriolar level. With the onset of exercise, the resistance to blood flow through contracting muscles decreases significantly and results in a fall in peripheral vascular resistance. Other perfusion beds in nonworking areas, primarily the splanchnic, undergo significant vasoconstriction, thereby directing blood to working areas and away from nonworking areas. Constriction of the capacitance vessels on the venous side of the circulation aids in returning blood to the heart, thereby facilitating increased cardiac output by maintaining preload. Venous constriction is of prime importance in enabling cardiac output to rise normally in the face of a net reduction in total peripheral vascular resistance.[1] A rise in resistance to flow in the splanchnic circulation, skin, and nonexercising muscles also occurs. When the patient begins to exercise, the normal BP response is a gradual elevation of systolic pressure with increasing workloads and essentially no significant change in diastolic pressure. Near peak workload, the systolic BP levels off and often declines, only to rise again within 1 or 2 minutes after exercise is terminated. As the patient recovers, the pressure returns to control levels. Factors that alter BP response are reviewed in the following text, and their clinical significance is discussed.

Hypertensive Response

Hypertension at rest has long been known to be a risk factor for the development of coronary artery disease (CAD).[9] Significant elevation of BP during exercise higher than the expected normal response has been recognized as adding an additional metabolic burden, but until a few years ago it was not thought to have any other clinical significance. Published reports indicate that subjects with normal resting pressure who develop an abnormally high systolic pressure with exercise have an increased risk of developing clinically significant hypertension in the future.[10–13] Miller-Craig and colleagues[14] suggest that exercise-induced hypertension is a better predictor of eventual clinical hypertension than elevated BP at rest, although Kannel and associates[15] report that labile hypertension in young adults also has definite predictive value. A recent presentation by Kjeldsen and colleagues[16] from Oslo reports that a hypertensive response in normal middle-aged men who exercised on the treadmill is also a predictor of subsequent mortality from CAD.

BP Response with Age

As patients grow older, although the cardiac output with exercise increases at about the same ratio as in younger subjects, the peripheral resistance is greater so that the systolic pressure is higher. As exercise increases, however, resistance drops, as in younger subjects, but not enough to lower the pressure to the range seen in youth. The normal maximal systolic pressure in older subjects is higher as age progresses, it suggests that cardiac function is good and that cardiac output can increase (Fig. 18–3).[17]

BP Response in Patients with Resting Hypertension

Exercise BP in most hypertensive patients increases at about the same rate as it does in normals, but starting from a higher baseline, the maximum systolic BP is usually greater. There are some, however, who as exercise progresses,

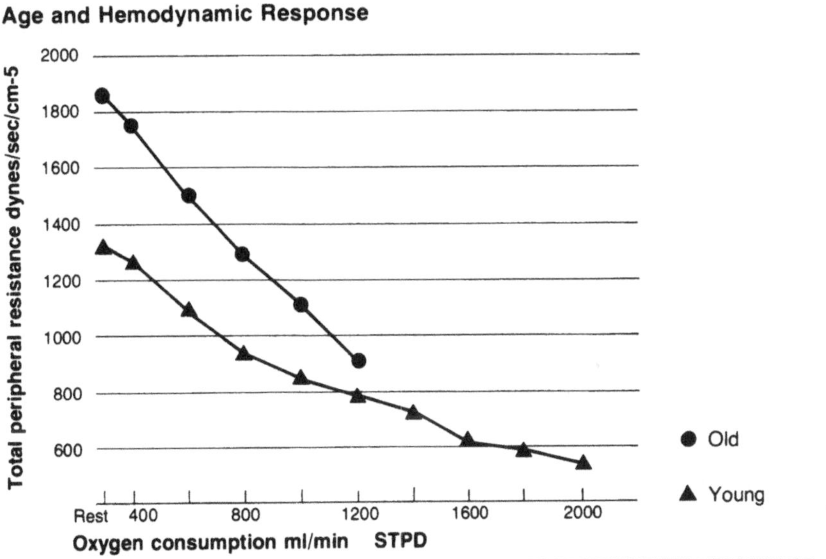

FIGURE 18–3. The drop in peripheral resistance with increased work in older subjects is similar to that in younger subjects, although it always remains somewhat higher. (From Julius,[17] with permission.)

have less of a rise, and their peak pressure may be similar to that of a normal age-matched subject. This indicates that the peripheral resistance drops in a more normal manner and responds more like that in a nonhypertensive subject. This may suggest that exercise would be a good therapeutic measure. Others not only have a steep rise during exercise, but the pressure continues to climb for several minutes after exercise and stays high during the recovery. A subject with this kind of response to exercise probably also responds with an increase in peripheral resistance and would be a greater risk. Such a patient might be expected to receive little benefit from an exercise program; in fact, it could be detrimental. I have not seen any data to confirm this however.

Effect of Left-Ventricular Hypertrophy on Myocardial Function During Exercise

The increase in coronary flow has been termed *flow reserve*, and its magnitude is important in providing adequate perfusion to the working myocardium. When hypertrophy due to hypertension has occurred, the capacity to increase flow to adequately meet the demands of this hypertrophied muscle is often markedly reduced.[18–20] There is evidence from studies with animals that decreased capillary density and extravascular compressive forces combine to predispose the hypertrophied myocardium to ischemic damage during exercise.[21] Hypertrophy has been shown to occur not only in the myocardium but also in the vascular smooth muscle.[22] Studies in hypertensive humans, even without left-ventricular hypertrophy, have revealed an attenuated vasodilator reserve and at times angina with a trial pacing.

There is evidence that these changes are in part due to a reduction in endothelin-mediated vasodilatation, which has been demonstrated in both animals and humans. This defect has also been found in arteries of the forearm in hypertensive humans.[23]

With this new information available, it is easy to understand why patients with hypertension may have ST depression and angina during exercise testing, even when they have normal epicardial coronary arteries. These changes may then reflect true ischemia, not really a false-positive test.

Hypertensive Response in CAD Patients

An exercise rise in systolic BP (well over 200 mm Hg) has been used as a reason to terminate exercise in some centers or hospitals. We have never done this because we have failed to see any complications related to a rising BP. There is a general tendency for the pressure to rise more in older subjects and those who are deconditioned. We followed up a large group of patients who had a maximum systolic BP response of more than 200 mm Hg for up to 8 years.[24] These patients were selected because they had ST-segment depression as well as an abnormal increase in BP response. When they were compared with patients with ST-segment depression and a normal BP response, the incidence of subsequent coronary events (death, myocardial infarction, and new angina) was reduced. This suggested to us that the increased BP response identified a cohort who had good left-ventricular function and could thus generate higher pressures. The possibility that the increased pressure also provided better coronary perfusion during exercise has to be considered. Irving and colleagues[25] found similar data in the Seattle Heart Watch subjects. They found a decrease in the rate of sudden cardiac death per year as maximum systolic BP increased. Morris and associates[26] correlated peak systolic BP with the number of coronary vessels obstructed and also with the ejection fraction. They found that the higher the pressure, the less disease, thus providing an anatomical explanation of our findings (Fig. 18–4).

Sheps and coworkers[27] found that when the diastolic pressure increased with exercise, it identified a subset of patients with a higher probability of CAD. This was confirmed by Paraskevaidis and associates[28] and by Akhras and colleagues,[29] who recorded BP by the intra-arterial method. It is of interest that the former investigators were unable to detect these changes when the pressure was measured by the standard cuff method. They also found that those who had an increase in diastolic pressure (20%) had a lower ejection fraction and stroke volume.

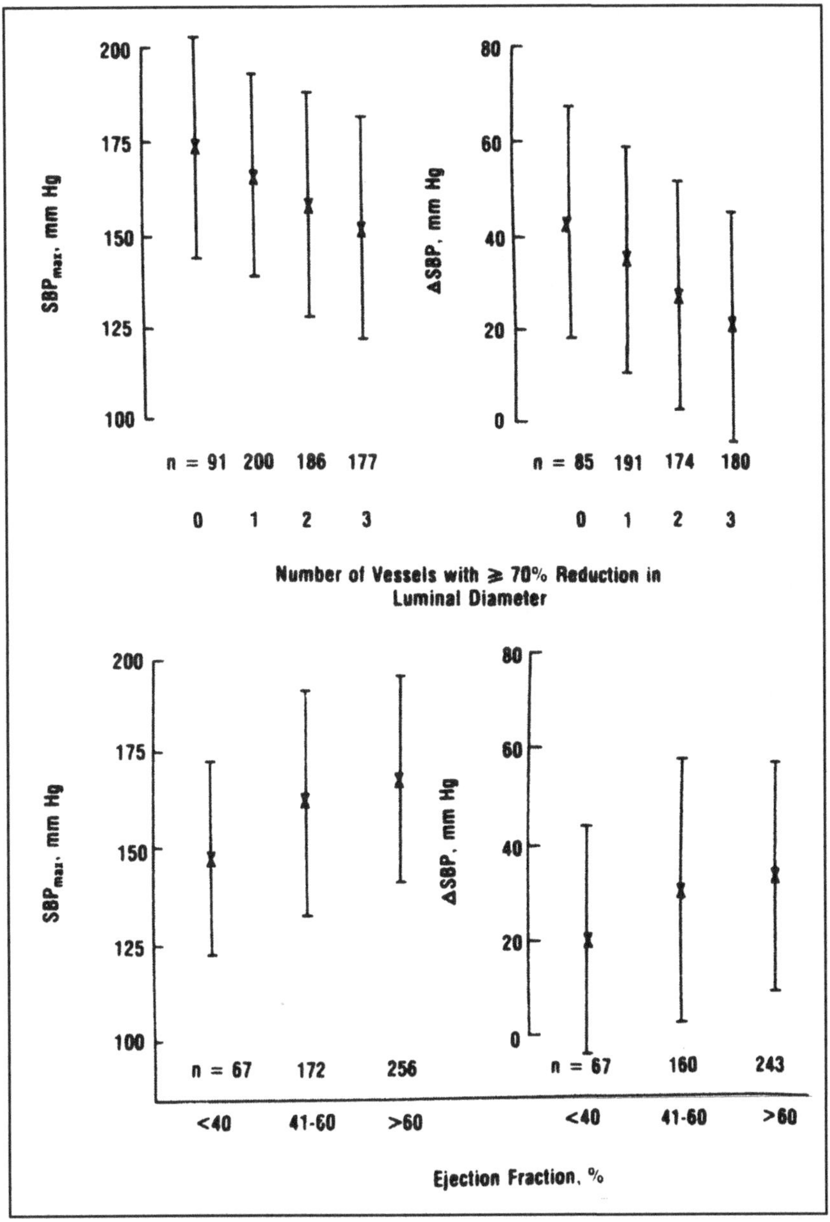

FIGURE 18–4. The peak systolic blood pressure (SBP_{max}) and change in systolic blood pressure with exercise (Δ SBP) are correlated with the number of significantly narrowed vessels on angiography (*upper graph*), and ejection fraction (*lower graph*). The higher the peak systolic blood pressure and change in SBP, the less severe the myocardial impairment. Conversely, patients with lower SBP with exercise tended to have more severe vessel involvement and lower ejection fractions. SBP = systolic blood pressure. (From Morris et al,[26] with permission.)

Hypotensive Response

Systolic hypotension during exercise occurs under a number of circumstances that must be clearly identified in order to assess its significance. The mechanism was once ascribed to very severe ischemia, but recent studies by Iskandrian and associates[30] suggest that it may be due to activation of mechanoreceptors, mechanisms similar to other types of neurally mediated hypotension. Lele and associates,[31] from Brisbane, Australia, have supported this concept by demonstrating a paradoxical drop in forearm vascular resistance in ischemic patients with exercise-induced hypotension. They also found that their ejection fraction increased instead of decreased, as usually occurs in ischemic patients.

Late in Exercise

Many normals as well as those with cardiac pathology extend exercise beyond their aerobic threshold. At this point, which is usually about 60% or more of their maximum capacity, they have a more rapid increase in heart rate and ventilation, and the systolic BP levels off and begins to fall because of increasing acidosis. This is probably due to the accumulation of lactic acid, which causes a drop in peripheral resistance as well as a decrease in myocardial contractility. When exercise is stopped, this decrease rapidly abates and the systolic pressure rebounds to a point considerably greater than that recorded at the end of exercise. This response has no predictive value in our experience except to indicate that the patient has exercised past anaerobic threshold and probably has done about as well as he or she is capable (Fig. 18–5).

Early in Exercise

Anxious patients occasionally have a sudden rise in BP for 1 or 2 minutes and then a drop of 10 or 20 mm Hg even as the exercise progresses, followed by a gradual increase again. This is probably due to an excess of norepinephrine, the effect of which is quickly dissipated by the increased metabolic demands. This can be differentiated from a more serious decrease in cardiac output by the vigor of the patient, the respiratory rate, and the absence of signs of ischemia. The BP does not go lower than the control in this situation.

BP Response with Ischemia

As early as 1959, Bruce and colleagues[32] reported that failure to increase the systolic BP greater than 130 mm Hg was a risk factor for subsequent coronary events; Thompson and Kelemen[33] in 1975 and Irving and Bruce[34] in 1977 emphasized the correlation of severe ischemia with a drop in pressure early in the exercise protocol. Hammermeister and associates[35] believe that

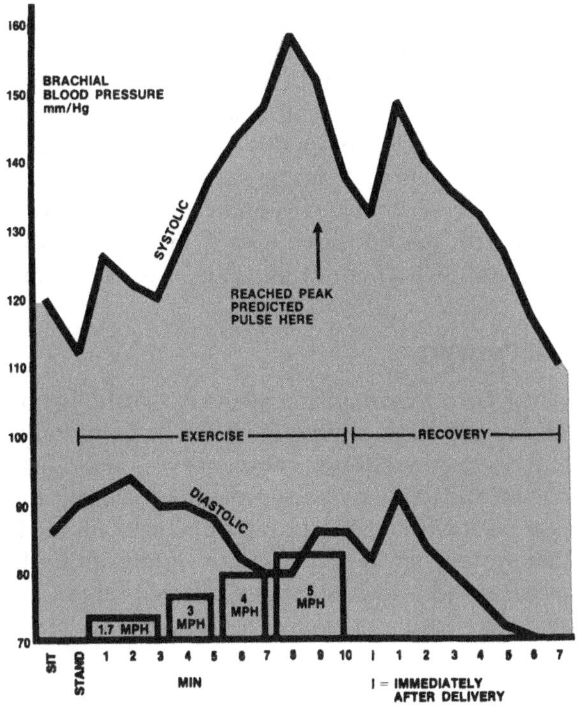

FIGURE 18–5. A typical BP change as seen during our exercise protocol recorded with an aneroid manometer on the arm. Systolic pressure rises as the workload increases until it gets near the peak capacity of the subject. At this point, it tends to drop sharply, probably because of a decrease in peripheral resistance or a drop in cardiac output, or both. The rebound phenomenon then occurs shortly after exercise is terminated.

in true ischemic hypotension, the pressure must drop below the resting level during exercise. Their report has been supported by Dubach and associates.[36] This drop can be associated with deep ST-segment depression, and at times it may identify patients likely to have left main CAD or severe three-vessel disease. San Marco and associates[37] found that exertional hypotension was as reliable as marked ST-segment depression in predicting severe three-vessel disease or left main CAD.

Weiner and colleagues[38] studied more than 400 consecutive patients with exercise testing and cardiac catheterization. Forty-seven patients manifested a fall in BP with exercise. Of this group, about 50% were randomized to medical therapy and 50% to surgical therapy. Cardiac catheterization revealed three-vessel disease or left main CAD in 55% of the patients. Repeat exercise testing verified the reproducibility of this BP response in the medical group. Repeat exercise testing in the surgical group revealed normal BP response in all patients after successful coronary bypass surgery. A number of reports have claimed that a drop in pressure during exercise reflects severe ischemic left-ventricular impairment. In some patients, the pressure changes are correlated with other findings, such as an appearance of reduced vitality, skin pallor, and other signs of inadequate perfusion (Fig. 18–6).[35,39] In some patients, the activation of ventricular baroreceptors may be initiated by the ischemic syndrome. Although this activation is more likely to be associated with severe ischemia, it can be seen with narrowing in relatively small nondominant vessels.[30] Exercise-indiced hypotension has been reported in women with false-positive tests,[39] in healthy athletes,[40] and in healthy older subjects.[41] Thus it is not always a predictor of coronary disease.

Recovery Blood Pressure

The rate of the systolic BP drop during recovery is usually fairly rapid after maximum exercise, although a rebound with a temporary rise about 1 minute after exercise termination is common.[42] As previously mentioned, this is believed to be due to the recovery from the anaerobic metabolism that has occurred near peak workload. A group from San Antonio led by Amon[44] has reported that systolic BP in patients with significant CAD fails to drop as fast as in normal subjects and has suggested that this response may help to differentiate those with ischemia. Hashimoto and associates,[45] from

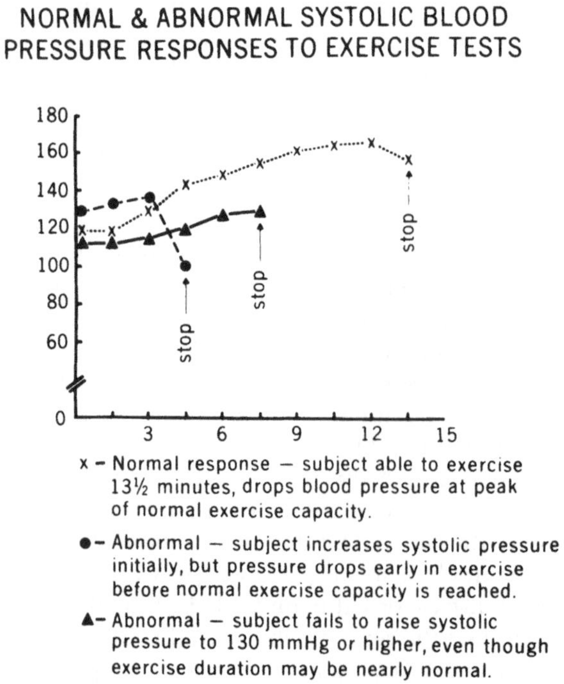

FIGURE 18–6. Normal and abnormal SBP responses to exercise tests. (From Sheffield and Roitman,[43] p 622, with permission.)

Hiroshima City, have recently studied this concept and found that 7 (20%) of 35 subjects had an increase in systolic pressure after bicycle exercise. This group had a reduced ejection fraction, a greater increase in plasma norepinephrine, and a greater increase in peripheral resistance. Acanfora and colleagues[46] also found the increase in systolic BP during recovery to be of diagnostic significance.

Because the recovery BP is so dependent on the magnitude of exercise and because the systolic BP at high workloads is so difficult to record accurately, I am somewhat skeptical of the clinical usefulness of the recovery systolic BP. We have been unable to verify Amon's work by retrospective analysis of our own data (Fig. 18–7). However, it appears that if a more accurate measure of BP could be devised, it would have diagnostic value. A review of the systolic BP data in Appendix I will suggest to the reader that normals often exhibit a delayed decrease in pressure.

Cardiomyopathies

Any process that reduces left-ventricular function may cause exertional hypotension with exercise testing. The common denominator of this clinical event appears to be that the upper limit of cardiac output cannot continue to meet the increased peripheral demands of the working tissues when the peak cardiac output is reached. The increasing demand of the peripheral tissues results in a rise in lactic acid and a generalized drop in pH, which causes a progressive decrease in peripheral vascular resistance and in BP. Cardiomyopathic processes, both hypertrophic and congestive, produce this effect.[47] Decreases in pressure with obstructive cardiomyopathies are likely to be more abrupt than in other conditions and may be associated with syncope and serious arrhythmias. Because these patients are often suspected of having CAD because of anginal pain, special care should be exercised when angina is found in a patient with a murmur of undetermined etiology. Frenneaux and associates[48] from London have reported on the exercise BP response in 129 patients with hypertrophic cardiomyopathy, 33% of whom had a hypotensive response to exercise. These patients were found to be younger and to have an adverse family history of sudden death, and they are believed to have a greater potential for sudden vascular collapse, either during or after exercise.

The Effects of Medications

Various types of medications have been shown to produce a fall in BP with exercise testing; the most common are antihypertensives.[49,50] Various classes of these agents such as the sympatholytic drugs, beta blockers, or peripheral vasodilators all have been implicated in abnormal BP response to exercise. These responses may be mediated either by a central mechanism inhibiting sympathetic outflow (such as with beta blockers or sympatholytics) or by a

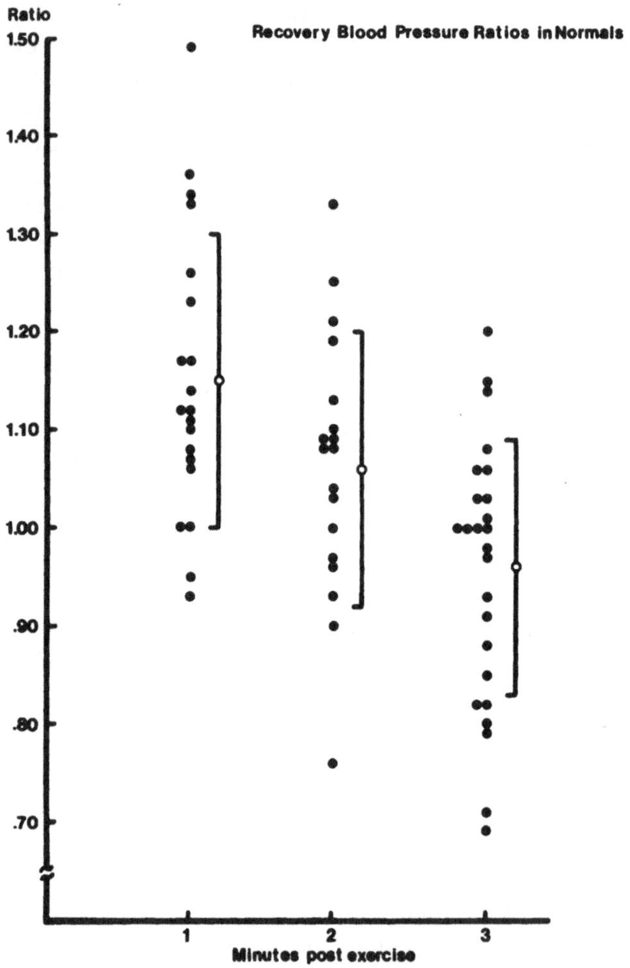

FIGURE 18–7. SBP as a percent of BP at end of exercise. The SBP during recovery was plotted in a group of normal subjects studied in our laboratory during the first 3 minutes. Most were higher than a ratio of 0.9 and would have been classified as abnormal using the criteria of Amon and coworkers.[44]

decrease in the ability of peripheral vasculature to respond to sympathetic activity. The peripheral vasodilators are notoriously likely to produce sudden drops in pressure. Diuretics do not produce much exertional hypotension; their major effect seems to be on the resting pressure. The psychoactive drugs—either major or minor tranquilizers—have been shown to cause moderate BP changes through both central and peripheral mechanisms. The effects of various drugs and metabolic processes on stress testing are covered in more detail in Chapter 22.

CONCLUSIONS

Careful observation of BP during exercise can yield important information not only about the peripheral resistance but also about the contractile state of the left ventricle. A heart that can function well when ejecting against a very high resistance (BP greater than 200 mm Hg) is usually fairly well perfused, as well as being free from significant fibrosis.

When we observe a fall in pressure, despite continuing exercise early in the test, poor perfusion or inadequate function due to other causes is almost certainly the case. Death on the treadmill can occur in these patients.

It now seems well established that a BP response to exercise that is greater than normal in a young healthy person is likely to predict clinically significant hypertension in the future. Thus, careful monitoring of BP at each increment of workload and during recovery is an essential part of stress testing. If the inherent limitations of our manual method of BP recording could be overcome, both the systolic and diastolic pressures could well add more to our information about the patient's function.

REFERENCES

1. Russell, RP: Assessment of sphygmomanometer skills-the need for improvement [abstract]. National Conference on High Blood Pressure Control April 28–30, p. 71, 1985.
2. Golden, DW, et al: Development of Korotkoff processor for automatic identification of auscultatory events. Part 1: Specifications of optical preprocessing bandpass filters. Biomed Eng 21:114, 1974.
3. Ellestad, MH: Reliability of blood pressure readings. Aus J Cardiol 63:983, 1989.
4. Sears, FW, et al: University Physics, 4th ed. Addison-Wesley Publishing Company, 1957.
5. Thompson, RF: Introduction to Physiological Psychology. New York: Harper & Row, 1975.
6. Mountcastle, VP: Medical Psychology, 14th ed. CV Mosby, St Louis, 1980.
7. Guyton, A: The relation of cardiac output and arterial pressure control. Circulation 64:1079, 1981.
8. Wilcox, J: Observer factors in the measurement of blood pressure. Nurs Res 10(1):4, 1961.
9. Braunwald, E: Heart Disease: A Textbook of Cardiovascular Medicine. WB Saunders, Philadelphia, p 1246, 1980.
10. Olin, RA, et al: Follow-up of normotensive men with exaggerated blood pressure response to exercise. Am Heart J 106(2):316, 1983.
11. Wilson, NV and Meyer, BM: Early prediction of hypertension using exercise blood pressure. Prev Med 10:62, 1981.
12. Jackson, AS, et al: Prediction of future resting hypertension from exercise blood pressure. J Cardiac Rehabil 3:263, 1983.
13. Wilhemsen, I, et al: Thirteen-year follow-up of a maximal exercise test in a population sample of 803 men aged 50 at entry [abstract]. European Cardiology Symposium on Prognostic values of Exercise Testing, Vienna, April 2–5, 1981.
14. Miller-Craig, M, et al: Use of graded exercise testing in assessing the hypertensive patient. Clin Cardiol 3:236, 1980.
15. Kannel, WB, et al: Labile hypertension: A faulty concept? Circulation 61:1183, 1980.
16. Kjeldsen, SE, et al: Paper presented at the AHA council for Hypertension. Newspaper of Cardiology, November 1993.
17. Julius, S: Exercise and the hypertensive patient: A hemodynamic approach. In Krakoff, LR (ed): Mediguide to Hypertension, Vol 1, 3rd ed. Laurence DellaCorte Publications, New York, 1980.

18. Strauer, BE: Significance of coronary circulation in hypertensive heart disease for the development and prevention of heart failure. Am J Cardiol 65:34G, 1990.
19. Casale, PN, et al: Value of echocardiographic measurement of left ventricular mass in predicting cardiovascular morbid events in hypertensive men. Ann Intern Med 105:173, 1986.
20. Marcus, ML, et al: Effects of cardiac hypertrophy secondary to hypertension on the coronary circulation. Am J Cardiol 44:1023, 1979.
21. Gradman, AH: Hypertension and ischemia: Evolving concepts. J Am Coll Cardiol 19:816, 1992.
22. Vogt, M, et al: Coronary microangiopathy and cardiac hypertrophy. Eur Heart J 11(suppl B): 133, 1990.
23. Panza, JA, et al: Abnormal endothelial dependent vascular relaxation in patients with essential hypertension. N Engl J Med 323:22, 1990.
24. Schrager, BR and Ellestad, MH: The importance of blood pressure measurement during exercise testing. Cardiovasc Rev Rep 4(3):381, 1983.
25. Irving, J, et al: Variations in and significance of systolic pressure during maximal exercise (treadmill) testing. Am J Cardiol 40:841, 1977.
26. Morris, S, et al: Incidence and significance of decreases in systolic blood pressure during graded treadmill exercise testing. Am J Cardiol 41:221, 1978.
27. Sheps, DS, et al: Exercise-induced increase in diastolic pressure: Indicator of severe coronary artery disease. Am J Cardiol 43:708, 1979.
28. Paraskevaidis, IA, et al: Increased response of diastolic blood pressure to exercise in patients with coronary artery disease: An index of latent ventricular dysfunction? Br Heart J 69:507, 1993.
29. Akhras, F, et al: Increased diastolic blood pressure response to exercise testing when coronary disease is suspected. Br Heart J 53:598, 1985.
30. Iskandrian, AS, et al: Mechanism of exercise-induced hypotension in coronary artery disease. Am J Cardiol 69:1517, 1992.
31. Lele, SS, et al: Mechanism of exercise hypotension in patients with ischemic heart disease-Role of neurocardiogenically mediated vasodilatation. Circulation 88(4):I-214, 1993.
32. Bruce, RA, et al: Exertional hypotension in cardiac patients. Circulation 19:543, 1959.
33. Thompson, P and Kelemen, M: Hypotension accompanying the onset of exertional angina. Circulation 52:28, 1975.
34. Irving, JB and Bruce, RA: Exertional hypotension and post exertional ventricular fibrillation in stress testing. Am J Cardiol 39:849, 1977.
35. Hammermeister, KE, et al: Prognostic and predictive value of exertional hypotension in suspected coronary heart disease. Am J Cardiol 51:1261, 1983.
36. Dubach, P, et al: Exercise-induced hypotension in a male population. Circulation 78:1380, 1988.
37. San Marco, M, et al: Abnormal blood pressure response and marked ischemic ST segment depression as predictors of severe coronary artery disease. Circulation 61:572, 1980.
38. Weiner, D, et al: Decrease in systolic blood pressure during exercise testing: Its producibility, response to coronary bypass surgery and prognostic significance. Am J Cardiol 49:1627, 1982.
39. Tsuda, M, et al: Diagnostic value of postexercise systolic blood pressure response for detecting coronary artery disease in patients with or without hypertension. Am Heart J 125:718, 1993.
40. Taylor, A, and Beller, G. Postexercise systolic blood pressure response: association with the presence and extent of perfusion abnormalities on thallium-201 scintigraphy. Am Heart J 129:227, 1995.
41. Gibbons, RJ, et al: ACC/AHA guidelines for exercise testing: A report of the American College of Cardiology/American Heart Association task force on practice guidelines (committee on exercise testing). ACC/AHA, 1997.
42. Erikssen, J, et al: Blood pressure response to bicycle exercise testing in apparently healthy middle aged men. Cardiology 66:56, 1980.
43. Sheffield, IT and Roitman, D: Stress testing methodology. Prog Cardiovasc Dis XIX(1):33, 1976.
44. Amon, KW, et al: Value of post exercise systolic blood pressure in diagnosing coronary disease [abstract]. Circulation 6(suppl B):36, 1983.
45. Hashamoto, MO, et al: Abnormal systolic blood pressure response during exercise recovery in patients with angina pectoris. J Am Coll Cardiol 22:659, 1993.

46. Acanfora, D, et al: The diagnostic value of the ratio of the recovery blood pressure to peak exercise systolic pressure for the detection of coronary disease. Circulation 77:1306, 1988.
47. Weider, OA: Clinical significance of abnormal blood pressure response during exercise stress testing. Pract Cardiol 10:37, 1984.
48. Frenneaux, MP, et al: Abnormal blood pressure response during exercise in hypertrophic cardiomyopathy. Circulation 82:1995, 1990.
49. Pickering, TG: Immediate and delayed hypotensive effects of propranolol at rest and during exercise. Trans Assoc Am Physicians 92:271, 1979.
50. Franciosa, J, et al: Exercise performance in mildly hypertensive patients: Impairment by propranolol but not oxprenolol. Chest 78:291, 1980.

19
Silent Myocardial Ischemia

Prevalence
Autopsy Data
Epidemiological and Screening Studies
ST Depression and Normal Coronary Arteries
Mechanisms and Pathophysiology
Pain Perception
Detection
Analysis of the M.H.I. Database
Prognosis
Implications
Clinical Strategy
Comment
Angina Equivalent
ST Depression with Prior Negative Test
Therapy
Medical
Surgical

Although the absence of chest pain and other symptoms of coronary artery disease (CAD) were once believed to provide assurance that its presence was unlikely, this concept must now be laid aside.[1,2] Gordon and Kannel[3] reported that the first symptom of CAD was myocardial infarction or death in 55% of men in the Framingham study. Most of us will agree that these two end-points are unacceptable. There are two groups of asymptomatic patients commonly considered for stress testing. This chapter deals primarily with those who have never had symptoms recognized as being of cardiac origin. The other group, who have had recognized myocardial infarction but have been asymptomatic following this event, are commonly believed to be free of ischemia but limited somewhat by scar tissue replacing functional myocardium. In actuality, more than 50% of this group have other vessels significantly narrowed. The use of exercise testing in these patients is covered in Chapters 10 and 14.

PREVALENCE

There are a number of ways to estimate how many people have silent myocardial ischemia.

Autopsy Data

Allison and colleagues[4] found that only 19% of subjects dying of sudden death had a history of angina, although 66% had pathological evidence of infarction. Spickerman and associates[5] in a similar study found that 32% had angina. On the other hand, a review of autopsy findings on subjects dying of noncardiac causes reveals that a 6% mean prevalence in men (aged 30–69) and a 2.6% mean for women characterizes the amount of CAD in those who are truly asymptomatic.[6]

Epidemiological and Screening Studies

Diamond and Forrester[6] reviewed reports of patients undergoing catheterization for reasons other than chest pain (eg, valvular heart disease, abnormal ECGs) and found that 4.5% had coronary narrowing. Erikssen and coworkers[7] catheterized subjects with abnormal ST-segment response to stress testing and found that 3.4% of the total cohort had significant narrowing. We do not know how many in Erikssen's study group had CAD, however, because those with normal exercise tests were not offered an angiogram. Again, using ST depression with exercise as a case-finding method, Buckendorf and colleagues[8] found CAD in 6% of their asymptomatic military aviation personnel (mean age equals 36). The 5-year follow-up heart study by Bruce and associates[9] of 2365 asymptomatic subjects identified 2% who had a coronary event. If one assumes a 5% per year event rate in a CAD population, then 75% of those manifested would yet to be discovered during the 5-year period, resulting in a prevalence of 8% with coronary narrowing. Allen and coworkers,[10] however, reported that 5.4% of 888 subjects followed up for 5 years developed CAD, which by the above reasoning could suggest a prevalence in their material of at least 20%. Moreover, when the initial abnormal exercise tests were stratified by age and sex (see Table 14–5), the prevalence of CAD in a hospital-based study would be higher, with 25% of men older than aged 41 demonstrating ST depression. In this age range, estimating a 50% specificity, the prevalence of CAD would be approximately 12%. If the prevalence of CAD in asymptomatic men in a population older than 40 is only 10%, there are at least 4 million people in the United States at risk for this syndrome.

ST DEPRESSION AND NORMAL CORONARY ARTERIES

We all are also faced with the problem of dealing with those who appear to have ischemia on the ECG, but have normal coronaries. The follow-up reports of Erikssen and colleagues[11] on this group found them also at risk for a cardiac disability and death. This is discussed in Chapter 17.

MECHANISMS AND PATHOPHYSIOLOGY

When patients are referred for exercise testing because of a history of chest pain, a large percentage fail to have angina during the test, even though they have ST-segment depression. Are they having ischemia? Deanfield and Shea[12] have studied ischemia with rubidium, an isotope with a short half-life, using positron emission tomography; they report that ST depression has been associated with reduced myocardial perfusion in every case studied. On the other hand, we know that there are a number of causes of ST depression besides ischemia. The evidence is conclusive, however, that in patients with CAD, ST depression usually represents myocardial ischemia.[11] Data from Maseri,[13] as well as data from several studies using Holter monitoring techniques,[14,15] indicate that about 75% of the ischemic episodes in patients with typical angina are silent. These studies suggest that lesser degrees of ischemia and shorter time periods are more likely to be silent. On the other hand, Kunkes and associates,[16] using Holter monitoring, found that silent ischemia was more common in patients with multivessel disease. Shell and Penny[15] believe an average period of ischemia of 5 to 7 minutes is necessary before angina appears. My own angioplasty experience indicates that in many cases severe ischemia is followed by pain in as little as 10 to 15 seconds, when the vessel is completely obstructed. On the other hand, reduced myocardial perfusion, often before ST depression develops, causes wall motion abnormalities that almost always precede angina, if it does occur. The best data suggest that even patients who may never have had pain with their ischemia will get pain most of the time if their ischemia gets severe enough or if they have a myocardial infarction. Pain is usually a late event in the ischemic cascade; just how late depends on the patient's pain threshold.

PAIN PERCEPTION

The failure of the patient to perceive ischemic pain may be related to a number of factors. It has been stated that the transmission of pain is interrupted in some diabetic patients due to a neuropathy, and these patients have been reported to have a higher prevalence of silent myocardial infarction.[17] Droste and Roskamm[18] have reported that patients with silent ischemia have a higher pain threshold when their cutaneous perception of pain is measured.

Because endorphins are reported to mitigate pain under certain circumstances, we tested 10 patients with angiographically proven CAD who had never had angina during stress testing or during daily life.[19] Each patient had 2 mm or more of ST depression during the exercise test, but intravenous naloxone (an endorphin antagonist) failed to bring on pain or influence the exercise test in any significant way. Thus, it appears that high endorphin levels are not the primary cause for painless ischemia. Heller and associates[20] measured exercise-induced endorphin levels in patients with silent ischemia compared with levels of those with exercise-induced angina and found there was no difference between the two groups. Although this finding tended to support our study with naloxone,[21] it seems to contradict an earlier study in which we found that patients with angina on the treadmill had a worse prognosis than those who did not.[19]

We have repeatedly observed that conditioning reduces or abolishes exercise-induced angina. Sim and Neill[22] reported on eight patients with this phenomenon and found that when the angina was produced by atrial pacing, it was not influenced by training. They found that the double product at angina threshold was also increased, suggesting an increase in myocardial oxygen supply. However, when atrial pacing was used to increase cardiac work, the double product at the anginal threshold and lactate secretion was the same before and after conditioning. The reasons for this are yet to be explained.

DETECTION

The failure to detect with exercise testing those subjects in an asymptomatic population who will eventually have a coronary event is not surprising, considering the known false-negative rate (20% to 40%) and the propensity for atherosclerotic lesions to progress, sometimes rapidly. Little and associates[23] report that a myocardial infarction often occurs in muscle perfused by an artery, which just prior to the infarct had an obstruction of only 50% or less and was probably not "flow-limiting" during most exercise. This is because a fissure occurs in the surface of the plaque, which initiates clotting and then quickly occludes the artery. Patients who have had an out-of-hospital bout of ventricular fibrillation have also been reported to have exercise-induced silent ischemia.[24]

Cumming and associates[25] and Bruce and colleagues[9] emphasize that more than 50% of their patients who developed coronary events failed to manifest ST-segment depression on the initial exercise test. On the other hand, an abnormal exercise ECG, especially when combined with other risk factors, has been shown to identify a cohort of high-risk subjects for a subsequent coronary event, in spite of the application of the Bayes' theorem. Recall from Chapter 14 that the post-test probability in an asymptomatic subject with ST depression is low because of the low prevalence of disease. If the known risk factors are used in conjunction with stress testing, however, the predictive power becomes more acceptable. Giagnoni and coworkers[26] from Milan compared 135 asymptomatic subjects with ST depression with a group without ST depression controlled for age and other risk factors. They found that after 6 years, the risk for coronary events of those with ST depression was five times that of the controlled subjects. We found similar results when analyzing subjects who were referred to our laboratory for screening tests rather than for chest pain syndromes (Fig. 19–1).

Hopkirk and coworkers[27] studied 225 asymptomatic men from the Air Force who had undergone stress testing for various reasons. They found that 0.3 millivolts (3 mm) of ST depression, persistence of ST depression for 6 minutes into recovery, and total duration of exercise of less than 10 minutes

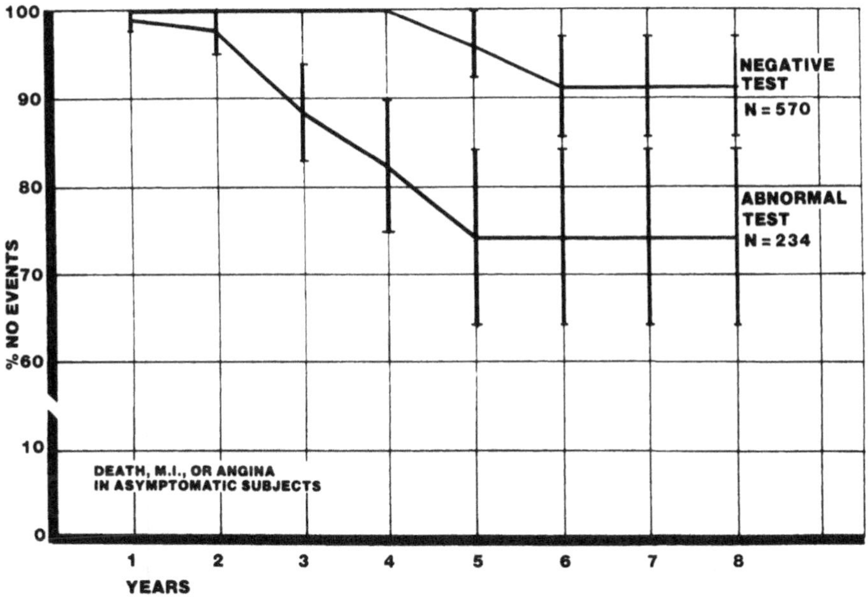

FIGURE 19–1. When only those who denied any symptoms were evaluated, the incidence of all coronary events was well below the incidence in all those reported in the study, in which 83% were symptomatic (see Fig. 14–7).

(equivalent to 7 minutes on the Bruce protocol) resulted in a high probability of disease. The investigators found that any two of the exercise variables were highly predictive (89%), but relatively insensitive (37%). When studying the false-positives, Hopkirk and coworkers[27] found that normalization of the ST-segment depression in the first 20 seconds of recovery was present in 18%. Yet, we have shown that rapid resolution of ST changes is not a very reliable indicator of normal coronary flow.[28]

When Allen and colleagues[10] analyzed their data on 888 asymptomatic subjects, they also needed a combination of findings for best results. ST-segment depression, R-wave increase, and a short exercise duration had reasonable sensitivity in 5 years and a very high specificity. Other markers for ischemia found useful in this population have been exercise thallium, coronary calcium detected on fluoroscopy or fast CT scanning, and prolonged P-wave duration. When any of these is abnormal in conjunction with an exercise test, the probability of CAD is more than 90%.[29]

ANALYSIS OF THE M.H.I. DATABASE

In order to study the reliability of exercise testing in patients with "silent ischemia" at Memorial Heart Institute we constructed tables on patients with a

Table 19–1. **Markers for Ischemia According to History of Angina Compared with No History**

	No History of Angina			*History of Angina*		
	Sensitivity	**Specificity**	**PPV**	**Sensitivity**	**Specificity**	**PPV**
Conventional Markers						
1) ST ↓ >1 mm (any lead)	0.64	0.51	0.57	0.69	0.51	0.70
2) ST ↓ >1 mm V_5	0.44	0.77	0.66	0.50	0.74	0.77
3) Downslope in recovery	0.64	0.51	0.57	0.69	0.50	0.70
4) Exercise time						
<3 min	0.07	0.95	0.60	0.76	0.93	0.64
>5 min	0.79	0.19	0.50	0.75	0.19	0.60
5) ST in males	0.66	0.51	0.67	0.69	0.55	0.75
6) ST in females	0.67	0.50	0.36	0.71	0.45	0.60
Unconventional Markers						
1) ST/R >0.1 mm	0.51	0.66	0.60	0.55	0.73	0.77
2) ST ↓ >1 + ST ↑ AVR	0.13	0.95	0.75	0.12	0.99	0.93
3) Δ HR <50	0.33	0.78	0.60	0.26	0.73	0.61
4) Δ T ↑ >2.5 mm V_2	0.18	0.84	0.53	0.23	0.81	0.66
5) Δ R >2 mm V_5	0.36	0.64	0.51	0.33	0.60	0.57
6) Δ R and ST ↓	0.28	0.78	0.56	0.26	0.84	0.72
7) ST ↑ >2 mm V_2 or V_3	0.15	0.91	0.63	0.07	0.92	0.57

history of chest pain as compared to no history of pain and on those who had pain during the tests as compared to those with no pain during the test (see Tables 19–1 and 19–2). Inspection of these tables will reveal that when angina is induced during the test the sensitivity is slightly better but not by very much. Some of the unconventional markers have a higher specificity regardless of the presence or absence of angina but usually a lower sensitivity. When some of the unconventional markers are combined, i.e. ST depression, ST depression in a precordial lead and ST elevation in AVR, the specificity becomes very good.

PROGNOSIS

Although many subjects with silent CAD have a sudden coronary event, the risk of an event is probably less than if ischemia is associated with typical anginal pain. Data from our files indicate that the risk of an event with asymptomatic ischemia is about 50% of that when classic angina accompanies the ECG findings during stress testing. Cohn[30] also found an improved survival in a small group of asymptomatic patients followed up for 7 years with CAD compared with those with anginal pain. The report by Droste and associates[31] should be reviewed by those who have a serious interest in this subject. These investigators have shown that prognosis is a function of how early ST depression occurs during the exercise test, how severe the CAD is on angiography, and the presence of chest pain in the patient's history. They also have reported that when subjects with silent ischemia are followed up

Table 19–2. **Markers for Ischemia Stratified as to History of Angina or Angina During Exercise Test**

	PPV		*Specificity*	
Markers	**No ex. Angina**	**No hx. Angina**	**No ex. Angina**	**No hx. Angina**
Conventional Markers				
1) ST ↓ >1 mm (any lead)	0.60	0.57	0.52	0.57
2) ST ↓ >1 mm in V_5	0.68	0.67	0.68	0.66
3) Downslope ST in recovery	0.60	0.57	0.51	0.60
4) Exercise time				
<3 min	0.65	0.60	0.65	0.95
>5 min	0.51	0.50	0.18	0.18
Unconventional Markers				
1) ST/R	0.65	0.60	0.65	0.66
2) ST ↓ >1 + ST ↑ AVR	0.80	0.75	0.96	0.95
3) Δ HR <50	0.61	0.53	0.78	0.78
4) Δ T ↑ >2.5 mm V_2	0.57	0.55	0.84	0.84
5) Δ R V_5 >2 mm	0.52	0.51	0.63	0.64
6) Δ R >2 mm and ST ↓ >1 mm	0.59	0.50	0.79	0.78
7) ST ↑ >2 mm V_2 or V_3	0.59	0.65	0.91	0.90

for 5 years, those who convert to classic angina have a poorer prognosis than those who remain asymptomatic.[31]

IMPLICATIONS

In spite of the apparent lower risk in this group of patients, the implications need some discussion. There appear to be three subsets of patients.

1. Those who never have pain. Cohn[30] has characterized this group as having a defective anginal warning system. Raper and associates[32] report patients with repeated massive infarction without chest pain and comment that these people are at risk because of the lack of pain. Our patients tested with naloxone were also in this category.[19] There is no doubt that angina in many is protective, and in this group its absence is a hazard and should be recognized as such. When we find patients before they are stricken by a catastrophe, they should be carefully evaluated for severity of disease prior to deciding on therapy.
2. Those who have pain with ischemia on some occasions, but not on others. This group comprises a majority of patients who are recognized with CAD. Factors that influence the variability are occasionally detectable, such as changes in myocardial work, magnitude of ischemic myocardium, coronary spasm, durations of ischemia, and so forth. Many, however, have angina or chest pain at different times and under different conditions that seem to defy categorization. As we learn more about the pathophysiology of CAD, some of these will be easier to understand.
3. Those who have chest pain with ischemia on most occasions. This group is a minority to be sure; yet a few years ago we believed most CAD patients fell into this group. Although we have learned a great deal about this process, there are many questions still unanswered.

CLINICAL STRATEGY

Esptein and coworkers,[33] Selzer and Cohn,[34] and others[35] have criticized the use of exercise testing in asymptomatic persons. There are probably also those who would be against the detection of asymptomatic prostatic cancer. On the whole, however, exercise testing is justified in asymptomatic subjects suspected of having an increased risk of disease. The presence of the classic risk factors in conjunction with the findings on an exercise test will go a long way toward determining the presence or absence of significant coronary narrowing. If clinically indicated, a patient should proceed to other noninvasive diagnostic measures after the exercise test is evaluated.

The following findings are usually associated with true-positive stress tests:

1. Short exercise time
2. Less than normal increase in heart rate or blood pressure during the test
3. Early onset of ST-segment depression with progression during exercise
4. Evolution to downsloping ST pattern during recovery
5. Persistence of systolic hypertension during the first 2 or 3 minutes of recovery
6. Marked increase in R-wave amplitude
7. Reduction in amplitude of the septal Q, if present
8. Widening of the QRS with exercise
9. High post-test probability on multivariate analysis or likelihood ratio
10. Confirmation with radionuclide stress testing

The flow chart shown in Figure 19–2 might serve as a guide when encountering an asymptomatic man with exercise-induced ST depression. Clinical findings not shown will shade the decision to follow a more aggressive or conservative pathway. These might include the family history, hypertension, smoking, cholesterol, cooperativeness of the patient, degree of denial, and many others.

Comment

We often explain to the patient that the abnormal stress test findings are another risk factor, which along with other findings influence the clinical course to follow. In this situation, I believe education of the patient and family is one of the most important aspects of good patient care. If the patient understands the problem, a major step will have been made in the direction of initiating a sensible course of management.

ANGINA EQUIVALENT

Even though the patient may come in with a story of no chest pain, any type of chest discomfort, upper abdominal gas or bloating, inordinate dyspnea with exercise, or just increasing fatigue, may be an angina equivalent. Frequently, when the possible implications of the test are explained, the patient may then report symptoms withheld prior to the test. The need for denial of possible illness is a powerful force in many men; yet when they find a friend who understands their problem, they may let go and fill in some of the blanks heretofore withheld.

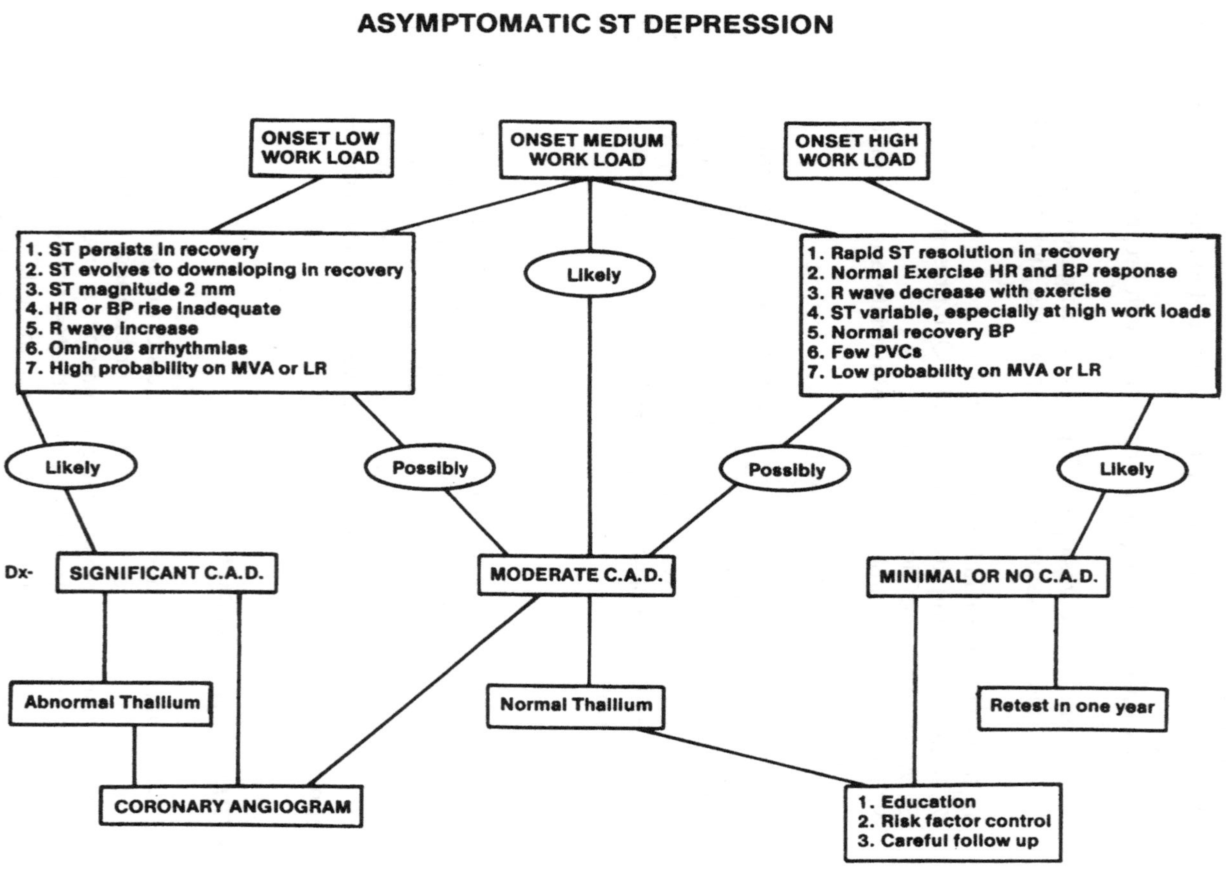

FIGURE 19–2. *Asymptomatic ST depression:* Diagnostic flow chart. Those patients with findings in the right-hand box may not need angiography if they can be followed up on a regular basis.

ST DEPRESSION WITH PRIOR NEGATIVE TEST

These patients usually manifest ST-segment depression at high workloads and can be managed as if it were the first test. However, now the patient is identified as having an increased risk. If the ST changes are manifested at low workloads, the implications are more serious. Men who convert from a normal to an abnormal ST-segment response almost invariably have coronary narrowing and are rarely false-positive.

THERAPY

Medical

There is evidence that repeated episodes of ischemia may cause myocardial cell death and ultimately permanent reduction in left-ventricular function. We know that this happens in aortic stenosis and hypertensive heart disease. Evidence is accumulating that it may also occur in CAD.[36–38] A recent randomized prospective trial (ASIST) of 2037 patients at 30 study sites was reported.[39] Those who developed ischemia during Holter monitoring during daily life (306 patients) were assigned to either atenolol or placebo. Repeat Holter monitoring after 4 weeks revealed that the number of ischemic episodes in the atenolol-treated patients was markedly reduced. Events such as infarction and death were also reduced, and the relative risk ratio in those treated was 0.56. There were 39 events in the controls and 17 in those treated with atenolol. A study by Nikutta and colleagues[40] from Hannover, Germany, reported that therapy—that is, medical therapy, percutanous transluminal coronary angioplasty, or bypass surgery—had a beneficial effect on prognosis in 103 patients with silent ischemia followed up for 38 months.

Previous reports also suggest that medical therapy to some degree reduces the percentage of ischemic episodes and decreases their severity.[41] The beta-blocker trials indicate that in postinfarction patients, mortality will also decrease.[42] Also, beta blockers have been shown to result in favorable redistribution of blood flow in the ischemic myocardium.[43] The Oslo randomized trial in healthy men clearly demonstrates that diet and risk factor control also reduce mortality and morbidity.[44] Is this enough? No one can be sure. When dealing with individual patients, physicians will probably act on their own experiences and, it is hoped, with a sound knowledge of pathophysiology and familiarity with the recent literature.

At this time, I tend to be more aggressive in patients with multivessel high-grade stenosis or very proximal left anterior descending artery disease who demonstrate severe ischemia or other signs of limited left-ventricular performance. Evidence that justifies this approach is now accumulating. On the other hand, the salutory results now occurring with statins may soon favor more conservative approaches in patients without symptoms. There are also patients who have angina for a time, which then totally disappears—even at maximum exercise—without any detectable change in myocardial perfusion or medical program. We do not yet know if this is accompanied by a change in prognosis.

Surgical

A brief discussion about management of patients with silent ischemia brings our thinking into focus. There is little hard scientific data to direct us. A number of studies,[45,46] including the CASS study,[47] suggest that surgery on an asymptomatic patient, unless the patient has left main artery disease, does not increase longevity.

On the other hand, Cohn,[30] Kent,[48] and others[47] who have had an active interest in this subset of patients for some time favor an invasive approach in certain circumstances. Severe three-vessel disease, low exercise tolerance, early onset of ST-segment depression, and other signs of major ischemia are reliable predictors of a more serious prognosis in asymptomatic or mildly symptomatic patients.[50] In fact, ST depression in the asymptomatic postinfarction patient is the most reliable predictor of subsequent coronary events.[51] If we had evidence that these subjects would eventually have angina prior to infarction, thus warning us to intervene, it would make sense to wait for the onset of symptoms. The fact is that most patients with infarctions do not have angina as a warning.[1] Therefore, we can either wait for the ax to fall or try to develop criteria for intervention. Thurer and associates[52] and others[53] have documented that bypass surgical mortality in this group is almost zero in the best surgical centers. As the long-term results with angioplasty continue to improve this may be the treatment of choice in many patients.

Few would argue that open coronaries are not preferable to stenotic ones. The real issue is, "What price should we pay?" or "What risks should we take to open them up for a time at least?" A NHLBI sponsored study in 1959 patients designed to determine how best to control angina and/or ischemia found that revascularization gave better results than medical therapy, however this was not accompanied by aggressive statin therapy.[54]

CONCLUSION

In spite of those who oppose stress testing in asymptomatic patients, I firmly believe we will continue to search for ways to identify asymptomatic CAD. The use of exercise or other types of stress testing is by far the most practical approach we have, in addition to the possibility that coronary calcium may find an important role. Our data indicates that exercise testing is about as reliable in patients with silent ischemia as in those with angina. When all the data available are combined to calculate the probability of disease, we have an excellent tool that warrants continued application. With the information obtained, we can act to prevent infarction and death in an ever-increasing number of our patients. A book dealing with silent ischemia, edited by Shlomo Stern, is recommended reading.[55]

REFERENCES

1. Gordon, T and Kannel, WB: Premature mortality from coronary heart disease. JAMA 215(10):1617–1625, 1971.
2. Kemp, GL and Ellestad, MH: The incidence of "silent" coronary heart disease. Calif Med 109:363–367, 1968.
3. Gordon, T and Kannel, WB: Multiple risk functions for predicting coronary heart disease: The concept, accuracy, and application. Am Heart J 103(6):1031–1039, 1982.
4. Allison, RB, et al: Clinicopathologic correlations in coronary atherosclerosis. Circulation 27:170, 1963.
5. Spickerman, RC, et al: The spectrum of coronary heart disease in a community of 30,000. Circulation 25:57, 1962.
6. Diamond, GA and Forrester, JS: Analysis of probability as an aid in the diagnosis of CAD. N Engl J Med 300:350, 1979.
7. Erikssen, J, et al: False positive diagnostic tests and coronary angiographic findings in 105 presumably healthy males. Circulation 54:371–376, 1976.
8. Buckendorf, W, Warren, SE, and Vieweg, WVR: Suspected coronary artery disease among military aviation personnel. Aviat Space Environ Med October:1153–1158, 1980.
9. Bruce, RA, DeRouen, TA, and Hossack, KF: Value of maximal exercise tests in risk assessment of primary coronary heart disease events in healthy men. Am J Cardiol 46:371–378, 1980.
10. Allen, WH, et al: Five year follow-up of maximal treadmill stress test in asymptomatic men and women. Circulation 62:522–527, 1980.
11. Erikssen, J, et al: False suspicion of coronary heart disease: A 7 year follow-up study of 36 apparently healthy middle-aged men. Circulation 68(3):490–497, 1983.
12. Deanfield, J and Shea, M: ST segment change as a marker of ischemia. Circulation 68(suppl 111):22, 1983.
13. Maseri, A: Pathogenic mechanisms of angina pectoris expanding views. Br Heart J 43:648, 1980.
14. Armstron, WF and Morris, SN: The ST segment during continuous ambulatory electrocardiographic monitoring (editorial). Ann Intern Med 98:249, 1983.
15. Shell, WE and Penny, WF, Jr: Mechanisms and therapy of spontaneous angina: The implications of silent myocardial ischemia. Vasc Med Apr/June 85–96, 1984.
16. Kunkes, SH, et al: Silent ST segment deviations and extent of coronary artery disease. Am J Heart 100:813, 1980.
17. Faerman, I, et al: Autonomic neuropathy and painless MI in diabetics. Diabetes 26:1147, 1977.
18. Droste, C and Roskamm, H: Experimental pain measurement in patients with asymptomatic myocardial ischemia. J Am Coll Cardiol 1(3):940–945, 1983.
19. Ellestad, MH and Kuan, P: Naloxone and asymptomatic ischemia: Failure to induce angina during exercise testing. Am J Cardiol 54:982–984, 1984.
20. Heller, GV, et al: Plasma beta-endorphin levels in silent myocardial ischemia induced by exercise. Am J Cardiol 59:735–739, 1987.
21. Cole, JP and Ellestad, MH: Significance of chest pain during treadmill exercise: Correlation with coronary events. Am J Cardiol 41:277, 1978.
22. Sin, DM and Neill, WA: Investigation of the physiological basis for increased exercise threshold for angina pectoris after physical conditioning. J Clin Invest 54(3):763–770, 1974.
23. Little, WC, Constantinescu, M, and Applegate, RJ: Can coronary angiography predict the site of a subsequent myocardial infarction in patients with mild-to-moderate coronary disease? Circulation 78:1157–1166, 1988.
24. Sharma, B, et al. Demonstration of exercise-induced painless ischemia in survivors of out-of-hospital ventricular fibrillation. Am J Cardiol 59:740–745, 1887.
25. Cumming, GR, et al: Electrocardiographic changes during exercise in asymptomatic men: 3-year follow-up. Can Med Assoc J 1112:578–581, 1975.

26. Giagnoni, E, et al: Prognostic value of exercise EKG testing in asymptomatic normotensive subjects. N Engl J Med 309(18):1085–1089, 1983.
27. Hopkirk, JAC, et al: Discriminant value of clinical and exercise variables in detecting significant coronary artery disease in asymptomatic men. J Am Coll Cardiol 3(4):887–894, 1984.
28. Ellestad, MH, et al: The predictive value of the time courses of ST segment depression during exercise testing in patients referred for coronary angiograms. Am Heart J 123:904–908, 1992.
29. Laslett, LJ, Amsterdam, EA, and Mason, DT: Evaluating the positive exercise stress test in the asymptomatic individual. Chest 81(3):364–367, 1982.
30. Cohn, PF: Asymptomatic coronary artery disease. Mod Concepts Cardiovasc Dis 50(10):55–60, 1981.
31. Droste, C, et al: Development of angina pectoris pain and cardiac events in asymptomatic patients with myocardial ischemia. Am J Cardiol 72:121–127, 1993.
32. Raper, AJ, Hastillo, A, and Paulsen, WJ: The syndrome of sudden severe painless myocardial ischemia. Am Heart J 107(4):813–815, 1984.
33. Epstein, SE, et al: Strategy for evaluation and surgical treatment of the asymptomatic or mildly symptomatic patient with coronary artery disease. Am J Cardiol 43:1015–1025, 1979.
34. Selzer, A and Cohn K: Asymptomatic coronary artery disease and coronary bypass surgery. Am J Cardiol 39:614–616, 1977.
35. Redwood, DR, Epstein, SE, and Bover, FS: Whither the ST segment during exercise. Circulation 54:703–706, 1976.
36. Braunwald, E and Kloner, RA: The stunned myocardium: Prolonged, postischemic ventricular dysfunction. Circulation 66(6):1146, 1982.
37. Geft, IL, et al: Intermittent brief periods of ischemia have a cumulative effect and may cause myocardial necrosis. Circulation 66(6):1150, 1982.
38. Hess, OM, et al: Myocardial structure in patients with exercise induced ischemia. Circulation 77:967, 1987.
39. Pepine, CJ: Is treatment of silent ischemia beneficial? J Myocard Ischemia 5:47, 1993.
40. Nikutta, P, et al: The unfavorable prognosis of silent ischemia can be improved by appropriatetherapy [abstract]. Am J Coll Cardiol 21(2):46A, 1993.
41. Schang, SJ and Pepine, CJ: Transient asymptomatic ST segment depression during daily activity. Am J Cardiol 39:396, 1977.
42. Wilhelmsson, C, et al: Reduction of sudden deaths after myocardial infarction by treatment with alprenolol: Preliminary results. Lancet 2:1157, 1974.
43. Kalischer, AL, et al: Effects of propranolol and timolol on left ventricular volumes during exercisein patients with coronary artery disease. J Am Coll Cardiol 3(1):210, 1984.
44. Hjermann, I, et al: Effect of diet and smoking intervention on the incidence of coronary heart disease. Lancet 44:1301, 1981.
45. Norris, RM, et al: Coronary surgery after recurrent myocardial infarction: Progress of a trial comparing surgical with nonsurgical management for asymptomatic patients with advanced coronary disease. Circulation 63(4):875, 1981.
46. Murphy ML, et al: Treatment of chronic stable angina: A preliminary report of survival data of the randomized VA Cooperative Study. N Engl J Med 297:621, 1977.
47. Weiner, DA, et al: Significance of silent ischemia during exercise testing in patients with coronary disease. Am J Cardiol 59:725, 1987.
48. Kent, K: Silent ischemia, pathophysiology still a mystery. Heart Lines 4:4, 1983.
49. Myerberg, RJ and Sheps, DS: Evaluation of management of the asymptomatic patient with ECG evidence of myocardial ischemia. Pract Cardiol September 113, 1978.
50. McNeer, JF, et al: The role of the exercise test in the evaluation of patients for ischemic heart disease. Circulation 57:64, 1978.
51. Theroux, P, et al: Prognostic value of exercise testing soon after myocardial infarction. N Engl J Med 301:341, 1979.
52. Thurer, RL, et al: Asymptomatic coronary artery disease managed by myocardial revascularization.Circulation August, 39, 1979.
53. Loop, FH: Personal communication.
54. Rogers, WJ, et al. Asymptomatic Cardiac Ischemia Pilot (ACIP) study: Outcome at one year for patients with asymptomatic cardiac ischemia randomized to medical therapy or revascularization. J Am Coll Cardiol 25:594, 1995.
55. Stern, S. Silent Myocardial Ischemia. Martin Dunitz, Ltd. 1998.

20
Sports Medicine and Rehabilitation

Performance of Athletes Versus Nonathletes
Risks of Coronary Events in Sports
Rhythm Disturbances
Sudden Death
Infarction
Health As Related to Previous Athletic Efforts
Environmental Factors
Quantity and Quality of Exercise to Maintain Fitness
How Much Is Enough?
Type of Exercise Test in Sports
Findings in Athletes
Duration and Intensity
Heart Rate and Blood Pressure
ECG Changes at Rest
Ventricular Hypertrophy
Rhythm and Conduction Disturbances
Exercise-Induced Abnormalities
ST-Segment Depression
Duration of ST-Segment Depression
Septal Q Waves
T Waves
ST Elevation
Use of Exercise Testing in Sports
Alerting the Patient and Physician to Occult Dysfunction
Following Progress in Known Disease
Effects of Exercise Training on ST Depression and Exercise Capacity
Evaluating Drug Regimens
Comment
Exercise Testing in Cardiac Rehabilitation
Discharge Exercise Test After a Coronary Event
Exercise Testing Prior to Formal Outpatient Rehabilitation
Exercise Prescription
Confirmation of Improvement or Detection of Progression

Although the performances of the fit athlete and the cardiac patient needing rehabilitation lie at opposite ends of the spectrum, many of the concepts in exercise physiology apply to both. Each person is involved in an attempt to improve function using the same basic mechanisms. Coronary patients under the supervision of Kavanaugh and colleagues[1] in Toronto were able to train vigorously enough to complete the Boston Marathon, which dramatically demonstrates that sports and coronary artery disease (CAD) are no longer incompatible.

The use of exercise testing in each case provides us with a way of detecting dysfunction if present as well as a measure of conditioning and a tool for prescribing a subsequent exercise program in evaluating progress. This chapter presents some of the special problems that arise when dealing with each group and suggests guidelines that we have found useful.

PERFORMANCE OF ATHLETES VERSUS NONATHLETES

Blackburn[2] claims that the modern affluent human is a species of animal who shortly after maturation, is confined in special cages. One is a mobile steel and plastic cage with exposure to complex decisions, frustration, and danger. The atmosphere is high in carbon monoxide while the subject is being transported to other stationary cages. There, the subject is required to sit motionless most of the day while conditioned to self-administer 20 potent doses of the poison nicotine and at least five doses of caffeine alkaloids.

This commentary on our modern lifestyle dramatizes how far we have come from the environment for which our evolution has prepared us. In these artificial, unhealthy surroundings, disease can be far advanced, as well as undetected and unsuspected. On the other hand, in persons who regularly stress their cardiovascular systems to near-maximum capacity, dysfunction is less likely to occur and more likely to be detected earlier if present. Thus, besides the benefits mentioned in Chapters 1 and 2, earlier awareness of declining function is another benefit of an active lifestyle. Although changes in cardiovascular function are of chief interest to us, improvement in bones, muscles, tendons, lungs, and other organs can be achieved with regular activity.

Because we have, through custom, considered the sedentary human to be normal, which may not be the case, it is important to recognize the common cardiovascular changes seen in athletes. These include reduced heart rate, increased sinus arrhythmia, second-degree heart block, larger cardiac volume, some degree of ventricular hypertrophy, and the ECG patterns that are listed later in this chapter.[3] Static exercise produces fewer cardiovascular alterations but may be associated with significant hypertension; therefore, left-ventricular hypertrophy may be greater than with dynamic exercise.

RISKS OF CORONARY EVENTS IN SPORTS

Rhythm Disturbances

Rhythm disturbances are more common if warm-up is inadequate, isometric exercise is sustained, and isotonic exercise is near maximum capacity, and they are also found during the early recovery period. Scherer and Kaltenbach,[4] however, reported no mortality in 353,000 exercise tests done in sports centers for evaluation of fitness. The risks usually come with older subjects and in patients with occult disease.

Sudden Death

As much as 25% of primary infarctions occur during exercise.[5] Contributory factors include excitement, excessive pressure to continue when exhausted, and sustained isometric activity. The immediate risk of sudden death is threefold to fourfold during exercise.[6] Some believe that the increased risk during exercise is balanced by a decreased risk between bouts. Sudden death during marathon running, however, is fairly common.[7] The death of Jim Fixx,[8] a well-known runner, writer, and lecturer, dramatized the risk of exercise and placed another hole in the theory that marathon running provides a dispensation from coronary artery disease (CAD) (Bassler hypothesis).[9] Bassler's claim that he had never known nor heard of any published reports of coronary death in a patient who had finished a marathon was published as a letter to the editor in *Lancet* in 1972. In 1973, Green and associates[10] reported on a 44-year-old experienced marathon runner who had cardiac arrest in the 24th mile of the Boston Marathon. Since then there have been many more such published reports.[11,12] Corrado and associates[13] reported on 22 cases in northern Italy in which autopsy data were available. In 10 cases, sudden death was the first sign of disease. In the rest, the athlete was aware of a problem but either ignored it or failed to accept advice given to follow a treatment regimen or alter the exercise program. An authoritative treatise by Noakes and colleagues[14] reviews this subject in detail. Sudden death during or immediately after exercise is especially common in cardiomyopathies—usually unrecognized hypertrophic cardiomyopathies in young asymptomatic athletes.[15] This is probably due to ventricular tachycardia and ventricular fibrillation occurring most commonly immediately after exercise.

Infarction

Infarction, arrhythmias, and sudden death often coexist and can be initiated by exercise. In younger runners, infarction occasionally occurs even with normal coronary arteries.[16] The cause of this is poorly understood, but some theories are presented in Chapter 17.

HEALTH AS RELATED TO PREVIOUS ATHLETIC EFFORTS

There is little evidence that athletic performance in a person's youth has a substantial effect on cardiovascular health in later years. On the other hand, life expectancy may be increased slightly in those who persist in strenuous sports for many years. Karvonen and associates[17] reported a maximum gain in longevity of 3 years in 396 Finnish championship male skiers. Of interest is that 37% of these skiers continued to ski regularly into their 60s. Soviet athletes have been reported to have a shorter life expectancy unless they reach aged 64, after which they also manage to live longer. These data are hard to evaluate because we know so little of the lifestyle of Russian athletes. Certain types of sports seem to be associated with different risks. Middle-aged British rugby players are believed to have the highest risk and marathon runners the lowest risk for death from CAD.[18]

ENVIRONMENTAL FACTORS

Cold has long been recognized as an initiating factor in angina and myocardial infarction in persons with CAD. Presumably, peripheral resistance increases in cold weather and thus myocardial work is greater with moderate activity. As the time and intensity of work increase, however, this increased peripheral resistance disappears in normal subjects. Every long-distance runner knows that exercise during times of increased heat and humidity presents problems. If occult disease is present, these factors constitute serious hazards, because low cardiac function is associated with a reduced capacity to eliminate heat and to overcome increased peripheral resistance. Thus, the risk of serious cardiac events increases when people push themselves in climate extremes.

QUANTITY AND QUALITY OF EXERCISE TO MAINTAIN FITNESS

Because a training effect is so dependent on the level of fitness at the onset of the program, it is difficult to give rigid guidelines. In a person who is very sedentary or who has been on bed rest, minimal exercise will increase fitness. On the other hand, the more fit a person is, the more that is needed to improve or maintain this level. This was established by the classic study of Saltin and associates[19] in Dallas in which they found that normal subjects on bed rest had a rapid increase in $\dot{V}O_2$ max in a short time after they resumed training. However, as they progressed, the benefits and percentage of change per unit of work steadily declined. Their function finally reached a plateau after about 6 weeks of training. It appears that, on the average, the higher the intensity and the longer the exercise intervals, the faster the training effect will progress—that is, as long as excessive fatigue does not limit the program, which may constitute a sign of overtraining.

HOW MUCH IS ENOUGH?

How much exercise is enough depends on the goals of the individual. If a person correctly believes that exercise is good for general health and will decrease the likelihood of developing CAD, he or she should probably exercise for 30 to 45 minutes at least 3 days per week. This regimen was recommended by Pollock[20] after evaluating a number of training schedules as to their ability to increase $\dot{V}O_2$ max as well as their likelihood of causing an injury. The earlier work of Paffenbarger and coworkers[21] suggested that about 2000 kcal/wk give maximum protection against CAD. Recent data on the same cohort of Harvard alumni, however, identified a subgroup of men involved in a moderately vigorous program expending at least 3500 kcal/wk who had considerably more protection than those who were less vigorous.[22] Hambrecht and associates[23] have also reported on a small series of men with known CAD randomized to a control program or a vigorous leisure time program and followed up by coronary angiography. Those expending greater than 1400 kcal/wk experienced stabilization of their coronary lesions, and those expending 2200 kcal or more experienced regression. The recent reports that regular exercise improves endothelial function explains at least one of the mechanisms responsible for the benefit.[24]

The exercise program should be carried out at an intensity of at least 60% to 80% of the individual's maximum capacity. These guidelines are for both sedentary subjects planning to engage in sports and CAD patients who would improve their function. If the sport envisioned requires a high level of fitness, increased intensity and training time will be required. Although there is a dose related benefit in that more exercise is better than a little, those who are sedentary can improve their health, fitness and well being by becoming even moderately active. Exercise reduces the risk of all-cause and cardiac mortality and is also beneficial in obesity, hypertension, diabetes and even breast and colon cancer.[25]

TYPE OF EXERCISE TEST IN SPORTS

The design of the exercise test may need to be specific for evaluation of certain activities; on the other hand, if only the aerobic capacity or maximum oxygen uptake is to be evaluated, a progressive exercise test—either on a treadmill or bicycle—is appropriate. We often use the same protocol for analyzing athletes as for patients. However, it is necessary to markedly extend the speed and grade for those who are highly conditioned. If research work requires knowledge of $\dot{V}O_2$, direct measurement of the oxygen consumption must be done. There are many approaches to this, depending on the experience of the examiner and the facilities available. In our laboratory, we use the Beckman metabolic cart. If less accuracy is deemed satisfactory, there are a number of formulas and nomograms that allow fairly reproducible estimates of oxygen capacity from the speed and grade or the time on the treadmill protocol or the watts achieved on the bicycle (see Chapter 6).

FINDINGS IN ATHLETES

Duration and Intensity

As expected, endurance-trained athletes can perform at high levels for longer periods. Those who train isometrically, such as weight lifters, may have little increase in their aerobic capacity.

Heart Rate and Blood Pressure

The lower resting heart and the average lower heart rate at any given workload is a recognized result of conditioning and has led to a method of predicting $\dot{V}O_2$ max from submaximal performance.[26] Maximum heart rate is also occasionally moderately reduced compared with the value predicted for age.

The expected increase in blood pressure is often lower in highly trained athletes, but this effect is frequently absent in the older age groups.

ECG Changes at Rest

As early as 1954, it was recognized that the ECG of athletes may be different from other subjects, and findings correlated with pathology in nonathletes may be the result of a normal response to vigorous training.[27,28] These include left- and right-ventricular hypertrophy, abnormalities in repolarization (T- and ST-segment changes), sinus bradycardia, and atrioventricular conduction disturbances[3] (Fig. 20–1).

Ventricular Hypertrophy

Both right- and left-ventricular hypertrophy are common as estimated by R-wave criteria. ST-T wave changes are seen but are less common. The incidence of these abnormalities in 42 professional basketball players reported on by Roeske and colleagues[29] is illustrated in Table 20–1. Right-axis deviation is common, and right-ventricular hypertrophy is frequently seen as well as left-ventricular hypertrophy. ST elevation in the lateral precordial leads, termed *early repolarization,* is also frequently seen. Echocardiography has demonstrated that the ECG changes are associated with left-ventricular dilatation and sometimes myocardial hypertrophy. It seems well established that this type of hypertrophy is simply work-related and has no untoward implications.

Rhythm and Conduction Disturbances

Sinus bradycardia is common and correlates to some degree with the level of fitness. Resting heart rates in the 40s are frequent, and occasionally less than

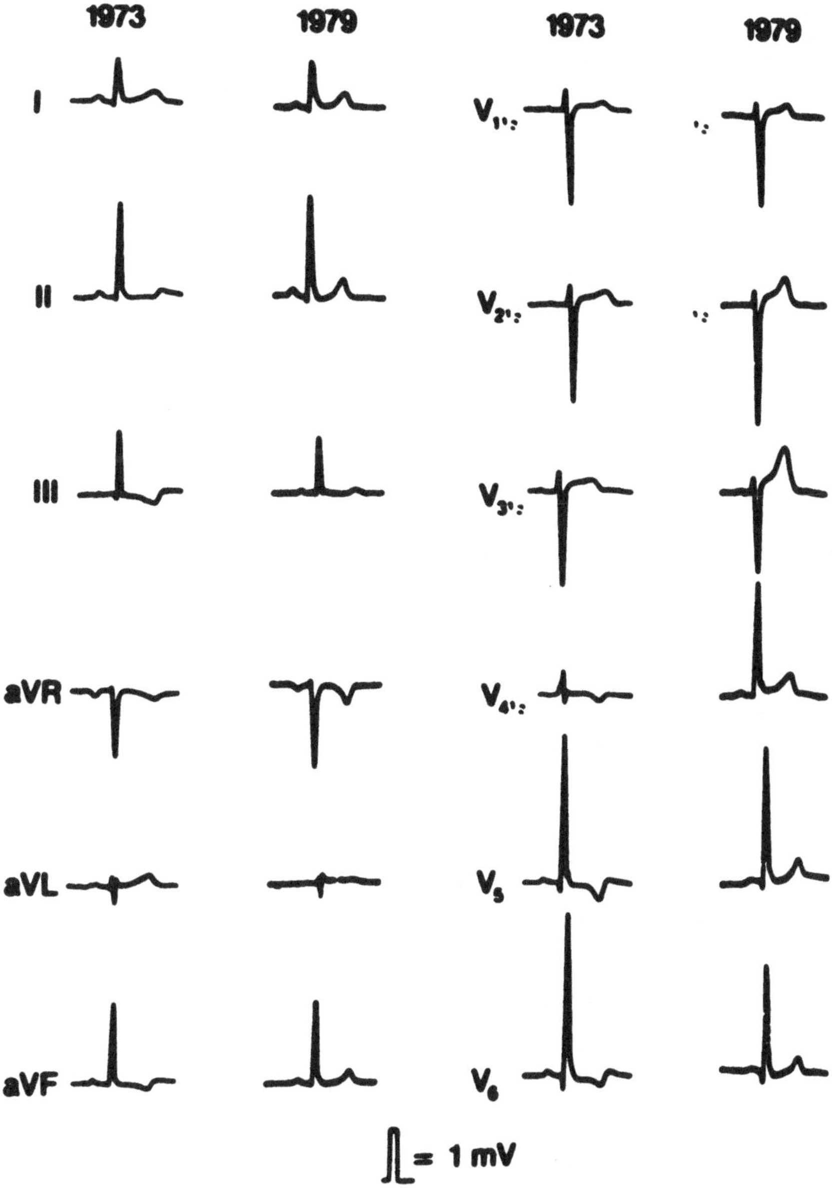

FIGURE 20–1. ECG of an Olympic walker prior to and 6 years after stopping training. Note loss of voltage and normalization of the T waves in V_5 and V_6. (From Oakley,[28] with permission.)

Table 20–1. Incidence of Left- and Right-Ventricular Hypertrophy by ECG and VCG in 42 Professional Basketball Players

	LVH		*RVH*	
	No.	%	No.	%
ECG	11	26	29	69
VCG	12	29	18	43
Both	9	21	16	38
Neither	28	67	11	26

LVH = left-ventricular hypertrophy; RVH = right-ventricular hypertrophy; VCG = vectorcardiogram.

40 beats per minute may be seen. Atrioventricular junctional rhythm and first- and second-degree heart block occur in 1% to 5% of subjects.[3] These conduction disturbances seem to be invariably normalized by exercise and are believed to be due to increased vagal tone. Occasional examples of Wolff-Parkinson-White syndrome and other varieties of preexcitation syndrome have also been described.[3] Ventricular ectopic beats initiated by exercise have been a worry because in CAD patients they may signal more severe rhythms, especially ventricular tachycardia (see Chapter 13). In athletes, these types of beats are rarely of concern if the subject has good ventricular function. Palatini and associates[30] have reported a 5-year follow-up in 52 professional endurance athletes who were found to have frequent premature ventricular contractions (PVCs) with exercise. None had any adverse events, and 23 who were still training continued to have frequent PVCs without significant problems.

Exercise-Induced Abnormalities

Most endurance athletes have normal ECG complexes during exercise. In fact, it is even common for senior runners to have patterns similar to those seen in very young subjects.

ST-Segment Depression

Rogers and colleagues[31] studied 43 boys aged 12 to 15, none of whom had exercise-induced ST depression. A significant number of young, symptom-free athletes do have ST depression with exercise, although this may be no more common than in nonathletes.[28] When ST depression occurs in young athletic men, it can be safely ignored as long as hypertrophic cardiomyopathy, right ventricular dysplasia, congenital long QT syndrome, and severe hypercholesterolemia can be ruled out.

In those about 40 years of age, it is a different story. Lie and colleagues[12] from Oslo, Norway, compared 21 athletes ranging from 31 to 69 years old with exercise-induced ST depression with 21 age-matched men without ST depression. After a 3-year follow-up, the investigators found that only 3 of the 21 athletes had cardiovascular disease and only one had coronary heart disease. They concluded that the ST depression was due to the left-ventricular hypertrophy caused by their athletic endeavors and possibly represented reduced subendocardial perfusion. Lie and colleagues[12] found that the patients had reduced diastolic compliance, especially as they aged. Their systolic function remained intact, even as their diastolic function decreased, in relationship to the degree of left-ventricular hypertrophy.

Is there a way to differentiate those who have CAD from those who don't? If the resting ECG shows hypertrophy, benign ST depression is more likely, although those with CAD may have this finding also. An exercise echocardiogram usually shows a wall motion abnormality in those who also have CAD and can be used as a second noninvasive test when the ST depression is suspected of being a false-positive. Some athletes with CAD may have a very high aerobic capacity, but usually report a decrement from previous performances.

Duration of ST-Segment Depression

During exercise, ST depression may occur at a moderate workload and evolve to a lesser magnitude at higher levels of work. This is almost always a sign that there is no coronary narrowing. ST depression may appear only at maximum workload and disappear within a few seconds into the recovery, which is a more reassuring finding but, as previously mentioned, not always a sign of normal coronary arteries. When significant ST depression occurs during exercise, remains for several minutes during recovery, and evolves to a downsloping pattern, it is more likely to be caused by true ischemia.

Septal Q Waves

Because of hypertrophy of the heart wall with training, the septal Q wave in the lateral precordial leads is often prominent at rest. If this increases with exercise and is associated with ST depression, ischemia is rarely present.[32] Septal Q waves are more common in younger patients and in endurance-trained athletes.

T Waves

Inverted T waves are seen in the resting ECG and usually become upright with exercise. This has no clinical significance. Very tall T waves in the immediate recovery period are common and probably represent an increased stroke volume (see Chapter 12).

ST Elevation

Resting ST elevation (early repolarization) in the precordial leads invariably disappears with exercise. This process is poorly understood but has no special significance. ST elevation induced by exercise is rare in the absence of ischemia.

USE OF EXERCISE TESTING IN SPORTS

Alerting the Patient and Physician to Occult Dysfunction

In today's fitness-conscious society, many individuals who have a number of coronary risk factors decide to mend their ways. Engaging in a regular fitness program may aggravate ischemia or predispose them to serious arrhythmias. Part of a complete examination in this group should include an exercise test. (Jim Fixx would probably be alive today if he had been tested.[8]) In individuals older than aged 40, a large percentage of sedentary subjects have hypertension. Therefore, it is important to determine the blood pressure response to exercise, because this response may provide information as to the risk of hypertension in the future as well as help in determining the need for present treatment.[33] In those who are serious about improving performance, the exercise capacity, maximum $\dot{V}O_2$ and blood pressure response to exercise, and anaerobic threshold may be of interest. We have found that demonstrating to the patient that his heart rate at a given workload is lower than when he started the program is an incentive to continue. Guidelines as to the mode of training may be made more intelligently with this information in mind.

Following Progress in Known Disease

In patients with recognized cardiac disability, the exercise prescription has traditionally been based on the treadmill or bicycle performance. The safety of exercise is predicted by adjusting its intensity after observation of the response to known workloads and extrapolating this to the daily regimen. Details of this approach have been provided in a number of monographs and texts.[12,34,35]

Effects of Exercise Training on ST Depression and Exercise Capacity

Training in cardiac patients increases exercise capacity and decreases heart rate for any given workload. This is usually apparent within 3 months and can be augmented by persisting for longer intervals. When the heart rate and usually the double product are reduced at a target workload, the magnitude of the ST depression at that level is reduced compared with the preexercise training period. If exercise is prolonged or increased so that the double product at the onset of ST depression is equivalent to that prior to the training period, ST depression may again be manifested,[34] although there have been some reports that the onset of ischemia will occur at a greater double product than prior to training.[36] If this is observed, it provides evidence of improved myocardial perfusion,[37] probably from increased collaterals, or improved endothelial function.[24]

Not infrequently, after retesting patients who have been on exercise programs, we have determined that they should stop exercising and consider an invasive procedure to improve coronary flow. This decision is usually based on the onset of ST-segment depression or anginal pain at an earlier workload than previously. The occurrence of ominous ventricular arrhythmias or a marked decrease in exercise heart rate or blood pressure would also be of concern. In this case, progression of the severity of coronary narrowing is very likely.

Evaluating Drug Regimens

A large number of drugs are now available to treat ischemia, hypertension, and cardiac arrhythmias. Only by exercise testing can we determine how our patients are responding to whatever regimen has been prescribed. All too often, clinicians base their estimates of effects on resting performance, only to find out later that during exercise, the program is ineffective and may not be providing the desired result. Because there is often some day-to-day variation in exercise capacity, two tests taken before and after the therapeutic regimen can provide more certainty that the change seen is significant.

Comment

Exercise testing was first used almost exclusively as a method of evaluating athletes. As more and more of the population engages in various types of sports, and as people engage in sports at older ages, exercise testing is becoming more important. It will continue to be an essential tool in the management of those engaging in sports, especially those with known or suspected disease, as well as in research on the effects of exercise on our health and well-being.

EXERCISE TESTING IN CARDIAC REHABILITATION

Although there is widespread disagreement as to the use of exercise testing in apparently healthy people prior to the institution of an exercise program, it is generally agreed that it plays an important role in the patient with known CAD.

Discharge Exercise Test After a Coronary Event

Discharge exercise testing is discussed extensively in Chapter 10, but its value is emphasized here because it provides guidelines regarding the likelihood of problems induced by exercise after the patient has experienced a coronary event. When a low-level test is completed on discharge without abnormalities, it is usually safe to allow rapid return to moderate activity. Within 4 to 6 weeks, a near-maximum test should be done to plan activity for the next few months.

Exercise Testing Prior to Formal Outpatient Rehabilitation

This type of test provides the following:

1. Patient reassurance
2. Risk prediction
3. Triage to various types of therapy
4. Formulation of an exercise prescription

Exercise Prescription

Most dynamic exercise programs are based on the concept that a heart rate of 60% or more of maximum is necessary for the training effect to occur. Because there is so much individual variation in heart rate and exercise capacity, the exercise test is an ideal way to arrive at the proper workload geared to each individual. If the patient can reach maximum predicted heart rate without symptoms or signs of ischemia or arrhythmias, the optimum heart rate for training can then be selected. If, on the other hand, the patient develops ST displacement, anginal pain, or arrhythmias during the test, a heart rate of approximately 10 beats less than that necessary to initiate the aberration is usually a safe level to maintain during a regular workout. At times, monitoring the patient during the workout is desirable to confirm the original level selected. As the patient gains experience, the patient can often perceive the level of exertion necessary to judge the amount of work prescribed.

After a time (usually about 4 weeks), the patient will be able to increase the work level without increasing the heart rate, a sign of improved aerobic capacity or conditioning.

Confirmation of Improvement or Detection of Progression

After the rehabilitation program has been instituted, a repeat exercise test either will document the improvement, providing a new safe level of performance, or occasionally will indicate disease progression. The latter is extremely important to alert the physician and the patient that some change in therapeutic plans may be in order. By this time, the patient will have a better understanding of the mechanisms of the disease process and the validity of the determinations made during exercise as well as the signs of cardiac dysfunction. Objective evidence is very important, since we have seen many patients who have no angina but more ischemia as determined by the onset of ST depression at a workload lower than during the previous test. This is particularly significant if it occurs after a good training effect has been obtained.

In summation, the exercise test in rehabilitation is a yardstick that is useful in measuring exercise capacity and the severity of disability, and in demonstrating to the patient the signs of progress. As more evidence that demonstrates the benefits of exercise is accumulated, estimates of fitness become increasingly useful.

REFERENCES

1. Kavanaugh, T, et al: Marathon running after myocardial infarction. JAMA 229:1602, 1974.
2. Blackburn, H: Disadvantages of intensive exercise therapy after myocardial infarction. In Ingelfinger, FJ, et al (eds): Controversy in Internal Medicine, ed 2. WB Saunders, Philadelphia, 1974, pp 169–170.
3. Hanne-Paparo, N, et al: Common ECG changes in athletes. Cardiology 61:267–278, 1976.
4. Scherer, D and Kaltenbach, M: Frequency of life-threatening complications associated with stress testing. Dtsch Med Wochenschr 104:1161, 1979.
5. McHenry PL, Phillips, JF, and Knoebel, SB: Correlation of computer-quantitated treadmill exercise electrocardiogram with arteriographic location of coronary artery disease. Am J Cardiol 30:747, 1972.
6. Shephard, RJ: The cardiac athlete: When does exercise training become overexertion? Prac Cardiol 6(2):39, 1980.
7. Milvy, P: Statistics, marathoning and CHD. Am Heart J 95(4):538–539, 1978.
8. Jim Fixx ran a risky race. Med World News, August 27, 1984, p 27.
9. Bassler, TJ: Athletic activity and longevity. Lancet 2:712, 1972.
10. Green, LH, Cohen, SI, and Kurland, G: Fatal myocardial infarction in marathon racing. Ann Intern Med 84(6):704–706, 1976.
11. Burke, AP, Farb, A, and Virmani, R: Sports-related and non sports-related sudden cardiac death in young adults. Am Heart J 121:568–575, 1991.
12. Lie, H, Ihlen, H, and Rootwelt, K: Significance of a positive exercise test in middle aged and old athletes as judged by echocardiography, radionuclide and follow-up findings. Eur Heart J 6:615–624, 1985.
13. Corrado, D, et al: Sudden death in young competitive athletes: Clinicopathologic correlations in 22 cases. Am J Med 89:588–596, 1990.
14. Noakes, TD, Opie, LH, and Rose, AG: Marathon running and immunity to CHD. Clin Sports Med 3:527, 1984.
15. Maron, EJ, Epstein, SE, and Roberts, WC: Hypertrophic cardiomyopathy: A common cause of sudden death in the young competitive athlete. Eur Heart J 4(suppl):135–144, 1983.
16. Franklin, BVA: Clinical exercise testing. Clin Sports Med 3:295, 1984.
17. Karvonen, MJ, et al: Longevity of endurance skiers. Med Sci Sports 6:49, 1974.
18. Crawford, MH and O'Rourke, RA: The Athlete's Heart: Year Book of Sports Medicine. Year Book Medical Publishers, Chicago, 1979, p 311.
19. Saltin, B, et al: Response to exercise after bed rest and after training. Circulation 37(7):VII–1, 1979.
20. Pollock, ML: How much exercise is enough? Phys Sportsmed 6(6):31, 1978.
21. Paffenbarger, RS, et al: Epidemiology of exercise and coronary heart disease. Clin Sports Med 3:297, 1984.
22. Paffenbarger, RS, Robert, PH, and Hyde, T: The association of changes in physical activity level and other lifestyle characteristics with mortality among men. N Engl J Med 328:538–545, 1993.

23. Hambrecht, R, et al: Various intensities of leisure time physical activity in patients with coronary artery disease: Effects on cardiorespiratory fitness and progression of coronary atherosclerotic lesions. J Am Coll Cardiol 22:468–7, 1993.
24. Kromhout, D, et al: Prevention cross-cultural, cohort, and intervention studies. Circulation 105:893, 2002.
25. ACIM Guidelines for Exercise Testing and Prescription, 6th ed. Franklin, B. (ed). Lippincott, Williams & Wilkins, 2000.
26. Naughton, JP and Hellerstein, HK: Exercise testing and exercise training in CHD. Academic Press, New York, 1973.
27. Beckner, G and Winsor, T: Cardiovascular adaptations to prolonged physical effort. Circulation 9:835, 1954.
28. Oakley CM: Treatment of primary pulmonary hypertension. In Sobel, E, Julian, DC, and Hugenholz, PG (eds): Perspectives in Cardiology. Current Medical Literatures Ltd, 1984.
29. Roeske, WR, et al: Non-invasive evaluation of ventricular hypertrophy in professional athletes. Circulation 53:286, 1976.
30. Palatini, P, et al: Prognostic significance of ventricular extrasystoles in healthy professional athletes: Results of a 5-year follow up. Cardiology 82:286, 1993.
31. Rogers, JH, Jr, et al: The exercise electrocardiogram in trained and untrained adolescent males. Med Sci Sports 9(3):164, 1977.
32. Famularo, M, et al: Identification of septal ischemia during exercise by Q wave analysis: Correlation with coronary angiography. Am J Cardiol 51(3):440, 1983.
33. Schrager, B and Ellestad, MH: The importance of blood pressure measurement during exercise testing. Cardiovasc Rev Rep 4(3):381, 1983.
34. Long, C: Prevention and Rehabilitation in Ischemic Heart Disease. Williams & Wilkins, Baltimore, 1983.
35. Fletcher, GF: Exercise in the Practice of Medicine. Futura Publishing, Mt. Kisco, NY, 1982.
36. Meyers, J, et al: A randomized trial of the effects of 1 year of exercise training on computer measured ST segment displacement in patients with coronary artery disease. J Am Coll Cardiol 4:1094, 1984.
37. Sasayama, S and Fujita, M: Recent insights into the coronary collateral circulation. Circulation 85:1197, 1992.

21
Pediatric Exercise Testing

Reasons for Clinical Exercise Testing
Equipment
Exercise Protocols
Measured Responses During Exercise Testing
Congenital Heart Disease
Valvular and Discrete Subvalvular Aortic Stenosis
Supravalvular Aortic Stenosis
Coarctation of Thoracic Aorta
Aortic Valve Insufficiency
Pulmonary Valvular Stenosis
Tetralogy of Fallot
Other Complex Congenital Anomalies
Arrhythmia with Normal Heart
Complete Congenital Heart Block
Congenital Long QT Syndrome
Kawasaki Disease
Sickle Cell Anemia
Hypertension
Hypertrophic Cardiomyopathy

In pediatrics, exercise testing is routine in evaluating working capacity, and adaptation to external work, growth, and level of fitness in normal subjects and in patients with cardiovascular or other disease processes. Modern technology has aided further development and the rediscovery of noninvasive or innocuous invasive procedures to do functional assessment of young subjects with different clinical problems of varying severity.

With estimates of working capacity, pulmonary ventilation, cardiac performance and function, myocardial perfusion, and rhythm and conduction of the heart, the oxygen transport system can be assessed under standardized conditions with low risk in children. The interpretation of the exercise study revealing the impact of specific diseases on the cardiovascular system, provides the clinical information for rational use in diagnosing and treating patients. Test results showing common response patterns that suggest a specific diagnosis often occur but must be accepted as a bonus because some physiological or pathophysiological pattern of exercise responses are common to several diagnoses.

This chapter presents current uses of exercise testing in pediatric cardiovascular medicine, and identifies additional needs for further investigational study. Cardiovascular responses due to the presence of a specific car-

Research for this chapter supported in part by Grant 5 RO1 HL184454-05 and Grant T32-HL07417-15 from National Heart, Heart, Lung, and Blood Institute; Grant 76853 from American Heart Association Southwestern Division.

diac defects or clinical situations show the potential and benefits of using exercise testing in clinical pediatrics. Studies such as nuclear imaging, echocardiography, or cardiac catheterization combined with exercise are omitted. These combined procedures, which are rapidly entering into routine clinical practice, are yielding important data and deserve separate consideration.

REASONS FOR CLINICAL EXERCISE TESTING

The results from exercise testing are used to supplement a rational approach in clinically managing patients. In children and young adults, clinical exercise testing, used to record responses to controlled external work, offers the opportunity to explore signs and symptoms suggestive of cardiopulmonary problems, assess results of specific surgical and medical treatment, and assist in determining prognosis and functional capacity of children with or without disorders, for reasonable participation in vocational, recreational, and athletic activities.

EQUIPMENT

A clinical exercise laboratory should be able to measure working capacity, blood pressure, heart rate, and record and view multiple ECG leads continuously during exercise.[1,2] For these requirements, a cycle or treadmill ergometer, an apparatus for measuring peripheral blood pressure indirectly, a multichannel recorder for the ECG, and an oscilloscope are needed. Other measurements such as cardiac output, systolic time indices, percent shortening fraction and ejection fraction enhance the assessment of cardiac performance and function but require additional electronic systems using ultrasonography, nuclear imaging, and mass spectrometry.

EXERCISE PROTOCOLS

Several cycle protocols both individualized and fixed, are available for routine clinical use in children and young adults.[1–4] Chantal and colleagues[4] performed progressive exercise testing, which was individualized for children aged 5 to 17 years with various cardiac and respiratory diseases. In the absence of a plateau of oxygen uptake, the criteria for a maximal test using the individualized protocol, were clinical exhaustion and a maximal heart rate. The individualized exercise protocol was well tolerated by all children with 66% of them reaching the predicted maximal VO_2, and 68% satisfying the criteria for a plateau of VO_2 at peak exercise. We use a fixed continuous, progressive exercise protocol, which is suitable for subjects of different sizes, ages, and clinical problems of varying severity[3] (Table 21–1). This fixed pro-

Table 21–1. **James Protocol**

	Body Surface Area (m^2)		
Levels	**<1**	**1–1.19**	**≥1.2**
1	200	200	200
2	300	400	500
3	500	600	800
Increments	100	100	200

Workload in kg-m/min; 3 min per level.
Adapted from James, et al.[1]

tocol appears to safely strike a comfortable balance of managing the challenge to leg power and endurance while attempting to reach at or near maximal exercise in a reasonable average time in the laboratory. Clinical exhaustion or predetermine end-point(s) are the primary reasons for ending a clinical exercise test. Treadmill protocols are also available, but normal data are limited in children.[1,2] In measuring many variables during exercise, the cycle ergometer has the advantage of allowing a stable upper body for obtaining fidelity recordings as compared to the treadmill.

MEASURED RESPONSES DURING EXERCISE TESTING

Physical working capacity has been estimated by using PWC170.[5] highest rate of work required to produce a heart rate of 170 beats per minute and respiratory rate of 30 or less (breaths per minute). Other estimates of working capacity are made by determining the highest rate of work in which oxygen uptake fails to increase,[6] and by calculating accumulative work accomplished or total exercise time to a finite end-point such as exhaustion.[3,7] Using the James protocol,[3] working capacity is estimated by calculating total work performed to exhaustion or to any adverse end-point such as those listed in Table 21–2 and by recording the highest rate of work (maximal

Table 21–2. **Indications for Exercise Test Termination**

Development of serious arrhythmia (eg, ventricular tachycardia or supraventricular tachycardia)
Failure of ECG monitoring system
Pain, headache, dizziness, syncope, excessive dyspnea, and fatigue precipitated by exercise
Pallor, clammy skin, or inappropriate affect
Excessive rise in systolic pressure exceeding 240 mm Hg and in diastolic pressure exceeding 120 mm Hg
Progressive fall in blood pressure
ST-Segment depression or elevation greater than 3 mm during exercise
Recognized type of intracardiac block precipitated by exercise
Increase in premature ventricular contractions during exercise

Adapted from James, et al.[1]

power output) maintained for 1.5 minutes or more during progressive continuous exercise. In this protocol, total work and maximal power output are directly related to body height, with the steepest slope in subjects with body surface area (BSA) of 1.2m.[2] or more (Fig. 21–1). Both boys and girls with BSA of less than $1.2m^2$ performed similar amounts of work during exercise. In normal subjects with BSA of $1.2m^2$ or more, boys performed more work and reached higher rates of work than girls.

Oxygen uptake (VO_2) is positively related to the intensity of work. Figure 21–2 illustrates the relationship between VO_2 and submaximal work rate in 48 normal subjects from our laboratory and 27 normal subjects studied by Bengtsson[8] several years earlier. The linear regression lines derived from the two studied populations are almost identical. We recommend measuring submaximal and maximal oxygen uptakes during clinical testing and representing each oxygen uptake value as a percentage of maximal oxygen uptake. In our laboratory, we calculate a predicted maximal oxygen uptake for each subject. When the measured maximal oxygen uptake is less than the predicted value (based on height and rate of work), the predicted value is used to calculate the percentage of each oxygen uptake value.[3]

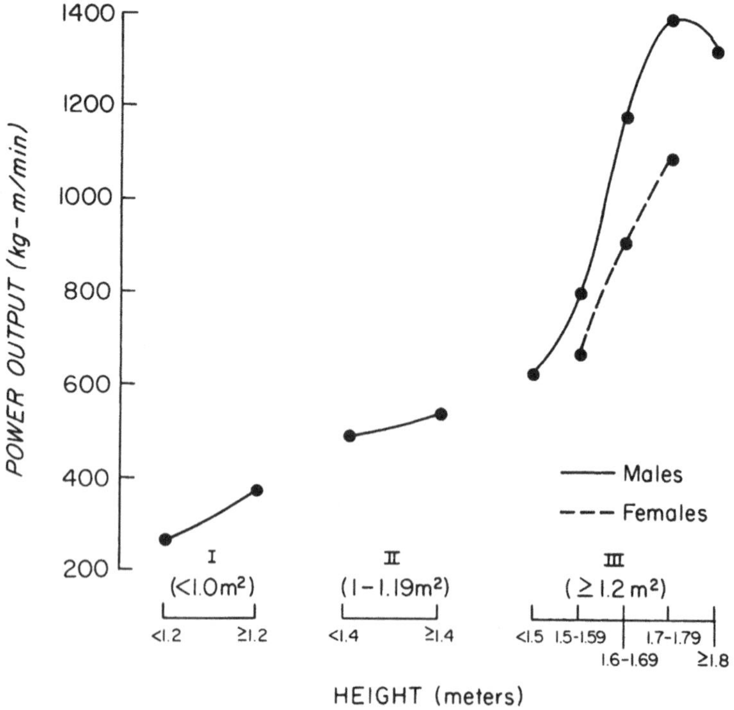

FIGURE 21–1. Maximal power output in healthy subjects by height within each subdivision of the James protocol. The measurement is similar in male and female patients with body surface area less than 1.2 m^2. For healthy subjects with body surface area greater than 1.2 m^2, male patients exceeded the females. (From James,[22] p 231, with permission.)

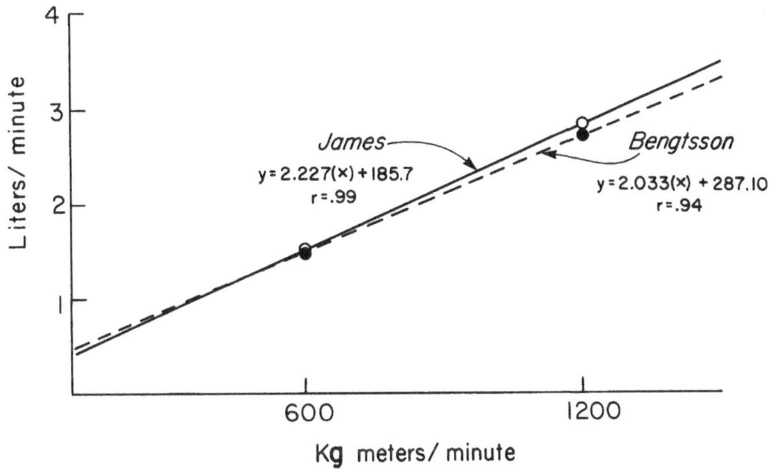

FIGURE 21–2. Regression data from James[22] and Bengtsson[8] describing similar relationship of oxygen uptake to work during submaximum exercise in healthy children. (From James,[22] p 232, with permission.)

Carbon dioxide production (VO_2) also increases with intensity of exercise to a level at which the slope changes markedly (Fig. 21–3). This change in slope is associated with an increase in minute ventilation and respiratory frequency, leveling of oxygen uptake, audible oral breathing, respiratory quotient (VCO_2/VO_2) greater than 1, and a serum lactate level difference before and after exercise of greater than 44.[9] In normal children, the ventilatory anaerobic threshold occurs when the minute ventilation: oxygen uptake increases without a simultaneous change in the minute ventilation: carbon dioxide production.[10]

Including gas analysis with clinical exercise testing, cardiac and pulmonary disorders in adults can produce differentiating responses in that cardiac patients may cross their anaerobic threshold and attain maximal oxygen uptake at 50% or less of maximal voluntary ventilation without desaturation. Pulmonary patients may not cross-anaerobic threshold or reach maximal oxygen uptake, but will have desaturation.[11] In children, these differentiating responses may not be as decisive, especially in pediatric patients with complex congenital heart disease with or without surgical treatment.[12] The gas analysis does provide an important link between the disease process and its effect on exercise performance. Peak oxygen uptake reported as a percentage of measured or predicted maximal oxygen uptake (whichever is greatest) allows meaningful interpretation of physical changes in children due to growth, level of physical training, age, disease, and treatment.

Systolic blood pressure increases promptly with progressive dynamic leg exercise. Diastolic and mean pressures increase to a moderate degree. The rise in arterial pressure reflects an increase in cardiac output greater than the

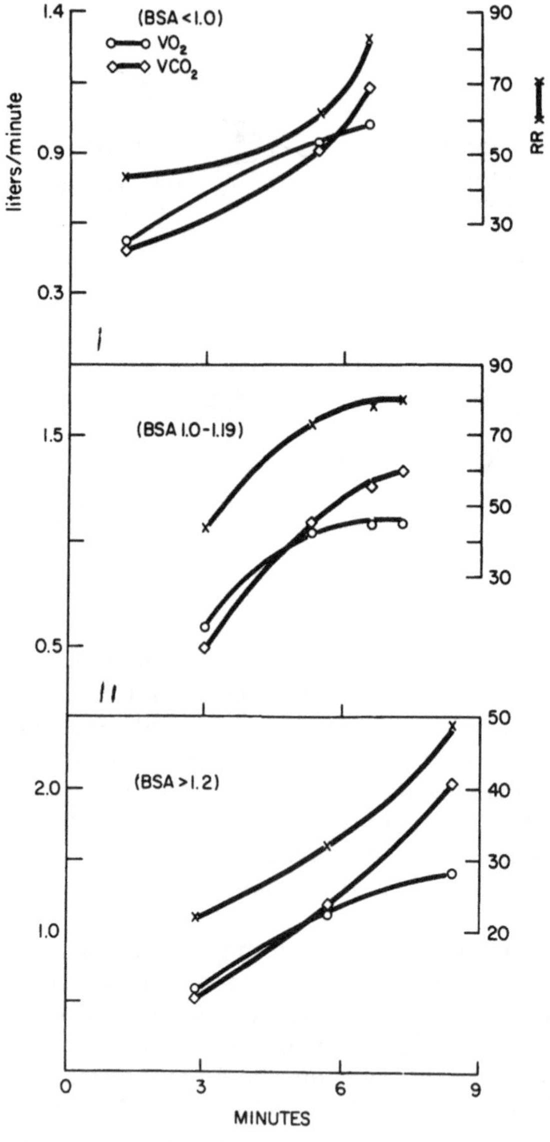

FIGURE 21–3. Oxygen uptake, carbon dioxide production, and respiratory frequency in a normal subject in each subdivision by body surface area of the James protocol.[1] $\dot{V}CO_2$ exceeded $\dot{V}O_2$ early during exercise in two subjects (*Middle and Bottom Panels*). $\dot{V}CO_2$ and respiratory frequency are tracking in each subject. (Adapted from James,[22] p 235, with permission.)

decrease in systemic vascular resistance. Exercise blood pressures yield essential information about pump performance (stroke volume and rate of ejection) and afterload (peripheral vascular resistance). Maximal exercise systolic pressure is directly related to height, workload, and level of resting systolic pressure. The absolute level of exercise systolic pressure is usually higher in boys (BSA of 1.2 m^2 or more) than in height-matched girls (BSA of 1.2 m^2 or more) and in those normal subjects with BSA of less than 1.2 m^2 (Fig. 21–4).

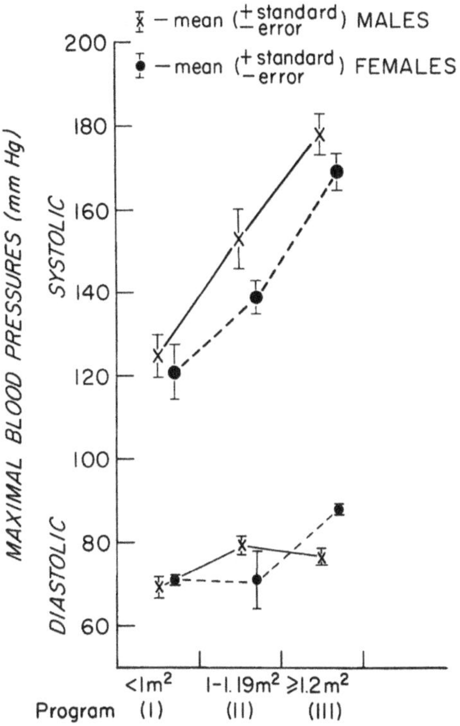

FIGURE 21–4. Relationship of maximum blood pressure to body surface area during exercise in healthy children. Maximum blood pressure increases with body size. Diastolic pressure changes minimally. (From James, FW: Exercise Testing in Children and Young Adults: An Overview. In Engle, MA (ed): Pediatric Cardiology. FA Davis, Philadelphia, 1978, p 187, with permission.)

Cardiac output is related directly to oxygen with linearity during submaximal exercise. The exercising muscle receives a large and increasing percentage of the cardiac output during progressive exercise compared with other tissues. Maximal cardiac output is a major determinant of maximal oxygen uptake. In a growing population, maximal cardiac output and maximal oxygen uptake, when predicted from the maximal power output (highest rate of work), have a similar relationship to height (Fig. 21–5). Anemia and cardiac disease can affect the normal relationship between cardiac output and oxygen uptake in a young patient of a specific size.

On the exercise electrogram (recorded at 50 mm/s), the RR interval shortens approximately 56% from rest to exercise (Fig. 21-6A). This average change in RR interval is due to shortened TP and QT intervals (-33%). The T wave shortens in duration by 18% in boys and 48% in girls. The QRS interval varies minimally in duration during exertion. The ST segment also decreases in duration and is sometimes encroached upon by the initial portion of the T wave. This finding may present difficulty in determining significant ST-segment changes in some subjects at peak exercise. Figures 21–6B and 21–7 illustrate the magnitude of changes for J-point, ST segment, and ST slope in normal young boys and girls at maximal exercise. The cri-

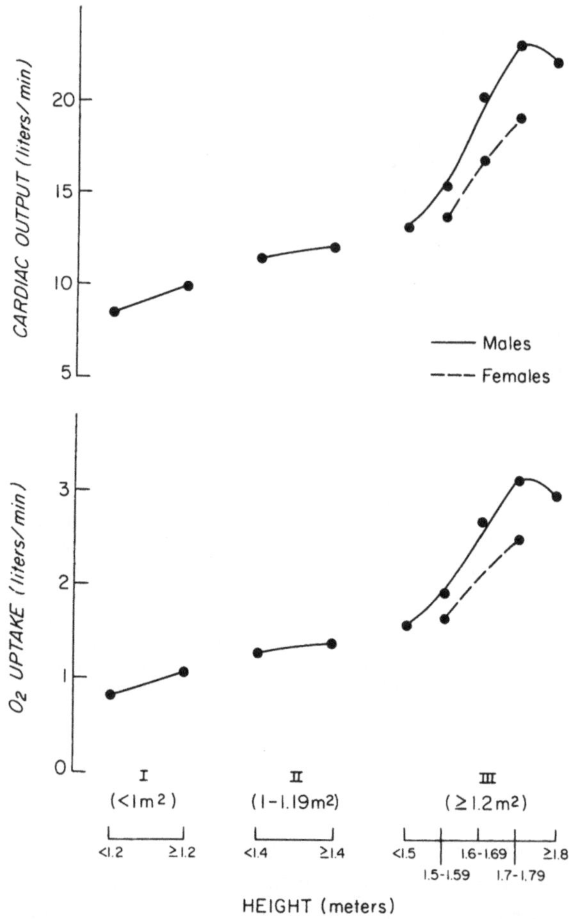

FIGURE 21–5. (*Top*) Maximum cardiac output and (*Bottom*) oxygen uptake in normal subjects by height within each subdivision (I, II, III) of the James protocol. The measurements are similar in male and female subjects with body surface area less than 1.2 m^2. For individuals with body surface area greater than 1.2 m^2, males exceeded the females. (From James,[22] p 237, with permission.)

terion for a positive ST-segment change is depression of 1 mm or more below the baseline of three to five consecutive QRS complexes extending for at lease 0.06 second after the J-point with a horizontal, upward, or downward sloping ST segment[1,3] (Fig. 21–8). Using this criterion, 7% of healthy normolipemic boys and 14% of normolipemic girls had 1 to 2 mm of ST segment depression at peak exercise.[13] The ST depression was recorded in at lease V5 in 9 (82%) of 11 healthy boys and girls. Exercise-induced rate or rhythm disturbances are rare in normal children who have no previously documented abnormalities.

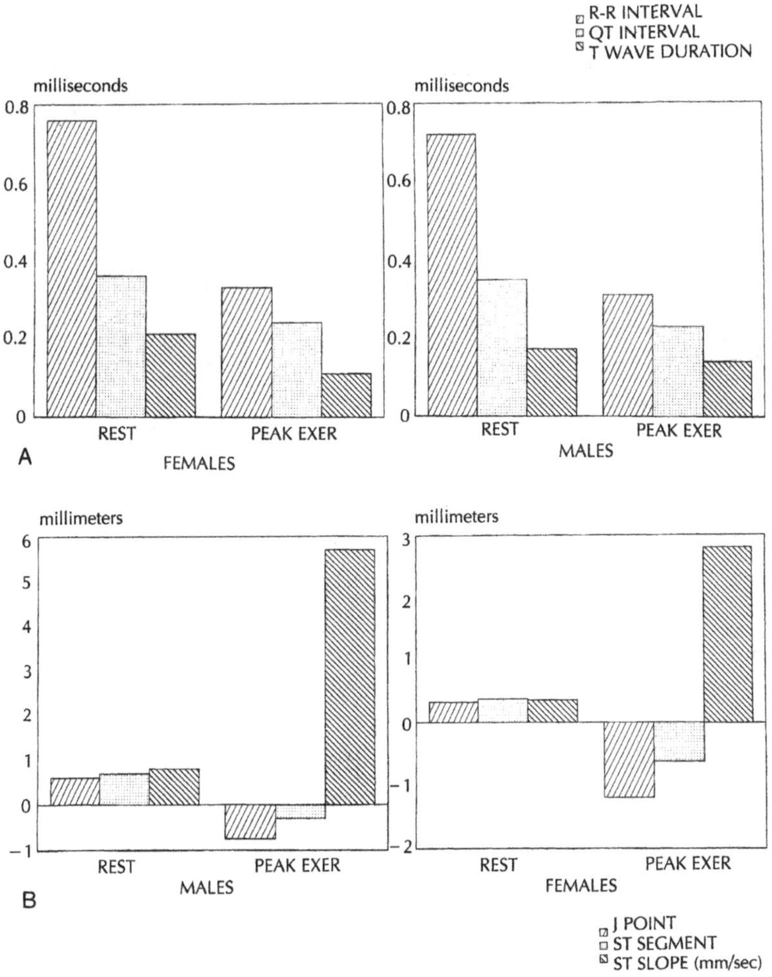

FIGURE 21–6. ECG intervals from rest to exercise in normal subjects. *(A)* Comparable changes are recorded in both sexes, except that the T-wave duration in female subjects decreased 50% from rest to exercise compared with male patients. *(B)* During exercise, average J-point depression exceeds 1 mm in females. Average ST-segment depression in female subjects also is greater than in males.

CONGENITAL HEART DISEASE

Valvular and Discrete Subvalvular Aortic Stenosis

Valvular obstruction to left-ventricular emptying occurs in 3% to 6% of patients with congenital cardiovascular disease.[14] The discrete subvalvular type of obstruction accounts for 8% to 10% of patients with congenital aortic

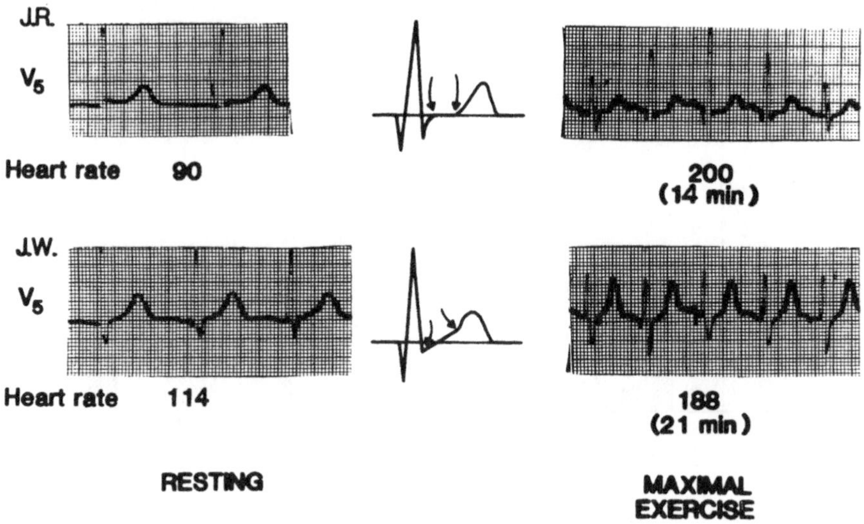

FIGURE 21–7. Normal ST-segment contours with schematic at rest and during exercise. ST-segment slope (*arrows*) may be horizontal or upward with J-point depression less than $-\pi 1$ mm. (From James, FW: Exercise Testing in Children and Young Adults: An Overview. In Engle, MA (ed): Pediatric Cardiology. FA Davis, Philadelphia, 1978, p 187, with permission.)

stenosis. Both valvular and discrete subvalvular aortic stenoses are progressive lesions; the most rapid progression occurs in the subvalvular type.[14,15]

Many physicians are concerned about the risk of sudden death, especially during physical activity, in patients with aortic stenosis. In the pediatric age group, patients with congenital fixed aortic stenosis who died suddenly during physical activity had symptoms, cardiomegaly, and abnormal ECGs showing left-ventricular hypertrophy with strain pattern.[16,17] In a prospective clinical study, Amato and Colleagues[18] reported sudden death in 6% of their patients. All patients had a positive exercise test, an aortic valve area ≤0.6 cm, and were asymptomatic in daily life. The recommendations of the Sixteenth Bethesda Conference[19] support full participation in athletics for patients who have resting peak systolic left-ventricular aortic gradients lower than 20 mm Hg and who have a normal ECG, 24-hour ambulatory ECG, and exercise test.

During standardized exercise testing, measuring blood pressure, estimating working capacity, ventilation, and cardiac performance, and recording of ECG contribute significant data for clinically managing pediatric patients with left-ventricular outflow tract obstruction.[20] Reduced exercise tolerance (Fig. 21–9), depressed ST segments (Fig. 21–10) and exercise systolic blood pressure, and prolonged left-ventricular ejection time are indices of significant obstruction and may signal impairment of left-ventricular performance.[20]

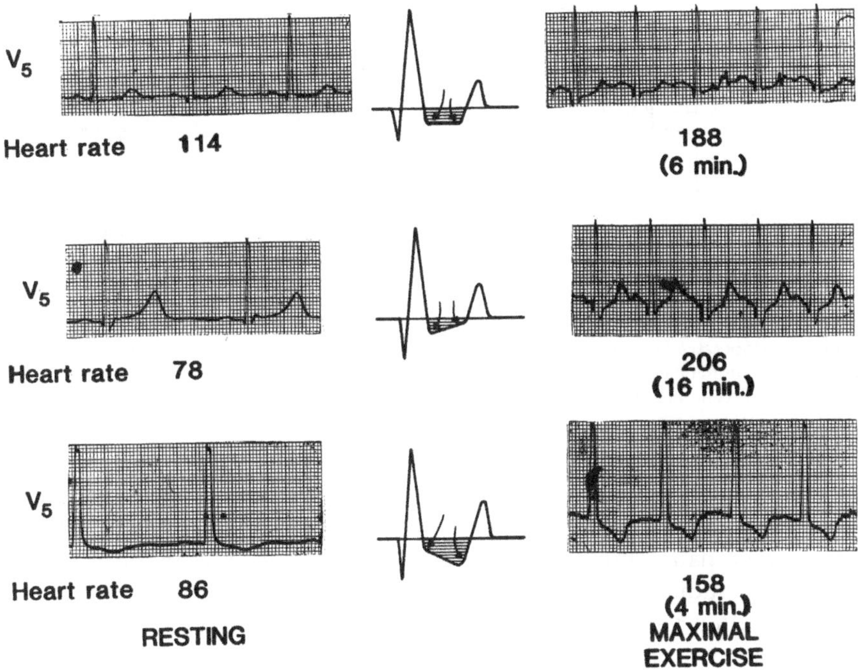

FIGURE 21–8. Abnormal ST-segment contours with schematic at rest and during exercise. ST segment (*arrows*) is depressed significantly with a horizontal, upward, or downward slope. (From James, FW: Exercise Testing in Children and Young Adults: An Overview. In Engle, MA (ed): Pediatric Cardiology. FA Davis, Philadelphia, 1978, p 187, with permission.)

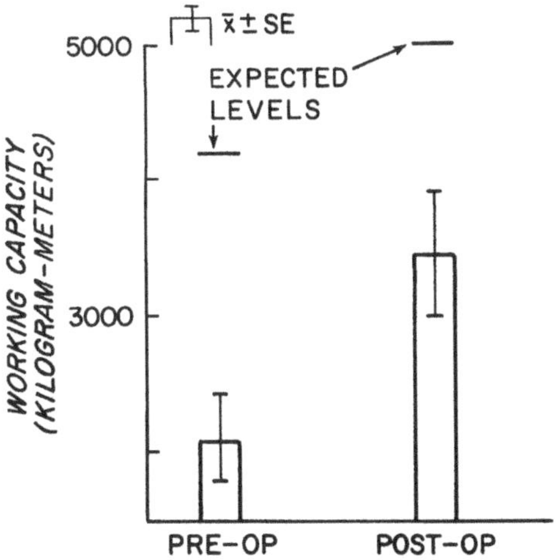

FIGURE 21–9. Working capacity in children with aortic stenosis. Working capacity increases after surgery but remains significantly lower than the expected normal level. (From James, FW: Exercise Testing in Children and Young Adults: An Overview. In Engle, MA (ed): Pediatric Cardiology. FA Davis, Philadelphia, 1978, p 187, with permission.)

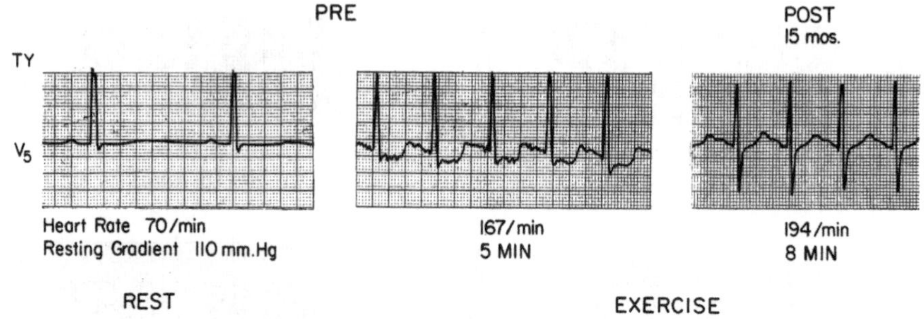

FIGURE 21–10. Horizontal ST-segment depression (preoperatively) and complete resolution by 15 months (postoperatively) in a patient with aortic stenosis and resting gradient of 110 mm Hg. At 15 months, maximum heart rate and exercise time are greater than the exercise results preoperatively. (Adapted from Whitmer et al.[24])

Working capacity correlates negatively with severity of obstruction and is markedly depressed in patients with left-ventricular aortic peak gradients at or greater than 70 mm Hg. Exercise systolic pressure rises modestly in patients with gradients higher than 30 mm Hg or may fall below resting levels in those with severe obstruction. Significant ST depression at submaximal exercise heart rates may imply serious obstruction compared with ST depression occurring at maximal exercise heart rates. A steeply negative ST heart rate slope indicating early onset and progression of ST depression during exercise suggests severe obstruction.[21] When measured immediately after exercise, the left ventricular ejection time is prolonged and lengthens further with increasing obstruction.[22]

Exercise-induced ST depressed of more than 2 mm is usually associated with a resting aortic gradient of 50 mm Hg or higher. An exercise profile including ST depression greater than 2 mm, blunted or decreased exercise systolic pressure, prolongation of left-ventricular ejection time, and severe reduction in working capacity are signs of severe left-ventricular outflow tract obstruction with subendocardial ischemia and left-ventricular impairment.[20] The reason for the ST depression is thought to be an imbalance between myocardial oxygen supply and demand, resulting in subendocardial ischemia of the left ventricle.[23] After effective relief of left-ventricular outflow tract obstruction, the ST depression is decreased and other abnormal cardiovascular responses progress toward normal[24] (Fig. 21–10 and 21–11). The rate and amount of improvement depend on the time period after surgery and the presence of residual defects.

Supravalvular Aortic Stenosis

In supravalvular aortic stenosis with significant narrowing of the aorta, systolic pressure is elevated in the right arm. Working capacity and ST depres-

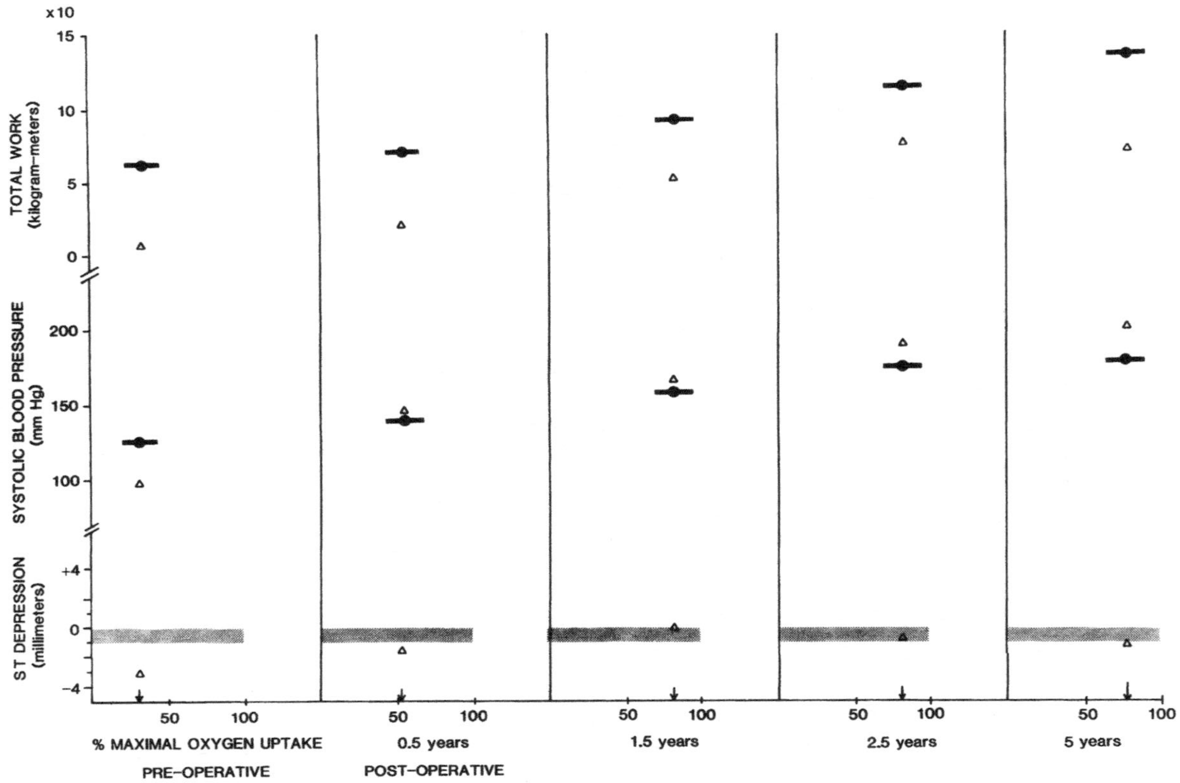

FIGURE 21–11. Longitudinal exercise data in a 12-year-old patient (Δ) after surgical relief of aortic stenosis. (*Top*) Total work increases but remains lower than normal up to five years postoperatively. (*Middle*) Systolic blood pressure increases above the expected mean, and ST segment returns to normal by 1.5 years after surgery. (From James,[20] with permission.)

sion measurements are similar to changes recorded in valvular or discrete subvalvular aortic stenosis.

Coarctation of Thoracic Aorta

Despite the availability of early surgery, some patients may present beyond childhood with systemic hypertension in the upper extremities and decreased pulses in the extremities, consistent with coartation of the aorta. During exercise, both systolic and diastolic hypertension persist, with ST depression occurring in some patients. Working capacity is decreased, usually without complaints of claudication in the legs.

After coartectomy, abnormal elevation of systolic blood pressure with normal or low diastolic pressure or ST depression may occur during submaximal exercise.[22] An abnormally elevated diastolic pressure at rest or during exercise is a clue to restenosis in a patient after coarctectomy. A residual resting gradient at the site of anastomosis often increases with exercise measured by intra-arterial catheters or noninvasively by a pneumatic cuff on the upper and lower extremities.

The surgical criteria for reoperation in patients who have systolic hypertension and a gradient at the site of anastomosis are still under investigation. Figure 21–12 is a reported management strategy based on measuring the arm-to-leg gradient at rest and during exercise to decide among three modes of treatment or combinations: antihypertensive medication, angioplasty during cardiac catheterization, or surgery.[25] According to the treatment strategy, patients with resting and exercise systolic hypertension and a

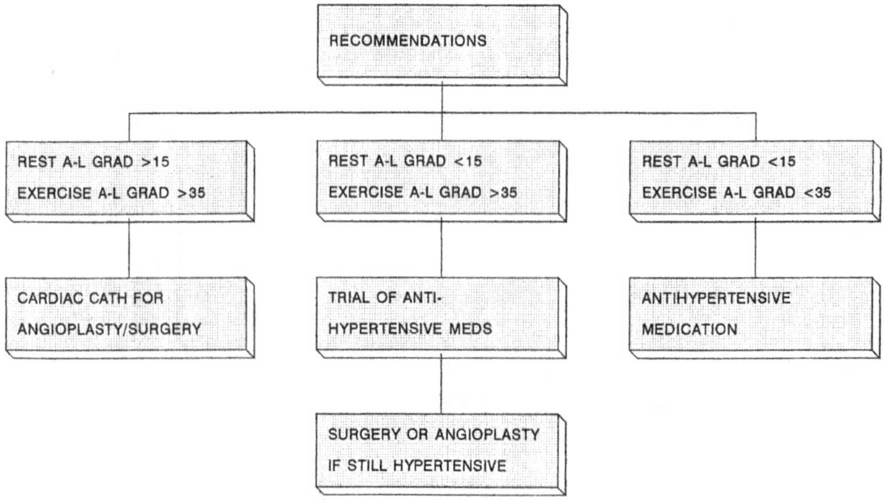

FIGURE 21–12. Management strategy for patients with hypertension after coarctectomy. A-L Grad = arm-to-leg gradient (in mm Hg). (Adapted from Rocchini.[25])

gradient of less than 35 mm Hg at the site of operation are candidates for antihypertensive therapy. The effectiveness of medical or surgical treatment should be assessed by exercise testing with repeated measurements of blood pressure, ST segments, and working capacity. Blood pressure should be controlled without reducing the ability to do work (Fig. 21–13). As we regain clinical experience with angioplasty and make better use of medications, repeat surgery may be unnecessary in some patients with residual gradients or restenosis.

Significant ST depression in multiple leads may occur during exercise in patients before and after coarctectomy. In a series of 48 patients, 28% of boys and 63% of girls had ST depression 1 mm or more in one or more leads.[26] Figure 21–14 illustrates significant ST depression and hypertension in a 15-year-old boy 6 years after coarctectomy. The resting gradient at the site of anastomosis is 25 mm Hg and most likely exceeds 35 mm Hg during exercise. Using the management strategy in Figure 21–12, this patient is found to be a candidate for cardiac catherizeration with angioplasty or surgery.

Premature atherosclerosis, intimal proliferation, and an enlarged caliber of the coronary arteries have been described in young patients with coarctation of the aorta. For patients with coarctation of the aorta who have exercise

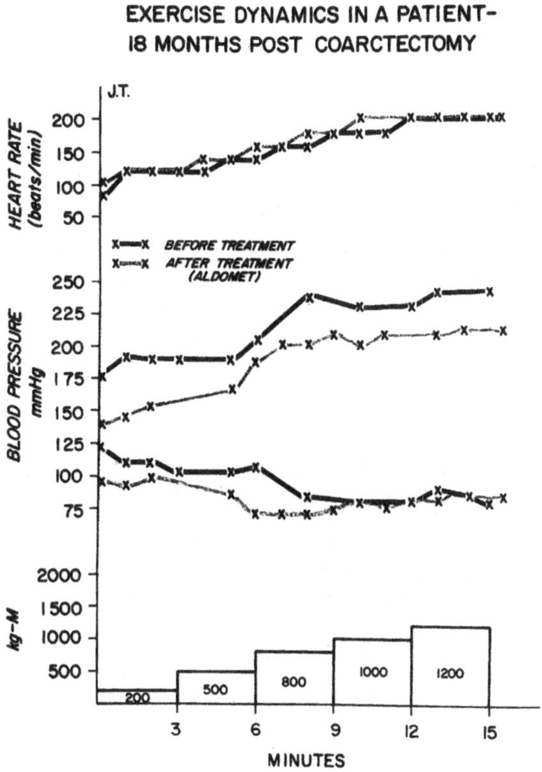

FIGURE 21–13. Exercise data before and after treatment in a patient 18 months postcoarctectomy. Blood pressure at rest and during exercise is reduced following treatment without a decrease in working tolerance. (From James, FW: Exercise Testing in Children and Young Adults: An Overview. In Engle, MA (ed): Pediatric Cardiology. FA Davis, Philadelphia, 1978, p 187, with permission.)

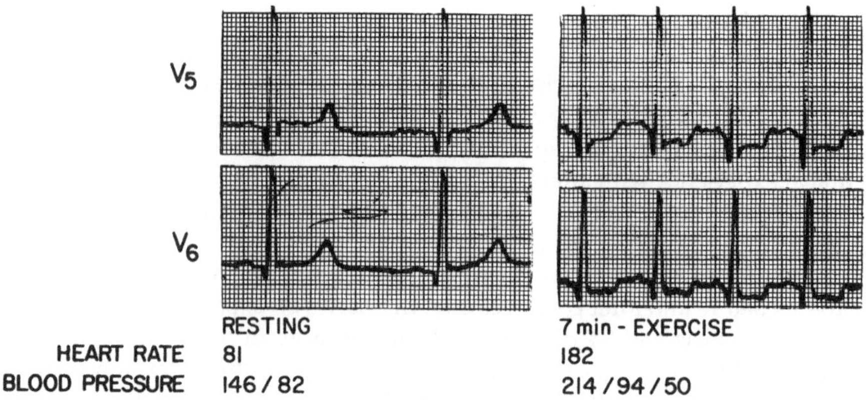

FIGURE 21–14. Exercise data in a 15-year-old patient after coarctectomy with ST depression and elevation of blood pressure. (From James, FW: Exercise Testing in Children and Young Adults: An Overview. In Engle, MA (ed): Pediatric Cardiology. FA Davis, Philadelphia, 1978, p 187, with permission.)

induced ST depression, coronary arteriogram is not recommended because of the risk and low sensitivity of the procedure. However, recent advances in intra-atrial ultrasonography may be less and may help to detect the presence of premature atherosclerosis and its relationship to exercise-induced ST depression in young patients.

Aortic Valve Insufficiency

Exercise systolic hypertension, ST depression at submaximal heart rate, and reduced exercise capacity are signs of significant aortic insufficiency and cardiac enlargement.[27] These abnormal exercise responses are potential exercise risk factors for identifying patients for valve replacement before irreversible damage and congestive heart failure occur. Figure 21–15 shows resting and

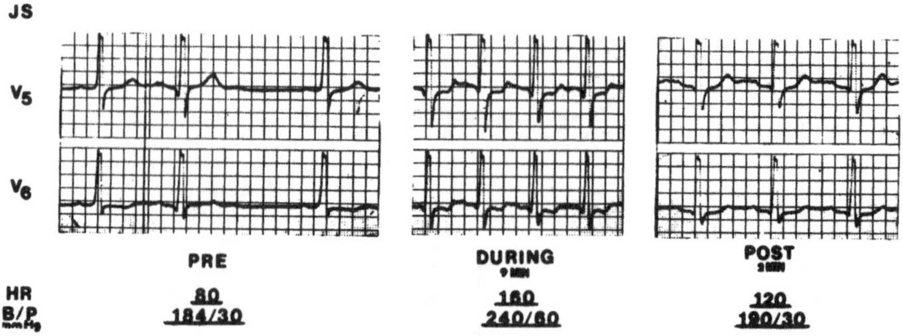

FIGURE 21–15. Sinus arrhythmia, systolic hypertension, and ST depression in a 22-year-old patient with aortic insufficiency.

exercise systolic hypertension and ST-segment changes in a 22-year-old patient with aortic insufficiency. The improvements in prosthetic valve technology have provided a better opportunity for considering early treatment in young patients with significant aortic valve insufficiency.

Pulmonary Valvular Stenosis

At rest or during exercise, severe pulmonary valvular stenosis can cause super systemic pressures in the right ventricle with a competent tricuspid valve and intact septum. Exercise testing can reveal significant abnormalities in many patients who are asymptomatic. During exercise, right-ventricular pressure can increase dramatically with peak levels as high as 300 mm Hg.[23] (Fig. 21-16). Elevated exercise systolic pressure and double product are somewhat common in patients with significant pulmonary stenosis (Fig. 21-17). As pulmonary valve area (less than 1.0 cm^2/m^2) decreases, right-

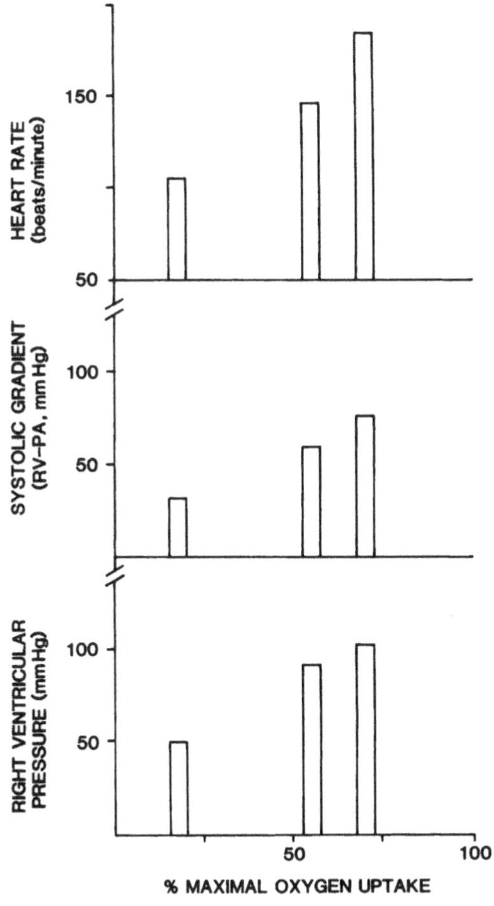

FIGURE 21–16. Exercise data in a 13-year-old patient with pulmonary valvular stenosis. Systolic gradient increases with peak right-ventricular pressure higher than 100 mm Hg during exercise.

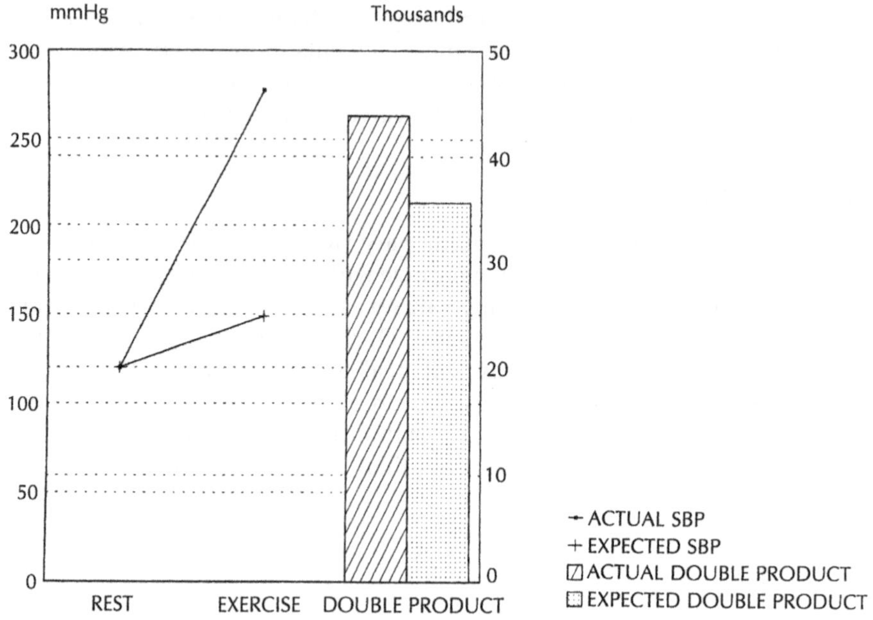

FIGURE 21–17. Exercise data in a 19-year-old patient with pulmonary valvular stenosis. Exercise systolic blood pressure (SBP) greatly exceeds expected normal, causing an elevated double product that suggests increased myocardial oxygen demand. Resting right-ventricular pressure (80/15) and gradient (51 mm Hg) probably increased above resting data during exercise.

ventricular end-diastolic pressure increases and stroke volume index decreases.[28] These changes can lead to reduced oxygen transport, reduced working capacity, and ischemic changes of the right ventricle. Several investigators[22,29,30] have found that working capacity is reduced in pulmonic stenosis and that significant ST depression may occur in the midprecordial (V2, V3) and inferior ECG leads (II, III, aVF), with ST elevation in aVR and aVL.[22] Surgical relief of the obstruction causes improvement in intracardiac pressures, and the working capacity approaches normal levels.[28]

Tetralogy of Fallot

Reduced oxygen transport and working capacity and exercise-induced ventricular arrhythmia are reported from exercise studies in pediatric patients after corrective surgery for tetralogy of Fallot.[31,32] Residual right-ventricular obstruction and/or incompetence of the pulmonary valve causing persistent hypertrophy and ventricular enlargement are commonly present following reconstructive surgery of the right-ventricular outflow tract. The residual defects are related to the type of surgery performed, the anatomy of the right-ventricular outflow tract, and the pulmonary arteries. The magnitude of these residual defects including the ventriculotomy and excision of tissue in the outflow tract can cause ventricular dysfunction, thereby affecting right-ventricular performance.

Maximal oxygen uptake levels are frequently low normal, corresponding to 80% to 85% of normal predicted values.[31] When hemoglobin level and oxygen binding capacity to hemoglobin are normal, the Fick principle reveals that oxygen transport is primarily related to the central determinants (heart rate and stroke volume), reflecting blood flow. Several studies have shown that maximal exercise heart rates and systolic blood pressure adjusted for age, sex, and size in postoperative patients are significantly less than in normal controls.[31,33] Furthermore, right-ventricular stroke volume is decreased or fails to rise normally during exercise. These changes suggesting right-ventricular dysfunction have occurred in the absence of significant residual obstruction to right ventricle or incompetence of the pulmonary valve. If these central changes in maximal heart rate and stroke volume are present, a decreased or low-normal cardiac output during exercise occurs with a negative influence on oxygen transport.[32]

Working capacity is normal in some postoperative patients and reduced in others. The reduced working capacity may be related to residual defects, reduced cardiac output, or lack of peripheral muscle fitness. Improvement in working capacity has occurred without much change in maximal oxygen uptake (Fig. 21–18). Additional studies are needed to help determine the training capacity of the cardiovascular and peripheral muscular systems in patients after surgery for tetralogy of Fallot.

Although complete right bundle branch block is common, some postoperative patients without the conduction change but with significant residual defects may develop exercise-induced ST depression in the midprecordial or inferior ECG leads (Fig. 21–19). Ventricular arrhythmia has been identified with sudden death in pediatric patients after corrective surgery for tetralogy of Fallot.[31,34] Exercise testing has provoked serious ventricular arrhythmia, with a high frequency in patients with significant residual defects.[34] In our laboratory, the arrhythmia is best detected immediately after strenuous effort in the supine position.

Pulmonary abnormalities, such as reduced diffusing capacity, high physiological dead space and airway obstruction, and an abnormal alveolar arterial P02 difference, are other central changes that can influence oxygen transport negatively and reduce working capacity.[31] Airway obstruction has been related to significant residual pulmonary valve incompetence, which may increase blood volume and interstitial water causing decreased alveolar compliance.[31] Further investigations are needed to identify the mechanism of these abnormalities and their relationship to the disease complex. Presently, the pulmonary reserve in patients after surgery for tetralogy of Fallot appears adequate and is not a significant limiting factor in oxygen transport and working capacity.

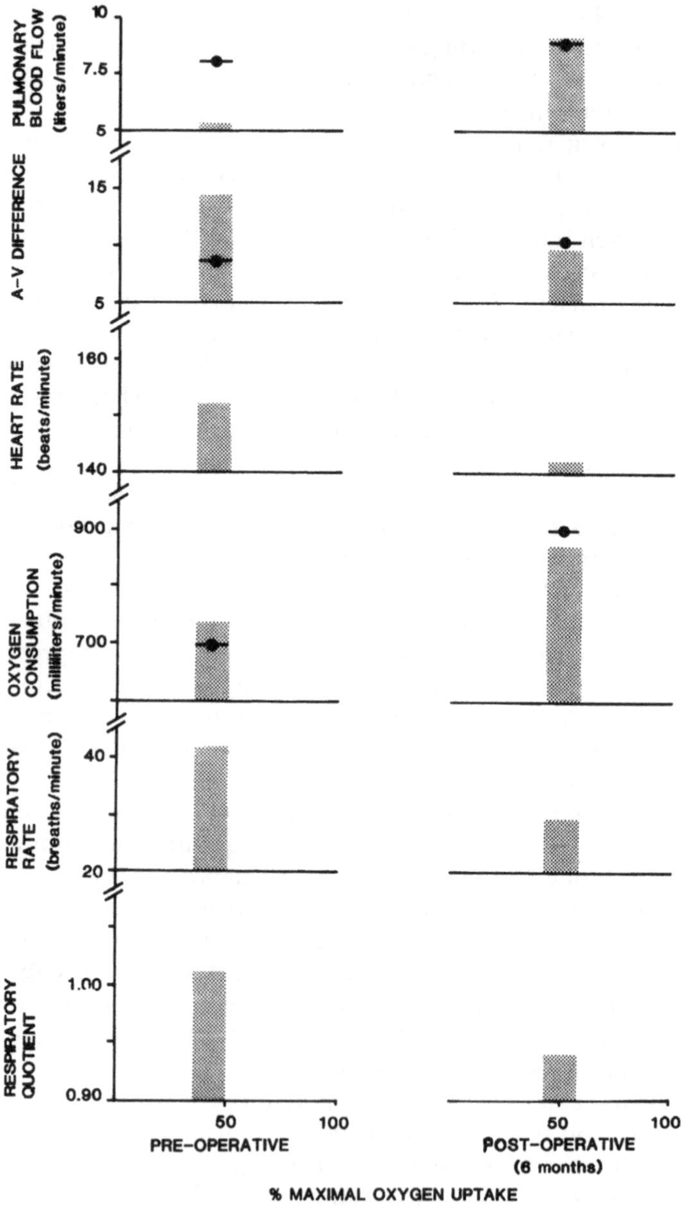

FIGURE 21–18. Preoperative and postoperative exercise data in an 11-year-old patient with surgical correction of tetralogy of Fallot. As shown from top to bottom, pulmonary blood flow increased and atrioventricular (AV) difference and heart rate decreased at 50% of maximum oxygen uptake. Respiratory rate and quotient decreased after surgery.

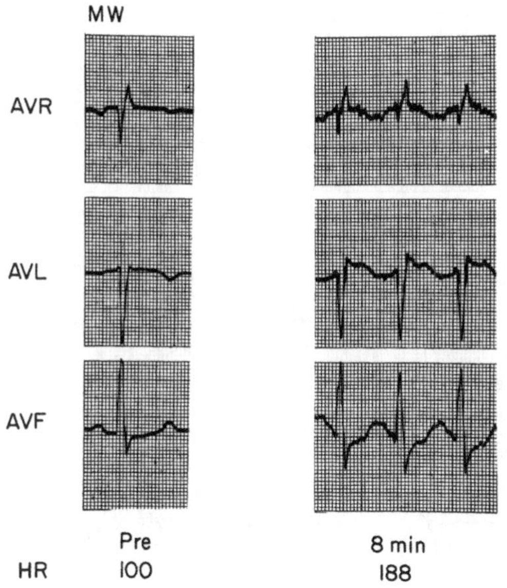

FIGURE 21–19. ST-segment elevation and depression during exercise in a 15-year-old boy, 8 years after corrective surgery for tetralogy of Fallot using a homograft. Resting residual right-ventricular outflow tract gradient = 50 mm Hg. Significant ST-segment changes are seen in aVR, aVL (elevation), and aVF (depression). (From James,[22] p 243, with permission.)

An exercise evaluation showing a markedly reduced or declining working capacity, ventricular arrhythmia, and ST depression identifies a patient who must be evaluated for residual defects, right-ventricular dysfunction, and possible surgical or medical treatment or both. Patients with serious ventricular arrhythmias and without significant residual defects are candidates for antiarrhythmic therapy to reduce the risk of sudden death (Fig. 21–20). A reduced or declining working capacity must not go unnoticed in young patients. These patients should be evaluated for excise therapy training to improve fitness, which will improve their quality of life.

Other Complex Congenital Anomalies

Ebstein's anomaly consists of an abnormal tricuspid valve with enlargement and elongation of the anterior leaflet and displacement of a portion of the septal and posterior leaflets from the tricuspid value annulus toward the right-ventricular apex. Each of the three leaflets may adhere somewhat to the endocardial surface of the right ventricle. An atrial septal defect is often associated. The right ventricle is usually dilated with thinning of the free wall and a reduction in right-ventricular mass. These structural defects result in enlargement of the right atrium due to an atrialized portion of the right ventricle and often to tricuspid insufficiency, right-to-left shunting, arrhythmias, and right-ventricular dysfunction.

Exercise studies have revealed that aerobic capacity, maximal heart rate, and arterial oxygen saturation are reduced in patients with Ebstein's anom-

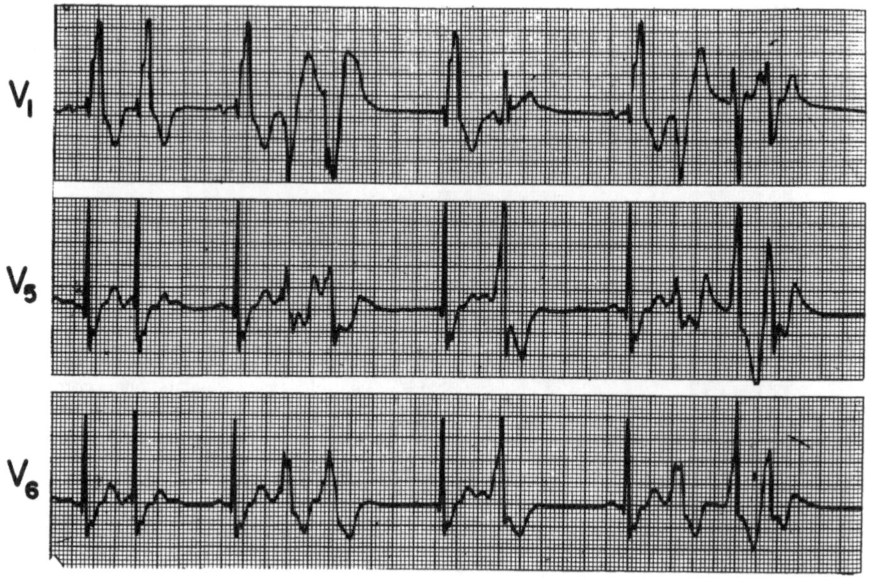

FIGURE 21–20. Postexercise arrhythmia in a patient after surgery for tetralogy of Fallot. Episodes of ventricular tachycardia were recorded. (Paper speed 50 mm/sec.) (From James and Kaplan: Unexpected cardiac arrest in patients after surgical correction of tetralogy of Fallot. Circulation 52:694, 1975, with permission of the American Heart Association, Inc.).

aly before surgical treatment.[35,36] Furthermore, an increased respiratory minute ventilation and ventilatory equivalent occur at rest and during exercise, especially in patients with right-to-left shunting. After surgical treatment, aerobic capacity and exercise capacity increase significantly toward normal, and arterial saturation remains normal, especially in patients whose interatrial shunting is eliminated.[35]

Close attention to cardiac rhythm is encouraged because of the relatively high risk of exercise-induced supraventricular tachycardia and frequency of ventricular arrhythmia.

The Fontan procedure has offered palliative treatment to many patients with complex cardiac anomalies with only a single functional ventricular chamber. The surgical approach is to connect systemic venous return from the right atrium to the pulmonary artery with or without a Glenn procedure. The single ventricular chamber is now dedicated to left-sided systemic function. Several modifications of the surgical procedure have taken place since the original description by Fontan and colleagues,[37] but these modified procedures are referred to as a Fontan operation.

In patients with a functionally single ventricle who are candidates for a Fontan procedure, aerobic capacity, maximal heart rate, cardiac output, and arterial saturation are reduced during exercise. Respiratory minute ventilation and frequency are increased as in other cardiac lesions with right-to-left

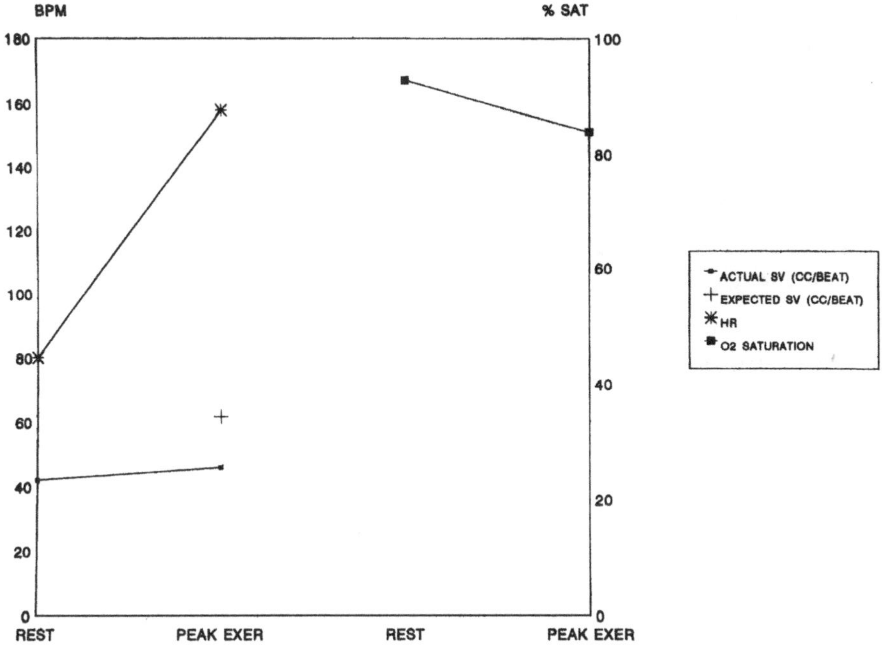

FIGURE 21–21. Average exercise data in 11 patients with functional single ventricle and Fontan procedure. At peak exercise, stroke volume is suppressed below expected (+), and arterial saturation decreased below resting level. (BPM = beats per minute; HR = heart rate; SV = stroke volume.)

shunting. After the Fontan procedure, these abnormal cardiopulmonary exercise responses improve significantly but may not completely normalize.[38] The frequency of arrhythmias and ST-segment depression is elevated in patients before and after operation. Progression of these ECG changes may reflect deterioration of the single ventricle. Figure 21–21 illustrates hemodynamic responses in 11 patients an average 4.7 years after a Fontan procedure. Cardiac output is low because of a subnormal stroke volume, and exercise-induced arterial desaturation is present. Cardiac arrhythmia was recorded in 7 of 11 patients (64%) with 2 having ventricular, 4 supraventricular, and 1 combined atrial and ventricular arrhythmia. Significant ST-segment depression was recorded in 6 of 11 patients (55%).

ARRHYTHMIA WITH NORMAL HEART

The occasional atrial or ventricular arrhythmia recorded in children with normal hearts is usually of no clinical significance. The working capacity, maximal heart rate, and blood pressure during exercise are usually normal in the young patient with occasional arrhythmia. Physical activity may pro-

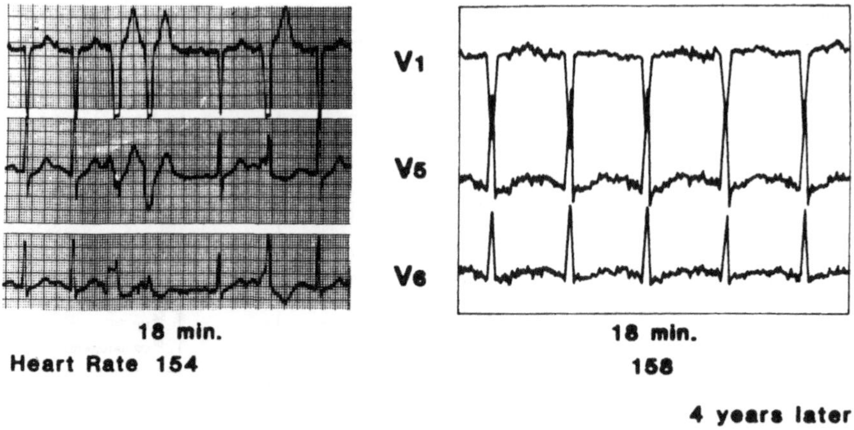

FIGURE 21–22. Exercise-induced arrhythmia in a 16-year-old swimmer with "normal" heart. The patient was asymptomatic during the episodes. Serial exercise tests revealed a decrease in frequency with complete resolution at follow-up in 4 years.

voke episodes of supraventricular tachycardia. When an episode is provoked during exercise testing, we have observed that measurements of cardiac output and blood pressure were maintained in the normal range during the early phase of the arrhythmia. The patients are usually unaware of the tachycardia during the active exercise period.

Exercise may induce ventricular arrhythmias or suppress or aggravate preexisting arrhythmia. From our experience, the exercise test is most useful in unmasking arrhythmia and determining any abnormal responses related to the arrhythmia. We have not found that just a suppressed or aggravated arrhythmia during exercise in an asymptomatic patient is indicative of severity. Antiarrhythmic therapy is withheld with close follow-up in asymptomatic patients with clinically normal hearts. The author has seen complete resolution of exercise-induced ventricular arrhythmia over time and has permitted subjects to participate in competitive sports after an appropriate evaluation, which includes exercise testing and echocardiogram (Fig. 21–22).

COMPLETE CONGENITAL HEART BLOCK

Patients with complete heart block demonstrate the enormous capacity of the cardiovascular system to adapt and maintain enough reserve so that some of these patients can participate satisfactorily in competitive sports. Atrial rate increases normally during exercise with a modest increase in ventricular rate. Cardiac output is normal at most levels during exercise because

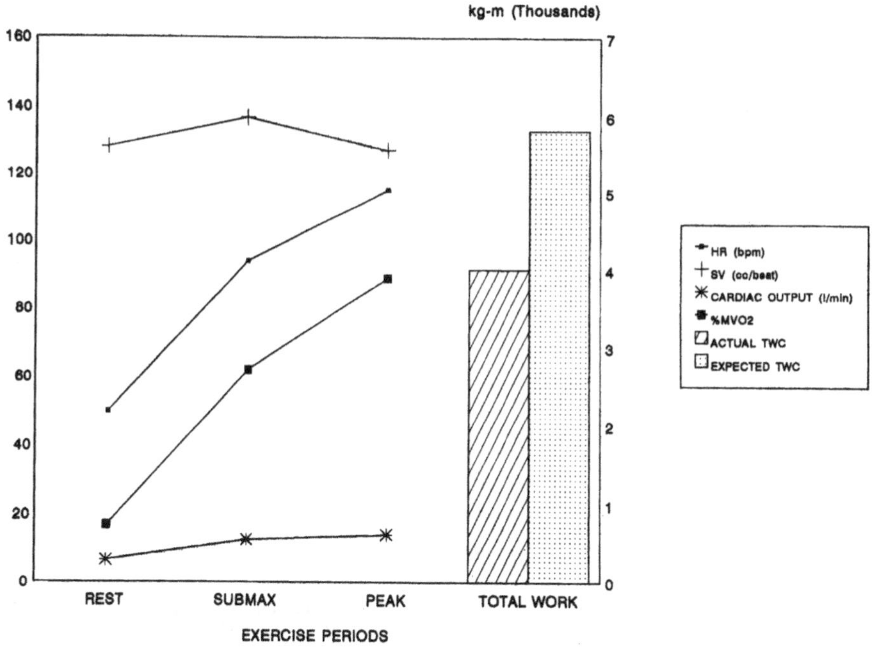

FIGURE 21–23. Exercise data in three patients with complete congenital heart block. Average stroke volume (+) is large with a modest increase in the ventricular rate. Total work is less than expected.

of the large stroke volume and modes increase in ventricular rate. Although cardiac output is often within normal limits, working capacity in the population of patients is generally low or below normal. Figure 21–23 and 21–24 depict the hemodynamic changes and working capacity in three patients with complete congenital heart block. The average stroke volume is large at rest and during exercise. The stroke volume pattern shows an increase from rest to exercise, then a decline at peak exercise. The patients were able to exercise only up to 85% VO2 max with average working capacity (total work) in low level of normal. In some patients, cardiac arrhythmia occurs during or after exercise.[26] In our experience, the arrhythmia has been primarily ventricular without any clinical symptoms in the patient. Menon and Colleagues[39] reported sinus node incompetence at peak exercise in eleven percent of a small series of patients with congenital complete heart block. Exercise testing is advisable for evaluating the chronotropic response of atrial and ventricular pacemakers, circulatory adaptation, ST-segment level, rhythm disturbance, and working capacity in congenital complete heart block. These exercise data will contribute to better clinical management and vocational guidance.

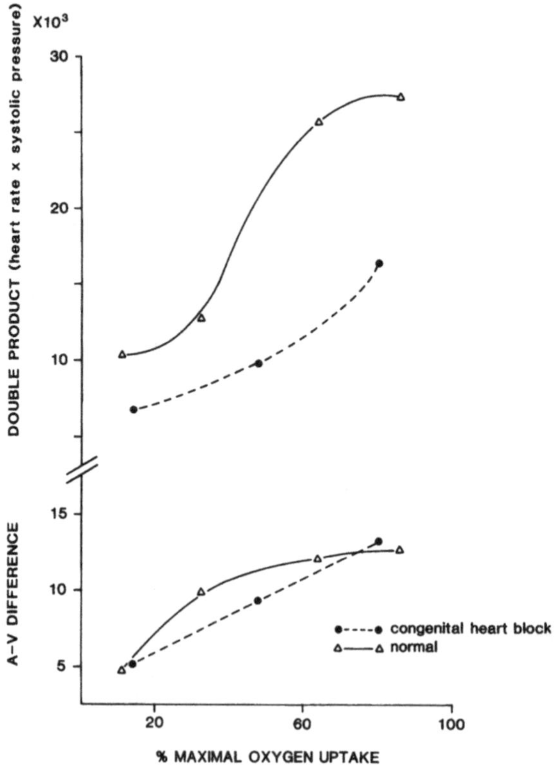

FIGURE 21–24. Double product and AV difference in three patients with complete congenital heart block at rest and during exercise. Double product in a patient is lower than normal because of low heart rate.

CONGENITAL LONG QT SYNDROME

The contribution of the exercise test in the clinical diagnosis of congenital long QT Syndrome is under study. A lengthening of the total QT interval during the immediate post-exercise period was observed in 61% of patients with congenital long QT Syndrome as compared to 12% of controls.[40] Dillenburg and Colleagues[41] demonstrated an increased sensitivity and specificity of the post-exercise QTc interval in identifying patients with long QT Syndrome as confirmed by the Schwartz score and ST-T-wave analysis. Further study in larger populations is needed to identify the true sensitivity and specificity of the exercise test in the clinical diagnosis of congenital long QT Syndrome.

KAWASAKI DISEASE

Since the reporting of Kawasaki disease in Japan more than 30 years ago, the original diagnostic clinical criteria as defined by Dr. Kawasaki are still authentic. Kawasaki disease is now being recognized as the leading cause of acquired heart disease in children in North America and Japan. Several epidemiologic and clinical observations suggest that the disease is caused by one or more infectious agents with each capable of producing clinical manifestation of the disease. Recent immunohistochemistry findings suggest many vascular growth factors that play a role in the formation of the coronary artery lesions. Advances have been made in the management of the disease with the introduction of aspirin and intravenous immunoglobulin (IVIG), which have reduced significantly the rate of coronary artery aneurysms and deaths in patients. It is estimated that 4% of children with Kawasaki disease will develop ischemic heart disease. In a series of 46 children, Paridon and Colleagues[42] reported normal maximal oxygen uptake, but stress-induced perfusion defects detected by Single-photon emission computed tomography in 37% of patients with no evidence of coronary artery lesions. The perfusion defects were observed in all patients with persistent coronary aneurysms, and 11% of the 46 children had exercise-induced ST segment changes. Jan and Colleagues[43] reported that a positive treadmill exercise test and/or ischemic finding on 201TI Single-photon emission computed tomography strongly indicate coronary angiography to detect possible stenotic lesions in the coronary arteries.

SICKLE CELL ANEMIA

Significant hemodynamic and ECG changes occur in patients with sickle cell anemia and without coronary artery disease. As hemoglobin level decreases, oxygen transport can be maintained by a compensatory increase in cardiac output. In 43 patients with sickle cell anemia, Figure 21–25 illustrates the magnitude of increase in cardiac output to maintain a satisfactory oxygen transport for a resting state between 10% and 19% of VO2 max and submaximal exercise state of less than 79% VO2 max. Patients with average hemoglobin of 7.9% mg% had cardiac output of approximately twice normal at rest but experienced a decline in cardiac performance during submaximal exercise. These patients with low hemoglobin have decreased myocardial oxygen supply, increased myocardial demand with elevated double product, and significant ST-segment depression during submaximal exercise.[44] Exercise testing can be used to identify the tolerance level, the risk of reduced cardiac performance and significant ST depression, suggesting myocardial ischemia in patients with sickle cell anemia. These data can potentially improve clinical management and assist patients to have a better quality of life.

HYPERTENSION

Several investigators have reported blood pressure responses during progressive cycle and treadmill exercises in normal children.[1,9] In the adoles-

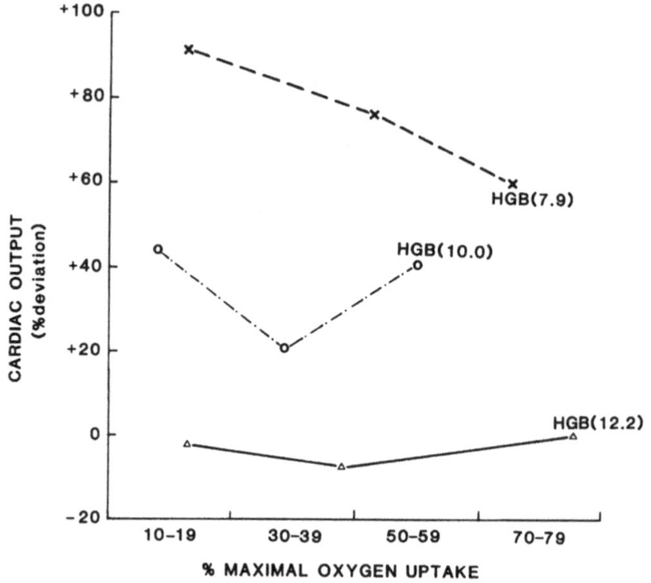

FIGURE 21–25. Cardiac output at rest and during exercise in patients with sickle cell anemia and different hemoglobin levels. As hemoglobin decreases, cardiac output increases for the same level of maximum oxygen uptake.

cent with the diagnosis of hypertension, we have seen three patterns of systolic pressure response emerge during progressive exercise on the cycle ergometer. Figure 21–26 illustrates three responses of systolic pressure from rest to exercise: (1) a normal systolic pressure at rest but elevated at peak exercise, (2) elevated systolic pressure at rest that normalizes at peak exercise, and (3) elevated pressure that remains elevated (Fig. 21–27). The patient whose systolic pressure normalized during exercise has the diagnosis of essential hypertension and was taking antihypertensive medication. Working capacity was reduced by more than 30% from the predicted level, a moderate reduction. Since blood pressure and cardiac output can be measured noninvasively in children, these measurements, performed during exercise can help to determine mechanisms and monitor the effectiveness of treatment.

HYPERTROPHIC CARDIOMYOPATHY

Hypertrophic cardiomyopathy is a well-recognized disease that can cause abnormal blood pressure,[45] myocardial ischemia,[26] and arrhythmia during or after exercise. These cardiovascular responses are related to the high incidence of syncope and sudden death that may occur in affected patients. In patients without a resting left-ventricular to aortic gradient, exercise systolic pressure may be elevated above normal, and stroke volume may rise only

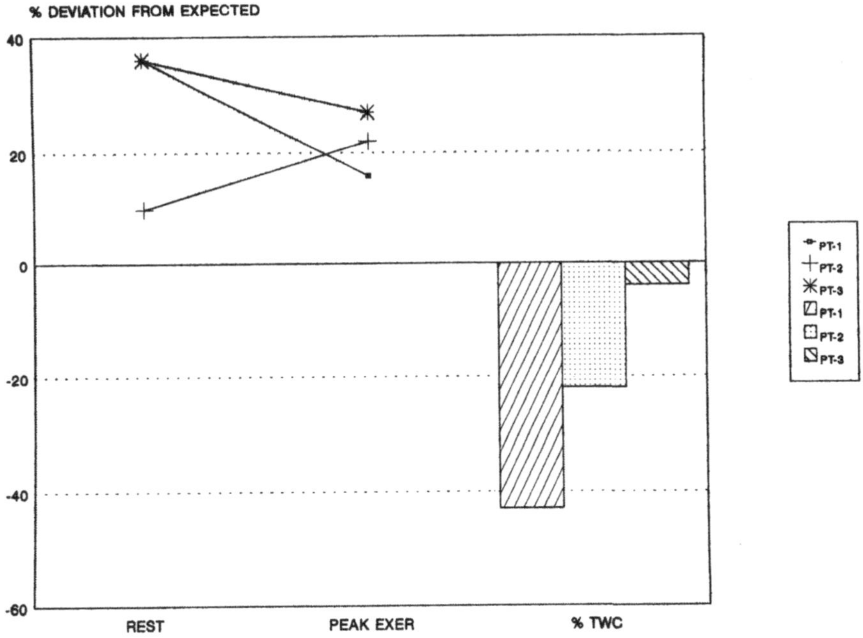

FIGURE 21–26. Systolic pressure and total working capacity (TWC) in three patients with hypertension. The normal range of systolic pressure is +20%. Patient 2 (+) has a normal systolic pressure at rest that increases abnormally at peak exercise. The other patients have elevated systolic pressures at rest, but during exercise Patient 1 normalizes and Patient 3's pressure remains elevated. Patient 1 is being treated for hypertension and has decreased working capacity.

moderately during exercise because of a hyperdynamic state at rest and a diminished left-ventricular end-systolic volume (Fig. 21–28). When there is exercise-induced hypotension, the risk of sudden death is high.[45]

In our laboratory, the measurements include cardiac output, blood pressure, systolic time intervals, multilead ECG, and careful monitoring of skin perfusion when testing patients with obstruction to left-ventricular outflow. We have found the exercise data to be useful in estimating severity and improving clinical management.

SUMMARY

A review of the clinical application of exercise testing identifies essential information that contributes to best practice of pediatric cardiovascular medicine. This discussion reveals the uniqueness of the cardiovascular defects as they affect the oxygen transport system in the young. An understanding of the pathophysiology responses revealed during testing permits maximal use of exercise data to combine with other clinical information for diagnosis, treatment, and counseling patients.

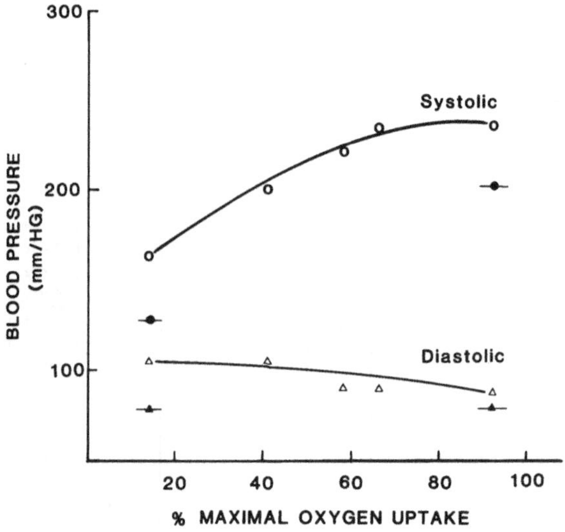

FIGURE 21–27. Resting and exercise blood pressure in a patient with hypertension. At rest, both systolic and diastolic pressures are elevated. At peak exercise, systolic pressure remains elevated, and diastolic pressure decreases to normal levels.

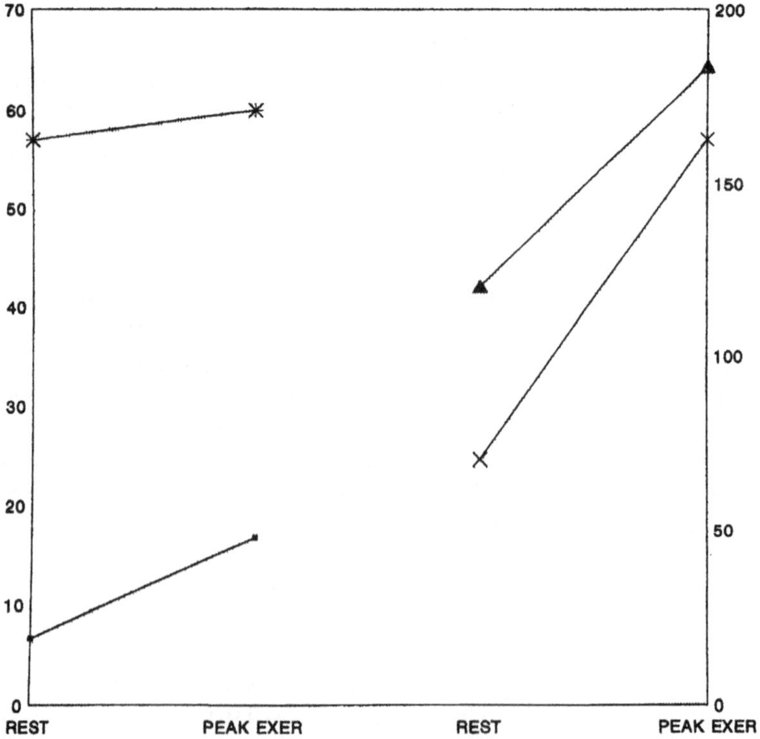

FIGURE 21–28. Exercise data in a patient with nonobstructive hypertrophic cardiomyopathy. Systolic pressure (▲, mm Hg), stroke volume (∗, mL/min), and cardiac output (•, L/min) increase during exercise, suggesting a lack of significant gradient and inadequate ventricular filling. X = heart rate in beats per minute.

ACKNOWLEDGMENT

The author appreciates the technical assistance of Wayne Mays and the secretarial assistance of Anthalena James Green.

REFERENCES

1. James, FW, et al: Standards for exercise testing in the pediatric age group. Circulation 66:1387A, 1982.
2. Washington, R, et al: Guidelines for Exercise Testing in the Pediatric Age Group: From the Committee on Atherosclerosis and Hypertension in Children, Council on Cardiovascular Disease in the Young, the American Heart Association. Circulation 90(4): 2166, 1994.
3. James, FW, et al: Responses of normal children and young adults to controlled bicycle exercise. Circulation 61:902, 1980.
4. Chantal, K, et al: Cardiopulmonary Exercise Testing in Children: An Individualized Protocol for Workload Increase. Chest 120(1): 81, 2001.
5. Wahlund, H: Determination of the physical working capacity. Acta Med Scand 215 (suppl):5,1948.
6. Astrand, PO and Rodahl, K: Textbook Physiology, 3rd ed. McGraw-Hill, New York, 1986.
7. Cumming, GR, et al: Bruce treadmill test in children: Normal values in a clinic population. Am J Cardiol 41:69, 1978.
8. Bengtsson, E: the working capacity in normal children evaluated by submaximal exercise on the bicycle ergometer and compared with adults. Acta Med Scand 154:91, 1956.
9. Issekutz, B Jr, et al: Use of respiratory quotients in assessment of aerobic work capacity. J Appl Physiol 17:47, 1962.
10. Washington, RL, et al: Normal aerobic and anaerobic data for North American school-age children. J Pediatr 112:223, 1988.
11. Singh,V: The role of gas analysis with exercise testing. Primary Care; Clinics in Office Practice. 28(1):159, 2001
12. McManus, A, et al: Maximising the Clinical use of exercise gaseous exchange testing in children with repaired cyanotic congenital heart defects: the development of an appropriate test strategy. Sports Med 29(4):229, 2000.
13. James, FW, et al: Maximal exercise testing in normal hyperlipidemic children. Atherosclerosis 25:85, 1976.
14. Friedman, WF and Kirkpatrick, SE: Congenital aortic stenosis. In Moss, AJ, Adams, FH and Emmanouilides, GC (eds): Heart disease in Infants, Children, and Adolescents, 2nd ed. Williams & Wilkins, Baltimore, 1977, p 178.
15. Mody, MR and Mody, GT: Serial hemodynamic observations in congenital valvular and subvalvular aortic stenosis. Am Heart J 89(2):137, 1975.
16. Doyle, EF, et al: Sudden death in young patients with congenital aortic stenosis. Pediatrics 53:481, 1974.
17. Driscoll, DJ and Edwards, WD: Sudden unexpected death in children and adolescents. J Am Coll Cardiol 5:118B, 1985.
18. Amato, M, et al.: Treatment decision in asymptomatic aortic valve stenosis: role of exercise testing. Heart 86(4):381, 2001.
19. McNamara, DG, et al: Task Force 1: Congenital heart disease. J Am Coll Cardiol 6:1200, 1985.
20. James, FW: Exercise responses in aortic stenosis. Prog Pediatr Cardiol 2(3):1, 1993.
21. James, FW, et al: Exercise, heart rate and S-T depression-A temporal relationship suggesting significant aortic stenosis in children. Circulation 72(suppl):III-96, 1985.
22. James, FW: Exercise Testing in Normal individuals and Patients with Cardiovascular Disease. In Engle, MA (ed): Pediatric Cardiovascular Disease. FA Davis, Philadelphia, 1981, p 227.
23. Kveselis, DA, et al: Hemodynamic determinants of exercise-induced ST-segment depression in children with valvar aortic stenosis. Am J Cardiol 55:1133, 1985.
24. Whitmer, JT, et al: Exercise testing in children before and after aortic valvotomy. Am Heart J 99:76, 1980.

25. Rocchini, AP: Exercise Evaluation After Repair of Coarctation of the Aorta, Pediatric Cardiovascular Exercise Responses: Part II. In Kaplan, S and Driscoll, DJ (eds): Prog Pediatr Cardiol, 2(3):14, 1993.
26. James, FW: Exercise ECG Test in Children. In Chung, EK (ed): Exercise Electrocardiography-Practical Approach, 2nd ed. Williams & Wilkins, Baltimore, 1983, p 132.
27. Goforth, D, et al: Maximal exercise in children with aortic incompetence: An adjunct to non-invasive assessment of disease severity. Am Heart J 108:1306, 1984.
28. Moller, JH: Exercise responses in pulmonary stenosis. Prog Pediatr Cardiol 2 (3):8, 1993.
29. Bar Or, O: Pulmonary Stenosis. In Katz, M and Stiehm, ER (eds): Pediatric Sports Medicine for the Practitioner. Springer-Verlag, New York, 1983, p 149.
30. Cumming, GR: Maximal exercise capacity of children with heart defects. Am J Cardiol 42:613, 1978.
31. Paridon, SM: Exercise response in tetralogy of Fallot and pulmonary artesia with ventricular septal defect. Prog Pediatr Cardiol 2(3):35, 1993.
32. Reybrouck, T, et al: Oxygen uptake versus exercise intensity: a new concept in assessing cardiovascular exercise function in patients with congenital heart disease. Heart 84(1):46, 2000.
33. Sarubbi, B, et al: Exercise capacity in young patients after total repair of Tetralogy of Fallot. Pediatric Cardiology 21(30):211, 2000.
34. James, FW, et al: Response to exercise in patients after total surgical correction of tetralogy of Fallot. Circulation 54:671, 1976.
35. Driscoll, DJ: Exercise responses in Ebstein's anomaly. Prog Pediatr Cardiol 2(3): 30, 1993.
36. Fredriksen, P, et al: Aerobic capacity in adults with various congenital heart diseases. Am J Cardiology 87(3):310, 2001.
37. Fontan, F, et al: "Correction" de l'artesia tricuspidienne: Rapport de deux cas corrigiges per l'utilization d'une technique chirurgicale nouvelle. Ann Chir Thorac Cardiovasc 10:39, 1971.
38. Driscoll, DJ: Exercise responses in Ebstein's anomally. Prog Pediatr Cardio 2(3):30, 1993.
39. Menon, A, et al: Chronotropic competence of the sinus node in congenital complete heart block. Am J Cardiology 82(9):1119, 1998.
40. Swan, H, et al: Rate adaptation of QT intervals during and after exercise in children with congenital long QT syndrome. Eur Heart J 19:508, 1998.
41. Dillenburg, R, et al: Is Exercise Testing Useful in Identifying Congenital Long QT Syndrome? Am J Cardiol 89(2):233, 2002.
42. Paridon, S, et al: Exercise capacity and incidence of myocardial perfusion defects after Kawasaki disease in children and adolescents. J Am Coll Cardiol 25(6):1420, 1995.
43. Jan, S, et al: Comparison of 201TI SPET and treadmill exercise testing in patients with Kawasaki disease. Nucl Med Commun 21(5):431, 2000.
44. McConnell, ME, et al: Hemodynamic response to exercise in patients with sickle cell anemia. Pediatr Cardiol 10:141, 1989.
45. Goodwin, JF: Exercise testing hypertrophic cardiomyopathy. Prog Pediatr Cardiol 2(2):61, 1993.

22
Radionuclide Techniques in Stress Testing

Radionuclide Angiography
- Diagnosis
- Prognosis
- Indications

Gated Cardiac Blood Pool
- Systolic Function
- Diastolic Function
- Interpretation of the Results
- Diagnosis
- Risk Stratification and Prognosis

Stress Myocardial Perfusion
- Tracers
  - *Thallium 201*
  - *Technetium-99m Labeled Tracers*
- Biologic Properties of Technetium 99m Labeled Agents
  - *Imaging Equipment*

Metabolic Imaging with FDG

Techniques
- Stress
- Vasodilators
- Adrenergic Agonists

Protocols
- Treadmill or Bicycle Stress
- Dipyridamole or Adenosine Infusion
- Dobutamine Infusion
- Nitrates

Image Acquisition
- Planar Imaging
- SPECT

Anatomic Correlation

Image Interpretation
- Preliminary Observations
  - *Misaligned Cuts*
  - *Verifying Correct Gating*
  - *Segmental Wall Thickening*
  - *Wall Motion*
- Quantitative Polar Map Displays
- Infarct versus Ischemia
- Significant Ancillary Findings in Ischemia
- Quantitation
- Reverse Redistribution
- Causes of "Reversible Deficits" Other Than Ischemia
  - *Left Bundle Branch Block*
  - *Other Causes of Reversible Perfusion Defects*

Uses of Myocardial Perfusion Imaging
- Diagnosis
  - *Results*
  - *Chronic Ischemic Disease*
- Acute Ischemic Syndromes
- Unstable Angina
- Prognosis
- Risk Stratification
  - *Post Acute MI*
- "Hibernating" Myocardium
- Metabolic Imaging for Defining Hibernating Myocardium
  - *Tracer Combinations for Defining Perfusion—Metabolic Mismatch*

Many factors influence selection of an appropriate stress test for a particular patient. These include the clinical question to be answered, the intended use of the data in decision-making, the patient's condition and institutional circumstances of expertise and resource availability. This chapter deals with the indications of diagnostic confirmation, assessment of severity, prognosis, risk stratification as well as selection and assessment of therapy in patients with chronic ischemic heart disease, unstable angina and acute myocardial infarction. Radionuclide cardiac stress testing has grown rapidly over the past two to three decades, so that all areas cannot be encompassed. For more detailed overviews, the reader is referred to several available monographs.[1–5] As currently widely performed, stress single photon emission computed tomography (SPECT) gated myocardial perfusion imaging (MPI) yields data not only with regard to relative myocardial perfusion for assessment of coronary reserve, but also analyzes wall motion, wall thickening and reliably provides measurement of post stress and resting ejection fractions. The images are acquired at various times after the stress during which the tracer has been injected, but the data reflect perfusion under the stress conditions during which the injection was made. It has largely replaced both stress radionuclide angiography and stress gated blood pool studies. These techniques are more cumbersome to adapt to the exercising patient and degraded by the motion accompanying the exercise state during which the data must be acquired in these techniques.

RADIONUCLIDE ANGIOGRAPHY

Radionuclide angiography (RNA) requires injection of a crisp bolus of activity into a central vein. Venous access should be secured with an indwelling venous line to avoid extravasation. Use of the external jugular vein avoids division of the bolus into cephalic and basilic pathways and retention by valves, providing a rapid transit time. Any of the technetium 99m labeled agents can be used, but use of Tc-99m DTPA permits a repeat injection for restudy after an interval of a few minutes. Data are obtained as the activity traverses the cardiac chambers during the first circulation. Fluctuating activity (counts) in the ventricular chambers accurately reflects relative volume change during the cardiac cycle, peaking at mechanical end diastole and reaching a nadir at end systole. The cycle can be divided into 16 equal portions based on the timing provided by the peak counts. Adding data from 3 to 4 consecutive cycles forms an average cardiac cycle with enough counts over these few seconds to yield data valid for measuring both right and left ventricular ejection fractions.[6] Since the bolus transits serially through the chambers, they are usually readily separated temporally. Wall motion can be accurately evaluated by visual analysis of the cine display of the 16 frames containing the left ventricular phase analogous to a left ventricular angiogram, although the ventricle is filled with radioactivity rather than contrast.

The RNA measures wall motion and EF at the single discrete point in time as the bolus transits though the chamber. In order to measure these parameters during exercise, a small camera is positioned over the precordium, usually in either an right anterior oblique (RAO) or anterior position as the patient attains peak stress level. Because several heartbeats are used for analysis, motion of the thorax and diaphragm degrade the study. Use of upright bicycle exercise provides better position stability than treadmill stress if this procedure is used. Small radioactive makers can be affixed to the thorax permitting computer realignment of the imaging data using these fiduciary markers to minimize the motion artifact.

In laboratories experienced with this technique the data provides very accurate assessment of ventricular motion and function.[7] Failure of the EF to increase absolutely by 5% over the resting value has proved a reliable means of detecting ventricular dysfunction, while the absolute value of the EF provides prognostic information.[8] The measured pulmonary transit time can be used as an index of ventricular function, but is affected by a number of factors, including poor bolus injection (detected by analyzing the bolus transit through the superior vena cava), tricuspid or pulmonary valve disease, right ventricular dysfunction, and processes affecting one or more components of the pulmonary circulation directly or indirectly, leading to increased pulmonary vascular resistance.

Left ventricular (LV) volume (V) can be calculated using the same method applied to single view x-ray studies.[9] The LV length (L), and short axis perpendicular diameter (D) measurements are obtained from calibrated first pass images, and the volume calculated as

$$V = \pi/6 \times L \times D^2.$$

We have found excellent correlation between radiographic cine ventriculography and radionuclide first pass studies. If a tracer that is retained in the blood, such as Tc-99m labeled red cells, is used, then forward cardiac output can be obtained using standard dye dilution curve techniques and either the measured blood volume or blood volume estimated from nomograms based on body surface area or weight.[10] Total cardiac output can be calculated using the stroke volume (SV), calculated from LV volume × EF, multiplied by the measured heart rate.

Diagnosis

RNA can be performed during the first pass of a Tc-99m labeled tracer that is injected to measure perfusion. Data collected during either injection at stress or rest can be analyzed for regional wall motion abnormalities as well as ejection fraction. The criteria for coronary artery disease (CAD) were based on fall in ejection fraction, development of wall motion abnormalities and increased end systolic volume during exercise compared with rest. Initial studies indicated high sensitivity and specificity.[7,11] In addition, quantitative regional ejection fractions as well as segmental wall motion abnormalities are highly predictive of perfusion abnormalities. The data can also help differentiate actual perfusion deficits from artifacts that may appear on the myocardial perfusion images.[12]

Study of less highly selected patients showed lower sensitivity for diagnosis of CAD. In part this depends on the prevalence of myocardial disease other than coronary artery disease in the group selected for study. Any disease process resulting in left ventricular dysfunction can yield an abnormal response to exercise. Wall motion abnormalities are in general less sensitive, about 60%, but more specific, about 85%, for diagnosing CAD than ejection fraction fall of 5%, which has a sensitivity of approximately 77% and specificity of approximately 58%. Overall specificity is lower in women, 45% as compared with men, 63%. For diagnosis of CAD, a group with a prior probability (prevalence) of 50% for CAD is likely to yield best results. By itself, radionuclide first pass angiography has neither the sensitivity nor specificity to serve as a screening test for CAD.[13]

Prognosis

The measurement of left ventricular function at maximum exercise provides critical, prognostic information in the patient with known CAD. In spite of its shortcomings as a diagnostic test, the exercise radionuclide angiogram fulfills this need well.[14] Follow-up of 1663 patients with CAD for a mean of 6.5 years showed an exercise ejection fraction of less than 50% was the best predictor of death and could be supplemented by other data obtained during the study including the resting EDV and the heart rate response to exercise.[15] Figure 22–1 is a first pass radionuclide angiogram that shows an

FIGURE 22–1. First pass radionuclide left ventriculogram obtained by summing 4 consecutive heart beats. As radioactive blood transits through the left ventricle, the count rate in the ventricle fluctuates directly related to chamber volume. End diastole is defined by the maximum count rate, end systole by the minimum. The time between consecutive beats is divided into 16 intervals, and each interval summed for the four beats so that quantitative data, including ejection fraction, volumes, volume curves, cardiac output as well as cine data can be readily obtained. The resting image *(A)*, obtained with the patient upright at rest during injection of Tc-99m MIBI for a resting MIBI study shows normal wall motion occurs between the end diastolic and end systolic frames with the outlines of the LV superimposed beneath the LV volume curve, lower right. Motion is best evaluated by viewing the cine presentation of the data. The parametric amplitude image, lower left coroner, represents the amplitude of the first harmonic term resulting from the Fourier transform of the original spatial-time data, that has periodic variation with time. It defines the aortic valve plane as a line of absent change. The phase image next to it is a means of assessing the coordination of chamber contraction. This program assumes the count rate change in each pixel representing a contracting blood filled chamber is defined by a cosine function. The computer color codes groups of pixels together according to where in the 360° cycle the peak, end diastole, occurs. The data obtained with injection made during the 9th minute *(B)* (6.3 METS) of maximum upright bicycle exercise. The patient achieved a heart rate of 149 beats per minute. Significant anterior wall hypokinesis can be seen. The LVEF is measured from count rate change, the volumes obtained from LV length diameter measurements using calibrated images.

While the end-diastolic volume, 136 ml, remained unchanged, an abnormal response to exercise is indicated by the increase in end-systolic volume from 61 ml to 83 ml. There is also a significant decrease in ejection fraction from 59% to 39%. The myocardial perfusion images were normal. The patient was a 67-year-old man who had taken up long distance running after coronary artery bypass grafting 10 years prior to this study. The angiogram showed patent grafts. The patient's symptoms responded to digoxin administration. (Original images were color-coded.)

A

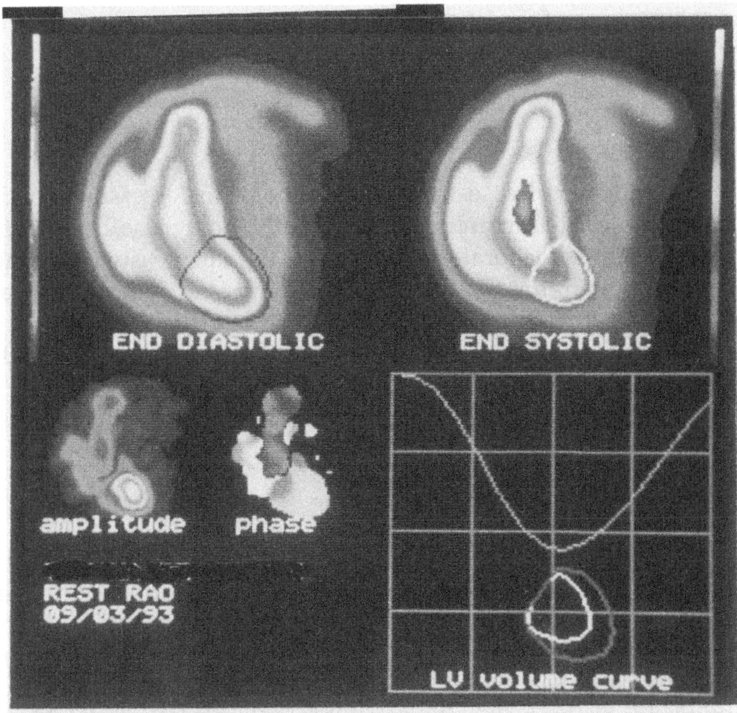
END DIASTOLIC
END SYSTOLIC
amplitude
phase
[redacted]
REST RAO
09/03/93
LV volume curve

B

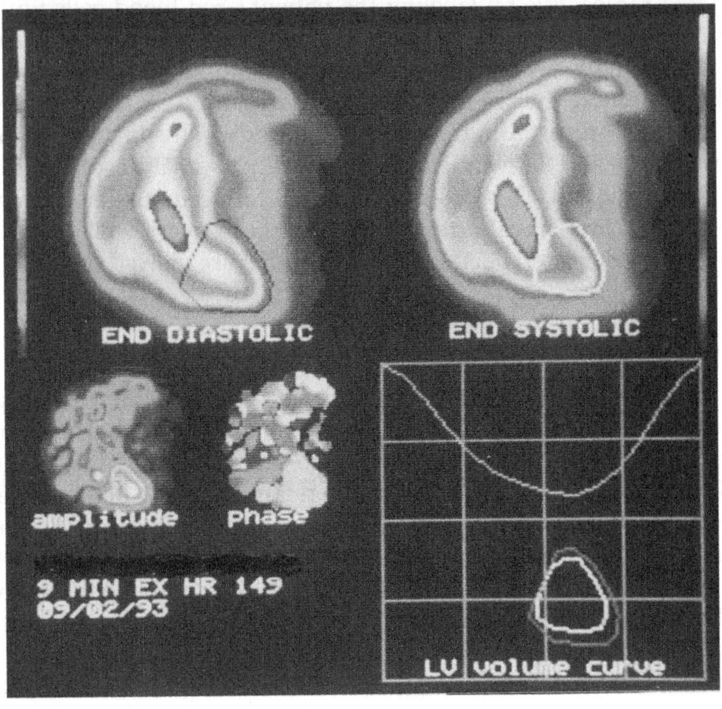
END DIASTOLIC
END SYSTOLIC
amplitude
phase
[redacted]
9 MIN EX HR 149
09/02/93
LV volume curve

abnormal response of the left ventricle to exercise in a patient with coronary artery disease, but patent grafts. He had heart failure.

Indications

(1) Resting study in risk assessment (2) prognosis and assessment of therapy after acute myocardial infarction (3) stress RNA may also be useful in appropriately equipped laboratories (4) may be used to measure baseline function in patients with unstable angina (5) diagnosis of symptomatic and selected patients with asymptomatic, chronic, ischemic heart disease at rest or during exercise, particularly in combination with a perfusion study performed from the same injection.

GATED CARDIAC BLOOD POOL

So-called MUGA (multiple gated acquisition) studies have also been used to measure ejection fraction (EF) and evaluate wall motion during graded phases of upright bicycle exercise. Initially, images were obtained only during end diastole and end systole,[16,17] but with availability of the minicomputer, a series of images could be accumulated throughout the cardiac cycle, permitting cine analysis of wall motion.[18,19] In this technique, the blood pool is rendered radioactive by labeling the patient's red blood cells with technetium 99m, so that activity remains in the ventricular chambers. An EKG signal is required to separate the cardiac cycle into 12–32 frames. Data is acquired for 1-minute intervals throughout the study. A small camera is positioned over the precordium throughout the study in the LAO view in order to separate right and left ventricles anatomically for analysis of ejection fraction and wall motion. This position, required for accurate determination of the ejection fraction, has shortcomings since it can't very well evaluate motion in the anterior lateral and inferior walls that are viewed only end on.

Systolic Function

Accurate measurement of the EF from gated blood pool images requires a regular, stable sinus rhythm. Computer correction to an equal total number of counts in each frame can aid when there is arrhythmia. The QT interval, critical for EF calculation, tends to remain relatively stable in the presence of small variations in heart rate. The EF measurement is count rate based, independent of any geometric assumptions. Wall motion analysis is obtained by viewing side-by-side cine presentations of the computer-reconstructed data obtained at different stages of stress, particularly peak stress, with rest. While the left ventricular volume can be obtained using either geometric or count-based methods,[20] the count based method using a calibrated pixel size is more rapid and less cumbersome, and, given the difficulties of edge detection on the images, just as accurate.[21]

Diastolic Function

Diastolic dysfunction can be appraised if the acquisition is obtained appropriately throughout the cardiac cycle, making sure the diastolic portion of the curve is not distorted by slight irregularities of rhythm.[22] This is accomplished with gating equipment that forms the diastolic portion of the curve by gating back from the QRS spike of the following beat and appropriately splicing this portion of the average cardiac cycle to the systolic portion of the cycle acquired from forward gating, forming a composite curve of the average cardiac cycle.[23] Alternatively, a histogram can be made in which beats are gated in pairs, so that the diastolic portion of an average cycle between beats can be analyzed. Diastolic function is evaluated by comparing the most rapid filling rate with the most rapid emptying rate, expressed as end diastolic volumes per second. Normally, the rates are relatively equal.

Interpretation of the Results

Criteria for abnormality include failure of the EF to increase absolutely by 5% with exercise, the development of wall motion abnormalities, and increase in the end systolic volume with exercise.[24] Like first pass RNA, the technique is cumbersome, requiring small cameras adaptable to being placed in front of the exercising patient. These have not been readily available, although a new generation of smaller, digital cameras is now emerging. Short data collection periods, preferably 1 minute in length, are required to accurately separate function at peak exercise from intervals leading up to, and particularly following this desired end point, when post exercise hyperemia and rebound enhanced systolic function may appear. Longer intervals smear the data and are less accurate. Figure 22–2 shows the gated images from serial 1-minute periods of an upright bicycle exercise study of a man with three-vessel coronary artery disease.

Diagnosis

While initial studies indicated high sensitivity for detection of coronary artery disease, these patient groups were highly selected. Many had prior infarcts. With increasing application to a wide variety of patients, sensitivity and, particularly, specificity declined, the latter partly related to post test selection bias whereby usually only patients with an abnormal test result went on to have further testing unless there was an overriding clinical suspicion of CAD.[25] The presence of wall motion abnormalities has a sensitivity of 73%, and specificity, 91%, for diagnosing CAD as compared with ejection fraction

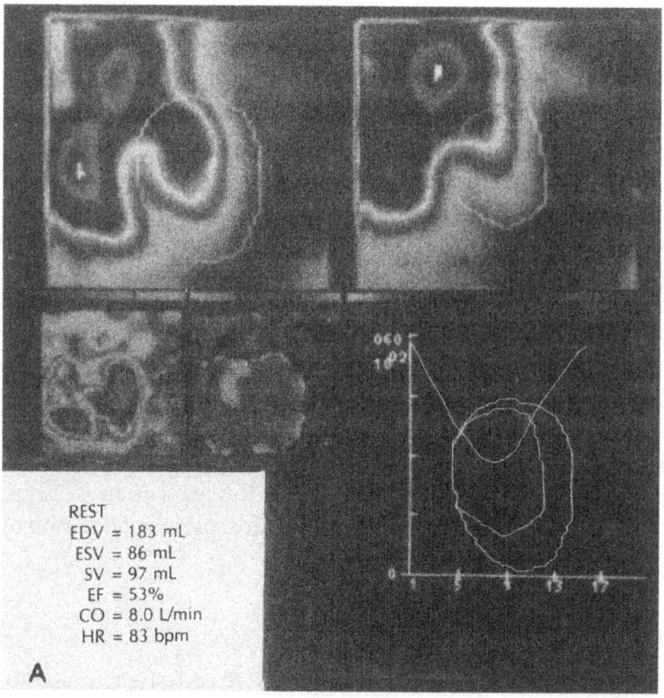
REST
EDV = 183 mL
ESV = 86 mL
SV = 97 mL
EF = 53%
CO = 8.0 L/min
HR = 83 bpm
A

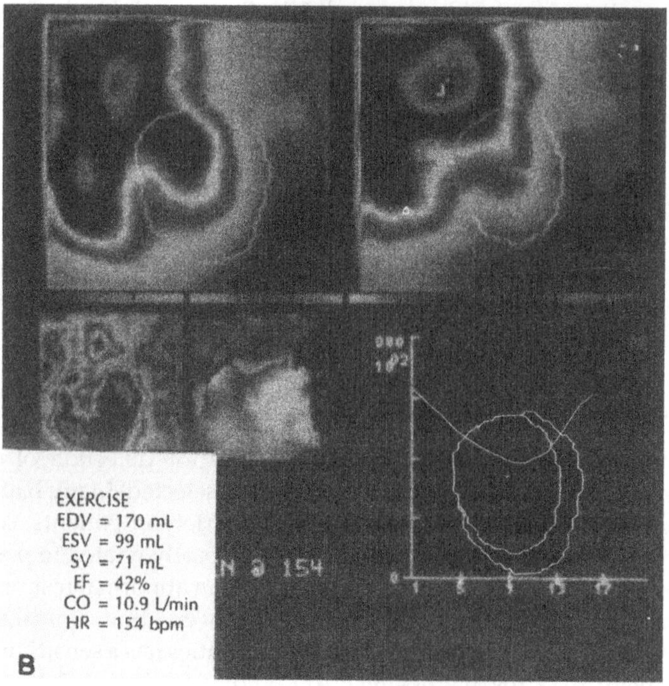
EXERCISE
EDV = 170 mL
ESV = 99 mL
SV = 71 mL
EF = 42%
CO = 10.9 L/min
HR = 154 bpm
B

fall of 5%, sensitivity 76%, specificity 80%.[26] It is of interest that infusion of a solution of insulin with glucose during submaximal dynamic exercise increases the ejection fraction response in normal controls, and to a lesser degree, in non insulin dependent diabetics.[27] Since the test measures parameters of left ventricular function and volume and not the presence of a particular pathologic process, it should not be surprising that it fails to discriminate between pathologic processes which ultimately lead to similar left ventricular dysfunction.

Risk Stratification and Prognosis

As a prognostic tool in patients with known CAD, the exercise gated blood pool image can sort selected, medically treated patients with known CAD into high and low risk groups.[28] The absolute fall in ejection fraction is related to the angiographically depicted extent of CAD, although there is a great deal of overlap between groups.[29] The largest survival discrepancy between medically and surgically treated patients with CAD occurs in those who have depressed systolic function in response to exercise. Others have confirmed these findings and have pointed out that with increasingly low ejection fraction on exercise, risk of cardiac events, including death, increases.[30,31] A resting ejection fraction of less than 30% is, by itself, a marker of poor prognosis in the individual with CAD.

Indications (1) resting EF and end systolic volume index following acute infarction to assess severity of disease (2) risk assessment and prognosis in patients with known CAD who have either received or not received reperfusion therapy.

STRESS MYOCARDIAL PERFUSION

Stress myocardial perfusion imaging (MPI) measures relative regional coronary reserve. It is determined by the additive effects of luminal stenoses in

FIGURE 22–2. One minute–gated blood pool images. The baseline resting image *(A)* shows end-diastolic image, upper left, and end-systolic image next to it. The left ventricular outline has been generated. Lower left image represents amplitude constant of the first harmonic term of the Fourier transform of the original object spatial-time data that has periodic variation (of counts) with time. It delineates areas, such as valve planes that have no periodic change. Adjacent to this is the phase image providing an estimate of the degree of contractile cordination. The LV volume curve is in the lower right corner, with superimposed LV outlines obtained from end-diastolic and end-systolic frames. The LV volumes can be estimated using Massardo's count rate method. They are increased for the patient's surface area. LVEF is at the lower limits of normal. Image *B* from the 8th minute of exercise (6.3 METS) shows moderate generalized hypokinesis from the LV outlines (best appreciated by viewing the study in cine format). End-systolic volume increases and ejection fraction falls, both indicators of an abnormal response to exercise. The patient presented with unstable angina, and, at cardiac catheterization had significant three-vessel coronary artery disease.

series and alterations in the resistance and vasodilatory capacity of the coronary microvasculature.[32–34] Quantitative measure of flow reserve requires invasive techniques to determine the driving pressure proximal to a stenosis compared with the driving pressure distal to it at conditions of maximum coronary bed vasodilatation. The myocardial distribution of the tracer injected at peak stress imaged at a later appropriate interval (10 minutes for thallium-201, 15 minutes to 90 minutes depending on the stress used, for ^{99m}Tc sestamibi) reflects myocardial perfusion at the time of injection. Comparing this distribution with that obtained with injection at rest estimates the relative coronary flow reserve, the regional ability of myocardial perfusion to increase in response to stress or pharmacological vasodilatation of the coronary vascular bed.

Tracers

The chief clinically used tracers that measure regional blood flow include: ^{201}Tl thallous chloride, a group IIIA potassium analog[35]; the isonitrile, ^{99m}Tc sestamibi, a monovalent cation with hydrophilic and hydrophobic components[36]; and, ^{99m}Tc Tetrofosmin, a lipophilic diphosphine that clears from the liver faster than sestamibi.[37] ^{99m}Tc teboroxime is a freely diffusible, neutral, lipophilic boronic acid adduct of a technetium dioxime complex (BATO) that has high initial myocardial uptake. Because of rapid washout, imaging must be performed within minutes of injection, best carried out with high speed multi-detector cameras.[38,39] No longer commercially distributed in this country, the more widespread availability of suitable imaging equipment may offer the opportunity to take advantage of its unique biological properties.

Radiopharmaceuticals have two sets of properties; one set related to the physical properties of the radioactive portion of the tracer, the other related to the biologic properties of the molecule.

Thallium 201

Thallium 201 thallous chloride is a cyclotron-produced product, which, in practical terms means it is manufactured at a site away from where it is used. It contains impurities (^{203}Pb and ^{202}Tl). Decay is via electron capture. The energetically unstable nucleus snags an unwary orbital electron to gain a more stable energy state, essentially converting a nuclear proton to a neutron resulting in the decay product ^{201}Hg. This process is accompanied by emission of 69, 71 and 83 keV mercury x-rays, which have relatively poor penetration of soft tissue. In addition, the decay transition results in emission of 135 and 167 keV photons that have better energies for clinical imaging, but are low in abundance providing little of the imaging data. Absorption of the photons by soft tissue produces apparent decrease in activity in the anterior lateral wall region in large-breasted women, inferior wall deficits related to diaphragmatic or subdiaphragmatic absorption, usually in stocky individuals, and generally poor images in morbidly obese individuals due to low count rate. Sometimes, if such an individual can stand, the heart can be placed closer to the detector for a series of planar images that have better diagnostic value than the SPECT image. These low energy photons are not well resolved as compared with the photon from ^{99m}Tc.

The relatively long half-life of 73 hours, while good for delayed images, artificially restricts the administered dose to 3–4 mCi to satisfy minimizing the radiation dose. The administered activity has been edging up with time, up from the 2–3 mCi listed in the last edition. Counts with current multiheaded cameras are sufficient to obtain gated myocardial single photon emission computed tomographic (SPECT) images. Gated images can be used to analyze regional wall motion, segmental myocardial thickening and measure ejection fraction at the time of imaging, based on volume calculations. A major problem with a paucity of useful photons is that it leads to longer imaging times and hence motion artifacts.

While image manipulation such as background subtraction and smoothing of these relatively low data density images may aid interpretation, improperly used, they may introduce artifact. Increasing the dose administered to gain better diagnostic information in a population more at risk from the effects of improperly diagnosed and treated CAD than the theoretical harm of radiation makes good sense. Per mCi, it delivers about 130 Gy to the kidney, 34 Gy to the myocardium, and 24 Gy to the whole body.

The initial distribution of an intravenously injected, rapidly diffusible tracer with a high net fraction of tracer transferred from the plasma to the myocardium during transit through the myocardial capillary bed serves as an indicator of myocardial blood flow.[40] Thallium, a group IIIA metal, has a hydrated ionic radius between that of K^+ and Rb^+. Myocyte uptake is chiefly an active process driven by the cellular membrane-bound adenotriphosphatase Na^+/K^+ pump that can be poisoned by the cardiac glycosides. A small portion of the extraction unaffected by oubain is related to the electrochemical gradient between plasma and the myocyte. The high rate of first pass extraction from the coronary circulation—more than 80%—remains linear over a wide range of physiological flow rates. Extraction depends upon the integrity of the cellular membrane. It is reduced by acidosis and hypoxemia. It becomes nonlinear at flow rates lower than 10% of the basal state. Linearity also falls off at flow rates greater than twice the basal level, a state achieved during pharmacologic vasodilatation dilatation.[35,41] When injection is made at peak stress, it is critical to maintain the stress for at least a minute following the injection to allow for localization reflecting peak stress conditions uncontaminated by post stress hyperemia.

Since thallium is not tightly bound intracellularly, it promptly begins to leak out, so-called "redistribution," as plasma levels fall. The rate of fall depends upon initial myocyte concentration, the gradient between the myocyte and plasma, the availability of the opportunity for equilibrium between myocyte and plasma and rate of redelivery of thallium to the myocyte. Plasma levels are affected by factors that influence the plasma/intracellular thallium distribution. Initial distribution is determined by the distribution of cardiac output at injection; e.g., high skeletal muscle uptake during exercise, in contrast to high gut uptake in the resting, non-fasting state.[42–46] By injecting thallium with the patient standing, gut uptake in the non-fasting patient may be reduced. Subsequent determinants of the plasma thallium levels include glucose and insulin levels that tend to drive thallium intracellularly along with glucose, making it unavailable for cardiac uptake. They also affect the rate of thallium washout from the myocardium. Dose infiltration or retention of thallium in the vein injected elevates plasma levels, artificially prolonging washout.

Technetium 99m Labeled Tracers

^{99m}Tc has a short half-life of 6 hours emitting a 140 keV photon that has less absorption in tissue and is more efficiently imaged with better resolution by current detectors as compared with the photons from ^{201}Tl. In busy laboratories, it is readily available as pertechnetate solution eluted from a molybdenum-99/technetium-99m generator. The short six-hour half-time means that comparatively large doses of the ^{99m}Tc agents may be administered without a large burden of radiation to the patient. For example, 30 mCi of ^{99m}Tc sestamibi delivers approximately the same whole body dose as 2 mCi ^{201}Tl. This yields relatively high information content images in a relatively short period of time, reducing the problem of motion artifacts as well as absorption artifacts.

The high count rate available with the ^{99m}Tc agents permits acquisition of radionuclide angiographic data during the first pass transit of the tracers through the cardiac chambers (RNA). With injection made in front of a camera, the data can be obtained during either rest or at peak stress permitting analysis of right and left ventricular ejection fractions, as well as left ventricular volumes and wall motion (Fig. 22–1). In addition, the relatively high count rate of the tracer retained in the myocardium, even though a smaller percent of the injected dose of sestamibi and tetrofosmin is retained as compared with thallium, permits acquisition of gated data while the myocardial perfusion data is also being acquired. Such data including wall motion, wall thickening, left ventricular ejection fraction and left ventricular volumes provide important ancillary data critical to the interpretation of the study. Because of time-consuming quality control procedures, some laboratories may elect to have the ready made, labeled technetium-99m agents delivered in a form ready for injection. This is not an inherent limitation of radiopharmaceutical availability, but reflects the availability of skilled personnel time. All of the ^{99m}Tc labeled myocardial perfusion agents can be made from kits containing the lyophilized precursor that can be stored, with reconstitution of the radiopharmaceutical by simple addition of ^{99m}Tc pertechnetate with appropriate steps for heating to form sestamibi and teboroxime.

Biologic Properties of Technetium 99m Labeled Agents

Like thallium, the myocardial uptake of the technetium-99m labeled agents is linear in the low and mid ranges of myocardial blood flow, but shows non linear correlation with flow at low values, less than 10% of baseline, where relative uptake is greater than the blood flow values it represents. The Tc-99m labeled agents, except for teboroxime, show a roll-off at blood flow levels exceeding twice baseline flow, values achieved with adenosine and dipyridamole testing. In this case, uptake is less than the value it represents, except for teboroxime which displays a linear relationship for high flow values and has high myocardial uptake behaving as a freely diffusible agent. Tetrofosmin exhibits loss of linearity at about twice baseline flow, whereas sestamibi exhibits loss of linearity as flow approaches three times baseline. Sestamibi has a moderate net myocardial extraction from the coronary circulation of approximately 40%, tetrofosmin about 30%. About 1.5% of the administered dose of sestamibi and 1.0%–1.2% of tetrofosmin are retained in the myocardium.

While about 30% of the technetium agent washes out from the myocardium over the first 3 hours, there is usually little redistribution of these agents, with the result that images several hours later reflect what was taking place at the time of injection. Thus injection can be made during an acute situation such as occurrence of chest pain in a patient with unstable angina, and the images performed later when the patient is more stable will reflect the circumstances at the time of injection. Another setting is prior to PTCA with imaging following the procedure reflecting the tissue at risk prior to the procedure. Follow up imaging will show the efficacy of the procedure in terms of reduction of the size of the perfusion deficit.[47] Clinically, the most problematic feature of sestamibi and to a lesser degree, tetrofosmin, is the high hepatic uptake and relatively slow hepatic clearance, faster for tetrofosmin than sestamibi, a property which may interfere with appropriate evaluation of inferior wall activity.

Table 22–1 indicates the clinically relevant properties of these tracers.[48]

Imaging Equipment

Protocols employing multiple planar images of the myocardium from different projections have largely given way to tomographic imaging (Single Photon Emission Computed Tomography-SPECT) which provides better separation of the anatomic distribution of the tracer between territories

Table 22–1. **Significant Properties of Common Myocardial Perfusion Imaging Radiopharmaceuticals**

	^{201}Tl **Thallium 201**	^{99M}Tc **Tc99m Sestamibi**	^{99M}Tc **Tc99m Tetrofosmin**	^{99M}Tc **Tc99m Teboroxime**
Chemical	elemental cation	cationic isonitrile	cationic diphosphine	neutral boronic acid adduct of Tc dioxime
Net myocardial first pass extraction	.60	.44	.40	.55
Percent myocardial uptake of injected dose	3–4	1.4	1–1.2	3–4
Advantages	Redisributes to measure ischemia and detect viability	Little redistribution; images later reflect events at injection time	Little redistribution; images later reflect events at injection time	Rapid washout—can do repeat studies after short time intervals—1/2 hour or less. Uptake linear with blood flow over very wide range
Disadvantages	Physical properties: Low energy photons result in absorption artifacts; long $T_{1/2}$ leads to low injected dose and low photon yield	Biological properties: Uptake in liver, gall bladder and intestine—clears slowly	Biologic properties: Uptake in liver, gall bladder and intestine—clears more rapidly than sestamibi	Biologic properties: Very rapid washout requires very rapid imaging devices

From reference 48, with permission of author and publisher.

subserved by the different coronary arteries. Planar imaging can supplement SPECT, particularly if the patient cannot lie down, if the patient cannot fit into the gantry, and if a standing image is necessary to separate cardiac from sub-diaphragmatic activity. In some patients only planar images can be obtained because of body habitus, inability to lie down, cardiac rotation with pneumonectomy, and overlying interfering structures such as an arm in a cast.

Single headed detectors can provide excellent clinical data performing either planar or SPECT imaging when used appropriately. When SPECT is used, a circular rather than contoured orbit around the anterolateral thorax is probably best to avoid attenuation artifacts. Multi-headed detectors can be used to shorten acquisition time without sacrificing resolution. A number of instruments obtain attenuation data using simultaneous transmission data, which, just as in CT, provides an anatomic attenuation map for the individual patient. Usually a linear gadolinium-153 source is used,[49] and acquisition of transmitted attenuation data obtained simultaneously with the emission data from myocardial activity. This is used to correct for attenuation. While this approach is strongly recommended,[50] there are many pitfalls, and results have as yet to be verified. New hybrid CT and SPECT imaging equipment might do this more accurately. Figure 22–4 shows a schematic view of the heart with sections corresponding to the SPECT images routinely obtained.

An EKG may be used to gate the SPECT images so that an average cardiac cycle can be reconstructed for measurement of the ejection fraction, for cine analysis of regional wall motion and regional myocardial wall thickening. In viewing the cine, the three-dimensional image of the beating heart may be turned and viewed from all projections. While the tracer injection may have been made at stress with the myocardial distribution reflecting relative perfusion at stress, the functional imaging data is obtained with the patient at rest. In cases of severe coronary disease, post exercise stunning may still be evident on images obtained even an hour after the stress (see Fig. 22–6).

Computer analysis of the reconstructed left ventricular myocardium may also be used to measure left ventricular volume, left ventricular mass and measure percentage of myocardium that is likely infarcted as well as that at risk from ischemic disease. Depending upon the program used, results may differ, but the measurements are reproducible permitting objective comparison of serial studies.

Indications: (1) triage of acute chest pain in patients with intermediate risk for having acute MI after standard testing; (2) assessing myocardium at risk prior to intervention in acute infarction, and for measuring completed infarct size and resting ventricular function; (3) ventricular function may also be measured during the first pass transit of the tracer that is used to measure myocardial perfusion (RNA-see above); (4) risk assessment, prognosis and assessment of therapy after acute infarction by evaluating the presence, extent and severity of stress-induced ischemia as well as detecting myocardial viability.

METABOLIC IMAGING WITH FDG

Metabolic imaging has become more readily available with the diffusion of positron emission tomography (PET) into the community and the availability of the glucose analog, 2-F-18 fluoro-2-deoxyglucose (F-18 FDG). Areas of hibernating myocardium that have markedly diminished blood flow exhibit loss of function although remaining viable. Such areas preserve metabolic function and, in the resting state, demonstrate preferential utilization of glucose rather than fatty acids as a substrate. This metabolic-perfusion mismatch provides a reliable marker for identifying, and also quantifying hibernating myocardium, factors critical to predicting the probability of functional benefit to be expected following successful revascularization.

The positron emitting perfusion agent, rubidium-82, measures regional myocardial perfusion. Detection of high-energy positrons is less subject to absorption artifacts as compared with routine SPECT agents that have lower energy and less penetrability of tissue. The half-life of Rb-82 is only 90 seconds. For clinical use, it must be obtained through continuous in-line elution of a strontium generator to supply a constant infusion of its decay product, rubidium-82, during resting and throughout stress maneuvers.

Specially designed imaging equipment can take advantage of the unique feature of positron decay in which the interaction of the positron with an electron results in the conversion of the mass of both into two back-to-back photons traveling at 180 degrees to one another. Detectors positioned opposite one another count an event between them if they both see a photon at the same time (in coincidence). A dedicated PET camera or a hybrid SPECT camera equipped with absorption correction programs can perform the coincidence detection imaging.

SPECT cameras equipped with high-energy collimators can provide excellent clinical information utilizing the standard single photon detection mode rather than coincidence mode imaging. Standard SPECT techniques allow simultaneous imaging of both F-18-FDG and ^{99m}Tc tracers that have been injected at sequential times, utilizing the different energies emitted by the tracers to separate the information provided by each tracer into its own unique image. The ^{99m}Tc tracer image represents perfusion, the FDG image, metabolism. This technique provides accurate regional correlation of perfusion and metabolism (see Figs. 22–14 and 21–15).

Indications: (1) identifying and quantifying ischemic regions and assessing prognosis in patients with chronic ischemic disease; (2) prediction of the functional outcome of successful revascularization of hibernating myocardium.

TECHNIQUES

Stress

Standard stress testing protocols are readily adapted to the use of radionuclide myocardial perfusion studies. Isotonic exercise as well as maneuvers that release catechol amines alter inotropic and chronotropic myocardial parameters. These include treadmill testing, upright or supine bicycle exercise, arm ergometer exercise, atrial pacing, pharmacologic stress with dobutamine or arbutamine and mental stress.[51–53] With treadmill stress testing, the increase in coronary artery blood flow is linearly related to the double product.[54] The increase in coronary blood flow that can be achieved with vigorous exercise (approximately doubling or tripling the baseline value) is less than that which routinely occurs with vasodilators. Isometric stress[55,56] and ice water immersion[57,58] increase after-load. Isotonic and isometric stress may be combined for additive effects.

With increasing myocardial oxygen demand and failure of the coronary vascular reserve to meet the demand, myocardial wall motion abnormalities develop, filling pressure increases, end diastolic volume increases and the ejection fraction fails to increase or, falls resulting in increased end systolic volume. Relative increase in preload during supine bicycle exercise may be more effective in inducing ischemia and altering cardiac function as compared with upright bicycle exercise and thus a more sensitive stress maneuver. Events at peak stress may last for only a short time. It is critical to capture the events occurring at this time uncontaminated by data reflecting conditions prior to or following those that obtain at maximum exertion.

Stress maneuvers that increase heart rate and substantially shorten diastole can lead to false-positive myocardial perfusion studies when conduction abnormalities cause regional delay in the onset of diastole. This is particularly common in left bundle branch block where there is apparent decrease in perfusion to the anterior and anteroseptal regions that may be unassociated with documented regional coronary disease. Spurious changes may also occur with right bundle branch block and in paced situations. In these patients it is best to use pharmaceutical vasodilatation such as dipyridamole or adenosine infusion that do not increase heart rate significantly. It is important to verify that the heart rate has not significantly increased at the time of injection.

Vasodilators

Dipyridamole[59] and adenosine[60] are effective agents for increasing coronary artery blood flow by reducing intra-myocardial vascular resistance of normal microvasculature. Dipyridamole exerts its effects by blocking cellular reuptake of adenosine produced in the cell and released into the extra cellular space. It has a serum half-life of approximately 20 to 30 minutes. Adenosine infusion results in direct increase of the extra cellular adenosine concentration. It has a very short half-life on the order of a few seconds. Accumulated extra cellular adenosine can bind to inhibitory A_1 receptors slowing the heart rate and prolonging A-V conduction. Binding to the stimulatory A_2 receptors increases adenosine cyclase and 3–5 cyclic adenosine monophosphate. This in turn leads to decreased trans-membrane calcium transport and results in vasodilatation of the intramyocardial resistance vessels if they are normal.[61] If there is no impediment to flow upstream, this results in a three- to five-fold increase in coronary blood flow.[62–65] Caffeine and other xanthines interfere with adenosine binding to and activating the cell surface receptors.

The vasodilators do not significantly increase myocardial oxygen demand, but depict differential increase in blood flow related to variable resistance related to proximal luminal obstruction or obstructions in series or to failure of dilatation in already compromised small resistance vessels. They are flow agents rather than stress maneuvers. Side effects are common, but rarely serious. Adenosine induces chest pain or tightness very commonly, which is distressing not only for the patient, but also for those administering the test. Both agents have excellent safety records in large, multi-center registries, especially when considering the patient population selected for study with these agents is elderly and debilitated, often with known coexisting severe peripheral vascular disease.[66–68] Death may occur in approximately 1 in 10,000 patients, while non-fatal infarctions occur with approximately the same frequency. Patients with unstable angina may sustain infarction with dipyridamole. Although dipyridamole increases cerebral blood flow under ordinary conditions, stroke and TIA have been associated with its use, presumably in the presence of severe, bilateral internal carotid and vertebral artery disease causing loss of cerebrovascular reserve, so that there is no compensatory mechanism to counter a drop in blood pressure. Dipyridamole may induce severe bronchospasm, and its use is contraindicated in patients with asthma.

Both may induce significant ischemia in the coronary vascular bed distal to a critical stenosis. Under baseline circumstances this territory is subserved by collateral circulation from another epicardial vessel with less significant stenosis. When driving pressure supporting collateral flow from the lesser affected artery is reduced related to the drop in distal vascular resistance in the territory of this vessel, increased run-off in the less severely affected territory results in reduced collateral flow to the more severely affected territory. Reduction in epicardial vessel pressure affected by critical stenosis may also reverse the net direction of flow that is from epicardial to endocardial at baseline to an endocardial to epicardial direction. This results in a steal pattern producing subendocardial ischemia. When an ischemic EKG change occurs with the use of dipyridamole or adenosine, it is highly predictive of severe, usually multi-vessel coronary disease.

Adrenergic Agonists

Dobutamine is a racemic mixture of the levo-isomer, a potent $alpha_1$ agonist and the dextro-isomer an $alpha_1$ antagonist opposing the levo form resulting in a net weak agonist effect. Both isomers are beta-receptor agonists with a strong $beta_1$, but weak $beta_2$ effect, resulting in prominent inotropic effects, and less prominent chronotropic effects on the myocardium. Infusion may result in net peripheral vasodilatation.[69] Like exercise, dobutamine infusion provokes increased myocardial oxygen demand resulting in a two to three fold increase of myocardial blood flow in areas that can respond normally.[70,71] Dobutamine has proven useful in tests that measure wall motion, as well as those that assess perfusion because it results in wall thickening and exaggerated motion in normal areas as compared with the failure of response in regions rendered ischemic. Such areas may be detectable even though reduced blood flow cannot be demonstrated.[72] Arbutamine has a strong $beta_1$ but weak $beta_2$ effects, and only mild $alpha_1$ tropism. Although it has the same inotropic and chronotropic effects as dobutamine, arbutamine results in less peripheral vasodilatation. It has been used with a relatively expensive, dedicated infusion feedback infusion system with good results.[73]

PROTOCOLS

There are many choices available. These include varying combinations of type of stress performed, tracer or tracers selected, use of a dual tracer protocol, selection of the type of imaging—planar or SPECT, patient positioning, and the use of a single day or more than one day protocol as well as the incorporation of delayed imaging when thallium is used. Each has advantages and disadvantages. Economic constraints as well as the clinical setting are critical determinants. The study should be tailored to the individual patient. Weight and body habitus are major considerations for selection of dose and protocol.

We prefer not to perform one-day protocol studies on very large patients who require increased dose to obtain a suitable count rate for a high-resolution study. When a single day protocol is used, thallium may be selected for the baseline rest study. This has the advantage that its relatively low energy gamma and x-ray emissions, using the appropriate window, may be effectively excluded from the exercise image data obtained with a ^{99m}Tc labeled agent. Because of energy differences, the reconstructed thallium image differs in size from the ^{99m}Tc agent image. This diminishes the ability to visually compare ventricular cavity size between the rest image performed with thallium and the stress image performed with the ^{99m}Tc agent. An important advantage of using thallium for the rest portion of the study is that imaging may begin 5 minutes following injection, whereas a low dose of Tc-99m sestamibi (MIBI) requires waiting an hour. When MIBI is used, drinking 450 ml of water 10 minutes prior to imaging reduces gastric fundal activity and speeds transit of activity through the gut,[74] although in those with gastric emptying problems, chiefly diabetics, retained fluid in the fundus may cause an absorption artifact with the patient imaged supine.

When using Tc-99m-MIBI and no same day imaging is to follow, we give a fatty liquid such as 150 ml of milk (or Lipumol® in those with lactose intolerance, prevalent in our population) 10 minutes after injection to promote emptying of the gallbladder, as well as 450 ml of water 10 minutes prior to imaging. Images with either Tl-201 or a Tc99m agent may be gated with modern equipment. In either case, it prudent to inspect the resting data prior to stress to select out those at risk during stress because of resting ischemia. These are patients with no history of infarct and a normal EKG, but with a large perfusion deficit on the resting image. Figure 22–3 indicates commonly selected protocols and their parameters.

We use ^{99m}Tc sestamibi routinely, except for selected cases in which viability is anticipated to be a critical question, chiefly in patients with known reduction in systolic function. When we do a treadmill stress study, we employ a 2-day protocol because of unpredictable time delays that may occur in the stress laboratory, disrupting the scheduling process. When we perform pharmaceutical "stress" studies we have more direct control of the traffic flow that permits a 1-day protocol. Unfortunately, when pharmaceutical stress is used alone, there may be significant accumulation of activity in the splanchnic circulation. Combining the pharmaceutical with mild isotonic up-right stress or isometric stress may reduce splanchnic uptake. When we choose a 2-day protocol, we perform the stress study first, and if it is normal we do not perform the rest study.

Preparation for stress radionuclide studies is the same as for standard stress testing when isotonic and isometric stress maneuvers are used. This includes discontinuing medications that interfere with cardiac response including beta-blockers and calcium channel blockers as well as long acting nitrates. Dobutamine and arbutamine also require cessation of these medications. They may be supplemented with the use of intravenous atropine 0.5–1.0 mg to overcome vagal inhibition that keeps the heart rate from rising.

FIGURE 22–3. Common protocols for stress rest myocardial perfusion studies. *A* is a protocol for doing stress and rest studies on two different days. The basic principle for a single day study is the use of a smaller dose for the first portion of the study followed by a larger dose used for the second portion of the study. The Rest–Stress sequence is shown in *B,* the Stress–Rest sequence in *E.* A dual isotope study *C* can be performed in a single day using thallium for the resting portion of the study and a Tc99m agent for the stress. Thallium can be used by itself, taking advantage of its unique redistribution properties *(D).* If Tc-99m sestamibi is used, infra-diaphragmatic activity should be allowed to clear before imaging begins. Injection made with the patient supine at rest or during supine vasodilator challenge, results in greater splanchnic activity that clears relatively slowly as compared with upright injection and injection made during exercise. Maneuvers to increase the rate of clearance from the liver include a fatty meal (using Lipumol® in our population which has a high prevalence of lactose intolerance), while 250 ml of water 10 minutes prior to imaging also seems to produce images with less interference.

A. Tc-99m Sestamibi/Tetrofosmin - 2 day protocol

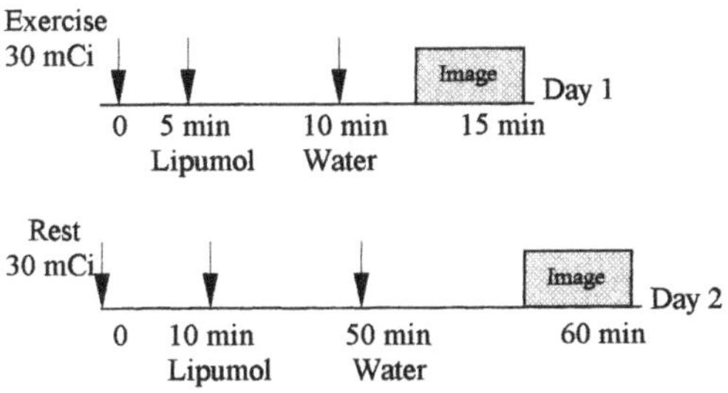

B. Tc99m Sestamibi/Tetrofosmin - 1 day protocol (Rest/Exercise)

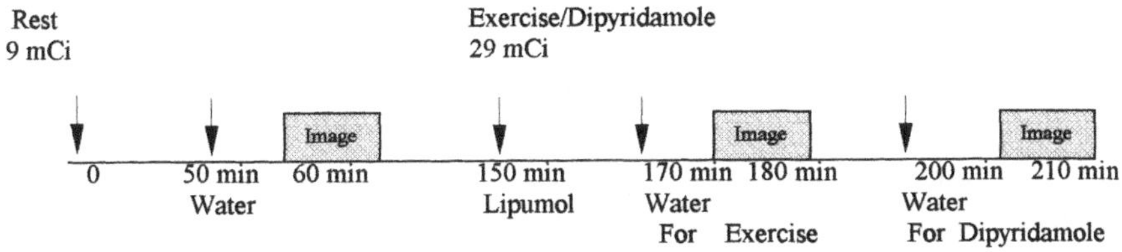

C. Dual Isotope (rest Thallium-201 - exercise Tc-99m Sestamibi/Tetrofosmin) same day protocol

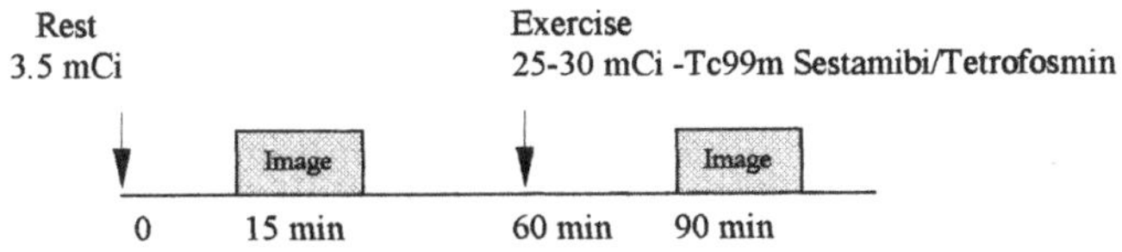

D. Thallium-201

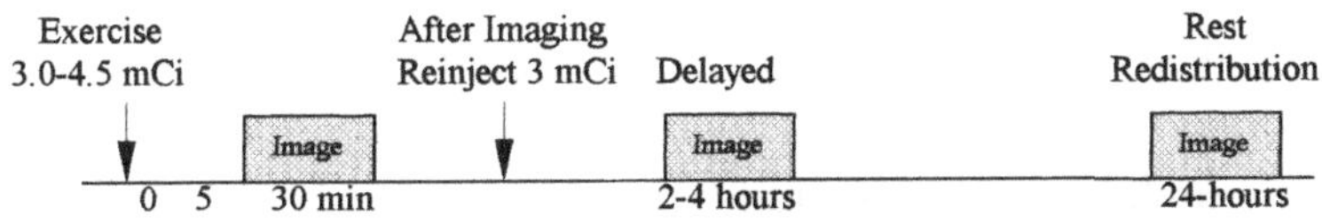

E. Tc -99m SestamibiTetrofosmin - 1 day protocol (Exercise/Rest)

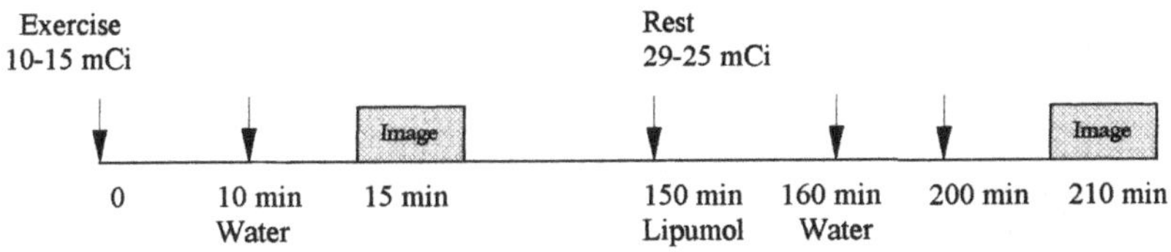

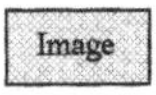

= Imaging

The use of the vasodilators, adenosine, and dipyridamole that do not depend on increasing myocardial demand may be effective without withdrawing these medications. Caffeine with a serum half-life of up to 8 hours competes with cellular surface receptors for adenosine. Products containing caffeine (coffee, decaffeinated coffee, tea, caffeine containing soft drinks, chocolate, cocoa, Exedrin) need to be withdrawn for 24 hours prior to performing a dipyridamole or adenosine study. A 36-hour withdrawal period for xanthine derivative medications is recommended.

Treadmill or Bicycle Stress

These routine isometric stress maneuvers are carried out as for routine stress studies, except that an intravenous cannula is placed in a large arm vein for injection of the perfusion tracer when peak exercise effort is reached. A relatively large peripheral vein should be cannulated, preferably the medial antecubital vein which leads relatively directly into the basilic vein so that bolus injection of a myocardial perfusion tracer can be made into the established line when the patient achieves the peak stress desired. It is critical that the patient continues to exercise for an additional minute when thallium is used (net extraction fraction of 0.6 during coronary transit), or an additional 2 minutes when one of the Tc99m agents is used (net extraction fraction of 0.4) so that imaging performed later reflects the evanescent events occurring at peak exercise and not post exercise changes.

If information is desired concerning regional wall motion and quantitative regional ejection fraction at peak exercise, then the injection must be made with the patient exercising in front of a camera. Small cameras are available for this purpose. The chief difficulty is ensuring stability of the chest during the 40 seconds required to collect the first pass transit data as detailed under the section for radionuclide angiography.

Dipyridamole or Adenosine Infusion

Unstable angina, aortic stenosis, hypertrophic cardiomyopathy, systolic hypotension (less than 90 mm Hg)–especially if accompanied by bradycardia, an infarct within the last 24 hours and a history of acute bronchospastic disease are contraindications to performing a dipyridamole stress study. Although dipyriamole is a cerebrovascular vasodilator, and has been used safely in a series of 400 patients with known cerebrovascular disease[75] infusion of dipyridamole has been associated with precipitating stroke or transient ischemic attack. This seems most likely to occur inpatients with stage II cerebrovascular insufficiency. At this point, maximum regional vasodilatation has exhausted cerebrovascular reserve as a compensatory mechanism, and cell survival is dependent upon an increased oxygen extraction fraction. These individuals often have severe, bilateral carotid artery disease as well as vertebral artery compromise. It is prudent besides obtaining a brief pertinent cardiac history and list of medications as well as inspecting the EKG, to elicit information that might be related to cerebrovascular insufficiency. For example we indicated that the risk of a dipyridamole study exceeded the benefit in a patient with known bilateral carotid artery occlusion and significant compromise of one vertebral artery who had had a stroke and was having transient ischemic attacks.

Dipyridamole should be infused at a rate of 0.142 mg/Kg/min (standard dose) or 0.213 mg/Kg/min (high dose) over a 4-minute period at a uniform rate to achieve a total dose of either 0.56 mg/Kg, standard dose or 0.84 mg/Kg, high dose. The higher dose may have greater sensitivity for detecting lesions with a lesser degree of stenosis with a safety similar to the standard dose, although there is not as much experience with this dose level compared with the standard dose.[68,76]

The dose can be made up in a standard volume of 20 ml in order to facilitate monitoring of injection at a rate of 5 ml/min. Infusion is performed through an in place venous catheter, preferably in a medial antecubital vein that has a direct pathway to the axillary vein via the basilic vein without the hang-up that may occur at the valve at the entry of the cephalic vein into the axillary vein when the lateral antecubital vein is selected. If a peripheral vein must be used, the patient often experiences a burning sensation since the solution is basic. Infusion, carried out under monitoring of blood pressure and EKG, should be at a steady rate using either a carefully timed hand injection or an infusion pump. To avoid pooling in the proximal arm vein which has at least a 15–20 ml capacity, it is best to use a Y-connection at the entrance of the dipyridamole solution into the intravenous cannula, continually flushing the dypiridamole with a saline drip that is carefully adjusted to keep flowing during and after the dipyridamole infusion.

Dipyridamole has a plasma half-time of approximately 30 minutes. The onset of maximum action occurs at 5 minutes. Due to systemic vasodilation, the systolic blood pressure usually falls 5–10 mm of Hg with a compensatory slight increase in heart rate. Occasionally, individuals will demonstrate an idiosyncratic increase in blood pressure. To decrease hepatic uptake when ^{99m}Tc sestamibi is used, some laboratories do the infusion and injection while the patient is walking on a level treadmill. Others have the patient perform handgrip squeeze at 1/3 maximum beginning immediately after the end of infusion lasting until 2 minutes after the injection of the myocardial perfusion tracer. Bolus injection of the myocardial perfusion tracer followed by a flush of 20 ml of saline is made at the fourth minute after infusion has been completed.

In response to dipyridamole infusion, most people will develop a headache or full feeling in the head and a sensation of warmth. Some will experience chest pain and some angina and some anxiety. Nausea is also common. A few will experience mid to lower abdominal pain and rarely leg pain. If angina-like symptoms or ischemic EKG changes develop prior to the administration of the tracer, oxygen may be administered without compromising the validity of the study. After waiting for myocardial localization of the tracer, 1 minute for ^{201}Tl, 2 minutes for ^{99m}Tc sestamibi or tetrofosmin, 75–100 mg of aminophylline are intravenously flushed in over 1 minute. If the symptoms do not abate, or, if ischemic EKG changes persist, nitroglycerine can be used. Some laboratories, including ours, routinely administer aminophylline at the conclusion of the study. It is probably best to err on the side of giving aminophylline rather than withholding it. At the conclusion of the test, we give the patient a cup of coffee or tea brewed by boiling the bag with the water adding cream or Lipumol® since caffeine has a longer plasma half-time than aminophylline (that is less than the plasma half-time of dipyridamole), and the fat speeds hepatic and gall bladder emptying.

Adenosine is infused intravenously 140 mg/Kg/minute over 6 minutes with administration of the myocardial tracer performed at the end of the third minute through a Y-tube or separate venous access in order not to interrupt the adenosine infusion, which continues another 2–3 minutes since adenosine has a very short half-time in the plasma, estimated on the order of 10–30 seconds. Because of the short half-life, constant infusion must be maintained, requiring an infusion pump. More than 80% of patients experience adverse side effects, including chest pain often indistinguishable from angina in more than half, jaw pain, flushing and nausea. In addition, about 10% develop A-V block that may or may not reverse after the infusion has ended. For this reason, in addition to the contraindications listed for dipyridamole, patients with a sick sinus syndrome or prolonged A-V conduction may best be studied by another method. Symptoms may be ameliorated by simultaneous low level exercise performed during the infusion.

Dobutamine Infusion

Dobutamine has the same physiologic effects as exercise. Its use lacks the additional prognostic power that is derived from functional parameters obtained during physical stress, including exercise duration and capacity and reproduction of symptoms. These are used in the Duke scoring system. Dobutamine has a half-time of about 2 minutes in plasma. Infusion is begun at a low rate of 5 μg/Kg/minute for 3 minutes, increased to 10 μ/Kg/min, and increased an additional 10 μg/Kg/min each three minutes until tolerance or a maximum of 40 μg/Kg/min is reached, at which point the myocardial perfusion tracer is administered and the infusion level continued for an additional 2 minutes. During this period, wall motion can be analyzed by ultrasound, or a first pass study that can be compared with baseline parameters. Some have used intravenous atropine to enhance the chronotropic response. EKG ST–T changes are common as are ventricular ectopy and chest pain. Headache, flushing and dyspnea are also frequent. Metoprolol, a selective $beta_1$ adrenergic antagonist, 5 to 10 mg, may be given intravenously for persistent ischemic symptoms, an exaggerated pressor response, increases in ventricular response due to enhanced A-V conduction or development of frequent ectopic ventricular beats.

Nitrates

Nitrates exert their main effect by producing vasodilatation, chiefly in the capacitance vessels, but also in the resistance vessels, reducing myocardial preload, and, to a lesser extent, after-load.[77] In addition, nitrates may dilate stenotic vessels, increasing flow through collateral vessels.[78–80] Although administering nitrates to normal individuals has no measurable effect on wall motion or systolic function, nitrates can improve wall motion and systolic function in those with CAD.[81–83] The magnitude of these effects may depend upon the development of an adequate collateral circulation that may carry additional flow. Intravenously administered nitrates have been used with tests that measure either wall motion or perfusion. Enhanced wall contractility or perfusion in response to nitrate administration predicts the presence of hibernating myocardial tissue that may have improved function if blood flow can be restored.[84–86] The study can also be performed by giving a single dose of sublingual nitroglycerine or spray, and monitoring blood pressure. If the systolic blood pressure decreases by 10 mm Hg, the myocardial perfusion tracer is injected obtaining a first pass RNA, followed 30–45 minutes later by myocardial perfusion imaging. If the target blood pressure drop does not occur after 4 minutes, a second tablet of nitroglycerine or spray is given and 4 minutes later the tracer administered. Figure 22–13 shows the application of this study in a patient with severely impaired LV function secondary to CAD. Following the study, he underwent successful CABG, resulting in considerably improved LV function. This is a relatively simple study to perform, that measures wall motion using a first pass study during injection as well as myocardial perfusion by imaging later. It appears to have the same ability as rest-redistribution thallium studies in predicting which segments will and which will not recover function following revascularization, approximately a 75% accuracy.[87]

IMAGE ACQUISITION

Correct quality control of instruments is essential to insure uniform camera response, linearity of data transfer, linearity of mapping in the field of view and best instrument resolution. High-count flood field data correction mapping is essential when SPECT is used, as is a rigorously maintained and verified center of rotation (COR) for the instrument.

Patient instruction and cooperation is critical for obtaining optimal studies. Gaining cooperation by fully informing the patient and answering all questions in straightforward language is essential for establishing a good relationship. While readying the patient for imaging, it is important to ascertain if there are any implanted devices which might interfere with imaging (pacemakers, breast implants), whether there is current or has been prior disease which might interfere or distort the anatomy (severe kyphoscolosis, situs inversus, pneumonectomy), to note the patient's size and weight, and, in women, to note bra size. In most women, it is best to remove the brassiere for imaging.

A few minutes spent in explaining why it is important to breathe in a quiet, normal pattern and not talk, sigh or yawn so as to limit diaphragmatic motion is well worthwhile. Every effort should be made to make the patient comfortable prior to beginning imaging so that restlessness will not degrade the imaging procedure. For supine positioning appropriate use of sponges to support the arms over the head can help. When imaging the patient prone, the head should be turned so the patient is comfortable, and the position noted so that it can be reproduced if another set of images is made.

Planar Imaging

Nuclear medicine images require an adequate number of counts from the organ of interest for best resolution. In the case of cardiac imaging, the count rates from thallium images are lower than those obtained from technetium labeled agents. On the other hand, the relative proportion of counts coming from the heart are higher in the thallium image than the technetium images that include relatively more counts from structures below the diaphragm. The count rate depends not only on the pharmaceutical, but also on the sensitivity of the camera, which is in part inherent in the instrument, but most related to the collimator selection. Usually, a low energy all purpose collimator is selected, but with more sensitive detectors, a high-resolution collimator can be used without significantly reducing the count rate. When the count rate is reduced, it takes longer to accumulate sufficient data and provides increased chance of patient motion. In general, ten minutes of data accumulation per view for thallium-201 and 5 minutes for technetium-99m suffice.

Using a fixed time rather than count for each image makes the views more comparable with one another, although differing amounts of tissue interposition lead to varying absorption effects on the different views. Three views are routinely obtained, but should be supplemented by additional views when necessary. These are the best left anterior oblique (LAO) view with the detector positioned between a 30 to 60 degree angle to the thorax to show the best perpendicular view of the septum. The anterior view is obtained by moving the detector 45 degrees counterclockwise from the best LAO view. Finally, a left lateral view is obtained with the patient lying right side down, which causes the left diaphragm to descend and have reduced motion. For this view, the detector is positioned perpendicular to the chest and not slanted to follow patient contour.

The anatomy of these images correlated with the usual coronary artery supply to these regions is shown in Figure 22–4. This figure also illustrates the utility of the right lateral decubitus view in defining the inferior wall. In this position, the left diaphragm that is "up," descends and moves very little, pulling away from the inferior cardiac wall and reducing motion artifact. The patient illustrated is morbidly obese, weighing 550 pounds and could not fit onto the table for SPECT imaging. The first three images were performed with the patient standing in front of the camera. The left lateral view was repeated with the patient in the decubitus position, lying on his right side on a mattress on the floor beneath the camera.

SPECT

Guidelines for standardizing SPECT myocardial perfusion imaging have been published[88] (down-loadable from www.asnc.org), but instrumentation

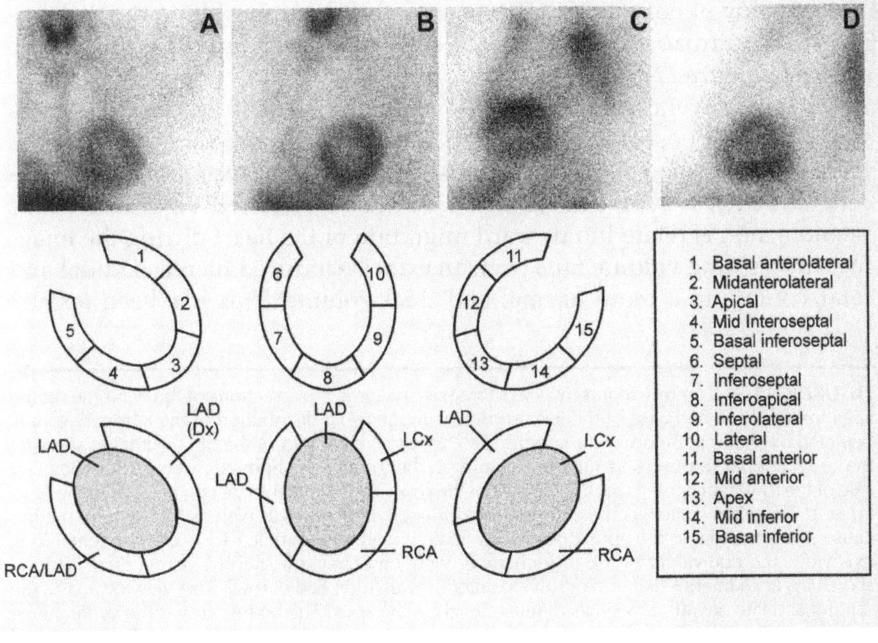

FIGURE 22–4. Planar thallium images in a 550-pound man who could not fit into the gantry for SPECT images. The best LAO view perpendicular to the septal plane, *B*, provides a guide for the anterior view, *A*, in which the camera head is rotated 45 degrees counterclockwise from the LAO position, followed by the left lateral view, *C*. In image *C*, the inferobasilar wall is attenuated by soft tissue. Since the patient could not fit under the camera for a right lateral decubitus view, the patient was imaged by having him lie in the right lateral decubitus position on a mattress placed on the floor, and lowering the camera to obtain the image in *D*. This shows the inferobasilar wall has normal activity. Beneath the images are diagrams of the wall segments as well as the coronary supply to them. (Diagrams after Wackers, 1992, by permission from the author and the publisher.)

and technique advances occur rapidly and are likely to outstrip the slower pace of collective committee opinion. SPECT imaging may be performed with the patient prone or supine. If possible, if the patient is short and obese with an overabundance of soft tissue, the right lateral decubitus position with the right side dependent may be best to minimize absorption artifacts. Each position has advantages and problems.

In the supine position large breasts overlying only portions rather than the entire heart can cause anterior wall attenuation artifact. In addition, there is frequently an absorption artifact in the proximal inferior wall related to attenuation from the diaphragm, which is relatively high with the patient supine, particularly in short, plump patients. This can be remedied by placing the patient prone, or in the right lateral decubitus position (Fig. 22–6). With the patient prone, absorption artifact related to the imaging table interposed between the patient and the detector may attenuate anterior wall activity, but the deficit is usually readily appreciated as an artifact because of its non-anatomic distribution. The right lateral decubitus position has some advantages, but most imaging tables are not designed for good support with the patient in this position so that its use requires a very cooperative patient. The anatomy of normal SPECT images and the relationship to the three dimensional cardiac anatomy as well as the coronary artery territories are shown in Figure 22–5.

To circumvent redistribution when thallium 201 is used for the stress study, prompt post stress imaging is important. Conversely, if imaging is performed too soon after exercise, a spurious inferior wall and basal inferoseptal deficit may appear in those that have exercised vigorously. This phenomenon is related to upward migration of the heart during the imaging time as lung volume falls from an exercise induced increased tidal and total volume to a more normal end tidal volume. This has been termed

FIGURE 22–5. *A.* Top row represents the short axis anatomic cross sections of the ventricles at the apex, mid-portion and base of the left ventricle with the usual distribution of the coronary supply depicted by shading. Below the anatomic sketches are the tracings of the SPECT images showing the usual arterial territories as different shadings. The top row is short axis views from apex (left side of the row of images) to base (right side of the row). The right ventricle can be seen in the basilar cuts. This view evaluates the anterior, inferior and lateral walls as well as the septum, but because it is tangential to the apex does not evaluate it well. The middle row is the horizontal long axis view, the equivalent of the four-chamber view on echocardiography, perpendicular to the short axis, from inferior (left end of row) to anterior wall (right end of row). This view evaluates the septum and lateral wall, as well as different levels of the apex. The bottom row is the vertical long axis view perpendicular to the other two axes from the septum (far left image) to the lateral wall (far right). This view allows direct comparison of the anterior and inferior walls as well as the apex. Note that it depicts the entire apex as being supplied by a wrap-around LAD, which is not always the case. The anterior (A), septal (S), lateral (L) and inferior (I) walls as well as the apex (AX) are indicated on the tracings. *B* is the actual images, presented as gray on black above and as color-coded images beneath. The color code changes abruptly at 54% of maximum counts. Because the color images are coded for counts and change abruptly, they are not capable of showing the nuances that can be appreciated on the continuous gray scale. In practice, both the gray scale, an inverted gray scale (black on clear backgound) and color images are viewed and interpreted directly from the computer display.

A

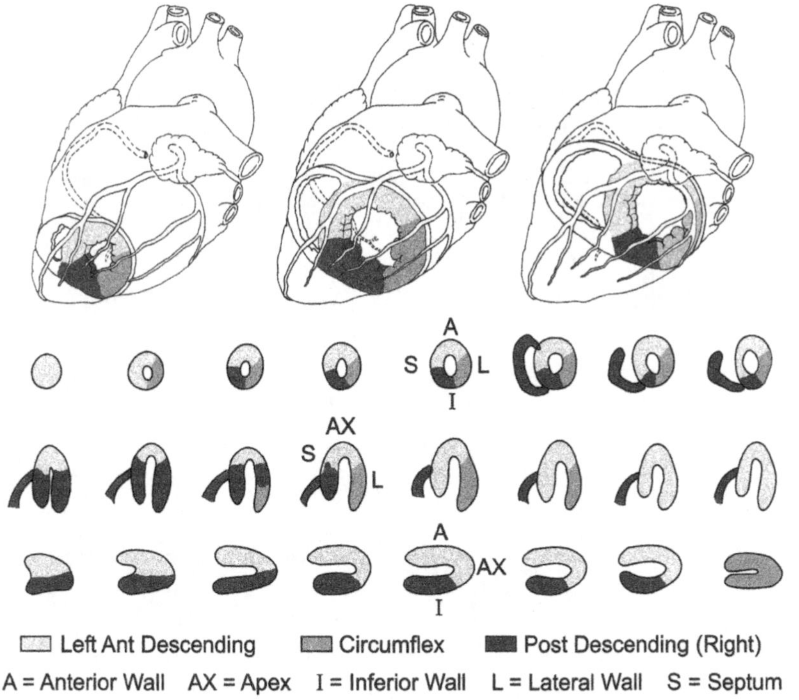
A
S
L
I
AX
S
L
A
AX
I
Left Ant Descending
Circumflex
Post Descending (Right)
A = Anterior Wall
AX = Apex
I = Inferior Wall
L = Lateral Wall
S = Septum

B

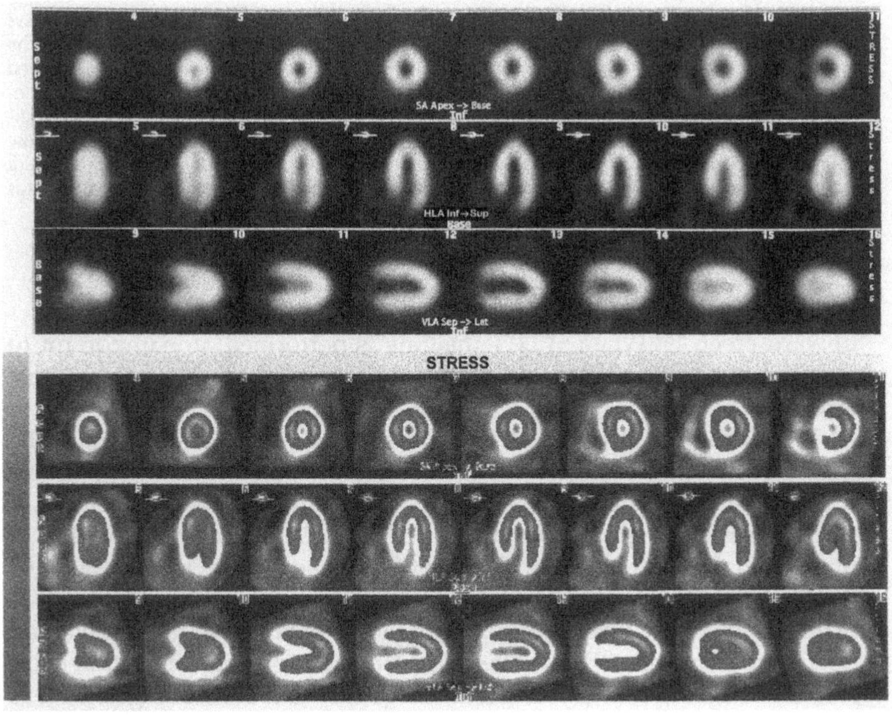
SA Apex -> Base
HLA Inf -> Sup
VLA Sep -> Lat
STRESS

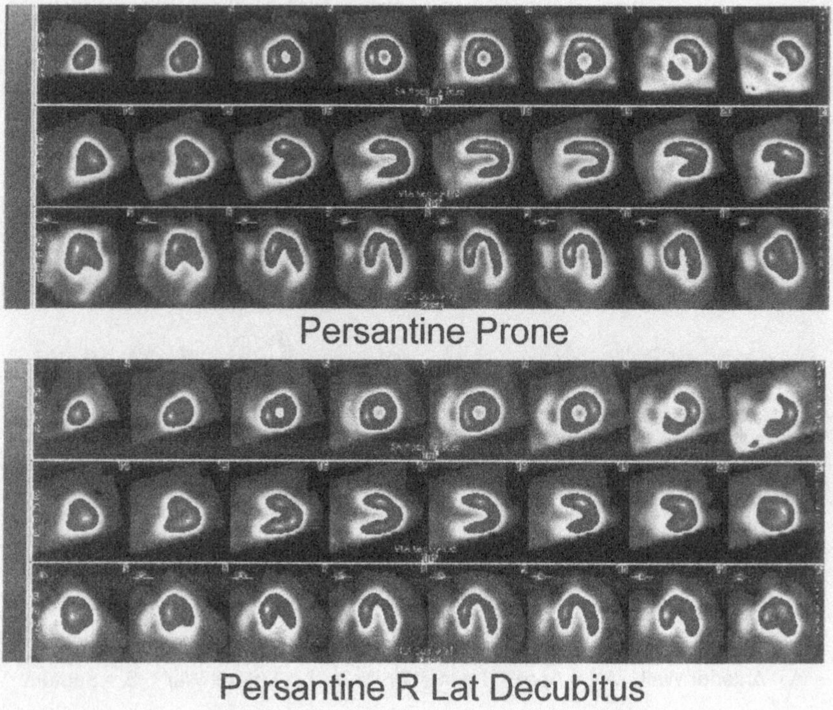

FIGURE 22–6. Comparison of prone (upper rows in the image sets) and right lateral decubitus views (beneath) from a study with injection made following persantine® infusion. The prone view is the one that we usually employ as the standard view since most patients find this comfortable. Placed in this position, patients tend to move less, but attentuation artifacts may occur in both the anterior wall due to table and soft tissue attenuation, and the inferobasilar area related to a high diaphragm. The decreased activity in the inferior wall seen at the base in the short-axis view (top row in both image sets) and in the vertical long-axis cuts (middle row in both image sets), in this patient who had a low likelihood of coronary disease, resolved when he assumed the lateral decubitus position.

"upward creep."[89] When SPECT imaging is performed, it is important to have planar images as well for purposes of quality control and anatomic correlation.

When thallium-201 is used, these images also allow assessment of the lung heart ratio, which, if elevated, indicates prolonged pulmonary transit accompanying left ventricular failure, and correlates with poor prognosis. If ^{99m}Tc-Sestamibi is used, the planar images should also be obtained within 10 minutes of injection for best evaluation of the lung uptake, and not 30 to 90 minutes later when the SPECT data is obtained. Initial data suggest that using this "immediate" image provides prognostic data similar to that obtained with thallium imaging.[90] No matter what technique is used, it is critical to inspect the images and verify the technical quality and positioning as well as ascertain the presence of artifacts, particularly motion, before dismissing the patient.

Whoever interprets SPECT images should review the rotating raw data presented on the computer monitor for motion and absorption artifacts to prevent interpretive errors. In addition, when gated SPECT is performed the moving slices that offer information concerning wall thickening and the volume rendered images that permit analysis of wall motion are best reviewed in cine mode from the computer presentation. Many laboratories, including ours, prefer to read the images directly from the computer. This permits ready adjustment of contrast over a continuously variable range as well as application of color scales as appropriate. Color scales may introduce artifacts smoothing out deficits so they are not perceived, or, exaggerating small differences in count rate making a normal area appear abnormal. While initially more difficult to interpret, a linear gray scale or inverted gray scale has the least propensity to introduce error. Great care should be taken to present images in a uniform and reproducible manner.

We use a linear gray scale, a linear inverted gray scale and a color-coded image in which the pixels with highest count rate are delineated in white so the high count rate can be easily measured. Warm red colors change abruptly to yellow at 54% of maximum when ^{99m}Tc sestamibi is used or 63% when ^{201}Tl is used. This directs the interpreter's attention to these areas on the linear gray scale images. The use of color images, while increasing the contrast between "normal" and "abnormal" tissue that has only 54% of the maximum uptake tends to obscure subtle abnormalities that are best appreciated on relatively linear gray scale images.

ANATOMIC CORRELATION

Figure 22–4 shows the views obtained with planar imaging: the anterior view, 45 degrees from the LAO view that best shows the septum separating the ventricles, and the left lateral view. This depicts the anatomic correlation of the images as well as the usual coronary artery supply. The myocardial wall parallel to the camera presents less activity to the detector than the walls more perpendicular to the plane of the camera. The detector sees the activity of the wall perpendicular to it stacked on end, while the wall furthest from the camera has its activity attenuated by distance and the non-radioactive cardiac blood pool. This leads to the appearance of visualization of the left ventricular cavity.

Normal areas of decreased activity occur at the left ventricular valve planes, in the region of the membranous septum and at the apex.[91] Artifactually decreased activity may occur in supine images in the inferior wall related to diaphragmatic attenuation as indicated above under the discussion of positioning. A thick right ventricle may also cause attenuation of the inferior wall on the anterior view. A common pitfall causing decreased activity in the anterior or anterior lateral wall is related to breast absorption artifact. In obese patients absorption by overlying tissue, including breast, abdomen and skin folds may cause a number of artifacts.[91] Occasionally, if the patient can stand, upright imaging can help by causing the diaphragm to descend and the heart to assume a more vertical position as well as allowing the abdominal bulge to descend permitting the patient to be positioned with the thorax closer to the detector. (Figure 22–4)

Figure 22–5 shows the standard SPECT views obtained. The anatomic correlation of the images as well as the usual regions supplied by the major coronary arteries are depicted. For quantitative analysis as well as condensation of a large amount of data, parametric presentation of the short axis views as a series of concentric circles, a so-called "bull's-eye" can be helpful. The apical region presents unique problems which have been dealt with in the Cedars Emory Quantitative Analysis program, CEQUAL®, by using two different images, one with evenly spaced concentric rings that presents a more accurate anatomic display, the other with fatter inner rings weighted for volume, emphasizing the apical contribution, represents a more quantitatively accurate display.

Anatomic correlation of arterial territories with the bull's-eye display assigns perfusion deficits to a particular coronary artery or overlapping distribution between two territories. Comparison with normal data bases permits reasonably accurate and reproducible quantitation of the perfusion deficit as well as helping to differentiate areas of decreased perfusion which do not change between stress and rest perfusion studies from those with normal or improved perfusion at rest. This kind of quantitation does not replace careful visual interpretation, but serves as a guide and aid.

IMAGE INTERPRETATION

Preliminary Observations

As indicated above, prior to interpreting the final SPECT image, the rotating raw data should be inspected for motion and absorption artifact. The planar images accompanying the SPECT study should be used to evaluate patient habitus, interposition of soft tissue, cardiac size and position as well as ancillary findings such as increased pulmonary uptake and noting any other areas of abnormal uptake that might represent non-cardiac abnormalities. The orientation of the heart should be noted. Horizontal hearts are subject to inferior wall artifacts. Counterclockwise or dextrorotaion of the heart may result in decreased lateral wall activity compared with the septum, while clockwise or levorotaion may have the opposite effect, causing a relative decrease in septal activity compared with the lateral wall.[92]

Misaligned Cuts

Small hearts with apparently thick walls are more likely to be seen in women rather than men. Inspection of the short axis transverse cuts offers the best opportunity for comparing the symmetry of uptake in the opposing walls, while the long axis views offer the best evaluation of the apex that is only tangentially imaged on the short axis views. The short axis images of the left ventricle should be circular. If they are elliptical, it usually means that the short axis has been selected in a non-perpendicular fashion to the long axis of the left ventricle. In addition, the septum should be oriented vertically and positioned the same in both stress and rest views. This can be ascertained by inspecting the position of the right ventricular wall in relationship to the left. The correctness of the long axis slices should also be verified. They should look like horseshoes. When the long axis is misaligned on the horizontal and vertical slices, one side of the horseshoe appears foreshortened and the apparent apical area is displaced. Incorrect selection of the vertical long axis plane causes apical displacement medially or laterally towards either the distal septum or distal lateral wall causing decreased activity in these regions. In the horizontal long axis views, off axis selection of the plane sections results in displacing the apex superiorly or inferiorly to cause apparent thinning of either the distal anterior or distal inferior wall.

Areas of normal thinning of activity include the apex and upper septum. Generally the septum has slightly less activity than the lateral wall no matter what tracer is used.[93] In some hypertensive patients, the lateral wall will have significantly more activity than the septum.[94] In the case of asymmetric septal hypertrophy, the septum appears thick. Occasionally increased activity occurs in the lateral wall in the region of the anterolateral and posterolateral papillary muscle. Sometimes apical hot spots occur. Often hot spots are the result of inappropriate application of filters in a patient whose study suffers from a low count rate. This is one of the reasons to increase the dose in obese individuals. Often the hot spots themselves are not so much the problem as is the fact that the images are scaled to the hot spot so that other areas appear to have decreased activity. Most quantitative data-bases were constructed from a relatively normal sized population and should be applied with caution to patients whose body habitus differs significantly from the usual.

Areas of decreased activity that do not correspond to an anatomic coronary artery distribution should be viewed with suspicion. For example, an isolated mid left ventricular wall deficit might be due to an abnormality in the distribution of a large diagonal branch, but with large breasts or large amount of soft tissue in the anterior chest wall interposed between the detector and anterior wall, or data obtained with the patient prone with the table interposed between the detector and anterior chest wall, it is more likely artifact.

Verifying Correct Gating

If a gating system is available, interpretation of perfusion deficits should be made in conjunction with wall thickening. The reconstructed LV curve should be examined for gating artifacts. If the LV volume curve does not follow the expected pattern, there most likely has been a gating problem.

Segmental Wall Thickening

Use of gated imaging can considerably aid in interpreting activity deficits. Failure of regional wall thickening in the area of concern bolsters the conclusion that the area is abnormally perfused. On the other hand, the preservation of wall thickening suggests artifact rather than decreased blood flow causing the decreased activity. Wall thickening should be assessed in cine mode. Both gray scale and a standardized color code can be used. Here the eye is looking for an increase in intensity with systole of the area in question. Areas that start as decreased intensity because of an absorption artifact will display an increase in the count rate and density with systole, although they will not achieve the same intensity as adjacent normal areas.

Wall Motion

Wall motion should also be evaluated in cine mode using a reproducible display and turning the 3-dimensional image to view the left ventricle from all aspects to gain best appreciation of the motion of the wall edge moving parallel to the image plane. Like any other cine projection of the left ventricle the presence or absence and degree of wall motion abnormality should be characterized and quantified. Except in very small volume hearts, in which the margin for error determination of LV endocardial surface is relatively large, the LVEF from the gated SPECT image is both reproducible and accurate. The EF corresponds very well to the LVEF obtained from the radionuclide angiogram first pass study obtained at rest. Since the data contains only eight points on the LV volume curve it tends to underestimate the EF when the heart rate is rapid.

Quantitative Polar Map Displays

Accurate interpretation requires knowledge of the usual coronary artery perfusion pattern and common variations. The key question is, "does this perfusion deficit fit into the usual coronary artery distribution pattern or a common variant?" This decision can often be aided with the use of a quantitative polar map program. These are usually presented as a bull's-eye display, with the center of the target representing the apex with the concentric rings depicting regions toward the cardiac base as the outer rings are reached. Using polar map patterns from patients with angiographically defined coronary artery disease, boundaries of the most probable distribution of vascular territories were defined.[95] The CEQUAL® program indicates the major coronary artery distribution.

A number of quantitative "normal" databases were assembled, presented in polar map coordinate form, and validated.[96–100] The images presented in this chapter are from the commercially available CEQUAL® program.[101] The SPECT visual anatomy should be confirmed, and attention directed to possibly abnormal areas, by information from the CEQUAL® image. The quantitative guide is not a substitute for careful visual assessment of the data. The CEQUAL® images are shown in the lower right corner of the illustrated cases presented in Figures 22–8 through 22–10 and Figure 22–12. The opinion concerning the likelihood of a region of decreased activity representing a perfusion deficit must be modified by observations concerning the presence or absence of absorption or motion artifacts.

Infarct versus Ischemia

Once the decision has been made that the decreased activity represents a perfusion deficit and its probable vascular distribution determined, the abnormality should be characterized with regard to size, and degree of decreased activity and whether or not there is significantly improved perfusion in this region on the resting images. The stress images must compared with the resting images with great care taken to ensure that the images correspond exactly in plane of cut as well as each individual image to its counterpart. Often the computer makes these alignment choices. They should be checked visually.

The distinction between infarction and ischemia causing decreased perfusion on the stress image rests upon whether or not the perfusion deficit persists on the rest image, indicating infarction; or whether it significantly improves or returns to normal, indicating ischemia. Although most perfusion deficits that don't change between stress and resting studies represent infarction, some, depending upon the clinical circumstances, will be due to stunned or hibernating myocardium. While some interpreters suggest that the interpretation of ischemia rests upon return of perfusion to nearly normal, smaller changes can also represent significant ischemia, particularly if large in extent. Areas of improved perfusion often exist adjacent to fixed perfusion deficits, representing peri-infarct ischemia, frequently in the regions of the borderland between two major coronary artery territories.

Figure 22–7 demonstrates a patient with LAD ischemia, Figure 22–8 a patient with circumflex ischemia and Figure 22–9, a patient with right coronary artery ischemia as well as the response to revascularization. Studies in patients post CABG may show non anatomic distribution of ischemia, that is, areas of proximal wall reversible deficits with more normal distribution in the wall distal to the area of ischemia. These findings relate to the placement and patency of grafts relative to significant native artery

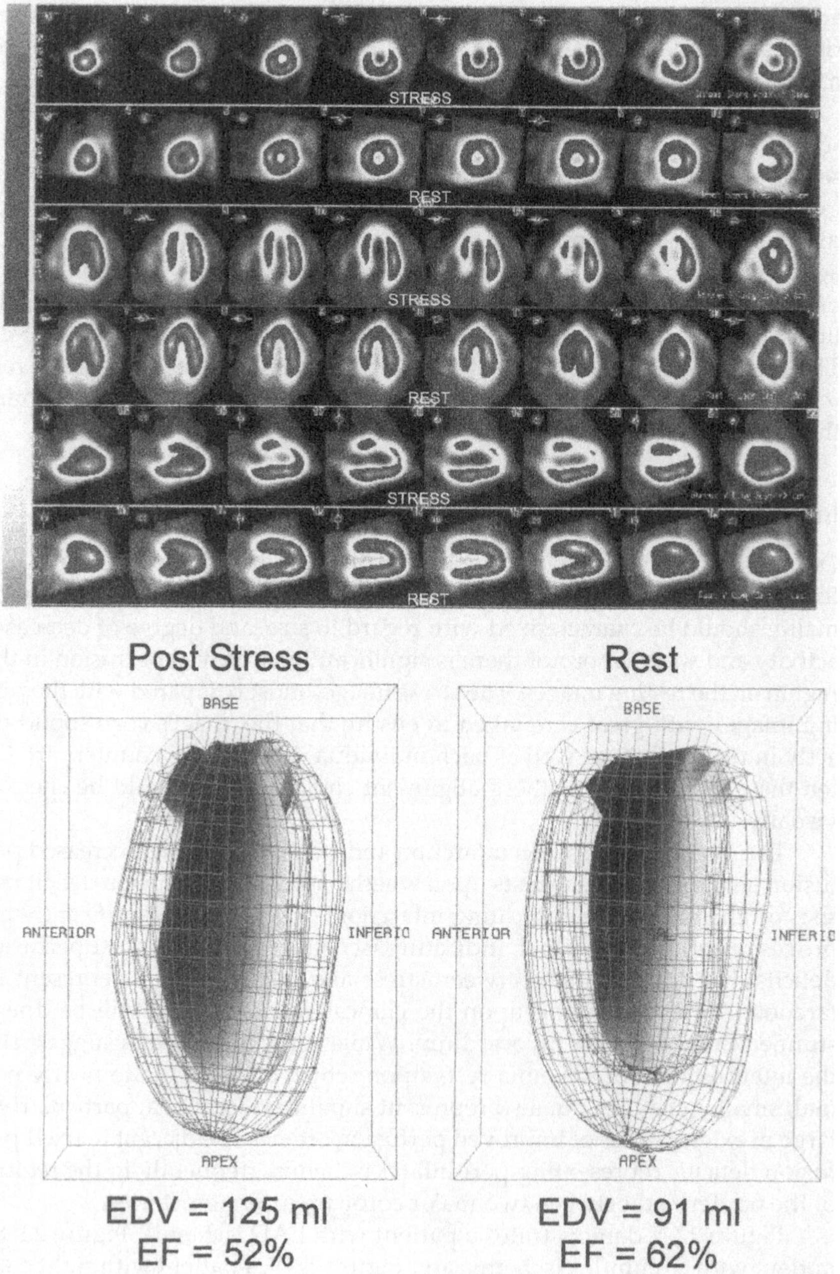
STRESS
REST
STRESS
REST
STRESS
REST
Post Stress
Rest
BASE
ANTERIOR
INFERIO
APEX
BASE
ANTERIOR
INFERIO
APEX
EDV = 125 ml
EF = 52%
EDV = 91 ml
EF = 62%

stenoses. Following successful PTCA and stenting, if no stunning has taken place, perfusion should promptly return to normal if the artery remains patent.

Significant Ancillary Findings in Ischemia

Wall motion and LV function in ischemic areas may provide significant prognostic information.[102] The post stress data using the ^{99m}Tc agents is accumulated at least 30 minutes following the stress procedure, during which period the patient is usually resting seated or recumbent. The presence of decreased wall motion and LV function in the post-stress image as compared with the resting image indicates post stress stunning, a marker for severe stenosis (Fig. 22–7, 22–9, 22–10).[103]

Increased pulmonary activity, usually related to prolonged pulmonary transit as a direct result of LV failure, is a marker for poor prognosis. Another ominous ancillary finding is transient ischemic dilatation. It is characterized by an apparent dilatation of the left ventricular cavity with an increase in diameter as seen on the post (either exercise or pharmacologic) stress image 1.2 times the diameter measured on the resting study image. Whether this is related to actual post stress LV dilatation due to stunning that persists up to an hour after the stress or represents an artifact of subendocardial ischemia producing an apparently larger LV cavity is uncertain. In any case, the finding is a marker of severe and extensive coronary artery disease and portends a poor prognosis. (See Fig. 22–10, 22–11 and 22–12.)

Quantitation

For purposes of reproducibility, diagnostic certitude and prognosis, a semi-quantitative approach using a segmental deficit approach has been

FIGURE 22–7. Post-stress stunning of the anterior wall due to severe LAD ischemic disease. Stress (top) and rest images (immediately beneath each stress row) of a 62-year-old hypertensive man who smoked. He experienced angina every time he played tennis. On the standard Bruce protocol he achieved 10 METS, developing angina and ST depression. The SPECT stress images show large anterior wall and apical deficits that have normal perfusion on the rest study performed the following day. The lower images represent selected views from the gated wall motion study obtained with the perfusion images. These are best viewed in cine mode. The outer cage represents the outside edge of the left ventricular wall at end diastole, while the inner cage represents the endocardial surface of the left ventricle at end diastole. The shaded, solid gray portion represents the left ventricle at end sysole, roughly equivalent to the left ventriculogram. On the post-stress study there is hypokinesis of the distal anterior wall and apex. On the study performed with injection made at rest, there is only apical hypokinesis. Note the significant difference in volume as well as decreased ejection fraction on the study performed about 1 hour following the injection with the patient on the treadmill. These indicators of post-stress stunning led to prompt intervention. At catheterization, there was occlusion of the proximal LAD, but wall motion was normal. A 3 × 18 mm stent was successfully placed across the occlusion.

A

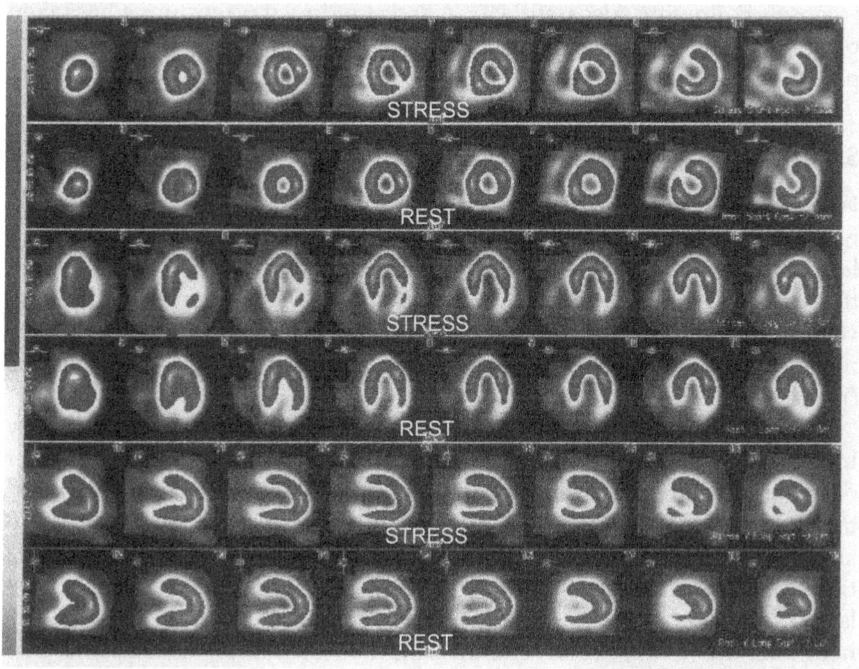

STRESS
REST
STRESS
REST
STRESS
REST

B

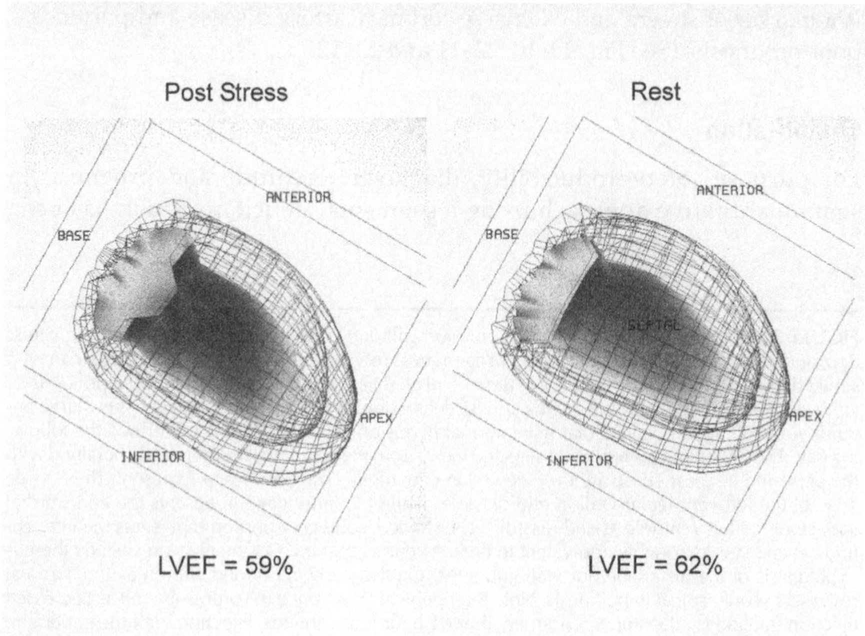

Post Stress
Rest
ANTERIOR
BASE
APEX
INFERIOR
ANTERIOR
BASE
SEPTAL
APEX
INFERIOR
LVEF = 59%
LVEF = 62%

C

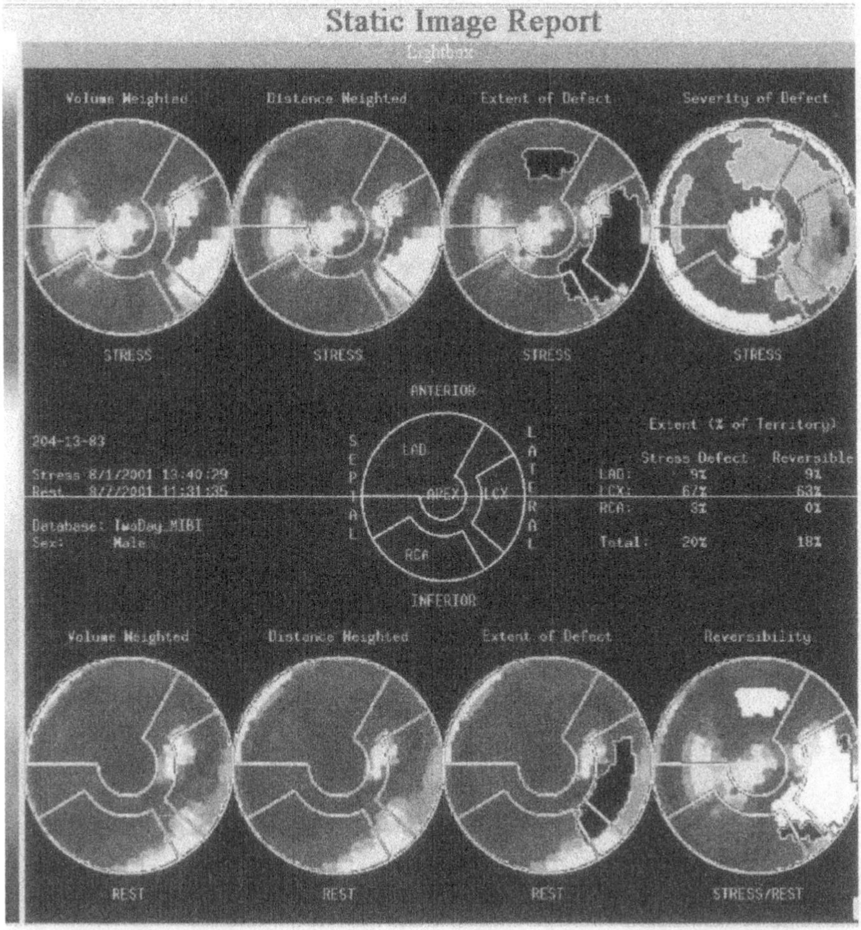

FIGURE 22–8. Lateral wall ischemia due to circumflex disease in a 64-year-old man with hypertension and elevated LDL cholesterol level. He developed 3mm ST depression during the 9th minute of a Bruce protocol treadmill stress study. The SPECT images, *A,* show a large perfusion deficit in the inferior lateral wall on the stress portion of the study that perfuses nearly normally on the resting images seen best on the horizontal long axis views. The RAO gated wall motion images, *B,* show moderate apical hypokinesis and a normal ejection fraction. The top row of polar map bull's-eye *(C)* plots based on the data from the stress images shows significantly decreased perfusion in the circumflex territory on the volume weighted (far left image that gives the best representation of ventricular mass involved) and distance weighted (the second map from the left that gives the best representation of anatomic area involved) while the extent of defect representation (map second from the right end) shows as black those areas that are two standard deviations below the normal database population. The severity map, far right includes not only the extent of the defect, but also indicates how much below 2 standard deviations the affected areas are. The deficit in the anterior wall on the stress polar maps was deemed insignificant, because it can be seen that the septum is not lined up vertically on the SPECT images so that the bull's-eye program misinterprets the upper septum as a portion of the anteroseptal wall. The bottom row of polar maps from the resting portion of the study shows a much smaller extent of the perfusion deficit. Finally, the bottom right polar map shows the degree to which the perfusion improves, and indicates that it is reversible. At catheterization, there was a proximal lesion of the posterolateral marginal branch of the circumflex artery.

A

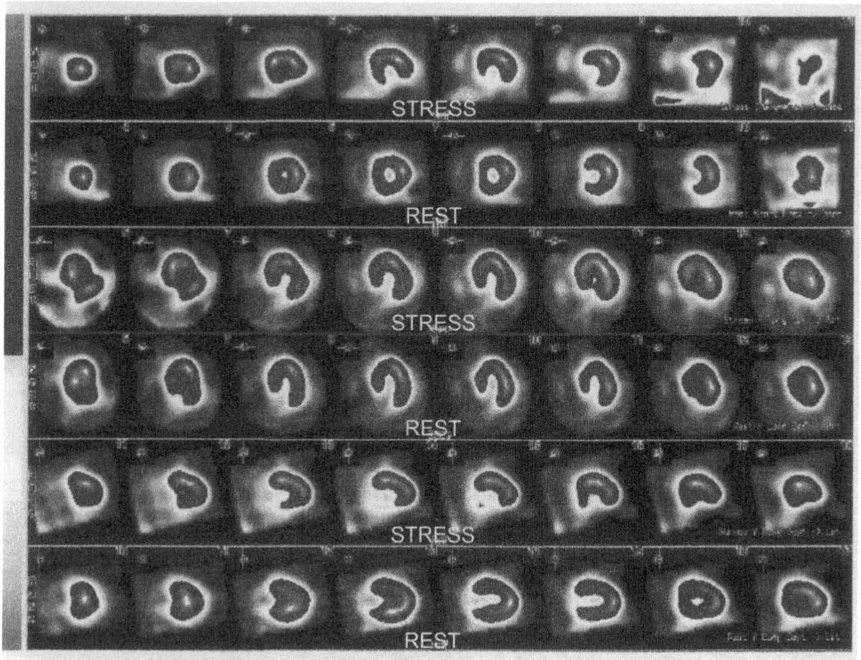
STRESS
REST
STRESS
REST
STRESS
REST

B

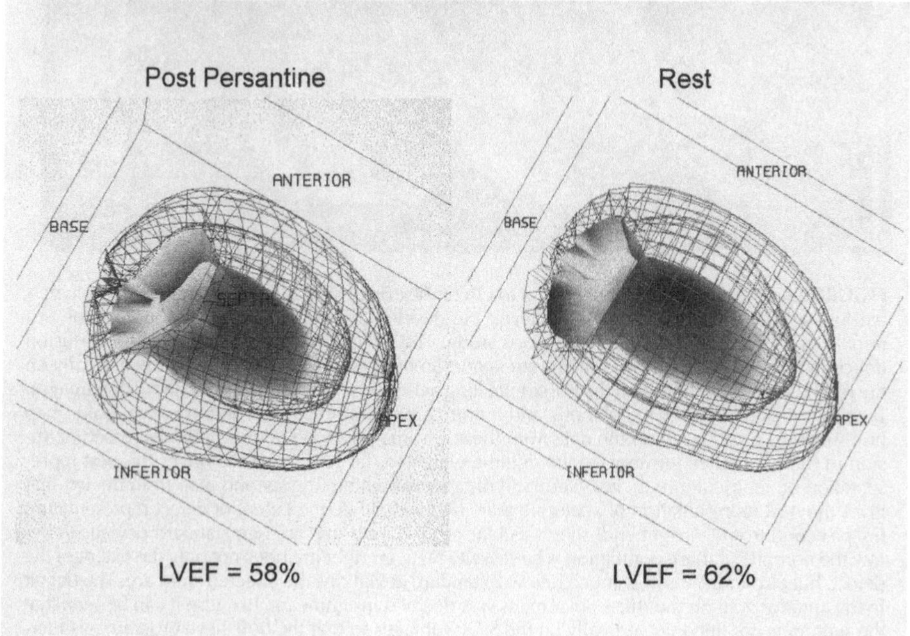
Post Persantine
Rest
ANTERIOR
BASE
SEPTAL
APEX
INFERIOR
ANTERIOR
BASE
APEX
INFERIOR
LVEF = 58%
LVEF = 62%

C

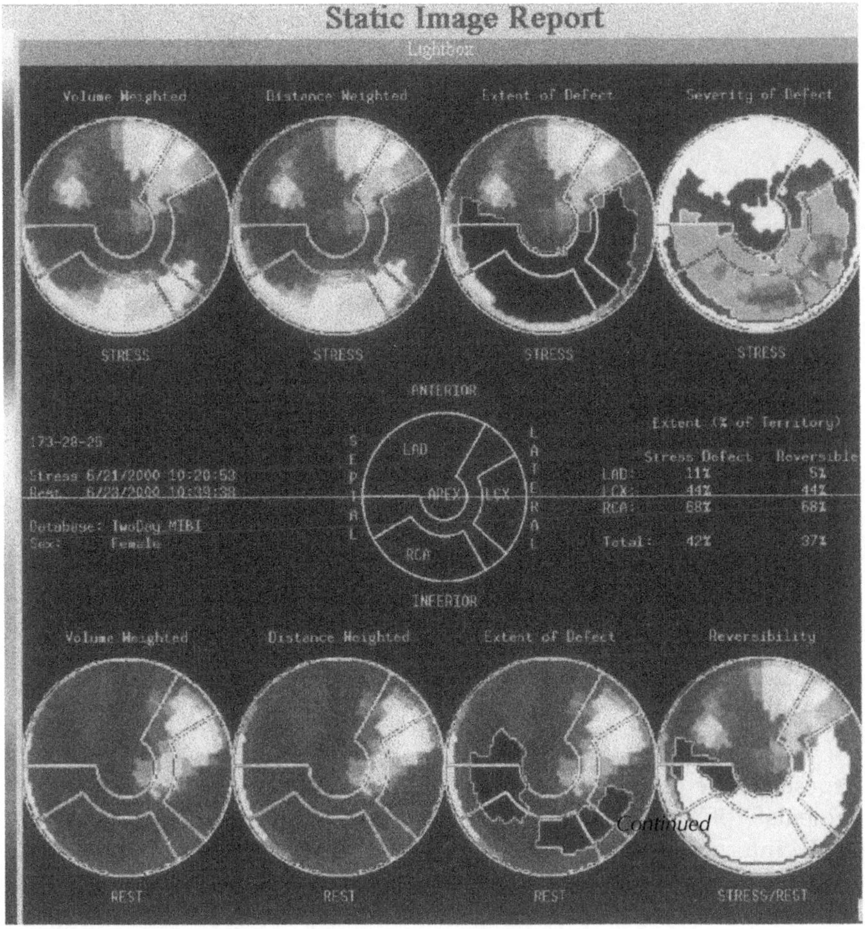

FIGURE 22–9*A–C.* Inferior wall ischemia due to right coronary artery disease in a 52-year-old woman who smoked and had a strong family history of coronary artery disease with two brothers who died from coronary artery disease before reading the age of 50. The SPECT persantine® and rest images, *A,* show a very large perfusion deficit in the inferior wall extending from the inferoseptal region to the lateral wall, abutting both the LAD and circumflex territories best seen on the short axis views. This region shows normal perfusion on the resting study. The RAO gated SPECT wall motion study, *B,* shows severe inferior wall hypokinesis after persantine, but only moderate inferoapical hypokinesis on the resting study, an ominous sign indicating post persantine® stunning, probably related to collateral flow steal. The bull's-eye images, *C,* show an extensive, severe, reversible inferior wall perfusion deficit involving the entire right coronary artery distribution. At catheterization, a 99% mid right coronary artery lesion was treated by angioplasty and stent placement leaving a small distal lesion and excluding a small right ventricular marginal branch. One year later, the repeat persantine® study, *D,* is normal. *Continued*

D

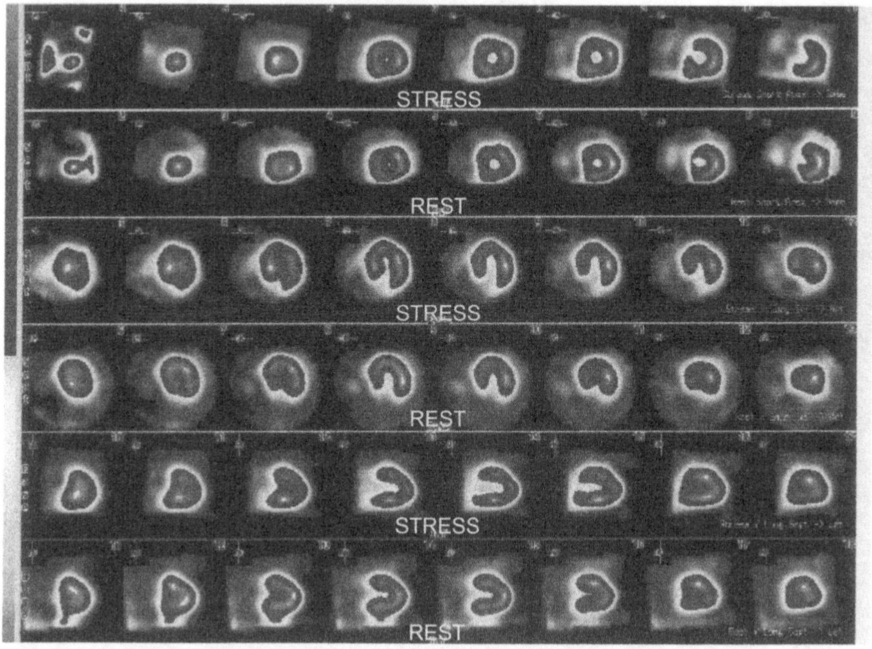

FIGURE 22–9*D*. *Continued.* One year later, the repeat persantine® study, *D,* is normal.

suggested. The templates proposed by the Cedars-Sinai group using 20 segments[104–106] or the ACC and ASNC using 17 segments can be used during the interpretation process. The score for each segment is entered as: normal = 0, slight reduction (probably normal) = 1, moderate reduction (probably abnormal) = 2, severe reduction of uptake = 3, and finally, absent uptake = 4. These templates as well as a template that can be downloaded from a website can be obtained from DuPont Pharmaceuticals (www.cardiolite.com) or from ASNC (www.ascn.org).[106] The higher the summed stress score, the more certitude there is that the study is abnormal, the worse the prognosis and the higher the risk group to which the patient can appropriately be assigned. The summed rest score can also be determined. The difference between the summed stress and rest scores provides a semi-quantitative assessment of the degree and amount of ischemia.

The same semi-quantitative approach can be applied to segmental wall motion analysis using a six point scoring system: 0 = normal, 1 = mild hypokinesis, 2 = moderate hypokinesis, 3 = severe hypokinesis 4= akinesis 5 = dyskinesis.[105]

A semiquantitative score may also be applied to wall thickening: 0 = normal, 1 = mild (equivocal) reduction, 2 = moderate-severe (definite) reduction, 3 = no detectable thickening.

Reverse Redistribution

Occasionally areas that show a small or no perfusion deficit on the post stress images will show the presence of a new or larger perfusion deficit on the resting injection study. This so-called "reverse redistribution" finding may represent the presence of a subendocardial infarct supplied by a patent coronary artery.[107] Under these circumstances, the increased blood flow achieved during the stress maneuver delivers enough tracer to obscure the partial wall thickness deficit which then becomes apparent on the resting study with less tracer deposition in the region compared with adjacent areas. After acute infarction, the finding appears on delayed resting studies done within the first week after intervention to open the artery. In this case, the initial rather than delayed resting image is more predictive of the final infarct size.[108] Sometimes with the low count rates encountered in thallium imaging, this finding may be artifactual when inappropriate background subtraction techniques are used. Some investigators think this finding represents ischemia, but the evidence is conflicting and not, for the most part, supportive of this hypothesis.

Causes of "Reversible Deficits" Other Than Ischemia

Left Bundle Branch Block

Reversible perfusion deficits appear with bundle branch block, particularly left bundle branch block (LBBB), in the absence of demonstrable significant CAD. Prognosis is excellent in patients with LBBB, no demonstrable significant CAD on angiography and an abnormal thallium perfusion study.[109] DePuey's group found that while thallium SPECT imaging was sensitive for the diagnosis of significant CAD in the presence of LBBB, defects in the septal area were common in the absence of significant CAD.[110] The preponderance of evidence indicates that there is lack of specificity of the finding of decreased septal perfusion in LBBB when the stress is associated with production of increased heart rate. Specificity is markedly improved, although less than in the absence of conduction abnormalities, when vasodilators are used.[111,112] It is of interest that experimental right ventricular pacing in an animal model which produces late, asynchronous contraction and reduced septal thickening results in decreased septal perfusion.[113] Such a model predicts this effect would become more important at higher heart rates with disproportionately reduced diastolic intervals. Right ventricular pacing can severely reduce left ventricular function and induce abnormal left ventricular wall motion.

Patients with right bundle branch block (RBBB) without left axis deviation and those with Wolff-Parkinson-White syndrome show no loss of specificity, although the latter group had an increased prevalence of slow washout of thallium in spite of achieving good exercise performance.[114]

A

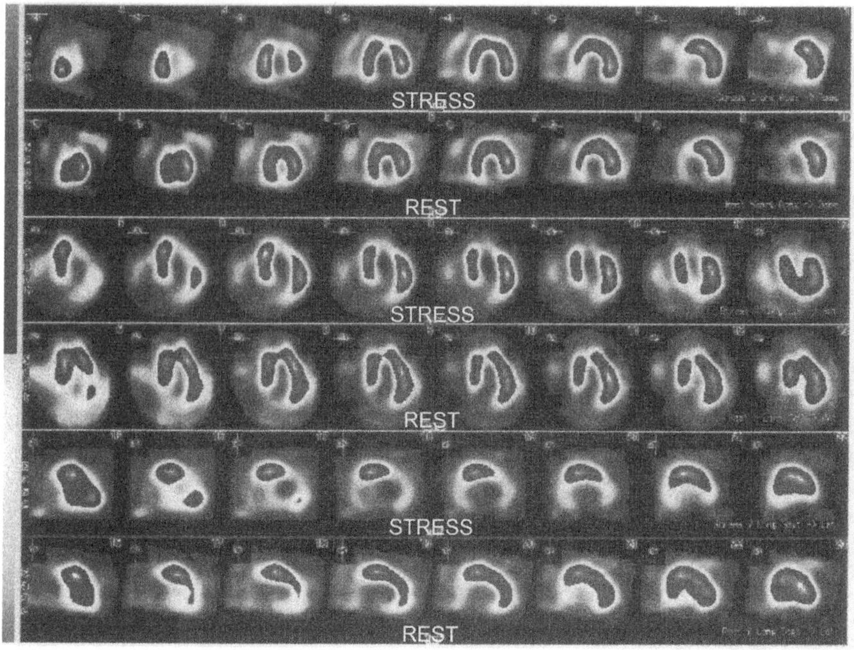
STRESS
REST
STRESS
REST
STRESS
REST

B

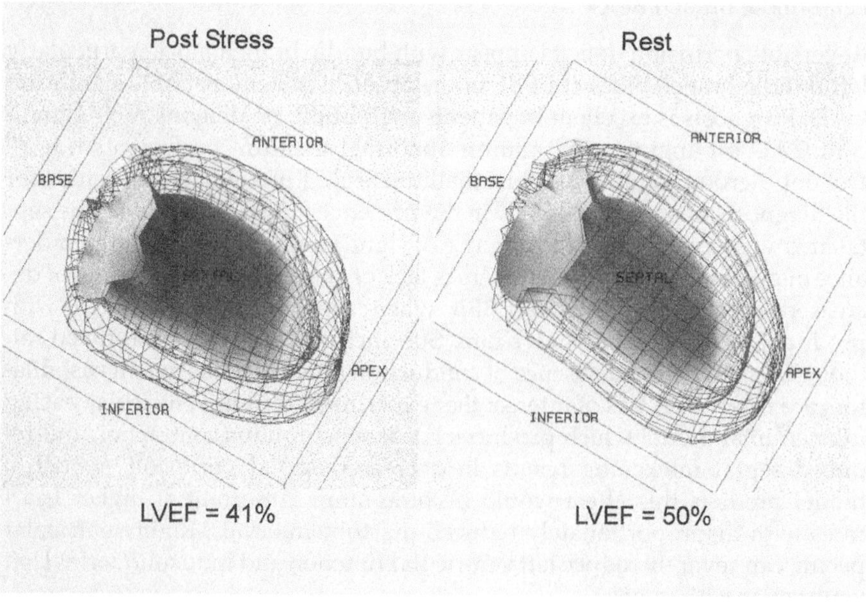
Post Stress
Rest
ANTERIOR
BASE
SEPTAL
APEX
INFERIOR
ANTERIOR
BASE
SEPTAL
APEX
INFERIOR
LVEF = 41%
LVEF = 50%

C

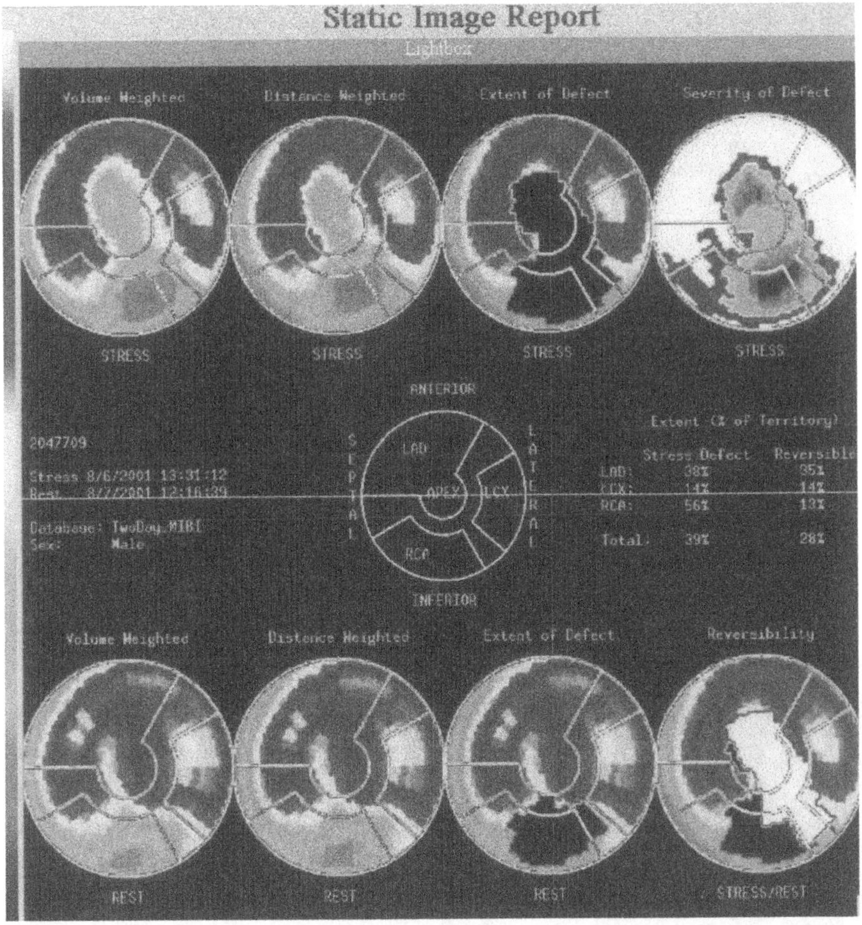

FIGURE 22–10. Transient ischemic dilatation of the left ventricle. This 62-year-old man had a large inferior wall infarct due to right coronary artery occlusion 10 months before this stress study which demonstrates post stress stunning due to severe LAD disease. SPECT images, *A*, show a large reversible anterior apical deficit at stress which has normal perfusion on the resting study. The large inferior wall perfusion deficit (infarct) persists on the resting study. The left ventricular cavity appears significantly larger on the post stress study when compared to the resting study, indicating transient ischemic dilation, a marker of multi-vessel disease and of poor prognosis. The post-persantine® RAO gated SPECT wall motion study, *B*, shows moderate anterior wall hypokinesis and severe inferior wall and apical hypokinesis with an ejection fraction of 41%. On the RAO gated image obtained following injection at rest, anterior wall motion is normal, while severe apical and inferior wall hypokinesis persist. The ejection fraction is 50%. The findings indicate post stress stunning of the anterior wall. The bull's-eye polar maps, *C*, indicate a large mid-anterior apical reversible deficit extending to the borderland territory between LAD, circumflex and right coronary artery distributions. In addition, there is a large inferior wall infarction. The polar map indicates approximately 30% of the myocardium is at ischemic risk, while approximately 20% (56% × 39%) has already been involved by an infarct. On catheterization there was severe triple vessel disease with a 100% occlusion of the LAD, a 90% occulsion of the proximal circumflex and a 90% occlusion of the distal right coronary artery with an ejection fraction of 43%. He underwent urgent coronary artery bypass grafting, but suffered a complete occlusion of the RCA graft one week later announced by ventricular fibrillation during an outpatient visit to the hospital pharmacy. He was resuscitated, but at angiography the graft could not be re-opened. He underwent cardiac rehabilitation.

A

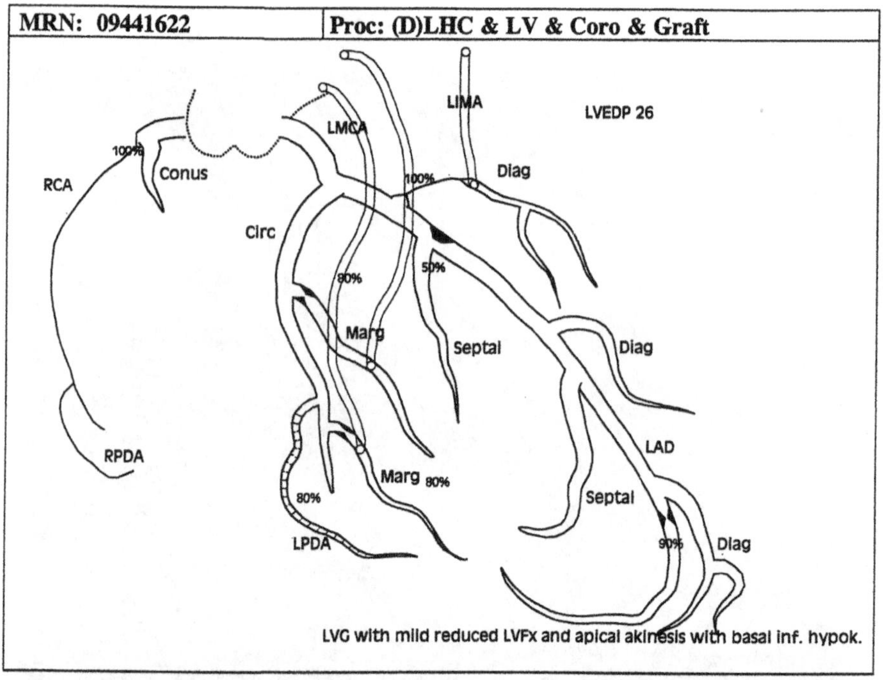

MRN: 09441622
Proc: (D)LHC & LV & Coro & Graft
LIMA
LVEDP 26
LMCA
100%
Conus
RCA
100%
Diag
Circ
50%
80%
Marg
Septal
Diag
LAD
RPDA
Marg 80%
Septal
80%
LPDA
90%
Diag
LVG with mild reduced LVFx and apical akinesis with basal inf. hypok.

B

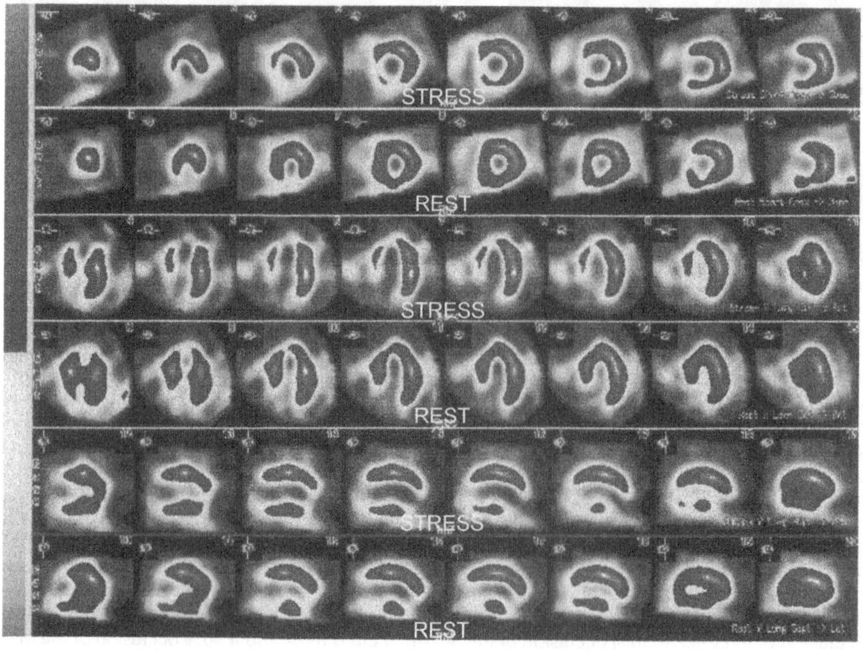

STRESS
REST
STRESS
REST
STRESS
REST

C

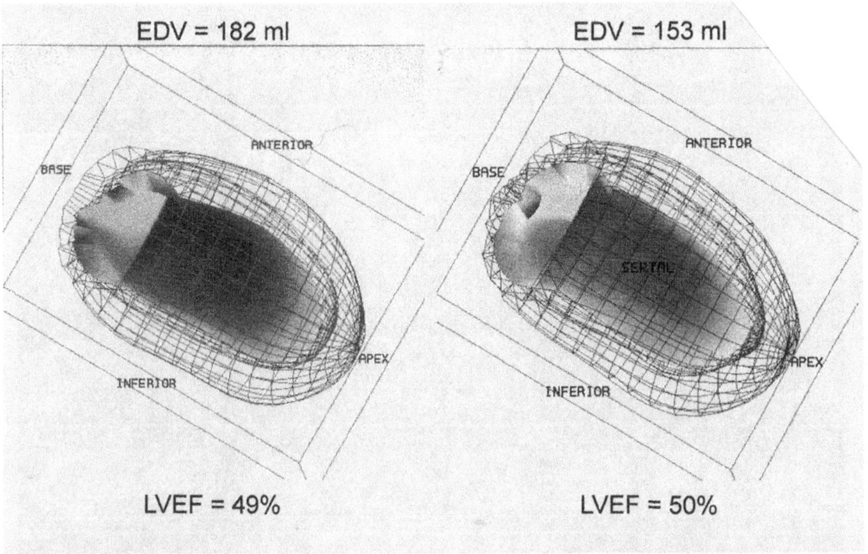

FIGURE 22–11. Unstable angina in a 63-year-old man who had undergone coronary artery bypass grafting for extensive multi-vessel disease after sustaining an inferior wall infarct, 5 years prior to this study. The results of coronary angiography diagrammed in *A,* did not explain his severe symptoms. The mid LAD stenosis was interpreted as only 50% by several reviewers, while the severe distal wrap around lesion was thought not worth intervention in this high-risk individual. The persantine®—rest SPECT study, *B,* shows a large area of anteroseptal, septal and inferior septal ischemia, as well as a moderate-to-large inferior wall infarct. There is transient ischemic dilatation of the left ventricle seen on the short axis views. The RAO gated SPECT study, *C,* shows moderate anterior wall hypokinesis post persantine® as well as severe inferior wall and apical hypokinesis. The rest portion of the study done the day before the persantine® study shows the ejection fraction is the same, but the anterior wall motion is nearly normal, and left ventricular end diastolic volume is significantly less, corresponding to the transient ischemic dilatation seen on the transverse sections. Because of the findings on this study and persistent symptoms, he had another catheterization during which a 99% stenosis of the proximal LAD, previously overlooked, was treated by stent placement. The ischemic areas resolved as did the post persantine stunning and transient ischemic dilatation on a study repeated 3 weeks after stent placement.

Other Causes of Reversible Perfusion Defects

Other pathological processes that have been associated with areas of reversible Tl-201 stress perfusion deficits in the absence of demonstrable significant CAD include aortic stenosis,[114] aortic regurgitation,[115] RBBB with left axis deviation,[111] anomalous origin of the left coronary artery,[116] and lesions confined to the secondary branches of the left main coronary artery.[117] The last is an expected finding with better, high-resolution equipment. About 5% of patients with mitral valve prolapse and normal coronary arteries demonstrate reversible, exercise-induced perfusion defects.[118] Reversible defects have also been reported with infiltrative myocardiopathies such as sarcoidosis.[119] Myocardial bridging of a major epicardial artery is usually associated with a normal thallium stress study, but there

A

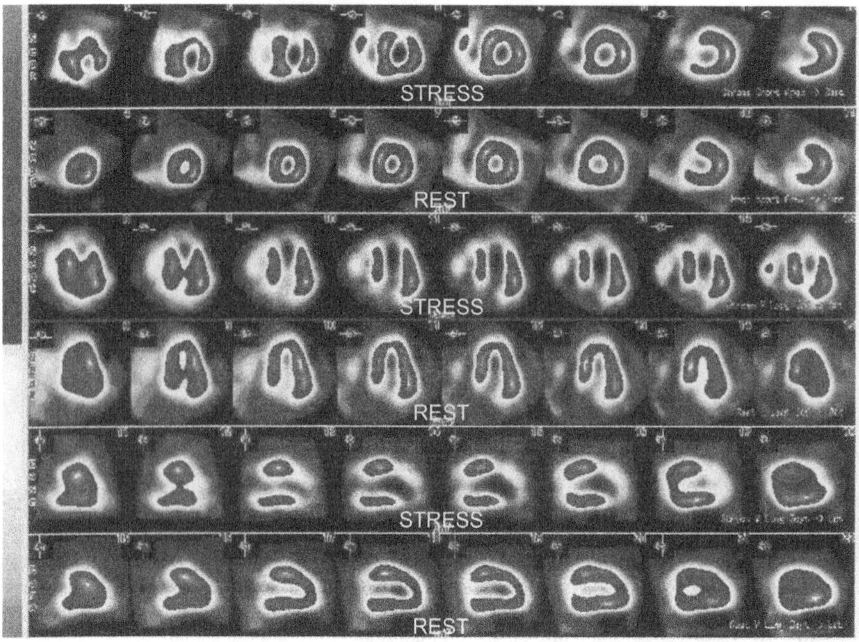
STRESS
REST
STRESS
REST
STRESS
REST

B

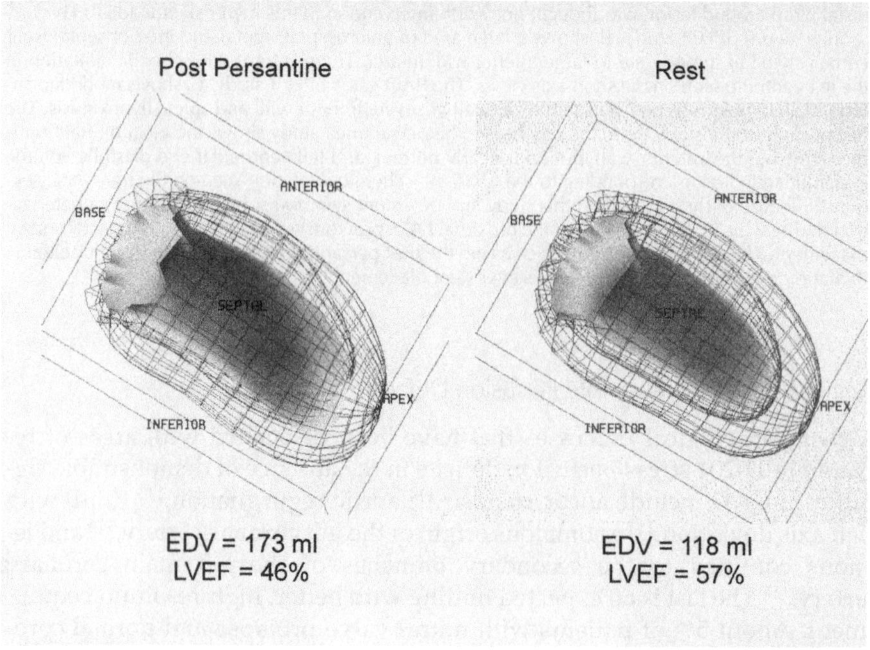
Post Persantine
Rest
ANTERIOR
BASE
SEPTAL
INFERIOR
APEX
ANTERIOR
BASE
INFERIOR
APEX
EDV = 173 ml
LVEF = 46%
EDV = 118 ml
LVEF = 57%

C

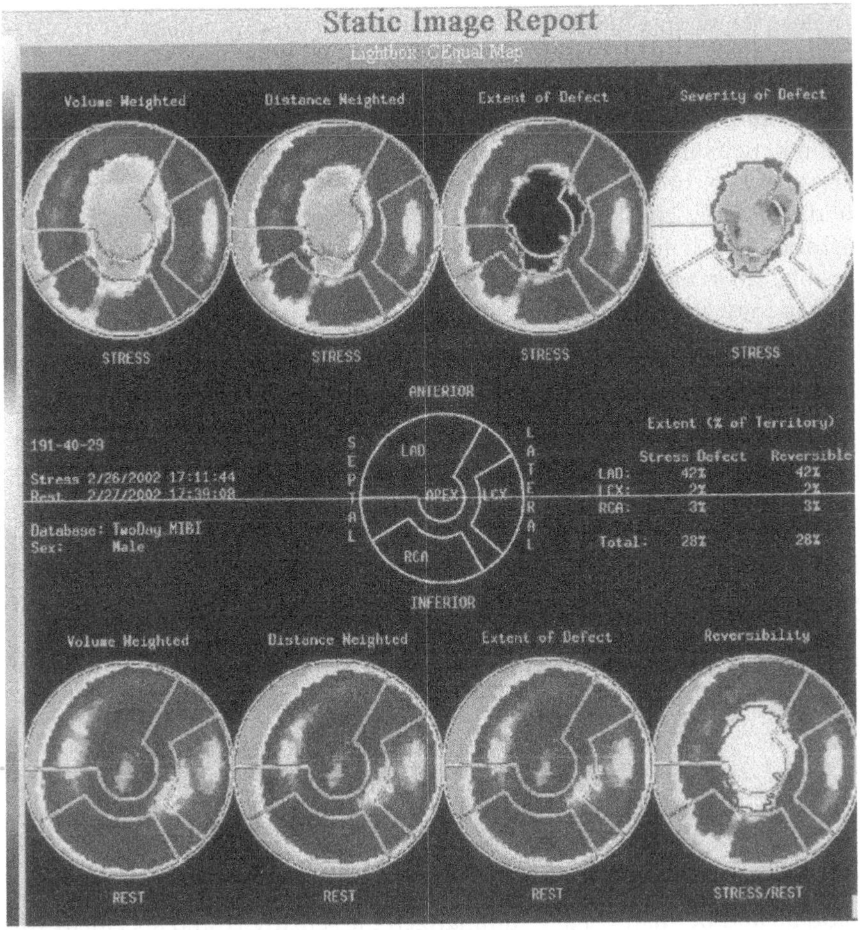

FIGURE 22–12. Post-persantine stunning, transient ischemic dilatation and increased right ventricular uptake as markers of poor prognosis in a 65-year-old man with atypical angina who complained of right parasternal chest pain when he walked, a precautionary exercise he took up after his brother underwent treatment for severe multi-vessel disease. During the persantine® study he developed ischemic ST changes. The post-persantine® SPECT study, *A,* shows a large mid to distal anterior wall and an apical deficit as well as distal inferior wall deficit best seen on the vertical long axis views (bottom rows). In addition the mid ventricular cuts on the short axis show increased right ventricular uptake. In comparison, the resting views show normal perfusion. The left ventricular cavity can be seen to be dilated, particularly in the distal apical portion on the post persantine® study as compared with the rest study. The gated SPECT images, *B,* show moderate distal anterior wall hypokinesis and apical akinesis one hour after receiving persantine®, regions which which have better, but not normal wall motion on the gated SPECT images made following injection at rest. Note the larger end diastolic volume and decreased LVEF on the post persantine study as compared with the resting study. The bull's-eye polar images, *C,* also support a completely reversible large anterior apical deficit affecting approximately 25%–30% of the left ventricular myocardium. Immediately upon the conclusion of this study, based on the results, the patient was admitted for urgent evaluation and therapy, but left against medical advice on the following day, and again 1 week later before catheterization could be performed. Three weeks later, while walking, he sustained a large anterior myocardial infarction, presenting for medical attention 24 hours after the onset of symptoms.

are exceptions, presumably related to obstructive physiology.[120–122] Cardiomyopathies resulting from other than ischemic processes may also demonstrate reversible defects.[123,124] Cocaine in the absence of significant demonstrable anatomic disease may also cause apparently reversible perfusion deficits in a pattern like unstable angina.[125] Exercise-induced coronary artery spasm may also produce reversible deficits.[126] Finally, some individuals with chest pain and patent epicardial coronary arteries on angiography, demonstrate abnormal coronary artery reserve and have reversible, stress induced perfusion deficits,[127] expected from a study that visually demonstrates the loss of coronary artery reserve while angiography defines anatomy, not physiology.

Table 22–2 indicates causes of fixed and reversible deficits unrelated to CAD that may be seen on stress myocardial perfusion studies. Some are the result of other causes of demonstrably decreased regional perfusion. Others result from a variety of artifacts related to the patient, the equipment or the technique.

In my opinion, it is best to read the studies initially without the bias of clinical information. But the final interpretation is offered only in conjunction with the clinical history, EKG findings, presence or absence of ischemic changes during stress at the time of injection of the perfusion tracer, the presence of conduction defects, left ventricular hypertrophy, and knowledge of stress parameters and the patient's response to them.

USES OF MYOCARDIAL PERFUSION IMAGING

Diagnosis

Maddahi and Berman[128] have summarized the sensitivity and specificity for visual analysis of planar thallium imaging as sensitivity 82%, specificity 88%, and for quantitative analysis, a sensitivity of 89% and a specificity of 68%. Referral bias results in reduced specificity. It results from using the myocardial perfusion image as a decision node for further work up; that is, patients with a normal study are unlikely to be referred for further evaluation unless there is a very strong clinical consideration supporting the presence of disease. Because of this the Cedars group has established the use of a normalcy rate. This term classifies as true normal those with a normal test result and supporting clinical data indicating a low likelihood of coronary artery disease but without confirming cardiac catheterization data. Employing the normalcy rate to correct for post-test referral bias,[25] results in a normalcy rate of 88%. The results using dipyridamole are the same as for exercise stress. The presence of a previous MI increases diagnostic sensitivity. Sensitivity also increases as the number of coronary arteries involved with more than 75% stenosis increases.

Table 22–2. **Causes of Defects on Myocardial Perfusion Scintigraphy**

Fixed Defects

- Acute myocardial infarction
- Old myocardial infarction
- Stunned myocardium
- Hibernating myocardium
- Myocardial fibrosis associated with
  - Cardiomyopathy
  - Sarcoidosis
  - Infiltrative cardiomyopathy
- Myocardial bridging
- Absorption effects
  - Breast tissue—implants
  - Changes in the thoracic wall
  - Increased pectoral musculature
  - Diaphragmatic (gastric) absorption
- Normal apical thinning
- Normal aortic valve plane
- Normal fibrous septum
- Artifact from incorrect scaling
- Artifact from incorrect background subtraction
- Artifact from absorption of photons by the scanning bed with patient prone

Reversible Defects

- Ischemic myocardium
- Left or right bundle branch block
- Mitral valve prolapse
- Aortic valve disease
- Dilated cardiomyopathy
- Hypertrophic cardiomyopathy
- Hypertensive cardiomyopathy
- Myocardial bridging
- Coronary artery spasm
- Cocaine
- Artifact from changing chest wall absorptive factors
- Artifact from upward creep with SPECT
- Artifact from variable gastric absorption between stress and redistribution or rest studies
- Artifact from patient motion
- Artifact from different positioning between stress and rest studies
- Artifact from incorrect axis choice in SPECT
- Artifact from incorrect background subtraction
- Artifact from incorrect scaling

SPECT—single photon emission computed tomography.

A summary of visual analysis of ^{201}Tl SPECT imaging yields a sensitivity of 92% and specificity of 77%. Quantitative SPECT analysis yields a sensitivity of 90% and specificity of 70% with a normalcy rate of 89%.

A summary of the sensitivity and specificity for detecting CAD with 50% stenosis using exercise myocardial perfusion SPECT with ^{99m}Tc agents indicates a sensitivity of 87%, and a specificity of 73%.[129]

Results in women have not been as good as in men. This may partly result from additional breast absorption artifact, and, when stress is performed, less ability to reach peak stress. Sensitivity of thallium and Tc-99m sestamibi for detecting coronary artery disease are similar, ranging in the 70% level for detecting 50% stenotic lesions to the 80% level for detecting 70% lesions; however, the specificity of the Tc-99m agent is significantly better than thallium, 92% as compared with 67%.[130] More recent meta analyses and large observational outcomes studies support the use of noninvasive testing to determine risk assessment in symptomatic women with an intermediate pre-test risk. In one large series, there was a stable decade long trend indicating that referral for testing was more liberal for women, they were more likely to have a normal result and they were less likely to be referred for cardiac catheterization.[131] The three year cardiac survival for women with no perfusion deficits on the myocardial stress perfusion study is 99% dropping to 85% with involvement of three vascular territories.[132]

Results

Meta-analysis of a number of large series of planar and SPECT studies for detecting CAD defined as 50% stenosis yield fairly similar results for SPECT studies with either ^{201}Tl or ^{99m} Tc sestamibi or tetrofosmin. Results of stress or pharmacological testing are also similar. Estimates from references 128 and 129 are given in Table 22–3.

Chronic Ischemic Disease

In patients with known coronary artery disease, myocardial perfusion imaging provides an independent means for risk stratification to guide therapeutic choices between conservative management and revascularization. A meta-analysis of the mortality rates in post CABG patients,[133] suggests that these patients may be categorized as low risk, less than 1% mortality per year, intermediate risk, 1%–3% mortality per year, and high risk, more than 3% mortality per year. While the low risk group most likely will not benefit

Table 22–3. **Results of Myocardial Stress Perfusion Imaging for the Diagnosis of Coronary Artery Disease**

	Sensitivity	Specificity	Normalcy Rate
Tl-201 planar	82%*	88%*	—
	89%**	68%**	88%
Tl-201 SPECT	90%	70%	89%
Tl-201 Dipyridamole SPECT	87%	81%	—
Tc-99m sestamibi SPECT	88%	73%	91%
Tc-99m tetrofosmin	92%	81%	97%

*Qualitative data analysis.
**Quantitative data analysis.
Summarized by permission from the authors and publisher.

from invasive intervention and the high risk group most likely would, the intermediate group can be cost effectively stratified by myocardial perfusion imaging into the low or high risk categories.

Acute Ischemic Syndromes

In patients presenting to the emergency department with acute chest pain suspected of having an ongoing acute myocardial infarction, the myocardial perfusion study can aid in triaging selected patients in whom routine diagnostic efforts including historical data, examination, EKG, chest film and blood studies result in an intermediate probability. A normal resting SPECT myocardial perfusion study correlates with a less than a 1% likelihood of the presence of an acute infarction. Even if an infarct later proved to be present, those with a normal resting myocardial perfusion study were most likely to have small, non-complicated infarcts.[134] Clinical data including history, risk factors and early changes in serum troponin levels, as well as the myocardial perfusion study have similar, high sensitivity, but the specificity of the myocardial perfusion image is higher. A negative myocardial perfusion scan has a 99% negative predictive value. In this setting, selective use of SPECT myocardial perfusion imaging proves cost effective in guiding who can safely be sent home, and who should be hospitalized.[135,136]

Myocardial perfusion imaging in acute coronary occlusive syndromes has been used to define areas of myocardium at risk.[47,98] In these settings, Tc-99m sestamibi can be injected prior to reperfusion therapy and imaging carried out several hours after therapy. Imaging at this time reflects myocardium at risk. Successful reperfusion therapy is reflected by improved myocardial perfusion on repeat perfusion studies performed as soon as the following day. Thereafter, follow up imaging often shows continuing improvement in myocardial blood flow over a several week period, perhaps reflecting recovery of stunned or ischemic tissue function so that these areas are able to take up sestamibi.

Unstable Angina

Selected patients presenting with unstable angina and a non-diagnostic EKG may be triaged effectively using myocardial perfusion imaging. The patient can be injected during pain with ^{99m}Tc sestamibi, treated and imaged up to 4 hours later to determine the status of myocardial perfusion at the time of injection. If the clinical situation permits, comparison of myocardial perfusion following a repeat injection made when the patient is without pain can help estimate the extent of the region at risk. Abnormal myocardial perfusion images are found in patients with unstable angina who are injected with a technetium 99m myocardial perfusion tracer during, or even shortly following an episode of chest pain related to unstable angina, even if unaccompanied by ischemic changes on the EKG. Such deficits are reversible and usually accompany severe three vessel disease.[137] The EKG is unlikely to demonstrate ischemic changes when the patient is pain free. Patients who have an abnormal EKG with pain are likely to demonstrate relatively large areas of ischemia on the perfusion study.

Prognosis

Studies of large numbers of patients with a normal outcome of myocardial stress perfusion studies have shown that the risk of myocardial infarction or cardiac death during the next year was 0.2%—0.5%.[138–144] Myocardial perfusion imaging provides a gain in incremental prognostic information in most groups of patients with known coronary artery disease, but the approach is cost effective only when applied to patients with a high risk for an adverse cardiac event. Parameters on the myocardial perfusion study directly related to an adverse myocardial event include the presence of ischemic defects, as well as the number and the extent of the defects. Other markers of poor prognosis include: increased lung uptake when thallium is used. Early planar imaging obtained 7 minutes following post-stress injection of Tc-99m sestamibi will provide similar information;[89] transient ischemic dilatation; increased right ventricular uptake; post-stress stunning evidenced by decreased regional wall motion on the post stress gated image as compared with the resting image; and ejection fraction <0.35. (See Fig. 22–7, 22–10, 22–11 and 22–12).

Risk Stratification

Post Acute MI

Risk stratification early following an acute myocardial infarction (AMI) can contribute significantly to clinical management and decision making. Traditionally an early sub-maximal stress study, including myocardial perfusion, performed just prior to discharge 6 to 12 days after AMI fulfilled this role. Studies using dipyridamole 2 to 4 days after AMI show that this procedure is not only safe, but has a superior ability to predict both early in-hospital and later post-discharge cardiac events as compared with the traditional approach.[145] The summed stress score seems to perform best in those patients receiving thrombolytic therapy. Significant independent predictors of the post discharge event rate included the summed stress score, the reversibility score, the rest score and an anterior AMI.

Following an acute, uncomplicated myocardial infarction, it is probably cost effective to use myocardial perfusion imaging to triage those patients who, on clinical grounds, have an intermediate risk for another acute cardiac event or for whom clinical indications for revascularization are not clear cut. This approach is effective whether or not therapeutic thrombolysis or stenting has been performed for the acute syndrome.

"Hibernating" Myocardium

Hibernating myocardium results from absence of coronary flow reserve leading to a persistent resting ischemic state or possibly myocardium that is repetitively stunned during routine daily activities because of insufficient blood supply to meet routine metabolic demands, or both. Whatever the cause, the result is decreased function in viable myocardium, that appropriately reperfused can regain function. Often patients with hibernating myocardium represent those with the most severe ischemic disease who have the highest risk for undergoing revascularization procedures, yet may have the most to gain in terms of improved survival with a successful procedure. Thus, accurate selection criteria are critical in this group.[146] Initial observations with thallium stress-redistribution imaging indicated that up to 30% of regions which appeared to have persistent, severe perfusion deficits on the three hour images appeared to be much better perfused on delayed imaging 18-24 later.[147] A more sensitive approach is the reinjection of thallium in the resting state after the 3 hour delayed images.[148,149] Reperfused areas have a high likelihood of regaining significant function in response to successful revascularization. If only the detection of hibernating myocardium is the issue, images three hours after resting injection of thallium-201 under fasting conditions likely to maintain relatively high levels of thallium in the plasma are suitable.[150,151] Such studies have approximately a 70% positive and negative predictive value for regional recovery, or lack of recovery of function.

Tc99m MIBI is predominantly a flow agent, and redistribution is not usually significant, although viable myocardial cells are required for its retention. The use of after-load reduction is simple to perform and can be helpful if the result is positive, but the negative predictive value of such a study is probably too low to be clinically valuable. The accuracy of this approach is probably about the same as for thallium-201 rest-redistribution studies.[152] Figure 22–13 shows the result of such a study in a man with severely impaired left ventricular function. The nitroglycerine study shown was performed by injecting Tc-99m sestamibi 4 minutes after a second sublingual dose of nitroglycerine. First pass data were obtained during injection. The study predicted good return of function that, in fact, occurred after successful revascularization.

Metabolic Imaging for Defining Hibernating Myocardium

The physiologic definition of hibernating myocardium is tissue with chronically reduced blood flow with resultant reduced contractile function that maintains metabolic capacity. The clinical availability of the glucose uptake tracer, F-18 fluorodeoxyglucose (F-18 FDG), permits the direct and accurate demonstration of this condition through a variety of imaging techniques. Myocardial areas with reduced perfusion and contractile function, maintain metabolic activity by utilizing glucose substrate in the resting state. The demonstration that such regions could regain function provided the clinical basis for defining hibernating myocardium as a perfusion-metabolic mis-

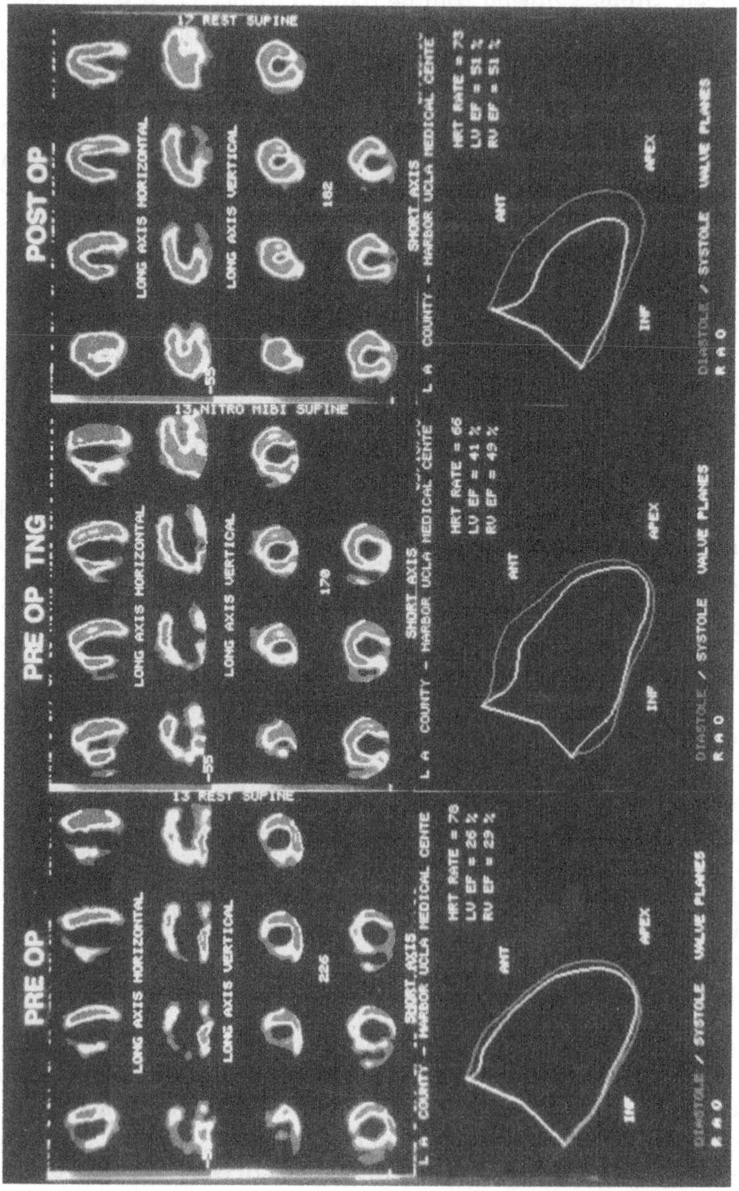
PRE OP
LONG AXIS HORIZONTAL
LONG AXIS VERTICAL
SHORT AXIS
225
13 REST SUPINE
L A COUNTY - HARBOR UCLA MEDICAL CENTE
HRT RATE = 78
LV EF = 26 %
RV EF = 29 %
ANT
INF
APEX
DIASTOLE / SYSTOLE VALUE PLANES
R A O
PRE OP TNG
LONG AXIS HORIZONTAL
LONG AXIS VERTICAL
SHORT AXIS
170
13 NITRO MIBI SUPINE
L A COUNTY - HARBOR UCLA MEDICAL CENTE
HRT RATE = 66
LV EF = 41 %
RV EF = 49 %
ANT
INF
APEX
DIASTOLE / SYSTOLE VALUE PLANES
R A O
POST OP
LONG AXIS HORIZONTAL
LONG AXIS VERTICAL
SHORT AXIS
182
17 REST SUPINE
L A COUNTY - HARBOR UCLA MEDICAL CENTE
HRT RATE = 73
LV EF = 51 %
RV EF = 51 %
ANT
INF
APEX
DIASTOLE / SYSTOLE VALUE PLANES
R A O

match.[153] Although a variety of metabolic tracers have been used, including acetate labeled with the very short half-lived positron-emitter, C-11,[154]and fatty acids with the single photon label I-123,[155] the current rapidly evolving clinical use and availability of F-18 FDG make it the favored tracer for measuring metabolism in ischemic segments.

Tracer Combinations for Defining Perfusion—Metabolic Mismatch

A variety of tracer combinations, instrumentation and protocols have been employed clinically. If positron emission tomomgraphy as well as cyclotron facilities are available, N-13 ammonia can be used as the flow tracer.[156] If the facility has no cyclotron, rubidium-82 obtained from a strontium-82—rubidium-82 generator with a useful life of 1 month can be used as the flow tracer.[157] Clinical imaging methods include dedicated PET instruments using a combination of F-18 FDG and either Rb 82 or N-13 ammonia; hybrid SPECT-PET coincidence detectors using F-18 FDG and either Tc99m MIBI or Thallium-201, or dedicated SPECT instruments imaging in a non-coincidence mode, but equipped with high-energy collimators that can image F-18 and Tc-99m agents simultaneously.[158] This last method has proven quite accurate used in a clinical setting. If a hybrid coincidence detection system is used for imaging, it should be equipped with attenuation correction. Otherwise, attenuation problems appear to affect the evaluation of the inferior and septal regions, particularly in bulky patients with a high mass index.[159]

The use of FDG requires careful patient preparation to enhance the myocardial utilization of the glucose substrate. This may be accomplished by oral glucose loading; or, by a combination of intravenous glucose, insulin and potassium; or, by reduction of fatty acid levels using nicotinic acid analogues. The use of glucose loading in the face of impaired glucose metabolism requires careful monitoring of blood glucose levels and can pose significant logistic problems unless a well-planned protocol is in place. It requires individuals available who are skilled in monitoring the diabetic patient. Several protocols have been proposed.[160–163]

FIGURE 22–13. Hibernating myocardium diagnosed using nitroglycerine. Use of sublingual nitroglycerine in conjunction with Tc99m MIBI for detecting hibernating myocardium in a man who was judged to have no reversible ischemia on persantine/rest studies. In this study the long axis vertical slices have the apex oriented to the reader's left. The pre-operative resting study (PRE-OP) shows very large anterior, septal and apical perfusion deficits. The first pass study obtained at the same time shows severe generalized hypokinesis with inferior wall akinesis, a right ventricular ejection fraction of 29% and a left ventricular ejection fraction of 26%. The SPECT images obtained from the injection performed 4 minutes after the second of two doses of sublingual nitroglycerine (PRE-OP TNG) show reperfusion of large portions of the anterior, and septal regions with fixed deficits in the apex and inferior wall. The first pass study obtained with the injection of Tc-99m MIBI for the perfusion portion of the study shows improvement of the anterior wall motion with the left ventricular ejection fraction rising to 41%, the right to 49%. Following coronary artery bypass grafting (POST-OP), the resting study shows resolution of the anterior, septal and apical deficits. Both left and right ejection fractions have risen to 51%. His New York heart association classification fell from class 4 to class 2.

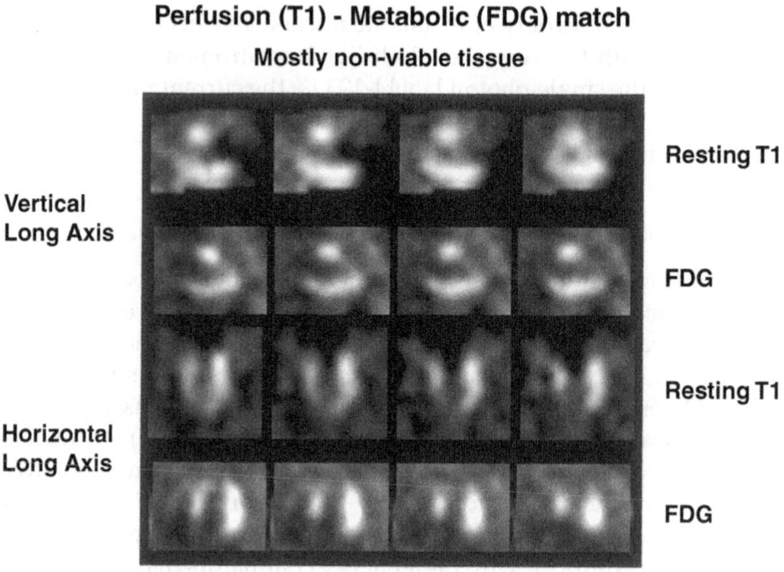

FIGURE 22–14. F-18 fluorodeoxyglucose (FDG) for detecting hibernating myocardium. The resting vertical long axis views performed with thallium show a large anterior apical perfusion deficit confirmed on the horizontal long axis views. The FDG images show minimal metabolism of glucose in the region of these perfusion deficits, a perfusion/metabolism matched deficit. This finding indicates largely non-viable tissue, unsuitable for reperfusion intervention. These images were obtained on the same hybrid three-headed SPECT system that performed all of the SPECT images that were used to illustrate this chapter. It may be rapidly converted for performing coincidence imaging. Its 3 large crystals have approximately a 33% increase in count rate advantage in obtaining coincidence data over dual crystal instruments. (Case courtesy of Fan-Ping Wang, M.D., and Lalitha Ramanna, M.D., LAC-USC Medical Center, Los Angeles.)

The recent introduction of the nicotinic acid derivative, Acipimax, promises a simpler, alternative method of patient preparation. Readily absorbed after oral administration and apparently free of significant side effects other than flushing, it is a potent inhibitor of peripheral lipolysis resulting in reduced plasma levels of free fatty acids. Two oral doses are given, one 3 hours and, the other, 1/2 hour, prior to injection.

This protocol yields good results for clinical imaging, comparable to using a euglycemic hyperinsulinemic clamp and better than using an oral glucose load.[164] Figure 22–14 shows the appearance of a metabolic perfusion match comparing the resting thallium study (perfusion) with metabolism (FDG) indicating an insignificant amount of hibernating myocardium in a large apical infarct. Figure 22–15 shows the appearance of a large inferior wall infarct on the thallium image performed 24 hours after injection of thallium at rest, while the FDG image indicates significant metabolic activity in this region, a metabolic-perfusion mismatch, supporting the presence of hibernating myocardium.

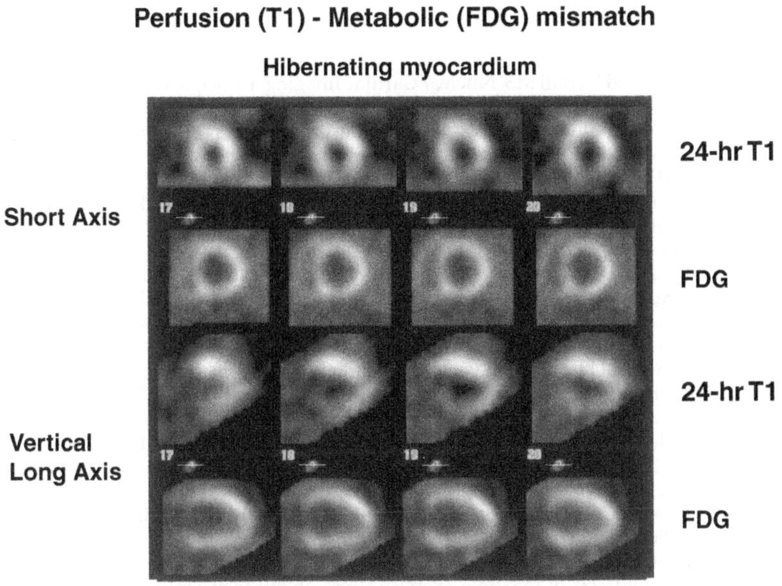

FIGURE 22–15. F-18-FDG for detection of hibernating myocardium. The 24-hour thallium redistribution study short axis and vertical long axis rows show a persistent large inferior wall perfusion deficit supporting the presence of non-viable myocardium in this region, unsuitable for revascularization. The FDG images (rows beneath the thallium images), however, show that this region actively metabolizes glucose. This indicates the region of mismatched decreased perfusion but active glucose metabolism is viable and might well benefit, in terms of improved function, from revascularization. (Case courtesy of Fan-Ping Wang, M.D. and Lalitha Ramanna, M.D., LAC-USC Medical Center, Los Angeles.)

A meta-analysis of 12 studies including 325 patients who underwent revascularization, indicated that FDG PET imaging yielded an average sensitivity of 88% and specificity of 73% for predicting the return or lack of return of contractile function to the areas that were revascularized.[165] An analysis of the FDG collimated SPECT method including 55 patients with ischemic left ventricular dysfunction who underwent revascularization indicated a sensitivity of 85% and specificity of 75% in predicting the return of function to the revascularized regions.[166] Both dedicated PET and SPECT F-18 FDG/perfusion imaging have demonstrated prognostic value in defining the cohort with ischemic cardiomyopathy which has the best improvement in event rate with surgical as compared with medical management. This is the group with viable myocardium, as opposed to non viable myocardium.[167] They had improvement in both contractile function and symptoms as well as performance. Validation of hybrid coincidence imaging requires further study.

Indications: (1) diagnosis of chronic ischemic disease; (2) diagnosis of hibernating myocardium; (3) prognosis in chronic ischemic cardiomyopathy.

REFERENCES

1. Iskandrian, AS and Verani MS. Nuclear Cardiac Imaging: Principles and Applications, 2nd ed. FA Davis Co., Philadelphia p 451, 1996.
2. DePuey, EG, et al: Clinical application of gated myocardial perfusion SPECT in Cardiac SPECT Imaging, 2nd ed, DePuey EG, Garcia EV, Berman DS (eds). Chapter 11, Lippincott Williams and Wilkins, Philadelphia, PA, 2001, p 211.
3. Wackers, FJ, et al: Nuclear Cardiology in Heart Disease: A Textbook of Cardiovascular Medicine, 6th ed, Chapter 9, Braunwld E, Zipes DP, Libby P. (eds) W.B. Saunders Co. Philadelphia, 2001, p 273.
4. Murray, IPC and Ell, PJ. (eds) Nuclear Cardiology in Nuclear Medicine in Clinical Diagnosis and Treatment, 2nd ed, Churchill Livingstone, Edinburgh, p 1305, 1998.
5. Sandler, MP, et al: Section IV. Cardiovascular in Diagnostic Nuclear Medicine, 3rd ed, Williams and Wilkins, Baltimore, p 329, 1995.
6. Jengo, JA, et al: Evaluation of left ventricular function (ejection fraction and segmental wall motion) by single pass radioisotope angiography. Circulation 57:326, 1978.
7. Jones, RH, et al: Accuracy of the diagnosis of coronary artery disease by radionuclide measurement of left ventricular function during rest and exercise. Circulation 64:586, 1981.
8. Jones, RH: Use of radionuclide mesurements of left ventricular function for prognosis in patients with coronary artery disease. Semin Nud Med 17:95, 1987.
9. Sandler, H and Dodge, HT: The use of single plane angiocardiograms for the calculation of left ventricular volume in man. Am Heart J 75:325, 1968.
10. Weber, PM, et al: Quantitative radioisotope angiocardiography. J Nucl Med 13:815, 1972.
11. Jengo, JA, et al: Effects of maximal exercise stress on left ventricular function in patients with coronary artery disease using first pass radionuclide ventriculography; a rapid noninvasive technique for determining ejection fraction and segmental wall motion. Circulation 59:60, 1979.
12. Borges-Neto, S, et al: Prediction of myocardial perfusion abnormalities by quantiative regional function using a radionuclide angiography database: A comparison with wall motion analysis. Clin Nucl Med 25:110, 2000.
13. Austin, EH, et al: Prospective evaluation of radionuclide angiocardiography for the diagnosis of coronary artery disease. Am J Cardiol 50:1212, 1982.
14. Pryor, DB, et al: Prognostic indicators from radionuclide angiography in medically treated patients with coronary artery disease. Am Cardiol 53:18, 1984.
15. Jones, RH, et al: Exercise radionuclide angiocardiography predicts cardiac death in patients with coronary artery disease. Circulation 84(1):1, 1992.
16. Zaret, BL, et al: A noninvasive scintiphotographic method for the detection of regional ventricular dysfunction in man. N Engl J Med 284:1165, 1971.
17. Strauss, HW, et al: A scintiphotographic method for measuring left ventricular ejection fraction in man without cardiac catheterization. Am J Cardiol 28:575, 1972.
18. Green, NW, et al: High temporal resolution ECG-gated scintigraphic angiocardiography. J Nucl Med 16:95, 1975.
19. Sneed, A, et al: Radionuclide cinecardiography using minicomputer generated sequential gated images. Br Heart J 39:982, 1977.
20. Massie, BM, et al: Radionuclide mesurement of left ventricular volume: Comparison of geometric and counts-based methods. Circulation 65:725, 1982.
21. Massardo, T, et al: Left ventricular volume calculation using a count-based ratio method applied to multigated radionuclide angiography. J Nucl Med 31:450, 1990.
22. Clements, IP, et al: determination of diastolic function by radionuclide ventriculography. Mayo Clinic Proc 65:1007, 1990.
23. Bonow, RO, et al: Improved left ventricular diastolic filling in patients with coronary artery disease after percutaneous transluminal coronary angioplasty. Circulation 56:1024, 1977.
24. Greenberg, PS, et al: Use of end-systolic volume changes with exercise to detect left ventricular dysfunction in patients with coronary artery disease. Clin Cardiol 5:409, 1982.
25. Rozanski, A, et al: The declining specificity of exercise radionuclide ventriculography. NEJM 309:518, 1983.
26. Diamond, GA, et al: A model for assessing the sensitivity and specificity of tests subject to selection bias. Application to exercise radionuclide ventriculography for diagnosis of coronary artery disease. J Chronic Dis 39(5):343, 1986.

27. Sasso, FC, et al: Effects of insulin-glucose infusion on left ventricular function at rest and during dynamic exercise in healthy subjects and non insulin dependent diabetic patients: A radionuclide ventriculographic study. Am Coll Cardiol 36:219, 2000.
28. Bonow, RO, et al: Exercise-induced ischemia in mildly symptomatic patients with coronary artery disease and preserved left ventricular function: indentification of subgroups at risk of death during medical therapy. NEJM 311:13390, 1984.
29. Bonow, RO, et al: Prognostic implications of symptomatic vs. asymptomatic (silent) myocardial ischemia induced by exercise in mildly symptomatic and in asymptomatic patients with angiographically documented coronary artery disease. Am J Cardiol 60:778, 1987.
30. Miller, TC, et al: Risk stratification of single or double vessel coronary artery disease and impaired left ventricular function using exercise radionuclide angiography. Am J Cardiol 65:1317, 1990.
31. Iskandrian, AD, et al: Prognostic implications of rest and exercise radionuclide ventriculography in patients with suspected or proven coronary artery disease. Int J Cardiol 6:707, 1984.
32. Gould, KL, et al: Coronary flow reserve as a physiologic measure of stenosis severity. J Am Coll Cardiol 15:459, 1990.
33. Donohue, TJ, et al: Assessing the hemodynamic significance of coronary artery stenoses: Analysis of translesional pressure-flow velocity relations in patients. J Am Coll Cardiol 22:449, 1993.
34. Miller, DD, et al: Correlation of pharmacological 99m Tc-sestamibi myocardial perfusion imaging with poststenotic coronary flow reserve in patients with angiographically intermediate coronary artery stenoses. Circulation 89:2150, 1994.
35. Lebowitz, E, et al: 201 TI for medical use. J Nucl Med 16:151, 1975.
36. Berman, DS, et al: Tc99m sestamibi in the assessment of chronic coronary artery disease. Semin Nucl Med 21:190, 1991.
37. Zaret, BL, et al; Myocardial perfusion imaging with ^{99m}TC-tetrofosmin: comparison to ^{201}Tl imaging and coronary angiography in a Phase III multicenter trial. Circulation 91:313, 1995.
38. Zelonka, JS: Multicenter trial of Tc99m teboroxime (cardiotec) a new myocardial perfusion agent. J Nuc Med 31:827, 1990.
39. Burns, RJ, et al: Exercise Tc99m-teboroxime cardiac SPECT: Results of a Canadian multicentre trial. J Nucl Med 32:919, 1991.
40. Sapirstein, LA: Regional blood flow by fractional distribution of indicators. Am J Physiol 193:161, 1968.
41. Weich, H, et al: The extraction of thallium-201 by the myocardium. Circulation 56:188, 1977.
42. Pohost, GM, et al: Differentiation of transiently ischemic from infarcted myocardium by serial imaging after a single dose of thallium-201. Circulation 55:294, 1997.
43. Beller, GA, et al: Kinetics of thallium distribution and redistribution: Clinical applications in sequential myocardial imaging. In Strauss, HW and Pitt, B (eds): Cardiovascular Nuclear Medicine, 2nd ed CV Mosby, St. Louis, p 225, 1979.
44. Beller, GA, et al: Effects of dipyridamole-induced vasodilation on myocardial uptake and clearance kinetics of thallium-201. Circulation 68:1328, 1983.
45. Ruddy, TD, et al: Myocardial uptake and clearance of thallium-201 in normal subjects: Comparison of dipyridamole hyperemia with stress. J Am Coll Cardiol 10:547, 1987.
46. Iskandrian, AS: Thallium-201 myocardial and radionuclide ventriculography: Theory technical considerations and interpretation. In Nuclear Cardiac Imaging: Principles and Applications. FA Davis, Philadelphia, p 81, 1987.
47. Gibbons, RJ, et al: Feasibility of tomographic 99m-Tc-hexakis-2-methoxy-2methylpropyl-isonitrile imaging for assessment of myocardial area at risk and the effect of treatment in acute myocardial infarction. Circulation 80:1277, 1989.
48. Taillefer, R: Radiopharmaceuticals in Cardiac SPECT Imaging, Second edition, DePuey EG, Garcia EV, Berman DS (eds). Chapter 8, Lippincott Williams and Wilkins, Philadelphia, PA p 117, 2001.
49. Galt, JR, et al: Attenuation and scatter compensation in mycocardial perfusion SPECT. Semin Nucl Med 29:204, 1999.
50. Hendel RC, et al: The value and practice of attenuation correction for myocardial perfusion SPECT imaging: A joint position statement from the American Society of Nuclear Cardiology and the Society of Nuclear Medicine. J Nucl Cardiol 9:135, 2002.

51. Becker, LC: Conditions for vasodilator induced coronary steal in experimental myocardial ischemia. Circulation. 57:1103, 1978.
52. Rozanski, A, et al: Mental stress and the induction of silent myocardial ischemia in patients with coronary artery disease. N Engl J Med 318:1005, 1988.
53. Stone, PH, et al: Relationship among mental stress-induced ischemia and ischemia during daily life and during exercise; the psychophysiologic investigations of myocardial ischemia (PIMI) study. J Am Coll Cardiol 33:1476, 1999.
54. Holmberg, S, et al: Coronary circulation during heavy exercise in control subjects and patients with coronary artery disease. Act Med Scand 190:465, 1971.
55. Kivowitz, C, et al: Effects of isometric exercise on left cardiac performance: The grip test. Circulation 44:994, 1971.
56. Helfant, RH, et al: Effect of sustained isometric handgrip exercise on left ventricular performance. Circulation 44:982, 1971.
57. Greene, MA, et al: Circulatory dynamics during the cold pressor test. Am J Cardiol 16:54, 1965.
58. Wasserman, AG, et al: Insensitivity of the cold pressor stimulation test for the detection of coronary artery disease. Circulation 67:1189, 1983.
59. Gould, KL: Noninvasive assessment of coronary stenoses by myocardial perfusion imaging during pharmacologic coronary vasodilatation. 1. Physiologic basis and experimental validation. Am J Cardiol 41:269, 1978.
60. Wilson, RF, et al: Effects of adenosine on human coronary arterial circulation. Circulation 82:1595, 1990.
61. Pennell, DJ: Cardiac Stress in Nuclear Medicine in Clinical Diagnosis and Treatment, 2nd ed. Chapter 100. Murray, IPC and Ell, PJ (eds) Churchill Livingstone Edinburg, p 1369, 1998.
62. Brown, G, et al: Intravenous dipyridamole combined with isometric handgrip for near maximal coronary blood flow in patients with coronary artery disease. Am J Cardiol 48:1077, 1981.
63. Wilson, RF, et al: Transluminal subselective measurement of coronary artery blood flow in patients with coronary artery blood flow velocity and vasodilator reserve in man. Circulation 72:82, 1985.
64. Rossen, JD, et al: Comparison of coronary vasodilation intravenous dipyridamole and adenosine. J Am Coll Cardiol 18:485, 1991.
65. Chan, SY, et al: Comparison of maximal myocardial blood flow during adenosine infusion with that of intravenous dipyridamole in normal men. J Am Coll Cardiol 20:979, 1992.
66. Cequeira, MD, et al: Safely profile of adenosine stress perfusion imaging: Results from the Adenoscn Multicenter Trial Registry. J Am Coll Cardiol 23:384, 1994.
67. Ranhosky, A, Kempthome-Rawson, J and the Intravenous Dipyridamole Investigators Group: The safety of intravenous dipyridamole thallium myocardial perfusion imaging. Circulation 81:1205, 1990.
68. Lette, J, et al: Safety of dipyridamole testing in 73,806 patients: the multicenter dipyridamole safety study. J Nucl Cardiol 2:3, 1995.
69. Hoffman, BB and Lefkowitz, RJ: Catecholamines and sympathominetic drugs. In Gilman, AG, et al (eds): Goodman and Gilman's The Pharmacological Basis of Therapeutics, 8th ed Pergamon Press, New York, p 187, 1990.
70. Pierard, LA, et al: Hemodynamic alterations during ischemia induced by dobutamine stress testing. Eur Heart J 10:783, 1989.
71. Pacold, L, et al: Effects of low-dose dobutamine on coronary hemodynamics, myocardial metabolism, and angina threshold in patients with coronary artery disease. Circulation 68:1044, 1983.
72. Martin, TW, et al: Comparison of adenosine, dipyridamole, and dobutamine in stress echocardiography. Ann Intern Med 116:190, 1992.
73. Kiat, H, et al: Arbutamine stress using a closed loop delivery system: a multicenter trial of diagnostic accuracy with thallium-201 SPECT. J Am Coll Cardiol 26:1159, 1995.
74. van Dongen, AJ and van Rijk, PP: Minimizing liver bowel and gastric activity in myocardial perfusion SPECT. J Nucl Med 41:1315, 2000.
75. Lette, J, et al: Safety of dipyridamole testing in patients with cerebrovascular disease. Am J Cardiol 75:535, 1995.
76. Picano, E, et al: Safety of intravenous high-dose dipyridamole exhocardiography. Am J Cardiol 70:252, 1992.

77. Murad, F: Drugs used for the treatment of angina: Organic nitrates, calcium channel blockers and beta-adrenergic blockers. In Gilman, AG, et al (eds): Goodman and Gilman's The Pharmacolgical Basis of Therapeutics, 8th ed. Pergamon Press, New York, p 764, 1990.
78. Abrams, J: Nitroglycerin and long-acting filtrate in clinical practice. Am J Med 74(Suppl):85, 1983.
79. Horowitz, LD, et al: Effects of nitroglycerin on regional myocardial blood flow in coronary artery disease. J Clin Invest 50:1578, 1971.
80. Brown, BG, et al: The mechanism of nitroglycerin action: Stenosis-vasodilatation as a major component of the drug response. Circulation 64:1089, 1981.
81. Salal, AF, et al: Radionuclide assessment of nitroglycerin influence on abnormal left ventricular segmental contraction in patients with coronary heart disease. Circulation 53:975, 1976.
82. Borer, JS, et al: Effect of nitroglycerin on exercise-induced abnormalities of left ventricular regional function and ejection fraction in coronary artery disease. Assessment by radionuclide angiography in symptomatic and asymptomatic patients. Circulation 57:314, 1978.
83. McNaulty, JH, et al: Improvement in left ventricular wall motion following nitroglycerin. Circulation 51:140, 1975.
84. Oudiz, RJ, et al: Nitrate-enhanced thallium 201 single-photon emission computed tomography imaging in hibernating myocardium. Am Heart J 138:369, 1999.
85. Bisi, G, et al: Technetium-99m sestamibi imaging with nitrate infusion to detect viable hibernating myocardium and predict postrevascularization recovery. J Nucl Med 36:1994, 1995.
86. Sciagra, R, et al: Influence of the assessment of defect severity and intravenous nitrate administration during tracer injection on the detection of viable hibernating myocardium with data based quantitative technetium 99m-labeled sestamibi single-photon emission computed tomography. J Nucl Cardiol 3:221, 1996.
87. Sciagra, R, et al: Comparison of baseline-nitrate technetium-99m sestamibi with rest-redistribution thallium-201 tomography in detecting viable hibernating myocardium and predicting postrevascularization recovery. J Am Coll Cardiol 30:384, 1997.
88. ACC/AHA/SNM Policy Statement: Statement: Standardization of Cardiac Tomographic Imaging: The Cardiovascular Imaging Committee, American College of Cardiology; The Committee on Advanced Cardiac Imaging and Technology, Council on Clinical Cardiology, American Heart Association; and Board of Directors, Cardiovascular Council, Society of Nuclear Medicine. J Nucl Cardiol 1:117, 1994. Post SC (ed): Imaging guidelines for nuclear cardiology procedures. Part 2. J Nucl Cardiol 6;649, 1999.
89. Friedman, J, et al: "Upward creep" of the heart: A frequent source of false-positive reversible defects during thallium-201 stress-redistribution SPECT. J Nucl Med 30:1718, 1989.
90. Choy, JB and Leslie, WD: Clinical correlates of Tc-99m sestamibi lung uptake. J Nucl Cardiol 8:639, 2001.
91. Wackers, FJ: Artifacts in planar and SPECT myocardial perfusion imaging. Am J Cardiac Imaging 6(1):42, 1992.
92. DePuey, EG: Artifacts in SPECT myocardial perfusion imaging in Cardiac SPECT Imaging. Second Edition, DePuey EG, Garcia EV, Berman DS (eds). Chapter 12, Lippincott Williams and Wilkins, Philadelphia, PA, p 231, 2001.
93. Naruse, H, et al: Quantitative comparison of planar and SPECT normal data files of thallium-201, technetium-99m-sestamibi, technetium-99m-tetrofosmin, and technetium-99m-furifosmin. J Nucl Med 37:1783, 1996.
94. DePuey, EG, et al: Alterations in myocardial thallium-201 distribution in patients with chronic systemic hypertension undergoing single-photon emission computed tomography. Am J Cardiol 62:234, 1998.
95. Maddahi, J, et al: Quantitative single photon computerized thallium-201 tomography for the evaluation of coronary artery disease: Optimization and propsective validation of a new technique. J Am Coll Cardiol 14:1689, 1989.
96. Van Train, KF, et al: Quantitative same-day rest-stress Tc-99m-sesetamibi SPECT: Definition and validation of stress normal limits and criteria for abnormality. J Nucl Med 34:1494, 1993.
97. O'Connor, MK, et al: In vitro validation of a simple tomographic technique for estimation of percentage of myocardium at risk using methoxyisobutylisonitrile technetium 99m (sestamibi). Eur J Nucl Med 17:69, 1990.

98. Lin, YH, et al: Validation of a new SPECT quantification method using computer simulation. IEEE Nucl Sci Symp Med Imaging Conf Rec 1506, 1995.
99. Ficaro, EP, et al: Development and clinical validation of normal Tc-99m sestamibi database: Comparison of 3-D-MSPECT to Cequal (abstract). J Nucl Med 5;125P, 1999.
100. Cerani, L, et al: Assessment of myocardial area at risk by technetium-99m sestamibi during coronary artery occlusion: Comparison between three tomographic methods of quantification: Eur J Nucl Med 23:31, 1996.
101. Garcia EV: Chapter 3 Quantiative Myocardial SPECT in Cardiac SPECT Imaging, Second Edition, E.G. DePuey, E.V. Garcia, and D.S. Berman (eds). Lippincott Williams & Wilkins, Philadelphia p 41, 2001.
102. Borges-Neto, S, et al: Prediction of severe coronary artery disease by combined rest and exercise radionuclide angiocardiography and tomographic perfusion imaging with technetium-99m labeled sestamibi: A comparison with clinical and electrocardiographic data. J Nucl Cardio 4:1, 1997.
103. Sharir, T, et al: Identification of severe and extensive coronary artery disease by post exercise regional wall motion abnormalities in Tc-99m sestamibi gated single-photon emission computed tomography. Am J Cardiol 86:1171, 2000.
104. Berman, DS and Germano, G: A guide to the interpretation and reporting of Cardiolite®, DuPont Pharmaceuticals Company Medical Imaging, 2000.
105. www.ascn.org
106. www.cardiolite.com
107. Weiss, AT, et al: Reverse redistribution of thallium-21: A sign of nontransmural myocardial infarction with patency of the infarct-related coronary artery. J Am Coll Cardiol 7:61, 1986.
108. Fujiwara, S, et al: Reverse redistribution of 99m Tc sestamibi after direct percutaneous transluminal angioplasty in acute myocardial infarction: Relationship with wall motion and functional response to dobutamine stimulation. Nucl Med Commun 22:1223, 2001.
109. Rothbart, RM, et al: Diagnostic accuracy and prognostic significance of quantitative thallium-201 scintigraphy in patients with left bundle branch block. Am J Noninvas Cardiol 1:197, 1987.
110. DePuey, EG, et al: Thallium-201 SPECT in coronary artery disease patients with left bundle branch block. J Nucl med 29:1479, 1988.
111. Rockett, JF, et al: Intravenous dipyridamole thallium-201 SPECT imaging in patients with left bundle branch block. Clin Nucl Med 15:401, 1990.
112. O'Keefe JH, et al: Adenosine thallium-201 is superior to exercise thallium-201 for detecting coronary artery disease in patients with left bundle branch block. J Am Coll Cardiol 21:1322, 1993.
113. Hirzel, HO, et al: Thallium-201 scintigraphy in complete left bandle branch block. Am J Cardiol 53:764, 1984.
114. Tawarahara, K, et al: Exercise testing and thallium-201 emission computed tomography in conduction disturbance. Am J Cardiol 69:97, 1992.
115. Pfister, ME, et al: Prevalence and significance of reversible radionuclide ischemic perfusion detects in symptomatic aortic valve disease with or without concomitant coronary artery disease. Am Heart J 103:92, 1982.
116. Verani, MS, et al: Demonstration of improved myocardial perfusion following aortic implantation of anomalous left coronary. J Nucl Med 19:1032, 1978.
117. Iskandrian, AS, et al: Exercise myocardial scans in patients' with disease limited to the secondary branches of the left coronary system. Clin Cardiol 2:121, 1979.
118. Greenspan, M, et al: Exercise myocardial scintigraphy with thallium 201: Use in patients with mitral valve prolapse without associated coronary artery disease. Chest 77:47, 1980.
119. Kinney, EL, et al: Thallium-scan myocardial defects and echocardiographic abnormalities in patients with sarcoidosis without clinical cardiac dysfunction. Am J Med 68:497, 1980.
120. Greenspan, M, et al: Myocardial bridging of the left anterior descending artery: Evaluation using exercise thallium-201 myocardial scintigraphy. Cathet Cardiovasc Diagn 6:173, 1980.
121. Rivitz, SM and Yasuda, T: Predictive value of dipyridamole thallium imaging in a patient with myocardial bridging but without fixed obstructive coronary artery disease. J Nucl Med 33:1905, 1992.
122. Ahmad, M, et al: Evidence of impaired myocardial perfusion and abnormal left ventricular function during exercise in patients with isolated systolic narrowing of the left anterior descending coronary artery. Am J Cardiol 48:832, 1981.

123. Glamann, DB, et al: Utility of various radionuclide techniques for distinguishing ischemic from nonischemic dilated cardiomyopathy. Arch Inten Med 152:769, 1992.
124. O'Gara, PT, et al: Myocardiomyopathy: Assessment with TI-201 emission computed tomography. Circulation 76:1214, 1987.
125. Kontoss, MC, et al: Myocardial perfusion imaging with technetium-99m sestamibi in patients with cocaine-associated chest pain. Ann Emerg Med 33:639, 1999.
126. Fuller, CM, et al: Exercise-induced coronary arterial spasm: demonstration, documentation of ischemia by myocardial scintigraphy and results of pharmacologic intervention. Am J Cardiol 46:500, 1980.
127. Legrand, V, et al: Abnormal coronary reserve and abnormal radionuclide exercise test results in patients with normal coronary angiograms. J Am Coll Cardiol 6:1245, 1985.
128. Maddahi, J and Berman, DA: Detection, evaluation, and risk stratification of coronary artery disease by thallium-201 myocardial perfusion scintigraphy in Cardiac SPECT Imaging, Second edition, DePuey EG, Garcia EV, Berman DS (eds). Chapter 9, Lippincott Williams and Wilkins, Philadelphia, PA, p 155, 2001.
129. Berman, DS, Hayes, SW and Germano, G: Assessment of myocardial perfusion and viability with Technetium-99m Perfusion agents in Cardiac SPECT Imaging, 2nd ed, DePuey EG, Garcia EV, Berman DS (eds). Chapter 10, Lippincott Williams and Wilkins, Philadelphia, PA p 179, 2001.
130. Taillefer, R, et al: Comparative diagnostic accuracy of T1-201 and Tc-99m sestamibi SPECT imaging (perfusion and ECG-gated SPECT) in detecting coronary artery disease in women. J Am Coll Cardiol 29:69, 1997.
131. Miller, TD, et al: Gender differences and temporal trends in clinical characteristics, stress test results and use of invasive procedures in patients undergoing evaluation for coronary artery disease. J Am Coll Cardiol 38:690, 2001.
132. Shaw, LJ, et al: Current evidence on diagnostic testing in women with suspected coronary artery disease: Choosing the appropriate test. Cardiol Rev 8:65, 2000.
133. Yusu, S et al: Effect of coronary artery bypass graft surgery on survival: Overview of 10-year results from randomized trials by Coronary Artery Bypass Graft Surgery Trialists Collaboration. Lancet 344:563, 1994.
134. Heller, GV, et al: Clinical value of acute rest technetium-99m tetrofosmin tomographic myocardial perfusion imaging in patients with acute chest pain and nondiagnostic electrocardiogram. J Am Coll Cardiol 31:1011, 1998.
135. Stowers, SA, et al: An economic analysis of an aggressive diagnostic strategy with single photon emission computer tomography myocardial perfusion imaging and early exercise stress testing in emergency department patients who present with chest pain but nondiagnostic electrocardiograms: Results from a randomized trial. Ann Emerg Med 35:17, 2000.
136. Abbott BG, et al: Selective use of single-photon emission computed tomography myocardial perfusion imaging in a chest pain center. Am J Cardiol 87:1351, 2001.
137. Bilodeau, L, et al: Technetium-99m sestamibi tomography in patients with spontaneous chest pain: Correlations with clinical, electrocardigraphic and angiographic findings. J Am Coll Cardiol 1:1684, 1991.
138. Stratmann, HG, et al: Exercise technetium-99m sestamibi tomography for cardiac risk stratification of patients with table chest pain. Circulation 89:615, 1994.
139. Stratmann, HG, et al: Prognostic value of dipyridamole technetium-99m sestamibi myocardial tomography in patients with stable chest pain who are unable to exercise. Am J Cardiol 73:647, 1994.
140. Berman, DS, et al: Incremental value of prognostic testing in patients with known or suspected ischemic heart disease: A basis for optimal utilization of exercise technetium-99m sestamibi myocardial perfusion Single-Photon Emission Computed Tomography. J Am Coll Cardiol 26:639, 1995.
141. Cequeira, MD, et al: Long-term survival in 618 patients from Western Washington Streptokinase in Myocardial Infarction trials. J Am Coll Cardiol 20:1452, 1992.
142. Vanzetto, G, et al: Long-term additive prognosis of thallium-201 myocardial perfusion imaging over clinical and exercise stress test in low to intermediate risk patients. Study in 1137 patients with a 6-year follow-up. Circulation 100:1521, 1999.
143. Olmos, LI, et al: Long-term prognostic value of exercise echocardiography compared with exercise ^{201}Tl, ECG, and clinical variables in patients evaluated for coronary artery disease. Circulation 98:2679, 1998.

144. Ladenheim, ML, et al: Extent and severity of myocardial hypoperfusion as predictors of prognosis in patients with suspected coronary artery disease. J Am Coll Cardiol 7(3):464, 1986.
145. Brown, KA, et al: Early dipyridamole ^{99m}Tc-sestamibi single photon computed tomographic imaging 2 to 4 days after acute myocardial infarction predicts in-hospital and post-discharge cardiac events: Comparison with submaximal exercise imaging. Circulation 100:2060, 1999.
146. Dilsizian, V, et al: The effect of coronary artery bypass grafting on left ventricular systolic function at rest: Evidence for preoperative subclinical myocardial ischemia. Am J Cardiol 61:1248, 1988.
147. Kiat, H, et al: Late reversibility of tomographic myocardial Tl-201 defects: An accurate marker of myocardial viability. J Am Coll Cardiol 12:1456, 1988.
148. Dilsizian, V, et al: Enhanced detection of ischemic but viable myocardium by the reinjection of thallium after stress-redistribution imaging. N Engl J Med 323:141, 1990.
149. Kayden, DS, et al: Thallium-201 for assessment of myocardial viability: Quantitative comparison of 24 hour redistribution with imaging after reinjection at rest. J Am Coll Cardiol 18:1480, 1991.
150. Berger, BC, et al: Redistribution of thallium at rest in patients with stable and unstable angina and the effect of coronary artery bypass surgery. Circulation 60:1114, 1979.
151. Iskandrian, AS, et al: Rest and redistribution thallium-201 myocardial scintigraphy to predict improvement in left ventricular function after coronary arterial bypass grafting. Am J Cardiol 51:1312, 1983.
152. Bisi, G, et al: Rest technetium-99m sestamibi tomography in combination with short-term administration of nitrates: Feasibility and reliability for prediction of post revascularization outcome of asynergic territories. J Am Coll Cardiol 24:1282, 1994.
153. Tillisch, J, et al: Reversibility of cardiac wall-motion abnormalities predicted by positron tomography. N Engl J Med 314:884, 1986.
154. Wolpers, H, et al: Assessment of myocardial viability by use of 11C-acetate and positron emission tomography. Circulation 94:1834, 1996.
155. Murrat G, et al: Metabolic cardiac imaging in coronary disease with severe left ventricular dysfunction: Assessment of myocardial viability with 123-I-iodophenylpentadecanoic acid imaged by a multicrystal gamma camera and correlation with transmural myocardial biopsy. J Nucl Med 33:1269, 1992.
156. Schelbert, HR, et al: Noninvasive assessment of coronary stenoses by myocardial imaging during pharmacologic vasodilatation. VI. Detection of coronary artery disease in man with intravenous N-13 ammonia and positron computed tomography. Am J Cardiol 49:1197, 1982.
157. Gould, KL, et al: Noninvasive assessment of coronary artery stenosis by myocardial perfusion imaging during pharmacologic coronary vasodilatation. VIII. Clinical feasibility of positron cardiac imaging without a cyclotron using generator-produced rubidium-82. J Am Coll Cardiol 7:775, 1986.
158. Sandler, MP, et al: Evaluation of myocardial ischemia using a rest metabolism/stress perfusion protocol with fluorine-18 deoxyglucose/technetium999m MIBI dual isotope simultaneous-acquisition single-photon emission computed tomography. J Am Coll Cardiol 26:870, 1995.
159. De Sutter, J, et al: Cardiac fluorine-18 fluorodeoxyglucose imaging using a dual-head gamma camera with coincidence detection. A clinical pilot study. Eur J Nucl Med 27:676, 2000.
160. Schelbert, H. Euglycemic hyperinsulinemic clamp and oral glucose load in stimulating myocardial glucose utilization during positron emission tomography. J Nucl Med 33:1263, 1992.
161. Gropler, RJ. Methodology governing the assessment of myocardial glucose metabolism by positron emission tomography and fluorine 18-labeled fluorodeoxyglucose. J Nucl Cardiol 1:S4, 1994.
162. Knuuti, MJ, et al: Euglycemic hyperinsulinemic clamp and oral glucose load in stimulating myocardial glucose utilization during positron emission tomography. J Nucl Med 33:1255, 1992.
163. Martin, WH, et al: A simplified intravenous glucose loading protocol for fluorine-18 fluorodeoxyglucose cardiac single-photo emission tomography. Eur J Nucl Med 24:1291, 1997.

164. Knuuti, MJ, et al: Enhancement of myocardial [fluorine-18]fluordeoxyglucose uptake by a nicotinic acid derivative. J Nucl Med 35:989, 1994.
165. Bax, JJ, et al: Accuracy of currently available techniques to predict functional recovery after revascularization in patients with chronic left ventricular dysfunction: comparison of pooled data. J Am Coll Cardiol 30:1451, 1997.
166. Bax, JJ, et al: Prediction of improvement of contractile function in patients with ischemic ventricular dysfunction by F-18-fluorodeoxyglucose SPECT. J Am Coll Cardiol 30:377, 1997.
167. Bax, JJ, et al: 18-Fluorodeoxyglucose imaging with positron emission tomography and single photon emission computed tomography: Cardiac applications. Semim Nucl Med 30:281, 2000.

23
Metabolic Abnormalities and Drugs

Metabolic Acidosis
Alkalosis
Thyroid Abnormalities
Hyperthyroidism
Hypothyroidism
Diabetes
Estrogens
Androgens
Carbon Monoxide
Nicotine
Digitalis
Quinidine
Class I_B Antiarrhythmic Drugs
Class I_C Antiarrhythmic Drugs
Amiodarone
Mechanism of Action of Antianginal Drugs
Nitrates
Long-Acting Nitrates
Dipyridamole
Beta Blockers
Mechanisms of Beta Blockade
Calcium Blockers
Atropine
Propranolol and Atropine
Catecholamines
Amphetamines
Isoproterenol
Psychotropic Drugs
Tricyclic Antidepressants
Lithium
Phenothiazines
Diazepam
Antihypertensive Agents
Diuretics
Methyldopa
Clonidine
Guanethidine
Vasodilators
Angiotensin Converting Enzyme Inhibitors
Angiotensin II Blockers
L-Arginine
p FOX Inhibitors (Partial Fatty Acid Oxidation Inhibitors)
Alcohol

Information on changes in cellular physiology, cardiopulmonary function, and exercise tolerance associated with metabolic abnormalities and various drug regimens is proliferating so fast that our knowledge today may be out of date tomorrow. Many drugs that we use can profoundly alter ischemia, afterload and preload, and the chronotropic and inotropic response. It is essential to consider these changes when undertaking exercise testing. New understanding of metabolic pathways and substances that interact with or alter the physiological processes controlling our cardiovascular system mandates constant study.

This chapter should help the physician to deal with most of the more common conditions and drugs in use. Careful study of newly introduced agents will be mandatory to determine their effects on patients during exercise testing.

METABOLIC ACIDOSIS

Acidosis depresses cardiac contractility, especially during exercise. The accumulation of lactic acid and the ability to tolerate this buildup constitute very important determinants of endurance in sports performance.[1] As the pH level drops with acidosis, the strength of myocardial contraction decreases, and the cardiac output also decreases. Individual susceptibility to this effect seems to vary, and conditioning and age may be factors in this discrepancy.[2] The same drop in pH level seems to have a protective effect against ventricular irritability. The only significant findings on the ECG may be some lowering of the T waves and slight prolongation of the QT interval, although these changes are nonspecific. If exercise is carried to maximum capacity, all subjects become acidotic, but this is quickly corrected during the recovery period.

ALKALOSIS

Carbon dioxide (CO_2) has long been recognized as having important vasoactive properties. The vasoconstrictive properties of a low PCO_2 and the dilatation in the vasculature of the brain seen with a high PCO_2 are the most notable.[2] More recently, the capacity of a low PCO_2 to cause intense coronary vasoconstriction with a resultant decrease in myocardial perfusion has been demonstrated by Case and coworkers.[3] Coronary vascular resistance increases with alkalosis, even when the arterial PO_2 is maintained in the normal range. Thus, ST depression following hyperventilation may actually represent myocardial ischemia.

Chronic hyperventilation is one of the most common types of alkalosis seen in ambulatory patients. This condition is common in emotionally labile women, who are often subject to vague chest symptoms and may be suspected of having coronary artery disease (CAD). Chronic alkalosis involves intracellular potassium depletion with a subsequent increase in urinary potassium loss. A lower than normal level of total body potassium may account for fatigue, loss of strength, and characteristic changes reflected in the ECG. The ECG of such a patient is illustrated in Figure 23–1. A 28-year-old woman was referred to our Pulmonary Rehabilitation Clinic because of suspected asthma or emphysema. Her spirometric measurements were normal, but the blood gas studies revealed a pH of 7.51 and a PCO_2 of 32; serum potassium was 3.2. The stress test disclosed ST-segment depression at rest, which was accentuated by hyperventilation. The results were considered by some observers to be suggestive of CAD. After potassium level correction, prolonged psychotherapy, and an exercise program, the patient became relatively free of symptoms, and her resting ECG returned to normal. This patient is an extreme example of the ECG changes seen in those who are chronically anxious and neurotic. One of the reasons for using a period of hy-

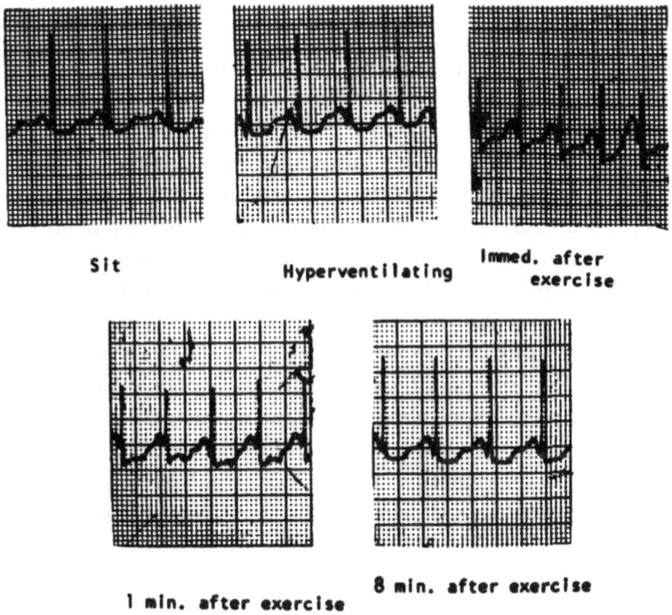

FIGURE 23–1. The CM_5 leads recorded from a 28-year-old woman with chronic hyperventilation, a low PCO_2, and a high pH. The tendency for the depressed ST segments to evolve toward normal immediately after exercise and then to assume a more pathological appearance during recovery is common in people with metabolic abnormalities.

perventilation prior to the stress test is to help identify such persons and distinguish the ST-segment changes caused by the metabolic defect from those resulting from ischemia due to coronary narrowing.

As discussed in Chapter 12, excessive diuretic use is another cause of alkalosis.

THYROID ABNORMALITIES

Hyperthyroidism

High levels of thyroid hormone (T_3 and T_4) profoundly influence cardiac function as well as the metabolism of all body tissues. The increase in heart rate, systolic blood pressure, ejection rate, and coronary blood flow is associated with a decrease in systemic resistance. Iskandrian and colleagues[4] studied 10 thyrotoxic patients with exercise radionuclide angiograms. They found the exercise capacity, heart rate, and blood pressure to be similar to those of normals, but at maximum capacity the ejection fraction was reduced. This supported the previous data indicating that hyperthyroidism is associated with cardiac dysfunction.[5,6] ST-segment changes are not usually seen in hyperthyroidism, however.

Hypothyroidism

A decrease in thyroid hormone is known to reduce cardiac output and to decrease myocardial contractility and heart rate. These changes are of sufficient magnitude that iodine 131 (I 131) was once proposed as a treatment for severe angina, even though it was known to be associated with acceleration of the atherosclerotic process. Hypothyroidism is often associated with T-wave flattening and ST-segment depression. Exercise has been reported to produce ST depression in about 50% of patients with severe myxedema. Thus, thyroid function should be taken into consideration when ST depression occurs, especially in a lethargic woman with a slow heart rate. Hylander and associates[7] studied the cardiovascular response to thyroid replacement and found that it took 12 weeks or more for the exercise-induced ST segments to return to normal, about the same amount of time it took for thyroid stimulating hormone to normalize. On the other hand, it took about 35 weeks for the exercise capacity to return to normal. They proposed that the heart returns to normal function before the peripheral response can recover.

DIABETES

Stress testing in diabetic patients requires some knowledge of the disturbances in metabolism and physiology brought on by this protean disease. Besides hypertension and hyperlipidemia, diabetes is known to be associated with alterations in the microvasculature and with deposits of mucopolysaccharides in the myocardium.[8,9] The latter changes may explain the report from the Framingham study that twice as many diabetic patients as age-matched controls develop congestive heart failure.[10] An inadequate insulin supply has been shown to inhibit the transport of glucose across the myocardial cell membrane,[11] and glucose phosphorylation by adenosine triphosphate is altered so that an excess of ammonium is liberated.[12] Not only does the ammonium decrease myocardial contractility secondary to the acidosis, but the increased use in free fatty acids also results in a decrease in glucose use and an excess deposit of glycogen in the heart muscle. These changes decrease both myocardial compliance and the contractile force and can best be identified by measuring the isovolumetric relaxation time, which is abnormally prolonged, especially after exercise.

Rubler[9] and Rubler and Arvan[13] have described a reduction in exercise capacity, higher systolic and diastolic pressures, and a lower maximum heart rate in asymptomatic diabetics. The latter finding may be an expression of the dysautonomia under study in diabetes[14] and is believed to be due to a generalized neuropathy.[15] Rubler,[9] however, failed to document a higher incidence of ST depression in diabetics when compared with that of patients of the same age in other studies.

On the other hand, Persson[16] studied 84 diabetic men with exercise and followed them up for 9 years. He found an increased prevalence of ST depression in the diabetic patients compared with controls, as well as a correlation with the duration of the diabetes. A similar increase in ST depression during exercise was also reported by Bellet and Roman[17] and Karlefors.[18]

It may be prudent to test diabetic subjects in a fasting state if they are on insulin, as reported by Riley and colleagues,[19] who found that intravenous glucose increases the incidence of ST-segment depression. It remains to be determined whether a glucose meal would have the same effect. When subjects on insulin are studied in our laboratory, we perform stress testing approximately 2 hours after either breakfast or lunch without altering either their diet or their insulin schedule. I am aware of no case in which this practice has resulted in a false-positive test or in any complications related to blood sugar levels.

ESTROGENS

Exercise-induced ST depression is often seen in women with normal coronary arteries.[20,21] Although there is still some question whether estrogen is a cause, the hormone has been reported to function as a vasoconstrictor.[22] In contrast, estrogen has also been reported to cause coronary dilatation by preventing constriction in CAD patients given acetylcholine.[23] Engel's group[24] has presented evidence of decreased myocardial perfusion in women taking estrogens. Various estrogens have been found to have an adverse effect on the incidence of myocardial infarction in subjects in the Coronary Drug Project,[25] and in men treated for carcinoma of the prostate.[26]

Jaffe[27] found that when treating patients with established CAD, 90% had more ST-segment depression after 2 weeks of treatment with 10 mg of conjugated estrogens or 5 mg of stilbestrol. When treating 10 patients (five men and five women) without CAD or ST depression, however, he failed to produce ST changes.[28] Because Jaffe used only the Master's test, we do not know whether ST depression would manifest at higher workloads. A recent report by Marmor and associates[29] clearly demonstrates that estrogens cause ST depression. Women with false-positive ST depression had a normal response after having their ovaries surgically removed. At this juncture, when patients taking estrogens have an abnormal ST response to exercise, the possibility of a drug-induced response should always be considered (Table 23–1), especially if the abnormal response occurs in a woman in the age group in which CAD is known to be rare. Because estrogens have some pharmacological similarity to digitalis, more careful studies need to be carried out to determine their role in myocardial metabolism.

ANDROGENS

Very few data are available on the influence of androgens on the heart. It seemed logical that after studying the effect of estrogens, Jaffe[28] would ex-

Table 23–1. **Agents Reported to Alter Exercise-Induced ST-Segment Changes**

False-Positive	False-Negative
Digitalis	Nitrates
Estrogens	Beta blockers
Diuretics	Quinidine
Catecholamines ?	Androgens ?
Lithium ?	Diazepam ?

tend the study to the evaluation of androgens. Because women have a lower incidence of infarction than men, it was long believed that estrogens protected against CAD and that androgens must have an adverse effect. The findings released by the Coronary Drug Project[25] implicating estrogen as a possible added risk factor were a surprise to most of us. The added evidence that estrogens aggravated exercise-induced ischemia, however, tended to confirm the concept that the physiological effect of this steroid has an adverse effect on cardiac function.

Jaffe[30] has reported that ethylestrenol, an anabolic steroid, and testosterone cypionate both reduce ST-segment depression in patients with CAD. When testosterone (200 mg intramuscularly) was compared with a placebo for 4 to 8 weeks, the treated subjects had a decrease in the sum of the ST depression in leads II, V_4, V_5, and V_6 immediately after a two-step test—32% after 4 weeks of treatment and 51% after 8 weeks of treatment. The reason for this improvement was not established, but the exercise heart rate was significantly lower in those who showed improvement. The blood pressure was not altered. Testosterone is known to improve muscle strength and to increase the sense of vigor, so that those treated actually may have needed less caloric expenditure because of increased muscle strength.[31] Androgens also increase the 2, 3-diphosphoglycerate in red blood cells, thus enabling them to carry more oxygen[11] and increase the concentration of hemoglobin.[32] The men in Jaffe's study, however, failed to have a measurable increase in hemoglobin.

Finally, a decrease in smooth muscle tone has been reported,[33] which might decrease coronary resistance. Holma[34] studied the hemodynamic changes in athletes following a 2-month oral dose of metandierone, an anabolic steroid. He found an increase in stroke volume, a reduction in heart rate, and improved peak forearm blood flow, which would also support the concept that smooth muscle relaxation is an important component.

At this point, the final mechanism for the improvement is unknown, but since angina was also decreased, there may actually be less ischemia after the administration of male hormones.

CARBON MONOXIDE

We are exposed to carbon monoxide daily in automobile exhaust and cigarette smoke. As early as 1973, it was reported that adverse effects from carbon monoxide could be detected in patients with CAD.[35] When exposure to carbon monoxide is chronic, the carboxyhemoglobin level increases, competes with oxyhemoglobin in our red blood cells, and produces relative hypoxia. Disagreement as to the importance of this potentially toxic substance was reported by Anderson and associates,[36] leading to a multicenter study in 63 men with CAD, funded by the Environmental Protection Agency.[37] Exposure to enough carbon monoxide to produce levels of both 2% and 3.9% carboxyhemoglobin was found to result in reduced treadmill time to the onset of ST depression and angina. These levels are commonly achieved by smokers or by those exposed to excessive automobile exhaust. This study suggests that a long ride on a crowded freeway or a day of smoking definitely increases ischemia and results in a greater magnitude of ST depression at a lower workload. Thus, exposure to carbon monoxide should be kept in mind when using exercise testing to evaluate the severity of ischemia.

NICOTINE

Although athletes and coaches always knew that nicotine impaired exercise capacity, the exact reasons were not clear. Also, it has long been known that smokers gain weight when they give up smoking. In about 1940, it was demonstrated that both dogs and humans increased their metabolism after smoking,[38] and in 1989 Perkins and colleagues[39] demonstrated that the modest increases in oxygen uptake were greatly accentuated by even mild exercise. These investigators also found that the increased work required to perform a given exercise load was not associated with an increase in perceived exertion.

The deleterious effects on respiratory function and the reduced oxyhemoglobin are therefore not necessarily the major causes of reduced performance. Nicotine has been shown to increase systolic and diastolic pressure and to reduce vagal tone, with its attendant increase in sympathetic drive.[40] The markers for this change are loss of RR variability, increased resting heart rate, and augmented response to Valsalva's maneuver. Blood flow to the skin is also reduced, resulting in a major increase in peripheral resistance. Kamimori[41] has shown that smoking decreases the diameter of epicardial coronary arteries in patients with coronary atheroma, as well as the velocity of blood flow. These changes have been shown to be due to endothelial cell dysfunction.[42]

Therefore, during exercise testing the heart rate and blood pressure will be greater for any given workload and ischemia will come on earlier. For all these reasons, it is wise to ask patients to refrain from smoking before their exercise test.

DIGITALIS

The alterations in ST segments produced by digitalis are well documented, and ischemic ST-segment changes can be accentuated when a patient who has taken the drug exercises. Digitalis also clearly produces exercise-induced ST-segment depression in persons with normal coronary arteries.

Oddly, even though digitalis has been used longer than any other drug in patients with cardiac disorders, doubt remains about some of its pharmacology. Some of its actions, however, are fairly well understood:

1. In the normal-sized heart, the inotropic effect is associated with an increased oxygen uptake.
2. In the failing heart, the size of the ventricle can be reduced, and thus the oxygen consumption is actually decreased.[43] Vogel and colleagues[44] have demonstrated with thallium 201 uptake that myocardial perfusion actually increases in the failing heart when a patient is given digitalis. These subjects have also been shown to have better left-ventricular function during exercise.[45]
3. A definite vasoconstrictor effect has been demonstrated both in coronary arteries and in peripheral tissue.[46,47] This seems to be due to a direct effect on the smooth muscles of both arteries and veins. In the heart, a reduction of flow to the subendocardium has been demonstrated by both rubidium 86 and radioactive microspheres.[48] When this happens, there is usually an increase in left-ventricular systolic and end-diastolic pressure associated with the drug. Evidence also suggests that at times the epicardium may be relatively overperfused and act as a physiological shunt.[49]
4. Even though the above decrease in subendocardial flow is present, the ST depression may not be due to significant ischemia[50]; although oxygen inhalation tends to correct the ST depression, nitroglycerin fails to have the same effect. Nitrates have been shown to dilate digitalis-induced coronary artery constriction, however.[51]
5. Digitalis has been demonstrated to cause an increase in intracellular calcium, a change also present in ischemia.[52]

Studies to elucidate the incidence and mechanism of digitalis-induced ST depression during exercise are numerous but still leave us with some uncertainties.[48,52,53] Reports that the administration of potassium reduces digitalis-induced ST depression may explain the reputed ST-segment improvement in some patients at high workloads, since this is when exercise causes a maximum increase in serum potassium. Also, as exercise progresses, serum digitalis decreases because of increased binding to working muscle.[49] Kawai and Hultgren[50] reported that approximately 50% of their normal subjects placed on a maintenance dose of digoxin and tested on a Master's protocol had significant ST depression, but that the changes could be minimized by oxygen inhalation or potassium infusion. Goldbarg[54] reported about the same incidence of ST depression in normal subjects taking digitalis. Tonkin and colleagues[55] reported that ST changes occurred in all subjects with digoxin levels higher than 0.5 mg/mL. They also found that when these patients reached a workload of over 75% of their maximum predicted heart rate, the ST depression disappeared, thereby enabling them to distinguish those subjects with ischemia from those with drug changes alone. They also found that most of their subjects had a J-point or upsloping pattern and that the depth of the ST depression and the serum digoxin level were roughly correlated ($r = .57$). A Swedish study by Sundqvist and colleagues[56] confirmed these findings using 11 healthy subjects. These volunteers had a mean age of only 28 years, however, and older subjects may have a different response.

Sketch and colleagues,[21] on the other hand, found that the ST depression continued to maximum workload in normal patients given digoxin and that the changes persisted in a few up to 6 minutes into recovery. They also reported that the incidence of ST depression increased with age. Although only 25% of the total cohort had ST depression, 100% of those older than aged 60 exhibited this finding. After 5 years, these researchers retested most of their subjects and found that those who originally had digitalis-induced ST depression were likely to have ST changes without the drug on follow-up. They postulate that digitalis unmasks ischemia and that some of those with ST depression after digoxin were really false-negative responders. This hypothesis, I believe, requires further verification.

Degre and associates[57] from Belgium reported that an increase in R-wave amplitude will differentiate those on digitalis. The specificity of the ST depression was 30% but increased to 70% when the increase in R-wave amplitude was added. Sensitivity was 100% and 50%, respectively. It has also been reported that ST depression due to ischemia is improved by nitroglycerin but that no change is seen if digitalis is the cause.

Our experience has been that ST depression of 4 to 5 mm almost always signals ischemia, even in patients who are taking digitalis. The maximum magnitude in the normal patients in Sketch and colleagues' study was 1.9 mm. A patient on digitalis who is tested and has no ST depression provides strong evidence against the presence of myocardial ischemia. Digitalis inhibits chronotropic response in patients with sinus rhythm as well as in those with atrial fibrillation.

Kawai and Hultgren[50] reported a normal QT interval in subjects with digitalis-induced ST changes, compared with prolonged QT intervals in those with ischemia. This important finding has not been confirmed. Davidson and Hagan[58] have proposed the use of stress testing in patients on digitalis with atrial fibrillation to assess the adequacy of the dose. When the drug level is adequate, the ventricular response to exercise will be similar to that of patients in sinus rhythm; when this is accomplished, exercise tolerance will improve.

QUINIDINE

Although it has been stated that the use of quinidine will bring about a false-positive stress test result, I have been unable to find a documented example and have never observed such a response in our laboratory. In toxic doses, quinidine may prolong conduction at any level in the conduction system, but when blood levels are in the therapeutic range, it is very useful as an antiarrhythmic agent during exercise. Gey and colleagues[59] gave quinidine gluconate to 29 subjects orally in doses of 10 and 15 mg/kg of body weight prior to a standard Bruce test. Some subjects were normal, whereas others had documented CAD. The investigators observed an excellent antiarrhythmic effect but were unable to identify a change in either heart rate or blood pressure, and no evidence of ST-segment depression was found. They reported that procainamide (Pronestyl), however, has been shown to produce significant ST depression during exercise.[60] Fluster and coworkers[61] reported that quinidine increases resting as well as exercise heart rate; this issue is unresolved at this time.

Surawicz and colleagues[62,63] have stated that the prolongation of phase 2 of the ventricular action potential by quinidine decreases the repolarization gradient during inscription of the ST segment and thereby diminishes the manifestation of ST depression even during ischemia. Friedberg and associates[64] have also reported that quinidine produces a false-negative stress test result.

CLASS I_B ANTIARRHYTHMIC DRUGS

The drugs in this class in common clinical use are lidocaine, phenytoin, tocainide, and mexiletine. Lidocaine is given intravenously only, so it is unlikely to be a problem with exercise testing. The other three agents, although not in wide use, may be given to ischemic patients who require exercise testing.

These agents cause small changes in conduction velocity, which may be augmented by an increased frequency of excitation. There is a decreased slope of phase 4 depolarization.[65] Ischemia causes a decrease in conduction velocity in patients taking these agents. The QT interval may shorten somewhat, but the QRS interval does not get wider. Both tocainide and lidocaine have been shown to cause a small decrease in left-ventricular function and an increase in peripheral resistance. No change in heart rate or any effect on ischemia has been reported.[66] Significant alterations are unlikely if patients taking these drugs are given an exercise test.

CLASS I_C ANTIARRHYTHMIC DRUGS

Flecainide and encainide, along with propafenone, are more potent agents than the class I_B drugs. Although flecainide and encainide have received some bad press because of their proarrhythmic effect, patients on these agents may require exercise testing. All these drugs suppress ventricular function, prolong conduction time, and are expected to reduce overall exercise capacity.[67]

The best information on the influence of class I_C drugs on exercising patients has been published on flecainide.[68] As exercise or heart rate increases, conduction slowing, probably due to the use-dependent sodium channel blockade, will prolong the QRS duration. In one case, this resulted in a monomorphic ventricular tachycardia at peak exercise. Thus, exercise in patients taking class I_C drugs will probably enhance their proarrhythmic effect, and one should be alert for exercise-induced prolongation of the QRS duration. If a resting tracing prior to the institution of flecainide is available, QRS prolongation can usually be observed even at rest after a therapeutic dose. The same effect is seen when the heart rate is increased by pacing, demonstrating that the effect is due to the rate rather than to the metabolic effect of exercise.

AMIODARONE

Amiodarone, a benzfuran derivative, was introduced as an antianginal agent in 1967 because of its depressant effect on sinus node function. It has emerged as a potent antiarrhythmic agent, especially for malignant ventricular tachycardia. A study by Rod and Shenasa[69] in Milwaukee found that it suppresses resting heart rate an average of 15 beats per minute and maximum exercise heart rate an average of 20 beats per minute. The systolic blood pressure at each heart rate prior to administration of the drug was the same as during the drug therapy, as was the functional capacity expressed in metabolic equivalents (MET).

The mechanism of heart rate suppression has been studied by Touboul and colleagues[70] and others.[71] They believe that an increase in action potential duration, a prolongation in sinus node recovery time, and a normal sinus node conduction time explain the findings. The increase in action potential duration, similar to that in I_C agents, rarely causes a problem because the drug supresses tachycardia. This drug, then, differs from beta blockers in that it does not have a negative inotropic effect, and that resting and exercise blood pressures are not reduced unless the patient is hypertensive.

MECHANISM OF ACTION OF ANTIANGINAL DRUGS

Simoons and Balakumaran[72] have claimed that antianginal drugs act through two primary mechanisms. Drugs that slow heart rate, such as beta blockers and alidine (a derivative of clonidine), characterize the first mechanisms.[73] The reduction in heart rate decreases myocardial oxygen demand and velocity of contraction and allows for a longer diastolic period, which favors an increased myocardial perfusion through compromised coronary arteries.[74] The second mechanism, illustrated by nitroglycerin, increases venous capacitance and decreases arterial resistance, thereby reducing inflow into the heart. This results in a decrease in left-ventricular volume and reduced wall stress and afterload. Calcium blockers may do both of the above. They may also have a direct effect on the myocardial cell membrane, but this is believed to be of lesser importance. As it turns out, a number of other important mechanisms come into play. Gaspardone and colleagues[75] have reported on the antianginal effect of a new xanthine, Bamiphylline, which, although increasing the time to angina during exercise testing, does not dilate coronary arteries, reduce heart rate, or reduce preload. The drug works by selective blockade of the A1 adenosine receptors, as does aminophylline. There is little doubt that adenosine is in some way linked to anginal pain.[76] There is evidence that aminophylline causes subepicardial constriction and therefore redirects blood to the subendocardium. The fact that adenosine produces a "coronary steal" is now well recognized by those using this agent to produce ischemia when recording thallium scintigrams to detect CAD.[77]

NITRATES

Although the reduction in arterial resistance is an important mechanism, a number of other mechanisms play a significant role. The simplistic concept that nitrates function as coronary dilators does not help in understanding this complex process. It is obvious that an agent that increases flow to a normal segment of myocardium might well shunt blood away from an ischemic area. Thus, the precapillary sphincters, believed to be under local metabolic control, are probably not significantly altered by these agents. It now is well established that nitrates serve to redistribute blood to the ischemic areas.[78] The mechanism of this redistribution is because of its direct effect on the microcirculation.[79] The demonstrated capacity of nitrates to reduce venous tone and thus allow the blood to sequestrate in the capacitance vessels, with the resultant decrease in cardiac filling,[80] must be an important part of the reduction in cardiac work. The drop in left-ventricular end-diastolic pressure (LVEDP) immediately after nitroglycerin administration is familiar to every catheterizing cardiologist.

One explanation for the favorable redistribution of blood may be related to the anatomical location of many collateral vessels. Fulton[81] has shown that in occlusive CAD, the major communications between normal and ischemic zones of myocardium are in the subendocardial plexus and are thus subject to cavity pressure. In subjects with a high diastolic pressure, which is common during an ischemic episode, this effect would be important. If the venous filling were to drop suddenly, the reduction of 10 to 20 mm of diastolic filling pressure might well favor a redistribution of blood to the ischemic areas through these pathways that are so vulnerable to the forces of compression present in the left-ventricular cavity. This mechanism has been attractively presented by McGregor[82] and supported by Vineberg and associates[83] and by others.[84] When Ganz and Marcus[85] injected nitroglycerin directly into the coronary arteries, they could not document an increased flow in the coronary sinus. On the other hand, other investigators have documented an increase in flow in both dogs[86] and humans[87] after nitroglycerin. It seems that even though nitrates have a demonstrated ability to provide smooth muscle relaxation, which in many cases affects the larger branches of the coronary tree, other mechanisms may be more important than the increase in flow.[88]

Long-Acting Nitrates

When the long-acting preparations, such as the stereoisomers of pentitol (Pentanitrate), isosorbide dinitrate (Isordil), and erythrol tetranitrate, are taken sublingually, they act much like glyceryl trinitrate but with longer activity.[89] Goldstein and colleagues[78] found that only a small percentage of their subjects had a favorable effect 1 hour after sublingual isosorbide dinitrate, and in most cases it was indistinguishable from those changes related to nitroglycerin.

When taken by mouth, there was some question as to the effectiveness of long-acting nitrates, but Russek and Funk[80] found 20 to 60 mg of pentaerythritol tetranitrate (Peritrate) to be effective in reducing the ST changes on a Master's test for up to 5 hours. Others have had difficulty confirming these findings, however.[90]

Wayne and colleagues[91] tested the responses on a treadmill of 19 patients with CAD while taking isosorbide dinitrate versus a placebo. They found that the drug delayed the onset of ST depression and reduced its magnitude; any ST depression was prevented in three patients. The data on long-acting nitrates can be summarized by concluding that when given prior to an exercise test, they may reduce the ST depression associated with exercise and possibly even prevent it in some cases. Thus, long-acting nitrates should be withheld for an appropriate interval. It has been my experience that in most subjects the ST changes are not eliminated but may appear at a higher workload than they would without a long-acting nitrate.

DIPYRIDAMOLE

Because of the widespread belief that nitrates owe their effectiveness to an increase in coronary flow, other agents with this capacity have been tried clinically.[92] Dipyridamole (Persantine) is one of these, but it falls far short of the nitrates in its ability to mitigate ischemic changes associated with exercise, even though it will increase coronary flow by 300% to 400%.[93] When dipyridamole is given, the coronary sinus oxygen concentration increases significantly, suggesting that perfusion of the myocardium may increase excessively without improving delivery to areas of ischemia. Its mechanism of action has been shown to be due to the stimulation of endogenous adenosine, which redistributes blood from the subendocardium to the subepicardium.[76] Reports of the ability of dipyridamole to produce collateral growth after long-term administration, as well as an alteration in platelet adhesiveness, may suggest its clinical usefulness in some settings.

Because of its propensity to redistribute blood away from areas of ischemia, intravenous administration has been used to initiate ischemia. Usually 0.75 mg/kg dipyridamole is administered intravenously in a 10-minute period during ECG monitoring. ST depression or anginal pain is a marker for ischemia, as it is in exercise testing. Tavazzi and coworkers[94] in Italy found a 74% sensitivity in patients with angina on effort, but there were no positive responders among those with angina at rest. Dipyridamole produced a positive test in 74% of those with an abnormal exercise test. None of the normal subjects had a positive test. Thus, dipyridamole provides a low sensitivity and possibly higher specificity in exercise testing. When given orally, it apparently fails to alter the ST segments or the response to exercise significantly. We have used dipyridamole extensively to initiate ischemia in patients undergoing nuclear studies who are unable to exercise for some reason.

BETA BLOCKERS

Although early on some denied the obvious benefits of beta blockers on the angina syndrome,[95] many clinicians began to use them to treat their patients with CAD soon after the drugs became available.

Mechanisms of Beta Blockade

It is now well established that beta blockers act by the following mechanisms:

1. Decrease in contractility. This is apparently due to their ability to isolate the beta receptors from the intrinsic catecholamines present in the circulation by reducing the metabolic demands associated with this stimulating hormone.

2. Decrease in heart rate. When the number of contractions per minute decreases, not only is the total energy per minute necessary to sustain contraction reduced, but also the longer diastole results in a better perfusion because of the known attenuating effect on coronary flow during systole. The ratio of the systolic pressure time interval to the diastolic pressure time interval is a very important parameter in the determination of the magnitude of coronary flow. The longer that diastole is sustained, the better the redistribution that takes place through the subendocardial collateral channels between the normal and ischemic areas, as mentioned in the previous section on nitrates.[96]
3. Depression of arterial pressure. This is due primarily to a reduction in cardiac output, which is a function of both heart rate and inotropism.
4. Change in myocardial intermediary metabolism. Evidence now suggests that oxidative catabolism is reduced and more glucose is used, resulting in a more efficient system.[97]
5. A shift in AV-O_2 dissociation curve. There are reports that propranolol shifts the hemoglobin dissociation curve to the right, thus facilitating a better release of oxygen as it perfuses the coronary bed. This is due to a redistribution of 2, 3-diphosphoglycerate in the red blood cell.[88]
6. Constriction of peripheral vessels, increasing total peripheral resistance.
7. Inhibition of lipolysis, thus decreasing the primary myocardial substrate, free fatty acids.
8. Further increase of serum potassium over the usual 1 mEq common with any sustained exercise.

It is well established that beta blockers are very useful in the treatment of ischemia, and a significant number of patients presenting for exercise testing will be taking a maintenance dose. Although it may limit the diagnostic value of the test somewhat, the practical approach is to test the patient without discontinuing the drug. The maximum heart rate will be decreased, but it has been reported that the drug will not obscure ischemic ST depression in patients with epicardial coronary narrowing.[98]

Not all the effects of beta blockers are beneficial. They increase the systolic ejection period, probably because of the reduction in velocity of ejection, they increase the LVEDP, and they cause some cardiac dilatation. Beta blockers also result in a higher plasma epinephrine in exercising subjects compared with those who are not blocked.[99] This is thought to be stimulated by the lower cardiac output and heart rate in exercising subjects and may be the cause for the higher peripheral resistance, probably because of the effect of epinephrine on the alpha receptors. Although all these factors increase myocardial oxygen uptake, they fail in most patients to outweigh the benefits, so that on balance, patients with CAD do better during exercise with beta blockers. Thus, in patients who have fairly severe ischemia, a higher workload can be achieved with an equivalent heart rate or double product after a beta blocker has been administered.[99,100]

Many patients not only exercise longer on the treadmill after having taken a beta blocker but also have less ST-segment depression and less angina. It is our feeling that this event can be predicted fairly well by knowing something about the patient's general cardiac function.Those with a large fibrotic left ventricle and a slow resting pulse are not usually benefited. On the other hand, if patients smoke, have a high resting pulse, and have never had an infarction, they are likely to be improved by this agent. Beta blockers have a more profound effect on older subjects, probably because of their reduced level of catecholamines.

A host of newer drugs with slightly different actions have followed the original beta-blocking agent, propranolol. The earliest were the so-called cardioselective agents such as metropolol, atenolol, and pindolol, by far the most potent, all of which had an effect on an exercising patients very similar to that of their predecessors. Since then, a number of modifications have been made, one of which is sotolol, designed to act primarily as an antiarrhythmic.[101] It has very little inotropic effect and functions much like the class III antiarrhythmic agents in that it prolongs the ventricular action potential, recognized readily by QT prolongation.[102] Sotolol also has a heart-rate–related effect: It prolongs the QT interval with slow heart rates but has very little effect on a heart rate higher than 120. Thus, exercise does not increase its proarrhythmic effect, as with the class I_C agents, although it could conceivably reduce its protective effect at high heart rates. Sotolol has very little, if any, hypotensive effect during exercise.[103]

Beta blockers also enhance the tendency for coronary arteries to develop spasm during exercise. This effect probably plays a role only when there is an increased propensity for vasoconstriction, as in Prinzmetal's angina. Asandi and associates[102] have reported that when ST-segment depression is variable from one minute to the next during an exercise test in a patient on beta blockers, one should be alert to the possibility that coronary spasm is occurring.

CALCIUM BLOCKERS

The mechanism of the antianginal effect of calcium blockers has been widely documented.[104] These agents reduce peripheral resistance, and compounds such as verapamil and diltiazem also reduce heart rate—two good reasons for their salutary effects. Inhibition of transmembrane calcium transport may not only have a peripheral effect but may also have a primary effect on the heart itself. This is due in part to the ability to dilate the epicardial coronary arteries, especially in the areas adjacent to stenotic segments, but also to the overall increase in flow to the capillary bed, probably because of an effect on the precapillary sphincters.[105] The inhibition of calcium overloading in ischemic myocardial muscle cells may also be important. As would be expected, when patients taking calcium blockers perform exercise tests, ischemia may come on at higher workloads, and systolic blood pressure and heart rate may be decreased for a given level of exercise.[106] If exercise is terminated by angina, work tolerance may also be increased by these drugs.

The first three drugs available in the United States provided a wide range of action. Verapamil has the most profound direct cardiac effect, with a lesser degree of action in the peripheral vasculature, whereas nifedipine has the least cardiac effect and the most profound action in the peripheral circulation.[107] Diltiazem has some of both effects and is intermediate between the other two. These drugs have been demonstrated to delay the time of onset of ST depression, but if the blood pressure drop is excessive, as may occur in some patients with nifedipine,[108] the reduced diastolic pressure may decrease myocardial perfusion and reduce exercise tolerance.[106]

A more recent group of calcium blockers, called second-generation dihydropyridine agents, has been released. Although they are similar to the first-generation agents, they do not produce tachycardia and have only a weak negative inotropic effect, if any.[109] Drugs in this category include felodipine, isradipine, nicardipine, amlodapine and several others. During exercise testing, the ischemic threshold is usually extended even though the heart rate may not be altered.[110]

ATROPINE

Atropine, which increases the heart rate in most patients, would be expected to make ST-segment changes more likely during exercise because of the increased metabolic demands associated with more contractions per minute. In fact, this rarely occurs, apparently because the patient's catecholamines normally play an important role in the increase in heart rate and the enhancement of ventricular contractility during exercise. The catecholamine changes override those due to the atropine. The patient's loss of ability to sweat after administration of atropine has a definite effect on heat elimination, however, so that if exercise lasts very long, exercise capacity definitely will be decreased. Atropine increases heart rate less in patients with poor left-ventricular function than in normals.

PROPRANOLOL AND ATROPINE

Jose and Taylor,[111] in their studies on intrinsic heart rate, proposed the administration of propranolol and atropine to obtain a medically denervated heart. The resultant resting heart rate seemed to correlate well with the contractility of the left ventricle. They termed this the *intrinsic heart rate.* Figure 23–2 illus-

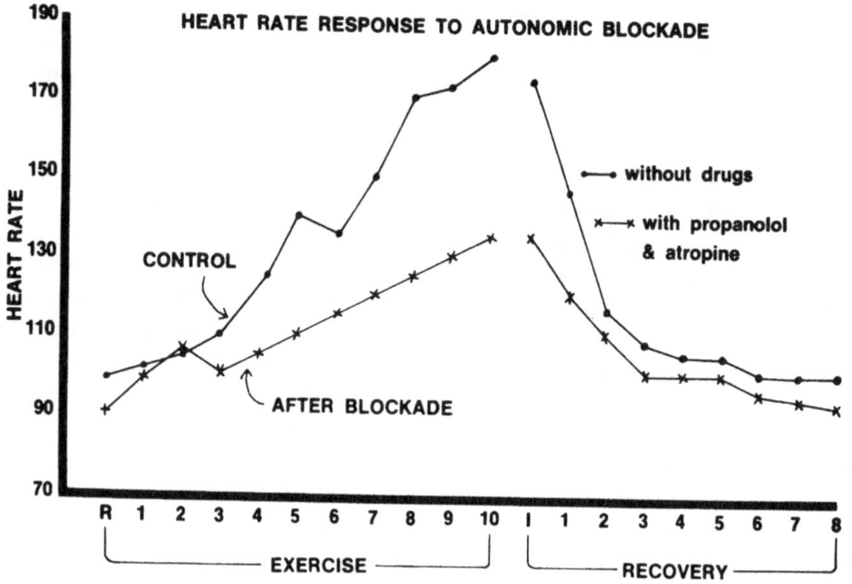

FIGURE 23–2. The heart rate response to a stress test before and after autonomic blockade by propranolol and atropine illustrates the magnitude of the catecholamine effect on heart rate during exercise.

trates the pulse response on our treadmill protocol before and after a blocking dose of these two agents was given intravenously. It can be seen that the exercise heart rate is considerably lower at the upper end of the scale, when the patient's intrinsic catecholamines are a major factor in acceleration. As would be expected, these pharmacological agents decrease the exercise capacity somewhat, along with the heart rate.

CATECHOLAMINES

The effect of catecholamines on the heart has been studied extensively.[63,108,109,112,113] Their well-known stimulatory effect on contractility, heart rate, and myocardial oxygen uptake suggests that they should be avoided by most subjects with suspected CAD, and thus they rarely present a problem in stress testing. In fact, one of the most common habits of CAD patients is smoking, which stimulates an increase in catecholamines[114] as well as a decrease in the oxygen carrying capacity of the blood to a variable degree, depending on the concentration of carbon monoxide fixed in the red blood cells. Cryer and colleagues[114] have shown a marked increase in both norepinephrine and epinephrine and the expected secondary hemodynamic changes associated with smoking two nonfiltered cigarettes. Aronow[115] has reported that ST-segment depression occurs at a low workload after smoking. We have urged patients to abstain from smoking for several hours prior to an exercise test; abstinence also helps to minimize arrhythmias associated with exercise.

AMPHETAMINES

Another family of agents in common usage, which may produce all the familiar changes associated with catecholamine ingestion, are the amphetamines. Not only do they cause the expected acute manifestations, but also they produce a chronic cardiomyopathy,[116] which might well be predicted in view of the well-known experimental cardiomyopathies associated with isoproterenol.[117]

ISOPROTERENOL

Because he wanted to produce a higher incidence of positive stress tests, Gubner[118] administered sublingual isoproterenol (Isuprel) prior to the Master's test. Daoud and associates[112] have studied the effects of catecholamines extensively and have reported that in subjects with inverted T waves, intravenous administration of isoproterenol corrects the inversion in a high percentage of subjects with normal hearts and also in some with CAD. We have found that exercise often results in the normalization of inverted T waves because of the catecholamine effect that normally comes with strenuous exercise. We have not used catecholamines to add an additional stimulus to stress testing because of our standard practice of using a maximum stress test. Gubner[118] was using a Master's test, which is often far from maximum, and there is no evidence that the use of an extra catecholamine stimulus might correct some of the false-negative results in those who do not reach a maximum heart rate.

PSYCHOTROPIC DRUGS

Tricyclic Antidepressants

Thirty million prescriptions are written in the United States each year for tricyclic antidepressants.[119] The Aberdeen General Hospital Group[119] studied the cardiovascular effects in 119 cardiac patients and found that 2.2% of patients in the wards were taking one or more of these antidepressant compounds and that the mortality rate in 40 months was 19% in treated patients compared with 12% in controls matched for age, sex, and cardiac diagnosis. The heart rate is higher and the T waves are lower with these drugs, and ST depression is common. The PR interval is prolonged, as is the HV interval when His' bundle recordings are performed. The QT_c and QRS intervals are increased as well in 15% of the patients, and a Mobitz type 2 atrioventricular (AV) block is not uncommon.[119] Vohra and colleagues[120] report an excellent correlation between the degree of prolongation of the QRS interval and the plasma concentration of the tricyclic antidepressants. There is good evidence that in patients with bundle branch block, a lower dose will produce a complete AV block compared with those with normal conduction.[115,117,119,121] Kantor and associates[122] and Bigger and colleagues[123] have reported that arrhythmias are very rare, and a growing body of evidence suggests that these agents have some antiarrhythmic properties. In fact, the pharmacological properties of tricyclic antidepressants are strikingly similar to those of quinidine. Muller and Burckhard[124] evaluated left-ventricular function with systolic time intervals and found a prolongation of the pre-ejection period and a decrease in the PEP/VET* ratio as well as a decrease in velocity of fiber shortening by echocardiography. The same finding has also been reported in rats by Thorstrand and coworkers.[125] These data and the reported cases of hypotension clearly point to a depression of left-ventricular function.

Although there have been no reports of exercise-induced ST depression due to tricyclic antidepressants, they are in such common use that it is important to be aware of their suppressive effect on the left-ventricular function and their tendency to produce both hypotension and increasing degrees of heart block. Caution should be the watchword for a physician called on to do stress testing in a patient taking this type of medication.

Lithium

Like the tricyclics, lithium for a time was a very popular agent, especially for treatment of depression. Its metabolic and cardiovascular implications are well documented. By interfering with the hormones mediated through cyclic adenosine monophosphate, it can cause[63]:

1. Diabetes insipidus
2. Hypothyroidism and goiters
3. Hypoglycemia-like symptoms
4. Replacement of intracellular potassium from the myocardium
5. Inhibition of the chronotropic effects of epinephrine
6. T-wave inversion
7. Conduction defects (ie, sinus node dysfunction with prolonged sinus recovery time[126,127])
8. Ventricular arrhythmias

In spite of all these changes, when Tilkian and colleagues[128] reported on 10 patients who underwent stress testing before and after a full therapeutic

*Pre-ejection period/ventricular ejection time.

dose of lithium, they found no decrease in exercise tolerance and no ST-segment depression associated with this drug. Some years ago, we tested a patient on lithium, who developed ST depression but had a normal response after the drug was withdrawn. Although T-wave inversion or flattening is common, ST changes caused by this agent are relatively rare, although a systematic evaluation including measurement of blood levels is yet to be done.

Phenothiazines

The pharmacological responses to phenothiazines are complex, owing to both a direct effect on the heart blood vessels and an indirect effect involving secondary central nervous system changes with resultant autonomic alterations. The following responses have been reported[129]:

1. A direct depressant effect on cardiac muscle.
2. A reduction in the rate of rise of phase 0 of the transmembrane action potential.
3. A decrease in the duration of phases 2 and 3 of the actual potential.
4. Antiarrhythmic properties similar to those of quinidine.[115]
5. These antiarrhythic properties result in prolongation of the RR and QT intervals, decreased amplitude, and prolongation of the QRS interval, and possibly ST depression.[130] (Linhart and Turnoff[131] have reported that a false-negative test was found in 5 of 13 subjects taking these drugs; they claimed that this was due to the quinidine-like action.)
6. Hypotension caused by both the alpha blockade and the direct effect on the smooth muscle of the vasculature,[132] as well as a reduction in cardiac output.

Although in small doses, phenothiazines have antiarrhythmic properties, toxic doses have been reported to cause ventricular ectopic beats, ventricular tachycardia, and ventricular fibrillation[133]; atrial fibrillation; complete heart block; and sudden death.[134]

Diazepam

Few psychotropic drugs enjoy the popularity of diazepam (Valium). Besides oral use, it is very popular in hospitals as a quick sedative when given intravenously. The cardiovascular effects are as follows:

1. Coronary vasodilatation lasting at least 30 minutes. When injected directly into the coronary circulation, vasodilatation results, but when the systemic and coronary circulations are isolated in an experiment so that systemic blood cannot enter the cardiac circulation, diazepam does not alter coronary flow.
2. Increase in left-ventricular contractility secondary to the aforementioned effect on coronary flow. When coronary flow is held constant in dogs, contractility is unchanged.

3. Augmentation of coronary flow in patients with CAD two or three times that of those with normal coronary anatomy.[135]
4. Slight reduction of aortic blood pressure.
5. Usually no change in heart rate and cardiac output.
6. Decrease in LVEDP suggesting dilatation of the capacitance vessels.[136]

Although an increase in coronary flow does not in itself establish diazepam as being useful in angina, the fact that it often improves angina, that it reduces LVEDP, and that it increases coronary flow more in patients with diseased coronary circulation suggests that redistribution to the ischemic area, as with nitrates, is very likely. This information then tells us that diazepam should be withheld prior to stress testing if the true picture of cardiovascular dynamics is to be documented. Although we know of no specific tests demonstrating an alteration in ischemic changes, it is likely that diazepam has the capacity to do so.

ANTIHYPERTENSIVE AGENTS

Because hypertension is commonly seen in CAD patients and because they are often under treatment when they come in for testing, a knowledge of the alterations to be expected with the various antihypertensive agents is important. Although physicians soon become familiar with the patterns of blood pressure alterations at rest in the supine and upright postures, they rarely consider the changes with exercise, which are probably equally as important.

Diuretics

Lund-Johansen[137] studied polythiazide, hydrochlorothiazide, and chlorthalidone at rest and during exercise when patients had taken a typical maintenance dose. The heart rate was not altered during exercise by these agents compared with that in controls. The thiazides caused a reduction in exercise blood pressure and peripheral resistance and a 7% reduction in plasma volume. The cardiac output, however, was not altered. The peripheral resistance was reduced 12% at rest, but only 7% at peak exercise. This was also reflected in a less dramatic decrease in blood pressure during exercise.

The chlorthalidone patients failed to show a drop in peripheral resistance; their decrease in blood pressure resulted from a decrease in cardiac output. The reason for the difference in mechanisms could not be determined. Ogilvie[138] found that exercise hypotension increased with dosage up to 100 mg/d with chlorthalidone. After this, the hypotensive effect began to be lost, and at 200 mg/d there was a paradoxical increase in diastolic blood pressure and heart rate. Thus, with chlorthalidone, at least, there seems to be a specific dosage beyond which the exercise effects are lost.

Diuretics may all induce ST-segment depression to a moderate degree if hypokalemia becomes significant.

Methyldopa

Methyldopa (Aldomet) along with guanethidine, reserpine, and clonidine, causes a reduction in heart rate during exercise but, unlike the others, no change is observed at rest. The primary hypotensive effect is caused by a decrease in peripheral resistance with no change in cardiac output. The decrease in resistance and in heart rate actually is associated with an increase in the stroke volume during exercise, compared with that in control patients. In some subjects studied by Sannerstedt and coworkers,[139] the resting blood pressure did not change, even though a significant drop was seen at peak exercise. Methyldopa, along with clonidine and the beta blockers, suppresses renin release, which may increase the amount of exercise-induced hyperkalemia usually seen; thus, these drugs should be used carefully when exercise is contemplated in patients with a precarious potassium balance.[140]

Clonidine

Clonidine, which is generically related to pentolamine and tolazoline, has been used successfully in hypertension. It produces a moderate decrease in both systemic resistance and cardiac output, thus resulting in a drop in pressure at all workloads as well as at rest.[96] Circulatory function seems to be well maintained, probably because the decrease in venous tone in the legs at rest seems to be compensated by an increase in resistance in the upper extremities during exercise. The circulatory dynamics seem a little better during exercise with clonidine than with either methyldopa or guanethidine.

When stress testing is planned, the previously mentioned effects of antihypertensive agents must be kept in mind. At this time, the cumulative effects of a number of drugs are not yet reported. It is almost certain that the response will vary according to whether the pressure is fixed or labile and will be especially dependent on the degree of ischemia or myocardial dysfunction, if present.

Guanethidine

Guanethidine is a classic sympathetic blocker used to treat hypertension. It is usually used only in severe cases in combination with diuretics, beta blockers, or both. Studies to evaluate the degree of peripheral vasoconstriction show a sharp drop in vasomotor tone when this drug is administered. There is not only a decrease in vasoconstriction in terms of the arterial circulation but also an increase in volume in the legs due to venous relaxation. Khatri and Cohn[141] believe that all patients taking guanethidine should undergo exercise testing for better determination of the degree of potential hypotensive response because of the marked tendency for postural changes to be masked until exercise demonstrates their presence. As might be expected, the cardiac output drops considerably when the patient is in the upright position owing to distal dependent pooling; however, with exercise, the decrease in peripheral resistance allows the cardiac output to rise more rapidly than would occur with a higher afterload. Because guanethidine produces a rather marked decrease in heart rate, the stroke output increases during exercise and the decrease in cardiac filling results in an increased contractile velocity and greater $\Delta P/\Delta T$.* No ST changes have been reported with methyldopa, clonidine, or guanethidine.

Vasodilators

Vasodilators are playing an increasing role in antihypertensive therapy. The first vasodilator to be used for the treatment of patients with hypertension, hydralazine, is now joined by prazosin and minoxidil.

Exercise can be augmented by the decrease in peripheral resistance, which causes some increase in heart rate with hydralazine. The heart rate increases less with prazosin and minoxidil.[142] This may explain the likelihood of an excessive drop in blood pressure with starting doses of these agents. All three vasodilators may improve exercise tolerance, especially if left-ventricular function is very limited.[143]

Angiotensin Converting Enzyme Inhibitors

Captopril was the first angiotensin converting enzyme (ACE) inhibitor to be released in the United States. Since then, a host of similar drugs have appeared, most of which are longer-acting but otherwise very similar. Except for one dissenting report,[144] evidence suggests that systolic blood pressure is lower during exercise in patients taking ACE inhibitors than in controls.[145] Little change in heart rate occurs. They have been reported to reduce exercise induced ischemia.[146]

Angiotensin II Blockers

In many ways the physiology of this class of drugs parallels that of the ACE inhibitors. They are becoming increasingly popular because of their low side effect profile. They are most commonly used in congestive heart failure patients but are often used in hypertension. These are the patients who often show up in the treadmill lab. The information available indicates that they will improve exercise capacity and prolong the time to ischemia.[147]

---

*Delta pressure over delta time.

L-Arginine

Although this agent is not marketed by a pharmaceutical company and can be obtained in any health food store it is becoming more popular and is an ingredient of a number of "energy foods".[148] Nitric oxide, the most important substance released by the endothelium is the end product of L-Arginine metabolism generated by Nitric oxide synthase. Evidence is now available that it will prolong exercise time on the treadmill and it will increase the time to the onset of ischemia.[149] It also has been used successfully to treat congestive heart failure.[150]

p FOX Inhibitors (Partial Fatty Acid Oxidation Inhibitors)

It has been demonstrated that although free fatty acids are the major substrate that drives myocardial metabolism when there is adequate oxygen available, as ischemia becomes manifested the heart switches to glucose.[151] The higher the concentration of free fatty acids, the less efficient this process becomes.[152] A number of drugs that facilitate increased glucose utilization during ischemia have been studied. The most useful appear to be Ranolazine,[153] glucose, insulin and potassium and carnatine.[154] Although the former has not yet been released by the FDA, it appears to improve exercise tolerance during ischemia. I would expect it will become available in the near future. Carnatine has also been shown to be beneficial but has never been used clinically in any quantity. Therefore, patients who are taking one of these agents will be able to increase the amount of exercise before becoming ischemic.[155]

ALCOHOL

Alcohol reduces cardiac output when taken in excessive amounts by normal persons, but in patients with significant CAD, only 3 to 4 oz can produce this effect. In a person with a normal heart, the acute effect of alcohol on coordination will be more evident than ECG changes associated with exercise. On the other hand, in patients with underlying heart disease due to hypertension or coronary narrowing, alcohol will reduce the cardiac output and therefore the exercise capacity of the patient. Patients with alcoholic cardiomyopathy may have ST-segment depression or may develop left bundle branch block with exercise as their ventricular filling pressure increases. Experimental studies on the isolated rat atrium have shown an almost linear decrease in contractility as the concentration of alcohol rises at levels commonly seen in human alcoholics.[156] The exact influence on the heart may be due to alcohol's effect on membrane permeability.[1] Thus, repolarization abnormalities would be expected if alcoholic cardiomyopathy is present or if the subject has recently ingested large amounts of alcohol, even if no underlying heart disease is recognized.

SUMMARY

It is apparent that the multiple pharmaceuticals used in cardiology can alter the physiological responses to exercise. It would be ideal to do exercise testing after the withdrawal of all drugs. This is rarely practical however and thus a knowledge of their influence is important when stress testing is planned. It has been my experience that a detailed knowledge of these agents is rare in physicians performing exercise tests. It is hoped that this chapter will shed some light in this dark corner.

REFERENCES

1. Simonson, E: Physiology of Work Capacity and Fatigue. Charles C Thomas, Springfield, IL, 1971.
2. Ganong, WF: Review of Medical Physiology. Lange Medical Publications, Los Altos, CA, 1973.
3. Case, RB, et al: Relative effect of CO_2 on canine coronary vascular resistance. Circ Res 42:410, 1978.
4. Iskandrian, AS, et al: Cardiac performance in thyrotoxicosis: Analysis of 10 untreated patients. Am J Cardiol 51:349–352, 1983.
5. Shafer, RB and Bianco, JA: Assessment of cardiac reserve in patients with hypertension. Chest 78:269–273, 1980.
6. Forfar, PG, et al: Abnormal left ventricular function in hyperthyroidism. N Engl J Med 307:1165, 1982.
7. Hylander, B, Ekelund, LG, and Rosenqvist, IN: The cardiovascular response at rest and during exercise in hypothyroid subjects to thyroxine substitution. Clin Cardiol 6:116–124, 1983.
8. James, TN: Pathology of small coronary arteries. Am J Cardiol 20:679, 1967.
9. Rubler, S: Cardiac manifestations of diabetes mellitus. Cardiovasc Med 2:823, 1977.
10. Kannel, WB, Hjortland, M, and Castelli, WP: Role of diabetes in congestive heart failure. Am J Cardiol 31:29, 1974.
11. Parker, JP et al: Androgen-induced increase in red cell 2, 3-diphosphoglycerate. N Engl Med 287:381, 1972.
12. Neely, TF and Morgan, HE: The relationship between carbohydrate and lipid metabolism and the energy balance of heart muscle. Ann Rev Physiol 36:413, 1974.
13. Rubler, S and Arvan, SB: Exercise testing in young asymptomatic diabetics. Angiology 27:539, 1976.
14. Ewing, DJ, et al: Vascular reflexes in diabetic autonomic neuropathy. Lancet 2:1354, 1973.
15. Bishu, SK and Berenz, MR: Circulatory reflex response in diabetic patients with and without neuropathy. J Am Geriatr Soc 19:159, 1971.
16. Persson, G: Exercise tests in male diabetics. Acta Med Scand 605(suppl):723, 1977.
17. Bellet, S and Roman, L: The exercise test in diabetic patients as studied by radioelectrocardiography. Circulation 36:245–254, 1967.
18. Karlefors, T: Exercise tests in male diabetics. Acta Med Scand 449(suppl):1943, 1966.
19. Riley, GP, Oberman, A, and Scheffield, LT: ECG effects of glucose ingestion. Arch Intern Med 130:703, 1972.
20. Ellestad, MH and Halleday, WK: Stress testing in the prognosis and management of ischemic heart disease. Angiology 28:149, 1977.
21. Sketch, MH, et al: Significant sex differences in the correlation of electrocardiographic exercise testing and coronary arteriograms. Am J Cardiol 36:196, 1976.

22. Pinto, RM, et al: Action of estradiol upon uterine contractility. Am J Obstet Gynecol 90:99, 1964.
23. Williams, JK, et al: Short term administration of estrogen and vascular response of atherosclerotic coronary arteries. J Am Coll Cardiol 20:452–457, 1992.
24. Engel, HJ, Hundeshagen, H, and Lichtlen, P: Transmural myocardial infarction in young women taking oral contraceptives. Br Heart J 39:477–484, 1977.
25. Coronary Drug Project Research Group. JAMA 214:1030, 1970.
26. Blackard, CE, et al: Incidence of cardiovascular disease and death in patients receiving diethylstilbestrol for carcinoma of the prostate. Cancer 26:249, 1970.
27. Jaffe, MD: Effect of oestrogens on post-exercise electrocardiogram. Br Heart J 38:1299, 1977.
28. Jaffe, MD: Effect of testosterone cypionate on post exercise ST segment depression. Br Heart J 39:1217, 1977.
29. Marmor, A, Zeira, M, and Zohar, S: Effects of bilateral hysterosalpingo-oophorectomy on exercise-induced ST segment abnormalities in young women. Am J Cardiol 71:1118–1119, 1990.
30. Jaffe, MD: Exercise testing in women with syndrome X. J Myocard Ischemia 4:61–62, 1992.
31. Murad, F and Gilman, AG: Androgens and anabolic steroids. In Goodman, LS and Gilman, AG, (eds): The Pharmacological Basis of Therapeutics, ed 5. Macmillan, New York, 1970, p 1451.
32. Shahidi, NT: Androgens and erythropoiesis. N Engl J Med 289:72, 1973.
33. Greenberg, S, Heitz, DA, and Long, JP: Testosterone-induced depression of adrenergic activity in the perfused canine hindlimb. Proc Soc Exp Biol Med 142:883, 1973.
34. Holma, P: Effect of an anabolic steroid (metandierone) on central and peripheral blood flow in well-trained athletes. Ann Clin Res 9:215, 1977.
35. Aronow, WS and Isbell, MW: Carbon monoxide effect on exercise-induced angina pectoris. Ann Intern Med 79:392–395, 1973.
36. Anderson, EW, et al: Effect of low-level carbon monoxide exposure on onset and duration of angina pectoris: A study in ten patients with ischemic heart disease. Ann Intern Med 79:46–50, 1973.
37. Allred, EN, et al: Short-term effect of carbon monoxide exposure on the exercise performance of subjects with coronary artery disease. N Engl J Med 321:1426–1432, 1989.
38. Henry, FM and Fitzhenry, JR: Oxygen metabolism of moderate exercise with some observations on the effects of tobacco smoking. J Appl Physiol 2:464–468, 1950.
39. Perkins, KA, et al: The effect of nicotine on energy expenditure during light physical activity. N Engl J Med 320:898–903, 1989.
40. Niedermaier, ON, et al: Influence of cigarette smoking on autonomic function. Circulation 88:562–571, 1993.
41. Kamimori, GH, et al: The effects of obesity, exercise, and nicotine on circulatory dynamics. Eur J Clin Pharmacol 31:595, 1987
42. Verma, S and Anderson, TJ: Fundamentals of endothelial function for the clinical cardiologist. Circulation 105:546, 2002.
43. Gross, GJ, et al: The effect of ouabain on nutritional circulation and regional myocardial blood flow. Am Heart J 93:487, 1977.
44. Vogel, R, et al: Effects of digitalis on resting and isometric exercise myocardial perfusion in patients with coronary artery disease and left ventricular dysfunction. Circulation 56:355,1977.
45. Glancy, DL et al: Effects of ouabain on the left ventricular response to exercise in patients with angina pectoris. Circulation 43:45, 1971.
46. Mason, DT and Braunwald, E: Studies on digitalis. X. Effect of ouabain on forearm vascular resistance and venous tone in normal subjects and patients in heart failure. J Clin Invest 43:532, 1964.
47. Ross, J, Jr, Waldhausen, A, and Braunwald, E: Studies on digitalis. Direct effects on peripheral vascular resistance. J Clin Invest 39:930, 1960.
48. Rudolph, AM and Heyman, MA: The circulation of the fetus in utero, methods for studying distribution of blood flow, cardiac output, and organ blood flow. Circ Res 21:163, 1967.
49. Gamble, WJ, et al: Regional coronary venous oxygen saturation and myocardial oxygen-tension following abrupt changes in ventricular pressure in the isolated dog heart. Circ Res 34:672, 1974.
50. Kawai, C and Hultgren, HN: The effect of digitalis upon the exercise electrocardiogram. Am Heart J 80:409, 1964.

51. Indolfi, C, et al: Digoxin-induced vasoconstriction of normal and atherosclerotic epicardial coronary arteries. Am J Cardiol 68:1274, 1991.
52. Katz, AM: Physiology of the Heart. Raven Press, New York, p 189, 1977.
53. Lewinter, MM, et al: The effects of oral propranolol, digoxin, and combination therapy on the resting and exercise electrocardiogram. Am Heart J 93:202, 1977.
54. Goldbarg, AN: The effects of pharmacological agents on human performance. In Naughton, J, Hellerstein, HK, and Mohler, LC (eds): Exercise Testing and Exercise Training in Coronary Heart Disease. Academic Press, New York, 1973, p 37.
55. Tonkon, MJ, et al: Effects of digitalis on the exercise electrocardiogram in normal adult subjects. Chest 72:714, 1977.
56. Sundqvist, K, et al: Effect of digoxin on the electrocardiogram at rest and during exercise in healthy subjects. Am J Cardiol 57:661, 1986.
57. Degre, S, et al: Analysis of exercise induced A wave amplitude changes in detection of coronary artery disease in patients on digitalis. Cardiology 68(suppl 2):178, 1981.
58. Davidson, DM and Hagan, AD: Role of exercise stress testing in assessing digoxin dosage in chronic atrial fibrillation. Cardiovasc Med June:671, 1979.
59. Gey, GO, et al: Quinidine plasma concentration and exertional arrhythmia. Am Heart J 90:19, 1975.
60. Gey, GO, et al: Plasma concentration of procainamide and prevalence of exertional arrhythmias. Ann Intern Med 80:718, 1974.
61. Fluster, PE, et al: Effect of quinidine in the heart rate and blood pressure response to exercise. Am Heart J 104:1244, 1982.
62. Surawicz, B and Lasseter, KC: Effects of drugs on the electrocardiogram. Prog Cardiovasc Dis 13:26, 1970.
63. Surawicz, B and Saito, S: Exercise testing for detection of myocardial ischemia in patients with abnormal electrocardiograms at rest. Am J Cardiol 41:943, 1978.
64. Freidberg, AS, et al: Objective evidence of the efficacy of medical therapy in angina pectoris. Am Heart J 22:494, 1941.
65. Gilman AG, et al (eds): Goodman and Gilman's The Pharmacological Basis of Therapeutics, 8th ed. Pergamon Press, New York, 1990.
66. Kupersmith, J, et al: In vivo electrophysiological effects on canine acute myocardial infarction. Circ Res 36, 1975.
67. Zipes, DP, et al: Current approach to management of arrhythmias: Role of propafenone. Cardiovasc Rev Rep 12 (June suppl):16, 1991.
68. Ranger, S, et al: Amplification of flecainide-induced ventricular conduction slowing by exercise. Circulation 79:1000, 1989.
69. Rod, JL and Shenasa, M: Functional significance of chronotropic response during chronic amiodarone therapy. Cardiology 71:7, 1984.
70. Touboul, P et al: Effects of amiodarone on sinus node in man. Br Heart J 42:573, 1979.
71. Melmed, S, et al: Hyperthyroxinemia with bradycardia and normal thyrotropin secretion after chronic amiodarone administration. J Clin Endocrinol Metab 53:997, 1981.
72. Simoons, ML and Balakumaran, K: The effects of drugs on the exercise electrocardiogram.Cardiology 68(suppl 2):124, 1981.
73. Kobinger, W, et al: N-allyl-derivative of clonidine, a substance with specific bradycardiac action at a cardiac site. Arch Pharmcol 306:255, 1979.
74. Fam, WM and McGregor, M: The effect of coronary vasodilator drugs on retrograde flow in areas of chronic myocardial ischemia. Circ Res 15:355, 1964.
75. Gaspardone, A, et al: Bamiphylline improves exercise-induced myocardial ischemia through a novel mechanism of action. Circulation 88:502, 1993.
76. Crea, F, et al: Role of adenosine in pathogenesis of anginal pain. Circulation 81:164, 1990.
77. Cannon, RA: Aminophylline for angina: The -Robin Hood Effect.+ J Am Coll Cardiol 14:1454, 1989.
78. Goldstein, RE, et al: Clinical and circulatory effects of isosorbide dinitrate: Comparison with nitroglycerin. Circulation 43:629, 1971.
79. Hoffman, JIE, and Spaan, JAE: Pressure-flow relations in coronary circulation. Physiol Rev 70:331, 1990.
80. Russek, HI and Funk, EH, Jr: Comparative responses to various nitrates in the treatment of angina pectoris. Postgrad Med 31:150, 1962.
81. Fulton, WF: The Coronary Arteries. Charles C Thomas, Springfield, IL, 1965.

82. McGregor, M: Drugs for the treatment of angina pectoris. In Lasagna, L, (ed): International Encyclopedia of Pharmacology and Therapeutics, Vol. 11. Clinical Pharmacology. Pergamon Press, Oxford, p 377, 1966.
83. Vineberg, AM, et al: The effect of Persantin on intercoronary collateral circulation and survival during gradual experimental coronary occlusion: A preliminary report. Can Med Assoc J 87:336, 1962.
84. Mautz, FR and Gregg, DE: The dynamics of collateral circulation following chronic occlusion of coronary arteries. Proc Soc Exp Biol 36:797, 1937.
85. Ganz, WM and Marcus, HS: Failure of intracoronary nitroglycerin to alleviate pacing induced angina. Circulation 46:880, 1972.
86. Essex, HE, et al: The effect of certain drugs on the coronary blood flow of the trained dog. Am Heart J 19:544, 1940.
87. Ross, RS, et al: The effect of nitroglycerin on the coronary circulation studied by cineangiography and xenon-33 myocardial blood flow measurements. Trans Am Clin Climatol Assoc 76:70, 1964.
88. Nickerson, M: Vasodilator drugs. In Goodman, LS and Gilman, A, (eds): The Pharmacological Basis of Therapeutics, 5th ed. Macmillan, New York, 1970, p 736.
89. Riseman, JEF, et al: Stereo-isomeric nitrates in the treatment of angina pectoris. Am J Cardiol 15:220, 1965.
90. Cole, SL, et al: Assay of anti-anginal agents: I. A curve analysis with multiple control periods. Circulation 15:405, 1957.
91. Wayne, VS, et al: The effects of isosorbide dinitrate on the exercise test. J Cardiopulm Rehabil 7:239–252, 1987.
92. Charlier, R: Coronary Vasodilators. Pergamon Press, New York, 1961.
93. Gregg, DE: Physiology of the coronary circulation. Circulation 27:1128, 1963.
94. Tavazzi, L, et al: Prognostic value of exercise hemodynamics after myocardial infarctions. Cardiology 68(suppl 2):53, 1981.
95. Aronow, WS and Kaplan, MA: Propranolol combined with isosorbide dinitrate versus placebo in angina pectoris. N Engl J Med 280:847, 1969.
96. Moir, TW: Subendocardial distribution of coronary blood flow and the effect of antianginal drugs. Circ Res 30:621, 1972.
97. Epstein, SE and Braunwald, E: Beta adrenergic receptor blocking drugs: Mechanisms of action and clinical application. N Engl J Med 275:1106, 1966.
98. Marcomichelakis, J, et al: Exercise testing after beta blockade: Improved specificity and predictive value in detecting coronary heart disease. Br Heart J 43:252, 1980.
99. Irving, MH, et al: Effect of beta adrenergic blockade on plasma catecholamines in exercise. Nature 248:531, 1974.
100. Jorgensen, CT, et al: Effect of propranolol on myocardial oxygen consumption and its hemodynamic correlates during upright exercise. Circulation 68:1173, 1973.
101. Funck-Brentano, C, et al: Rate dependence of sotolol-induced prolongation of ventricular repolarization during exercise in humans. Circulation 83:536, 1991.
102. Asandi, H, et al: ST Segment fluctuation during treadmill exercise in patients with angina pectoris. J Electrocardiogr 21:147, 1988.
103. Holmberg F, et al: Therapeutic and metabolic effects of sotolol. Clin Pharmacol Ther 36:174, 1984.
104. Pepine, CJ and Lambert, CR: Effects of nicardipine on coronary blood flow. Am Heart J 116:248, 1988.
105. Moskawicz, RM, et al: Nifedipine therapy for stable angina pectoris. Am J Cardiol 44: 811, 1979.
106. Rice, KR, et al: Effects of nifedipine on myocardial perfusion during exercise in chronic stable angina pectoris. Am J Cardiol 65:1097, 1990.
107. Deponti, C, et al: Effects of nifedipine, acebutolol, and their association on exercise tolerance in patients with effort angina. Cardiology 68(suppl 2):195, 1981.
108. Fox, KM, et al: The dose-response effects of nifedipine on ST segment changes in exercise testing: Preliminary studies. Cardiology 68(suppl 2):209, 1981.
109. Lund-Johansen, P and Omvik, P: Chronic effects of tiapamil and felodipine in essential hypertension at rest and during exercise. J Cardiovasc Pharmacol 8(suppl 4):S42, 1990.
110. Ardissino, D, et al: Usefulness of the hyperventilation test in stable exertional angina pectoris in selecting medical therapy. Am J Cardiol 65:417, 1990.

111. Jose, AD and Taylor, RR Autonomic blockade by propranolol and atropine to study intrinsic myocardial function in man. J Clin Invest 48:2109, 1969.
112. Daoud, FS, et al: Effect of isoproterenol on the abnormal T wave. Am J Cardiol 30:810, 1972.
113. Sano, T, et al: Mechanism of inotropic action of catecholamines and ouabain in cardiac muscle in relation to changes in action potential. Jpn Heart 111:269, 1970.
114. Cryer, PE, et al: Smoking, catecholamines and coronary heart disease. Cardiol Med 23:471, 1977.
115. Aronow, ES: The effect of smoking cigarettes on the apex cardiograms in coronary heart disease. Chest 59:365, 1971.
116. Smith, RR, et al: Cardiomyopathy associated with amphetamine administration Am Heart J 91:792, 1976.
117. Kohn, DE, et al: Isoproterenol-induced cardiac necrosis. Ann NY Acad Sci 156:286, 1969.
118. Gubner, RS: Newer developments in exercise electrocardiography and evaluation of chest pain. Trans Assoc Life Ins Med Dir Am 52:125, 1969.
119. Bassett, AL and Hoffman, BF: Antiarrhythmic drugs, electrophysiological actions. Ann Rev Pharmacol 11:143, 1971.
120. Vohra, J, et al: Assessment of CV side effects of therapeutic doses of tricyclic antidepressant drugs. Austr NZ J Med 5:7, 1975.
121. Smith, RR and Rusbatch, BJ: Amitriptyline and the heart. Br Heart J 3:311, 1967.
122. Kantor, SJ, et al: Imipramine-induced heart block: A longitudinal case study. JAMA 231:1364, 1975.
123. Bigger, JT Jr, et al: Cardiac antiarrhythmic effect of imipramine hydrochloride. N Engl J Med 287:206, 1977.
124. Muller, V and Burckhard, D: Die wirkung tri-und tetrazyklischer antidepressiva auf ilerz und Kreislauf. Schweiz Med Wochenschr 104:1911, 1974.
125. Thorstrand, J, et al: Cardiac effects of amitriptyline in rats. Scand J Clin Lab Invest 36:7, 1976.
126. Singer, L and Rotenberg, D: Mechanisms of lithium action. N Engl J Med 289:254, 1973.
127. Wellens, HJ, et al: Symptomatic sinus node abnormalities following lithium carbonate therapy. Am J Med 59:285, 1975.
128. Tilkian, AG, et al: Effect of lithium on cardiovascular performance: Report on extended ambulatory monitoring and exercise testing before and during lithium therapy. Am J Cardiol 38:701, 1976.
129. Jarvik, ME: Drugs in the treatment of psychiatric disorders. In Goodman, LS and Gilman, A, (eds): The Pharmacological Basis of Therapeutics, 5th ed. Macmillan, New York, 1970.
130. Crane, GE: Cardiac toxicity and psychotropic drugs. Dis Nerve Syst 31:534, 1970.
131. Linhart, JW and Turnoff, HB: Maximum treadmill exercise tests in patients with abnormal central electrocardiograms. Circulation 49:667, 1974.
132. Fowler, NO, et al: Electrocardiographic changes and cardiac arrhythmias in patients receiving psychotropic drugs. Am J Cardiol 37:223, 1976.
133. Giles, TD and Modlin, RK: Death associated with ventricular arrhythmias and thioridazine hydrochloride. JAMA 205:180, 1968.
134. Hollister, LE and Kosek, JC: Sudden death during treatment with phenothiazine derivatives. JAMA 192:1035, 1965.
135. Ikram, H, et al: Effect of diazepam on myocardial blood flow of patients with and without coronary artery disease. Br Heart J 35:626, 1973.
136. Cote, P, et al: Therapeutic implications of diazepam in patients with elevated left ventricular filling pressure. Am Heart J 91:747, 1976.
137. Lund-Johansen, P: Hemodynamic changes in long term diuretic therapy of essential hypertension: A comparative study of chlorthalidone, polythiazide and hydrochlorothiazide. Acta Med Scand 187:509, 1970.
138. Ogilvie, RI: Cardiovascular response to exercise under increasing doses of chlorthalidone. Eur J Clin Pharmacol 9:339, 1976.
139. Sannerstedt, E, Varnauskas, E and Werko, L: Hemodynamic effects of methyldopa (Aldomet) at rest and during exercise in patients with arterial hypertension. Acta Med Scand 171:75, 1962.
140. Lowenthal, DT, et al: Biochemical and pharmacodynamic responses to anti-renin, antihypertensives during exercise. Ann Sports Med 1:59, 1983.

141. Khatri, AM and Cohn, JN: Mechanism of exercise hypotension after sympathetic blockade. Am J Cardiol 27:329, 1970
142. Lund-Johansen, P: Hemodynamic changes at rest and during exercise in long-term prazosin therapy for essential hypertension. Proceedings of Postgraduate Medicine Symposium on Prazosin, New York, November p 45, 1975.
143. Nelson, GIC, et al: Haemodynamic effects of sustained treatment with prazosin and metoprolol, alone and in combination, in borderline hypertensive heart failure. J Cardiovasc Pharmacol 4:240, 1982.
144. Pickring, TG, et al: Comparison of antihypertensive and hormonal effects of captopril and propranolol at rest and during exercise. Am J Cardiol 49:1566, 1982.
145. Fagard, R, et al: Effects of angiotensin antagonism on hemodynamics, renin and catecholamines during exercise. J Appl Physiol 43:440, 1977.
146. Dickstein, K, et al: Comparison of the effects of losartan and enalapril on clinical status and exercise performance in patients with moderate or severe chronic heart failure. J Am Coll Cardiol 26:438, 1995.
147. Hamroff, G, et al: Addition of angiotensin II receptor blockade to maximal angiotensin-converting enzyme inhibition improves exercise capacity in patients with severe congestive heart failure. Circulation 99:990, 1999.
148. Maxwell, AJ, et al: Randomized trial of a medical food for the dietary management of chronic stable angina. JACC 39:37, 2002.
149. Thorne, S, et al: Early endothelial dysfunction in adults at risk from atherosclerosis: Different responses to L-Arginine. JACC 32:110, 1998.
150. Hirooka, Y, et al: Effects of L-arginine on impaired acetylcholine-induced and ischemic vasodilation of the forearm in patients with heart failure. Circulation 90:658, 1994.
151. Lopaschuk, GD, et al: Free fatty acids with myocardial ischemia. Am Heart J 128:61, 1994.
152. Oliver, FM, et al: Relation between serum-free fatty acids and arrhythmia and death. Lancet 1:710, 1968.
153. McCormack, JG, et al: Ranolazine stimulates glucose oxidation in normoxic, ischemic rat hearts. Circulation 93:135, 1996.
154. Brevetti, G, et al: Clinical utility of carnitines: Selected references. Circulation 77:767, 1988.
155. Pepine, CJ and Wolff, AA: A controlled trial with a novel anti-ischemic agent, Ranolazine, in chronic stable angina pectoris that is responsive to conventional antianginal agents.
156. Gimeno, AL, et al: Effects of ethanol on cellular membrane potentials and contractility of isolated rat atrium. Am J Physiol 203:194, 1962.

24
Computer Technology and Exercise Testing

Digital Computer Simulation of the Human ECG
Simulation of the Normal ECG, Hypertrophies, Bundle Branch Blocks, Infarct, and Ischemia
Validation Studies of Infarct Size and Regional Transmural Ischemia
Optimal ECG Lead Locations
Analog-to-Digital (A-D) Conversion
Digital Processing, Noise Reduction, and Measurement Accuracy
Advantages of Computerized Measurement in Exercise Systems
P-Wave Changes and Hemodynamic Changes with Myocardial Ischemia
More Complex Clinical and Exercise Test Variables
Sheffield ST-Segment Integral
Hollenberg Exercise Score
ST/HR Slope
ΔST/ΔHR Index
Screening of Asymptomatic Subjects for Ischemia
Significant Occlusive CAD in Asymptomatic Subjects
Future Strategies for Improving Quantitation of Myocardial Infarct and Ischemia
ECG Body Surface Maps and Exercise
Comprehensive Normal and Exercise ECG Database—A Pooled Global Resource
Improvement in Screening for Ischemia in Asymptomatic Subjects

This chapter deals with computerized exercise stress test systems, which have become the method of choice in most stress testing laboratories. The arrival of powerful high-speed desktop microcomputers has led to the development of potent data processing systems at an increasingly more reasonable cost. During the period represented by the four editions of this book, the rapid expansion in digital computer technology has provided the tools for developing large databases of exercise test parameters in subjects with and without coronary artery disease (CAD). Such databases are now readily accessible for comparison with other computerized clinical, ECG, hemodynamic, nuclear perfusion/angiographic, and cineangiographic databases. The resting standard 12-lead ECG is ideal for recording and accurately measuring times and voltages of all ECG waveforms with these systems. The body surface ECG is the time history of excitation of the four chambers of the heart. The excitation process (depolarization) spreads first across the atria (P wave), then through the atrioventricular (AV) node (PR interval), and through the His-Purkinje conduction system to the ventricles (QRS complex), stimulating the muscle fibers in these cells to contract and pump blood and nutrition to the whole.

Current is also generated as the recovery process (repolarization, seen as the ST-T) returns myocardial cells to the ready state to repeat this vital process. The electrical message from the heart itself is the basis and ground for preexercise assessment of prior infarct size, resting ischemia, intraventricular conduction, ventricular hypertrophy, and cardiac rhythm. The digital computer simulation of this process, which includes realistic cardiac and torso geometry and inhomogeneities, was the tool used to quantify these complex interactions at rest and as modified by the stress testing procedures.[1–8]

Computer systems for exercise stress testing generally control the workload. They also maintain a record of heart rate, time, and workload, displaying these data on a computer screen along with enlarged baseline ECG waveforms selected by the testor. Changes in these variables, including the ECG waveforms, are displayed for comparison with the baseline measurements and easily monitored throughout the stress test. The continuous stream of ECG waveforms, data, and computer measurements representing this test are stored on-line in the system. At the higher workloads and heart rates, the basic ECG tracing shows considerable additional electrical signal generated from exercising muscles and respiratory changes in the torso volume conductor, which are considered "noise" or artifact. The computer systems now process these signals on-line to minimize these artifactual effects. The processed, on-line "cleaned" data are a valuable addition to the test procedures, since decisions pertinent to the conduct of the test depend on these data. The cleaned data allow more accurate measurements of the exercise ECG, especially the low-amplitude signals such as the P wave, the PR segment, the junction of the QRS and ST (ST-J), and the ST-T segment. Having cleaned data has facilitated a more accurate interpretation of the response of these ECG parameters to the progressive workload during exercise testing. In the exercise test laboratory, the computerized systems now also perform a number of numerical chores in real time, which used to require laborious off-line review and measurements. The data also are easily entered directly into a database archive for comparison with other test data from the same subject and from other related population groups.

The computer has also been widely used in the application of Bayes' statistical models using prior risk factors, clinical data, treadmill performance, weighted combinations of all the ECG parameters and special algorithms that contribute independent information regarding the conditional post-test probability of significant CAD (see also Chapter 14). Each of the advances in adapting digital computers to the general area of exercise testing are discussed in more detail in the sections that follow.

DIGITAL COMPUTER SIMULATION OF THE HUMAN ECG

Simulation of the Normal ECG, Hypertrophies, Bundle Branch Blocks, Infarct, and Ischemia

Computer simulations of the heart's electrical activity (ECG) are introduced here because the resting ECG is the basic foundation on which the changes secondary to myocardial infarction and ischemia during stress testing are understood and their significance is interpreted and quantified. The complex interactions between atrial and ventricular hypertrophies, bundle branch blocks, and myocardial infarct and ischemia have been unraveled with the simulation. The simulation is composed of the geometry of a normal adult male heart at a 1-mm^3 resolution, embedded in a digitized normal male torso that includes all the factors known to influence the human ECG. These factors are the realistic anatomy of the His-Purkinje conduction system, myocardium, blood mass, lungs, and external torso geometry. Included also is a digital computer simulation of the sequence of the electrical excitation wave front driving the mechanical contraction of the heart that is based on measured geometry and electrical properties of this excitation wave.[2]

The advantage of using a simulation based directly on known anatomy and electrophysiology is that the results of numerical experiments with the model have immediate translation to this anatomy, geometry, and electrophysiology. Once such an anatomically and electrophysiologically based model was validated for typical hypertrophies, bundle branch blocks, fascicular blocks, and infarcts, a large number of experiments with combinations of infarct size, chamber enlargements, and conduction defects were performed in a few weeks, creating an archive of the combined effects of these interactions.

Validation Studies of Infarct Size and Regional Transmural Ischemia

Criteria for quantitation of infarct size (QRS score[4–7]) generated from the simulation have been validated in pathoanatomical studies.[9–13] The size of single infarcts as estimated by myocardial infarction (MI) size score summarized by Selvester and associates[3] correlated well ($r = .81$) with quantitative planometric pathoanatomical measured infarct size. A multiple regression model developed on 68 patients with single infarcts, 32 with multiple infarcts, and 229 normal subjects, predicted regional damage found in each of 12 left-ventricular segments ($r = .73$ to $.91$) by the same quantitative pathoanatomical methods.[13] Total MI as the percentage of the left ventricle infarcted for each patient was predicted by summing up the infarct in each segment and correlated as follows: single infarcts, $r = .81$; multiple infarcts,

$r = .73$; and all infarcts, $r = .80$. (For details on how to implement the QRS score for infarct size, see Selvester and associates.[6])

In clinical studies of patients with CAD and serial biplane angiograms and high-resolution ECGs using 18 simultaneous leads, it was demonstrated that ECG criteria generated from the model were 97% reliable in predicting serial angiographic change or lack of it.[18] It follows that a fundamental part of every person's basic health and medical database should be a digital, high-quality 12-lead ECG taken in early adulthood with at least four extra leads being desirable. Each person should carry a plasticized copy of this ECG for immediate comparison with a new one taken as part of a suspected new cardiac event.

Optimal ECG Lead Locations

Work with the total body ECG simulation revealed evidence that local segments of the heart were reflected on local torso locations with variable lead field strengths between heart regions and torso lead location.[19] These are usually related to the QRS amplitude at the torso location.[20,21] The study, described previously, of local coronary ischemia produced in man by balloon occlusion of individual coronary arteries at the time of coronary dilatation or angioplasty, was done using a commercially available 16-lead system (Marquette case II).[14] The four extra leads were located at V_{4R}, V_8, at the third intercostal space above V_4, and at the seventh below V_3. The study directly confirmed the predictions of the model regarding the type of ECG changes and their location on the torso produced by well-defined local regions of acute transmural ischemia. Acute transmural ischemia of the right ventricle and the inferior left ventricle from right coronary occlusion was optimally recorded in V_{4R}, in the seventh interspace below V_3, and aVF. For left-circumflex occlusion and acute posterolateral transmural ischemia, the optimal leads were V_6 and V_8. For diagonal coronary occlusion, the leads were aVL, and the third interspace above V_4. For left anterior descending occlusion, distal to the diagonal branch, the optimal leads are V_2 to V_4: for proximal occlusion also include aVL and the third interspace above V_4. For details of proposed lead sets and criteria for the evaluation of transmural ischemia, the reader may consult references listed at the end of the chapter, especially the USAFSAM and Armstrong Laboratory technical reports.[16, 17] Based on the computer modeling and validation studies and on the work of Kornreich and coworkers,[22–26] the presence of new and unique information in 6 to 10 extra leads beyond the standard 12 leads is expected to improve both the specificity and sensitivity of the ECG changes during exercise testing. A number of laboratories are working to establish the optimal number of leads and their location for computer-assisted exercise testing (see also "ECG Body Surface Maps and Exercise").

ANALOG-TO-DIGITAL (A-D) CONVERSION

The body surface ECG is a time-varying continuous analog signal of electrical current (dipole moment) generated at the cell boundary of myocardial cells in the atria and ventricles. The continuously varying electrical field resulting from this dynamic excitation/recovery process and detected by pairs of body surface electrodes is amplified and seen as continuous varying, or analog, voltage differences. These changing voltages can be traced by a galvanometer and displayed as a strip chart of recurring P-QRS-T complexes. The analog voltages can be measured very accurately (to the nearest 5 μ or 0.05 mm and 0.005 mV at the standard gain) in rapid sequence and stored as digits or numbers. This process is logically termed analog-digital (A-D) conversion. Digital computers can manipulate and store millions (megabytes) of these data bits or numbers incredibly fast and reliably. Most current digital processing ECG and exercise test systems sample the analog waveforms at a rate of 250 samples per second, or at 4-msec intervals. The digitized waveform, which is a series of stored digital voltages, appears as a series of dots at 4-msec intervals if plotted directly on a strip chart. When the dots are connected by lines, the digital-analog (D-A) reconstructed waveform is an A-D, D-A representation of the original analog signal, as shown in Figure 24–1. The slow-moving waveforms such as the ST and T are recorded very accurately by 4-msec sampling. On the other hand, rapidly moving waveforms such as the QRS may have the peak voltage occur between two 4-msec measurements, which produces a ± 5% error in peak amplitude measurements. In spite of this form of error, digital systems that measure Q, R, and S voltages to the nearest 0.005 mV or 0.05 mm at the standard ECG gain of 1 cm = 1 mV, are much more reliable and reproducible than manual measurements of these ECG records.

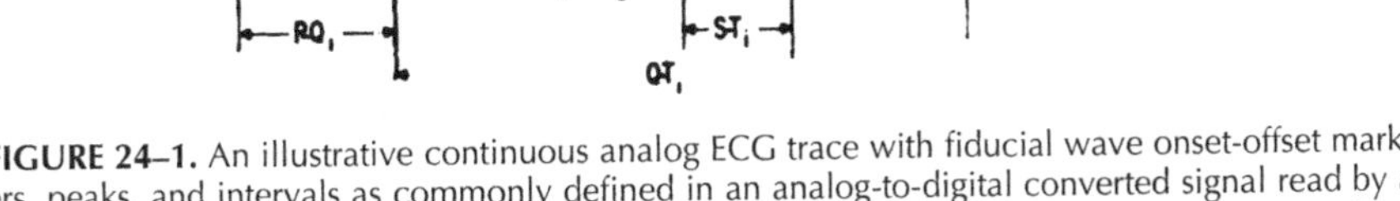

FIGURE 24–1. An illustrative continuous analog ECG trace with fiducial wave onset-offset markers, peaks, and intervals as commonly defined in an analog-to-digital converted signal read by a digital computer. The wave recognition algorithm identifies these waveform parameters and incorporates them into a measurement table for each of the 12 leads. It then compares the measurements to tables of values in each lead for normal and abnormal subjects and generates a diagnostic statement for each tracing. (From Caseres, CA and Rikli, AE: Diagnostic Computers. Charles C Thomas, Springfield, IL, 1969, with permission.)

DIGITAL PROCESSING, NOISE REDUCTION, AND MEASUREMENT ACCURACY

During exercise, skeletal muscle noise and respiratory variability in the baseline may disturb the recorded ECG so much that measurements of the original waveforms are unreliable. The bioelectrical signal of both skeletal muscle noise and respiratory noise are not systematically aligned in time with the heart's electrical signal. Thus, in recent years the common solution to the problem of noisy ECG signals has been to "time-align" related heartbeats with a dominant morphology and average them to reduce the effect of this unrelated noise. This is usually done by selecting, as a template, a typical or dominant beat and matching each new incoming beat to this template. Figure 24–2 illustrates the steps required for this process.

The first step in the matching process is QRS detection.[27, 28] The second is the classification of each QRS complex in a preliminary series and the selection of the dominant beat. In the presence of a great deal of ectopy, the narrow-complex normally conducted beat is selected. Time alignment around fiducial points common to succeeding typical or dominant QRS complexes is a crucial component of the template matching and signal averaging process. Premature ventricular beats, including ventricular fusion and aberrantly conducted beats, are rejected from the final averaged or median beat. During a stress test, if the dominant beat changes—for example, if a rate-dependent bundle branch block supervenes—a new template is formed, and the template matching and averaging process continues.

Although single-channel QRS detectors were initially used in exercise test systems to try to improve signal-to-noise ratios, all recent systems operate on simultaneous multichannel ECG recordings. Skeletal muscle noise and motion artifact are usually not synchronous in all leads. Multichannel QRS detection and time alignment are therefore more reliable than single-channel QRS detectors. It follows that in multichannel recording, computerized algorithms for QRS template matching and time alignment are more robust.

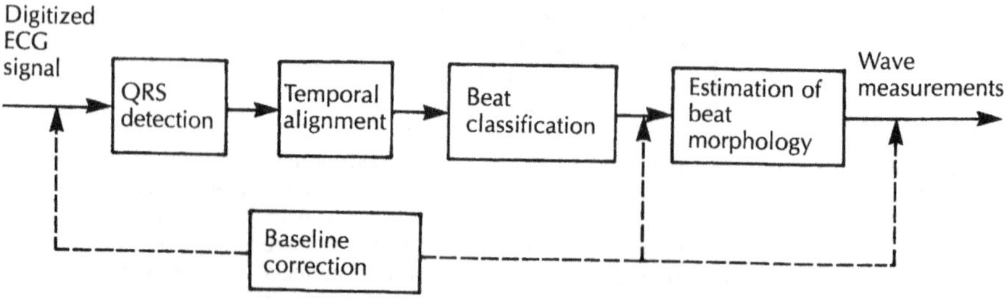

FIGURE 24–2. Algorithms used for noise reduction. Baseline correction can be performed at different stages in the processing. (From Pahlm, O and Sörnmo, L,[28] with permission.)

Wandering of the ECG baseline is due to changes in the volume conductor caused by respiration and also body movements, especially if there is poor skin-electrode contact (see Chapter 9). Motion artifact is accentuated at higher workloads during exercise. The 0.05-Hz low-pass filter used in current ECG systems is effective in attenuating slow baseline drifts due to temperature changes or normal respiration but not very effective at higher respiratory rates. A number of algorithms are currently in use that are generally effective in reducing the effect of baseline wander during exercise.[29–31] However, a number of investigators have pointed out the need for available unprocessed multilead ECG signals at each stage of the exercise protocol to provide quality control for artifact that may be produced by the algorithm.[32–34] Major error in interpretation and a significant increase in false-positive findings can result if this is not done.

ADVANTAGES OF COMPUTERIZED MEASUREMENTS IN EXERCISE SYSTEMS

With careful review of the onset-offset waveform fiducial markers on the signal-processed data and with the quality controls of the baseline wander artifacts just described, the digital measurements are generally more accurate and reproducible than manual measurements at the usual gain and paper speed. Over the years, at various stages of baseline, exercise, and recovery, trend plots of a number of test variables such as heart rate, STJ (defined as the junction of the QRS and the ST segment), STJ + 40, 60, 70, 80, and ST slope have been done post-test by hand measurements. Such plots are readily done on-line by computer-based systems. Detailed measurements of waveform duration (dur) and amplitude (amp) items such as P_{dur}, P_{amp}, Q_{dur}, and Q_{amp}, can also be evaluated for each lead and stored along with the waveforms at rest and at each stage of exercise and recovery. Such measurements, data tabulation, and storage are trivial tasks for current high-speed microcomputer digital systems. With careful overreading to quality control for automated choice of onset-offset fiducials, this essentially eliminates the tedium and human error of manual measurements.

P-WAVE CHANGES AND HEMODYNAMIC CHANGES WITH MYOCARDIAL ISCHEMIA

The available digital data exercise systems, with their concomitant improvement in the signal-to-noise ratio, now make it possible to study small waves such as the P and U waves during and after exercise. Myrianthefs and associates[35] explored the high probability that the known ischemic dysfunction, especially of the left ventricle during exercise, would produce measurable changes in the left-atrial component of the P wave in the exercise ECG. It has been known for years that left-ventricular end-diastolic pressure (LVEDP) is elevated during anginal episodes.[36] Heikkaila and colleagues[37] and Orlando and associates[38] had also demonstrated that the left-atrial component of the P wave was responsive to the LVEDP as reflected in the pulmonary wedge pressure during acute left-ventricular ischemic dysfunction. As documented in Myrianthefs' paper, a change in P duration during exercise and persisting into recovery was significantly more common in patients with documented ischemic heart disease than in normals. Based on the work of Heikkaila and Orlando and associates,[37, 38] one would expect the change in P duration and the magnitude of the left-atrial component to be proportional to the severity of the ischemic hemodynamic change (LVEDP). To our knowledge, none of the commercially available computerized exercise systems currently presents measurements of P or left-atrial P amplitude and duration or trend plots of these variables. However, it is reasonable to expect these systems to be able to do so in the near future. When this is done, yet another exercise ECG variable produced by computer signal processing can be expected to further enhance the diagnostic usefulness of the automated stress exercise ECG systems.

MORE COMPLEX CLINICAL AND EXERCISE TEST VARIABLES

Sheffield ST-Segment Integral

Early studies by Sheffield and associates[39] proposed that by recording the integral of the ST-segment depression with exercise, the maximum integral would be a more accurate measure of myocardial ischemia. To accomplish this with manual methods required off-line planimetry of enlarged QRS-T complexes at rest and at various levels of exercise and recovery. The availability of digital processing systems, once the major programming was done, led to an on-line method of making these complex integral measurements (Figure 24–3). When these studies were first proposed, they required large mainframe computers, but they can now be accomplished on desktop PC-based systems and in much less time. The measurements previously described, providing a picture of the ST change during exercise and in recovery, are provided as an option of many currently available commercial exercise test systems. Sheffield and associates[39] have reported that the integral of ST depression measured by computer was more stable and reproducible in serial studies than manual measurements of ST.

Hollenberg Exercise Score

The Hollenberg treadmill exercise score has also been incorporated into a number of commercially available exercise test systems.[40] It uses the sum of the ST shifts from baseline in two leads normalized to QRS amplitude and

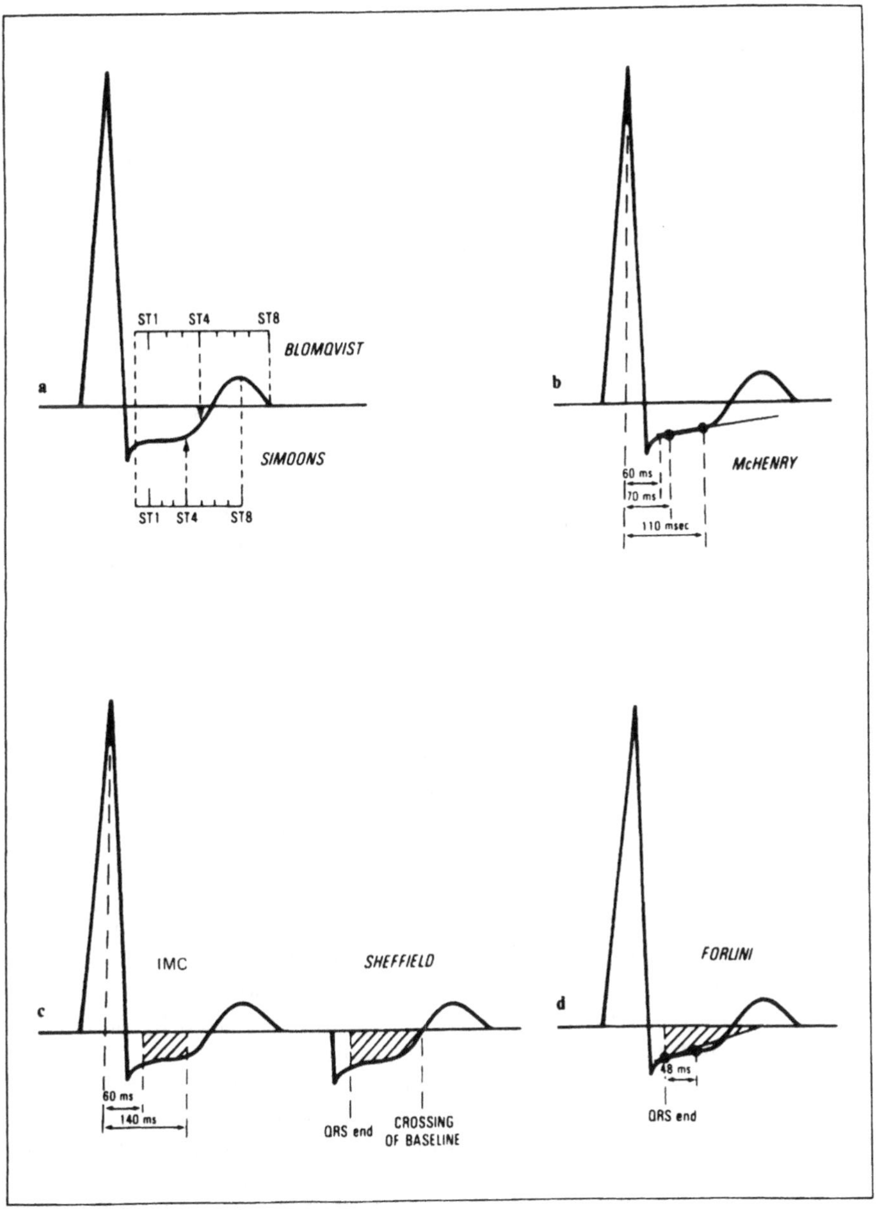

FIGURE 24–3. Computer measurements used to evaluate ST-segment depression.

a. Blomqvist and Simoons divided parts of the ST segment into equal units and measured depression at ST4.
b. McHenry calculated the ST index by multiplying slope in mvs by magnitude of ST depression.
c. The IMC described by Sketch and Sheffield method of calculating the integral.
d. Integral, as calculated by Forlini. (From Savvides, M and Froelicher, V: Non-invasive non-nuclear exercise testing. Cardiology 71:100–117, 1984, with permission.)

ST slope over time (from the start of exercise through recovery), exercise duration, and fraction of maximum predicted heart rate. Hollenberg and associates[40]originally reported a high sensitivity (87%) and specificity (92%) for the treadmill score in patients with a high prevalence of disease. They reported a significant improvement in the false-positive rate, reduced from 12% for conventional ST criteria to less than 1% for the treadmill score, in asymptomatic men with a low prevalence of CAD. The population studied consisted of 377 military officers (mean age 37), 294 with coronary high-risk profiles and 83 controls with low-risk profiles. Forty-five had a positive exercise ECG by conventional criteria, three of whom had a positive Hollenberg score. Two of the three had left-ventricular hypertrophy on ECG and were judged prospectively to be negative for CAD. With separate informed consent, coronary angiography was done on the 10 patients with the highest risk profile scores and the most positive exercise test by standard criteria. This also included the three patients with a positive treadmill score. Of these 10, 1 had single-vessel right coronary disease, and had been considered prospectively to have mild CAD. The sensitivity/specificity in the remaining 374 with a negative treadmill score or the 332 with a negative standard exercise ECG was not evaluated and is unknown, as is the number of subjects excluded with prior infarct or known CAD.

ST/HR Slope

Elamin and associates[41–42] of the Leeds group reported a remarkably improved accuracy of the exercise ECG during upright bicycle exercise for the detection and quantitation of the severity of CAD using linear regression analysis of the maximum rate-related change in ST-segment depression (maximum ST/HR slope). In highly selected hospital populations of patients with angina, documented CAD, and normal controls, the maximum ST/HR slope was 100% effective in distinguishing patients with one-vessel, two-vessel, and three-vessel disease from each other and from normals. Improved accuracy in similarly selected groups was reported by others.[43–49] None of the latter studies achieved 100% accuracy.

The performance of ST/HR slope was also shown to be sensitive to variations in methods, especially the rate of increase in the exercise load, which was carefully monitored in the Leeds protocol. On standard treadmill exercise protocols (ie, Balke-Ware, Bruce, Ellestad), the rate of increase in exercise load was so rapid that the maximum ST/HR slope could not be calculated by linear regression analysis in a significant number of patients because it was not linear for the last 3 minutes or more of exercise. It was also soon found that patients with chronic left-ventricular overloading from hypertension and aortic valve disease, those with myopathies, and those with conduction defects (Wolff-Parkinson-White syndrome, right bundle branch block, and left bundle branch block) had abnormal maximum ST/HR slopes similar to or higher than those with significant CAD without these abnormalities.[50–52] The clinical use of this technique was further limited by the time-consuming manual ST-segment measurements and calculator-based linear regression analysis after testing.

Kligfield, Okin, and associates[43–49] responded to these problems with a series of papers in which they suggested modification of the standard treadmill exercise protocols to a more gradual increase in exercise workloads and thus of heart rate. They collaborated with commercial vendors to develop a computer-based implementation of the maximum ST/HR slope measured during the last 3 minutes or more of exercise. The automated measurements were found to be highly correlated with the more tedious manual measurements (r = .99 to 1.00). The presence of automated measurements led to studies assessing the optimal measurement point for ST-segment depression; that is, STJ and STJ + 20 to STJ + 80 msec after the J-point. The studies used another highly selected population of normals and subjects with classic angina, documented CAD, or both. With specificities held at 96%, they reported sensitivities of 61%, 80%, 84%, 93%, and 79% for STJ and STJ + 20, 40, 60, and 80 msec, respectively. Thus, the STJ + 60 msec measurement point was found to be optimal.

ΔST/ΔHR Index

A modification of the maximum ST/HR slope was reported by Kligfield and colleagues[53] by a simple rate adjustment of the heart rate slope. This ΔST/ΔHR index* method could be applied to any maximum exercise test protocol. It did not require linear correlation of the ST/HR slope for the terminal 3 minutes or more of exercise and thus did not require modification of routine test protocols with a lower rate of change in exercise loads (Fig. 24–4). The ΔST/ΔHR index was found to have improved sensitivity to ischemic heart disease at fixed 96% specificities when compared with standard exercise ECG criteria (90% versus 60%). However, compared with the maximum ST/HR slope, the index was somewhat less sensitive (90% versus 93%) and also less discriminating in revealing the severity of disease, that is the number of vessels with severe occlusions.

Screening of Asymptomatic Subjects for Ischemia

In asymptomatic subjects, the application of the Hollenberg treadmill score, maximum ST/HR slope, and the ΔST/ΔHR index has significantly improved the incidence of false-positive exercise tests compared with that found in conventional exercise ECG criteria. In 377 military officers, the Hollenberg score reduced the false-positive rate from 12% to less than 1%.[40] In the 1174 factory workers of Leeds and York (UK) reported by Boyle and

---

*Overall change in ST segment divided by overall change in heart rate.

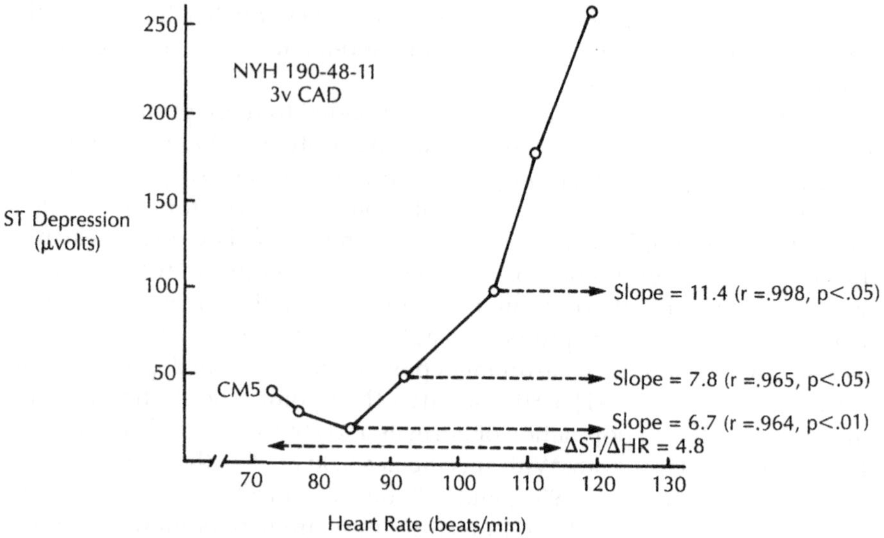

FIGURE 24–4. Relationship of ST-segment depression in lead CM_5 to heart rate during exercise in a patient with three-vessel CAD. The ST/HR slopes calculated from the final three, four, or five data points are each statistically significant but different. The highest significant value is selected as the test result for this lead. Note that other values, including the ΔST/ΔHR, do not accurately approximate the maximum value. Slope = ST/HR; ΔST/ΔHR = overall change in ST segment divided by overall change in heart rate. (From Okin, et al,[44] with permission.)

coworkers,[52] the false-positive rate was 5.8% for the maximum ST/HR slope. In 606 members of the Virginia National Guard reported by Okin and associates[54] the false-positive rate was 9% for a combination of positive standard treadmill and radionuclide cineradiography (RCNA). Determining ΔST/ΔHR index on the standard treadmill positives reduced this false-positive rate to 3% with no loss of true-positives. Finally, the ΔST/ΔHR index was studied in 3168 asymptomatic Framingham offspring by Okin and colleagues.[55] When 4-year new coronary events were taken as the "gold standard" marker for CAD, the age-adjusted relative risk (RR) of a positive test was 2.2 compared with 1.2 for a positive exercise test using conventional criteria. The ST depression with reference to heart rate during exercise and recovery was also used to generate the rate-recovery loop (see also Chapter 12). A positive rate-recovery loop had an independent RR of 2.1. With both ST/HR index and rate-recovery loop positive, the RR was 6.2; with both negative, the RR was 1.0. The incidence of CAD as defined by new coronary events was 65/3168 (2.1%) in a mean of 4.3 years. This projects to 5% in 10 years.

In all of these studies of screening of asymptomatic subjects, those with known recent or old infarct or classic angina pectoris had been excluded. The percentage excluded with known CAD ranged from unknown in the Hollenberg study of 377 military officers to 0.5% in the Leeds/York study, 2.1%

in the Virginia Guard study and 2.9% in the Framingham offspring. In each of these studies the combined prevalence of CAD, detected by both prior clinical infarct and angina pectoris in the excluded subjects, and by the screening protocols, ranges from less than 1% for the Hollenberg study of young military personnel to 7.9% for the Framingham offspring.

Because of appropriate ethical considerations, one major element not addressed by any of these studies is the incidence of significant (luminal occlusion of 50% or more) coronary obstruction in asymptomatic subjects with negative exercise tests or other screening procedures. The incidence of false-negatives in these studies ranged from 60% to 90% or more, as discussed in the following sections. On the other hand, noninvasive screening for asymptomatic myocardial ischemia has been greatly enhanced by the combined computerized techniques of exercise stress testing with ECG changes, radionuclide angiography, and scintigraphic myocardial perfusion imaging. When combined with the noninvasive detection of coronary calcium by ultrafast, ECG-gated, x-ray computed tomography (ultrafast-CT) as an invariate marker of CAD, the false-negative rate can be reduced even further.

SIGNIFICANT OCCLUSIVE CAD IN ASYMPTOMATIC SUBJECTS

Significant occlusive CAD (luminal occlusion of 50% or more) can be expected to be considerably more prevalent in asymptomatic subjects than actually detected by the screening protocols just described. Studies of Korean and Vietnam War casualty victims by Enos and associates[56] and McNamara and associates[57] and studies of young male victims of trauma by Joseph and colleagues [58] suggest that there was a significant false-negative rate in the screening protocols of ambulatory populations previously described. Janowitz, Agatston, and colleagues[59, 60] found coronary calcium by ultrafast CT in 11% of asymptomatic 20- to 29-year-olds, 23% of 35- to 40-year-old asymptomatic male factory workers, and 70% of an age-matched group of CAD patients. Significant coronary obstruction in the presence of coronary calcification was found in 75% of the latter group. It is well documented in the pathology literature that calcification of the coronary artery is an invariant marker of coronary atheroma, although the atheroma may be early and not high grade, especially in the younger adult.[61–63] As shown in Figure 24–5, the absence of coronary calcium in the presence of high-grade obstruction ranges from 30% in the younger adult men to less than 1% for those older than aged 60. From these data, the incidence of severe obstruction in the asymptomatic younger (31- to 48-year-old) officers studied by Hollenberg and associates[40] is projected to be 10% to 15%, compared with the less than 1% reported. In the Virginia guard, the Leeds/York factory workers, and the Framingham offspring, in which subjects are an average of 10 years older, the

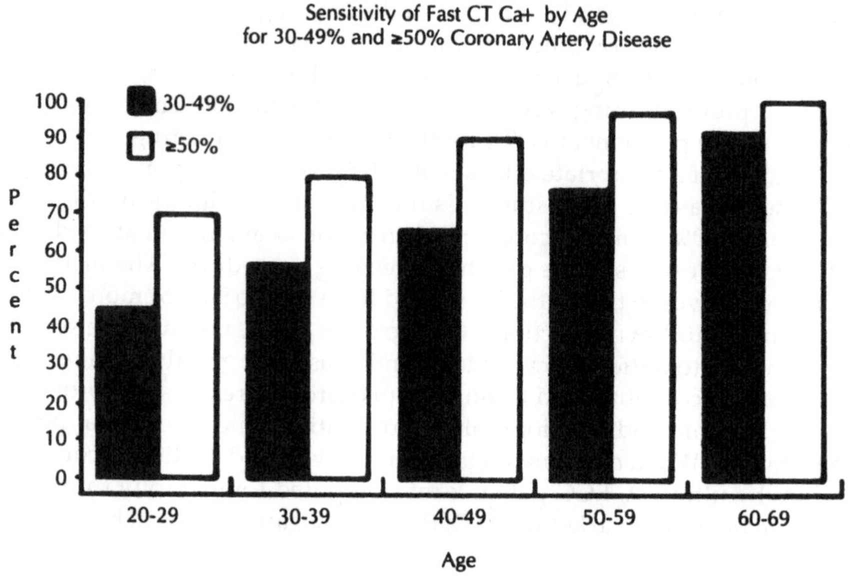

FIGURE 24–5. The percentage of coronary vessels with mild-to-severe coronary stenosis by age groups of asymptomatic subjects that show coronary calcium by ultrafast-CT. This bar graph is based on a survey of the literature (see text for details). No data were available for 20- to 29-year-olds; the projections for this age group were extrapolated backward from the data for the older subjects shown here.

projected rate of high-grade CAD is 20% to 23%, with coronary calcium found in 18% to 20%. When adjusted for those with known CAD, the detection rates from the combined screening procedures of 3.1%, 1.3%, and 7.9%, respectively, would increase to a sensitivity of 14%, 6%, and 37% for these low-incidence populations.

FUTURE STRATEGIES FOR IMPROVING QUANTITATION OF MYOCARDIAL INFARCT AND ISCHEMIA

ECG Body Surface Maps and Exercise

The availability of high-speed digital data acquisition systems has made possible the recording of a large number of simultaneous, signal-averaged body surface ECG leads and the processing of this large body of data into equipotential contour maps, or cine projection of prospective plots over time. A number of investigators have reported 87-lead to 120-lead ECG body surface maps (BSMs) at rest and during exercise in normals and in patients with documented ventricular hypertrophies or CAD.[25,26,64–67] Only Montague and associates[25] have recorded BSMs throughout the exercise and recovery period. The others have recorded the exercise BSMs early in the postexercise period. These workers have established 95% confidence limits of normal for ST depression (or elevation) over the torso surface. Predictably, they found that the breakpoint for the optimal separation of normal ST from abnormal was variable over the torso. One way of systematizing these results is to normalize each ECG lead for 2 standard deviations of normal ST, or alternatively for the lead field strength between the heart and the lead.

Ellestad and associates[20] and others[21] have shown that ST criteria are related at least in part to the QRS amplitude across a number of precordial sites. Expressing the ST depression as a percentage of the R amplitude improves sensitivity, especially in those with smaller R waves, with no loss of specificity. These data, along with computer simulations of the resting and ischemic heart, and rest and exercise multilead ECG databases, are the basic building blocks for increasing the accuracy of quantitative multilead ECG criteria for infarct and ischemia. Work on specific criteria and optimal lead sets is under way in several laboratories.

Comprehensive Normal and Exercise ECG Database—A Pooled Global Resource

The rapid increase in available digital data acquisition, signal processing, and databasing technology has opened the door to the development of a quantitative approach to exercise stress testing. The tedium of consulting manually designed tables of normal values during rest, exercise, and recovery for each of the wave amplitudes and durations for each of the 12 leads of the standard ECG and 4 extra leads is now relieved by the high-speed microcomputers of many available exercise ECG recording systems, for which it is an easy task. The acquisition, manipulation, and storing of numbers (numbers crunching) is accomplished by these machines with remarkable speed and dependability.

The development of comprehensive normal multilead ECG digital databases is well under way in a number of centers.[68–73] The ability to pool these resources for the good of all is well under way in Canada and Europe, as noted in the small sample of a much larger number of collaborative studies by Kornreich, Montegue, Rautaharju and associates,[22–26] but is lagging behind in the United States. The European Community is proceeding well toward this goal, as exemplified by the prodigious accomplishments of the Common Standards for Electrocardiology group.[68,69] In the near future, the definition of multilead specific criteria for P, QRS, ST-T, and U variables indicative of ischemia and fine-tuning of the data partitions used in each of the test procedures for optimal performance in the population being tested will rely heavily on these computer tools.

Improvement in Screening for Ischemia in Asymptomatic Subjects

There is an important need to develop a unified strategy combining the salutary role of the computer in the rest and stress testing ECG, in radionuclide angiography in scintigraphic myocardial perfusion imaging, and in the ultrafast-CT imaging of coronary calcium. The latter has a low sensitivity (40% to 50%) for significant CAD, but when present, the finding is an invariant marker for coronary atheroma. It would be especially important to improve screening to detect CAD and silent infarct/ischemia in certain asymptomatic, low-incidence groups involved in public safety (eg, airline pilots and military pilots of high- performance aircraft).

Loecker and colleagues[63] recently reported on the routine screening of US Air Force airmen after age 35 by a medical examination that included a resting 12-lead ECG. Those who had indications of health problems, such as serial ECG changes suggestive of ischemic heart disease, were referred to the School of Aerospace Medicine at Brooks Air Force Base, Texas, for comprehensive workup with maximum treadmill exercise testing with thallium scintigraphy and cinefluoroscopy for coronary calcium. Those who had documented prior infarct or classic angina were not included in this study. In the remaining asymptomatic airmen, if one or more of these tests suggested coronary ischemia, angiography was required for them to remain on flying status. Over the 5 years covered by the report, 1466 asymptomatic airmen were referred for further workup, and 669 were referred for angiography, of whom 56 declined and 613 had angiography. As shown in Figure 24–6, 325 (53%) had entirely normal coronary arteries, 80 (13%) had minimal intimal roughening involving less than 10% of the luminal diameter, 49 (8%) had 10% to 29% luminal narrowing, 55 (9%) had 30% to 49% luminal disease, and 104 (17%) had 50% or more of obstructive CAD. The mean age of the subjects screened was 40.2 ± 5 years (age range 26 to 65). The findings of Agatston and associates[60] for a group of patients of similar ages with suspected CAD who had simultaneous cinefluoroscopy and ultrafast-CT were projected by us to these airmen. The prevalence of calcium by ultrafast-CT, as shown by the regions with horizontal lines in Figure 24–5, included all those showing calcium by fluoroscopy. These data were also used to project the distribution of coronary calcium as related to the severity of CAD in asymptomatic ambulatory men described previously (see Fig. 24–6).

In summation, these data, when projected to segments of the population with a low incidence of CAD, suggest that a combination of screening with ultrafast-CT and treadmill testing with a gradual exercise increment and ST/HR rate slope determination and selective use of radionuclide angiography or myocardial perfusion scintigraphy would yield a major improvement in detection of ischemia. Cut points or diagnostic partitions for the various

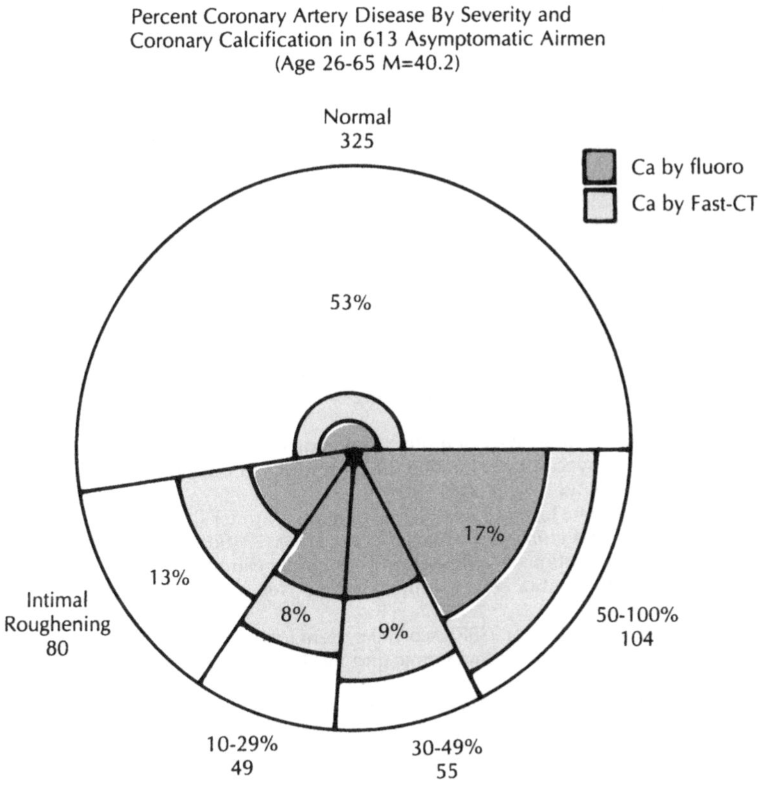

FIGURE 24–6. The distribution of angiographically abnormal coronary arteries in 40-year-old asymptomatic airmen. The occurrence of coronary calcium reported at fluoroscopy by Loecker and associates[63] is projected to what might be expected by ultrafast-CT. The projections are based on the ratio of coronary calcium at fluoroscopy compared with findings by ultrafast-CT in asymptomatic 40 year olds by Agatston and colleagues.[60] The shaded areas of the figure indicate the percentage of each subgroup with fluoroscopic coronary calcium. The radius of each sector is scaled to the percentage of subjects in each category with fluoro calcium, ultrafast-CT calcium, or no calcium.

methods previously described can be developed from studies in these populations that make the most of the diagnostic performance of the combined protocols. As we learn to decipher the signal that the heart is sending out, we will be using computers as basic tools to define the details of regional ischemia and infarct by answering the following: How severe is the dysfunction? How much is due to ischemia? How much is due to irreversible infarct? This information is basic to making the best use of stress testing in screening of healthy populations, in health maintenance, in early detection of ischemia, and in intervention in the care of heart disease.

REFERENCES

1. Selvester, RH, Solomon, JC, and Gillespie, T: Digital computer model of a total body ECG surface map: An Adult male torso simulation with lungs. Circulation 38:684, 1968
2. Selvester, RH, Kirk, WL, and Pearson, RB: Propagation velocities and voltage magnitudes in local segments of myocardium. Circ Res 27 (4): 619–625, 1970.
3. Solomon, JC and Selvester, RH: Simulation of measured activation sequence in the human heart. Am Heart J 85:518, 1973.
4. Selvester, RH and Solomon, JC: Infarct size and QRS changes (QRS criteria applicable to computer diagnostic programs). Proceedings Engineering Foundation Conference. In Tolan, GD and Pryor, TA (eds): Computerized Interpretations of the ECG, V. Engineering Foundation, New York, 1980, p. 69.
5. Palmeri, ST, Harrison, DG, and Wagner, GS: A QRS scoring system for assessing left ventricular function after myocardial infarction. N Engl J Med 306(1):4, 1982.
6. Selvester, RH, Wagner, GS, and Hindman, NB: The development and application of the Selvester QRS scoring system for estimating myocardial infarct size. Arch Intern Med 145:1877–1881 1985.
7. Selvester, RH and Solomon, JC: Computer simulation of the human electrocardiogram: Fascicular blocks and myocardial infarction. In Computers in Cardiology, Proceedings of the IEEE Computer Society, 1987, p. 215–218.
8. Selvester, RH, Solomon, Jc, and Tolan, GT: Fine grid computer simulation of QRS-T and criteria for quantitating regional ischemia. J Electrocardiol 20 (Supp): 1–8, 1987.
9. Ideker, RE, et al: Evaluation of a QRS scoring system for estimating myocardial infarct size. II. Correlation with quatitative anatomic findings for anterior infarcts. Am J Cardiol 49:1604–1614, 1982.
10. Ward, RM, et al: Evaluation of a QRS scoring system for estimating myocardial infarct size. IV. Correlation with quantitative anatomic findings for posterolateral infarcts. Am J Cardiol 53:706–714, 1984.
11. Bounous, EP, et al: Prognostic value of the simplified Selvester QRS score in patients with coronary artery disease. J Am Coll Cardiol 11(1):35–41, 1988.
12. Sevilla, DC, et al: Anatomic validation of electrocardiographic estimation of the size of acute and healed myocardial infarcts. Am J Cardiol 65:1301–1307, 1990.
13. Selvester, RHS, et al: ECG myocardial infarct size: A gender-, age-, race-insensitive 12-segment multiple regression. I. Retrospective learning set of 100 pathoanatomic infarcts and 229 normal control subjects. J Electrocardiol 27 (suppl): 31–41, 1994.
14. Wagner, NB, et al: Transient alterations in the QRS complex and ST segment during balloon angioplasty of the left anterior descending coronary artery. Am J Cardiol 62:1038–1042, 1988.
15. Saetre, HA, et al: Sixteen-lead electrocardiographic changes with coronary angioplasty: Location of STT changes with balloon occlusion of five arterial segments. Proceedings of the 16th ISCE Conference: Computer Applications in Electrocardiology. In Kligfield,P and Bailey, JJ. eds: J Electrocardiol 24 (suppl); 152:–162, 1991.
16. Selvester, RH and Solomon, JC: Optimal ECG electrode sites and criteria for detection of asymptomatic coronary artery disease at rest and with exercise: Update 1990. Technical Report of School of Aerospace Medicine, TR-AL-1991-0029, Brooks AFB, Texas, 1992.
17. Selvester, RH and Solomon, JC: Optimal ECG electrode sites and criteria for detection of asymptomatic coronary artery disease at rest and with exercise. Technical Report of School of Aerospace Medicine, USAFSAM-TR-85-47. Brooks AFB, Texas, 1985.
18. Selvester, RH and Sanmarco, ME. Infarct size in hi-gain, hi-fidelity serial VCG's and serial ventriculograms in patients with proven coronary artery disease. Proceedings of the 4th World Congress on Electrocardiography, Modern Electrocardiology, Zantaloczy, (ed): Akademiai, Budapest, and Exerpta Medica, Amsterdam, 1978.
19. Selvester, RH and Gillespie, TL: Simulated ECG surface map's sensitivity to local segments of myocardium. Proceedings, Vermont Conference Body Surface Mapping of Cardiac Fields. Advances in Cardiology, vol. 10. Lepeschkin, E and Rush, S (eds): S Karger, Basel, 1974 p 120.
20. Ellestad, MH, Crump, R, and Surber, M: The significance of lead strength on ST changes during treadmill stress test. J Electrocardiol 25 (suppl): 31–34, 1992.

21. Bonoris, PE, et al: Significance of changes in R wave amplitude during treadmill stress testing: Angiographic correlation. Am J Cardiol 41:846–851, 1978.
22. Kornreich, F, et al: Multigroup diagnosis of body surface potential maps. J Electrocardiol 22, (Suppl): 169–178, 1989.
23. Kornreich, F, et al: Identification of best electrocardiographic leads for the diagnosing anterior and inferior myocardial infarction by statistical analysis of body surface potential maps. Am J Cardiol 58:863–871, 1986.
24. Kornreich, F, Montague, TJ, and Rautaharju, PM: Location and magnitude of ST changes in acute myocardial infarction by analysis of body surface potential maps. J Electrocardiol 24 (suppl:) 15–19, 1992.
25. Montague TJ, et al: Exercise body surface mapping in single and multiple coronary disease. Chest 97:1333–1342, 1990.
26 Kornreich, F, Montague, TJ, and Rautaharju, PM": Body surface potential mapping of ST segment changes with acute myocardial infarction: Implications for ECG enrollment criteria for thrombolytic therapy. Circulation 87:774–784, 1993.
27. Mortara, D: A new pattern recognition approach to exercise analysis. In van Bennek, JH and Willems, JL (eds): Proceedings of Trends in Computer-Processed Electrocardiograms. North-Holland Publishers, Amsterdam, 1977, pp 404–410.
28. Pahlm, O and Sörnmo, L: Data processing of exercise ECGs. IEEE Trans Biomed Engl 34:158–165, 1987.
29. Meyers, CR and Keiser, HN: Electrocardiogram baseline noise estimation and removal using cubic splines and state-space computational techniques. Comput Biomed Res 10:459–464. 1977.
30. McManus, CD, et al: Estimation and removal of baseline drift in the electrocardiogram. Comput Biomed Res 18:1–9, 1985.
31. Watanabe, K, Bhargava, V, and Froelicher, VF: Computer analysis of the exercise electrocardiogram: A review. Prog Cardiovasc Dis 22:423–446, 1980.
32. Bhargava, V, Watanabe, K, and Froelicher, V: Progress in computer analysis of the exercise electrocardiogram. Am J Cardiol 47:1143–1151, 1981.
33. Chaitman, BR: The changing role of the exercise electrocardiogram as a diagnostic and prognostic test for chronic ischemic heart disease. J Am Coll Cardiol 8:1195–1210, 1986.
34. Miliken, JA, Abdollah, H, and Burggraf, GW: False-positive treadmill exercise tests due to computer signal averaging. Am J Cardiol 65:946–948, 1990.
35. Myrianthefs, MM, et al: Significance of signal-averaged P- wave changes during exercise in patients with coronary artery disease and correlation with angiographic findings. Am J Cardiol 68:1619–1624, 1991.
36. Wiener, L, Dwyer, EM Jr, and Cox, WH: Left ventricular hemodynamics in exercise-induced angina pectoris. Circulation 38:240–249, 1968.
37. Heikkaila, J, Heugenholtz, PG, and Tabakin, BS: Prediction of the left atrial filling pressure and its sequential change in acute myocardial infarction from the terminal force of the P wave. Br Heart J 35:142–151, 1973.
38. Orlando, J, et al: Correlation of mean pulmonary wedge pressure, left atrial dimensions, and PTF-V1 in patients with acute myocardial infarction. Circulation 55:750–752, 1977.
39. Sheffield, TJ, et al: On-line analysis of the exercise electrocardiogram. Circulation 40:935–944, 1969.
40. Hollenberg, M, et al: Comparison of a quantitative treadmill exercise score with standard electrocardiographic criteria in screening asymptomatic young men for coronary artery disease. N Engl J Med 313:600–606, 1985.
41. Elamin, MS, et al: Prediction of severity of coronary artery disease using slope of sub-maximal ST segment/heart rate relationship. Cardiovasc Res 14:681–684, 1980.
42. Elamin, M, Boyle, R, and Linden, RJ: Accurate detection of coronary disease by a new exercise test. Br Heart J 48:311–320, 1982.
43. Kligfield, P, et al: Correlation of the exercise ST/HR slope with anatomic and radionuclide cineradiographic findings in stable angina pectoris. Am J Cardiol 56:418–421, 1985.
44. Okin, PM, Ameisen, O, and Kligfield, P: A modified treadmill exercise protocol for computer-assisted analysis of the ST segment/heart rate slope: Methods and reproducibility. J Electrocardiol 19:311–318, 1986.
45. Kligfield, P, Ameisen, O, and Okin, PM: Relation of the exercise ST/HR slope to simple heart rate adjustment of ST segment depression. J Electrocardiol 20: (suppl): 135–140, 1987.

46. Okin, PM and Kligfield, P: Computer-based implementation of the ST-segment/heart rate slope. Am J Cardiol 64:926–930, 1989.
47. Okin, PM, Bergman, G, and Kligfield, P: Effect of ST segment measurement point of performance of standard and heart rate-adjusted ST segment criteria for the identification of coronary artery disease. Circulation 84:57–66, 1991.
48. Okin, PM and Kligfield, P: Identifying coronary artery disease in women by heart rate adjustment of ST-segment depression and improved performance of linear regression over simple averaging with comparison to standard criteria. Am J Cardiol 69(4):297–302, 1992.
49. Okin, PM and Kligfield, P: Population selection and performance of the exercise ECG for the identification of coronary artery disease. Am Heart J 127: 296–304, 1994.
50. Ameisen, O, et al: Predictive value and limitations of the ST/HR slope. Br Heart J 53:547–551, 1985.
51. Bishop, N, et al: The contribution of cardiac enlargement to myocardial ischemia—assessment using the maximal ST/HR slope in patients before and after aortic valve surgery. Clin Sci 12(suppl):55–63, 1985.
52. Boyle, RM, Adlakha, HL, and Mary, DASG: Diagnostic value of the maximal ST segment/heart rate slope in asymptomatic factory populations. J Electrocardiol 20 (suppl): 128–134, 1987.
53. Kligfield, P, Ameisen, O, and Okin, PM: Heart rate adjustment of ST segment depression for improved detection of coronary artery disease. Circulation 79:245–255, 1989.
54 Okin PM, et al: Heart rate adjustment of the ST-segment depression for reduction of false positive electrocardiographic responses to exercise in asymptomatic men screened for coronary artery disease. Am J Cardiol 62:1043–1047, 1988.
55. Okin, PM, et al: Heart rate adjustment of exercise-induced ST segment depression: Improved risk stratification in the Framingham offspring study. Circulation 83:866–874, 1991.
56. Enos, WF, Homes, RH, and Beger, J: Coronary disease among United States soldiers killed in action in Korea. JAMA 52:1090–1093, 1953.
57. McNamara, JJ, et al: Coronary artery disease in combat casualties in Vietnam. JAMA 216 1185–1187, 1971.
58. Joseph, SA, et al: Early manifestations of coronary atherosclerosis in trauma victims determined at autopsy. [Abstract] J Am Coll Cardiol 21(suppl):319A, 1993.
59. Janowitz, WR, et al: Differences in prevalence and extent of coronary artery calcium detected by ultrafast computed tomography in asymptomatic men and women. Am J Cardiol 72:247–252, 1993.
60. Agatston, AS, et al: Quantification of coronary calcium using ultrafast computed tomography. J Am Coll Cardiol 15:827–832, 1990.
61. Blankenhorn, DH: Coronary arterial calcification: A review. Am J Med Sci 242:1–9, 1961.
62. Eggan, DA, Strong, JP, and McGill, HC: Coronary calcification: Relationship to clinically significant coronary lesions and race, sex, and topographical distribution. Circulation 32:948–955, 1965.
63. Loecker, TH, et al: Fluoroscopic coronary calcification and associated coronary disease in asymptomatic young men. J Am Coll Cardiol 19:1167–1172, 1992.
64. Ikeda, K, et al: Non-invasive detection of coronary artery disease by body surface electrocardiographic mapping after dipyridamole infusion. J Electrocardiol 19:213–224, 1986.
65. Fox, KM, et al: Precordial electrocardiographic mapping in the identification of patients with left main stem narrowing. Int J Cardiol 3:315–323, 1983.
66. Yasui, S, et al: Quantitative evaluation of treadmill test induced ST-T changes using body surface mapping. Jap Circ J 45:1208–1211, 1981.
67. Mirvis, DM: Body surface potential distribution of exercise-induced QRS changes in normal subjects. Am J Cardiol 46:988–996, 1980.
68. Willems, JL (ed): Common Standards for Quantitative Electrocardiography. CSE Atlas Referee Results, First Phase Library—Data Set One ACCO. 1-655, Leuven 1983.
69. Willems, JL: For the CSE working party: Assessment of the performance of electrocardiographic computer programs with the use of a reference data base. Circulation 71:523–534 1985.
70. Selvester, RH: A comprehensive multilead ECG normal database for the next few decades. A position paper. Computer ECG Analysis: Towards Standardization. Willems, JL, van

Bemmel, JH and Zywietz, C. (eds): Proceedings, Third International Conference on Common Standards for Quantitative Electrocardiography. North Holland Publishing Company, Amsterdam, 1986.
71. Macfarlane, PW, and Lawrie, TDV: The normal electrocardiogram and vector cardiogram. In Macfarlane, PW and Lawrie, TDV (eds): Comprehensive Electrocardiology, Theory and Practice in Health and Disease, Appendix 1, vol 3. Pergamon Press, New York, 1989.
72. Rautahrju, PM, Zhou, SH, and Calhoun, HP: Ethnic differences in ECG amplitudes in North American white, black, and hispanic men and women: Effects of obesity and age. J Electrocardiol 27 (suppl):20–31, 1994.
73. De Bacquer, D, et al: Prevalence and correlates of ECG abnormalities in the adult Belgian population. J Electrocardiol 28:1–12, 1995.

Index

Note: Page numbers followed by "f" indicate figures; those followed by "t" indicated tables.

Abdominal thoracic pump, 13
Acute myocardial infarction (AMI), 466
Adenosine, 50–51, 429–430, 434–436, 492
Adenosine triphosphate (ATP), 32, 33, 60, 61, 66
Adrenergic agonists, 431
Adrenergic influences on coronary circulation, 23–24
Aerobic capacity, 320t
Aerobic metabolism, 32–33
Age
  and CAD, 309, 310, 310f–311f
  and conditioning, 21–22, 147, 148t
  effect of, 17, 18f, 19, 298–299, 298f, 299f
  and positive stress tests, 279t, 280
Alcohol, 505–506
Alkalosis, 482–483
Aminophylline, 492
Amiodarone, 491
Amphetamines, 499
Anaerobic metabolism, 33
Anaerobic threshold, 119–120
Analog-to-digital (A-D) conversion, 517–517f
Androgens, 485–486
Angina, 180, 196, 252f, 294, 295f, 361
  antianginal drugs, mechanism of action of, 492
  atypical, 333
  diagnostic value, 182
  and ischemia, 359, 359t. *See also* Ischemia
  microvascular. *See* Syndrome X
  myocardial infarction and, 328
  in post-MI testing, 172–173
  Prinzmetal's, 204–205, 328–329
  probable, 312, 313f
  progression, 287–288, 291f
  typical, 312, 313f, 333
  unstable, 458f–459f, 465–466
Anginal pain, 64–66, 65f, 282–283, 296–297, 297f. *See also under* Pain
Angiograms, coronary, 78, 273
Angiography, coronary
  ST-segment depression and, 281–283
Angioplasty, coronary
  percutaneous transluminal, 169, 170
  stress testing after, 179, 184–185
Angioplasty patients, evaluation of, 179–180
Angiotensin converting enzyme (ACE) inhibitors, 504
Angiotensin II blockers, 504
Antianginal drugs, mechanism of action of, 492
Aorta, thoracic
  coarctation of, 394–396, 394f–396f
Aortic murmur, 121
Aortic stenosis, 87, 121
  supravalvular, 392, 394
  valvular and discrete subvalvular, 389–390, 391f–393f, 392
  working capacity in children with, 391f, 392, 394
Aortic valve insufficiency, 396–397, 396f
Arbutamine, 431, 432
Arrhythmias, 241–242, 266, 368
  abolition by exercise, 251
  class I_B antiarrhythmic drugs, 490–491
  class I_C antiarrhythmic drugs, 491
  evaluation of, 81
  sinus, 396f
  supraventricular, 243–247, 244f–247f
  ventricular
    exercise-induced, 173, 248–249, 249f, 401, 402f, 403–404, 404f
    resting, 248
Arrhythrogenic right ventricular dysplasia, 254
Arteries. *See* Coronary arteries
Arteriovenous oxygen ($AV\text{-}O_2$), 19, 22
Astrand protocol, 142, 144f
  modified, 143f

Athens QRS score, 219, 220f
Athletes, 367
  duration and intensity of performance, 372
  ECG changes at rest, 372, 373f, 374, 374t
  exercise-induced abnormalities, 374–376
  heart rate and blood pressure, 372
  vs. nonathletes, performance of, 368
Athletic efforts, previous
  health as related to, 369–370
Atrial extrasystoles, 218, 244, 244f
Atrial fibrillation or flutter, 245–246, 246f–247f
Atrial premature beats, 244, 244f–245f
Atrial septal defect, 401
Atrial tachycardia, paroxysmal, 246–247
Atrioventricular (AV) block, 264
  first-degree, 255
  second-degree, 255
  third-degree, 264, 264f
Atrioventricular (AV) node, 255
Atropine, 497, 498f
Augmented V lead, left leg (AVF), 205
Augmented V lead, right arm (AVR), 203–205, 233
Auscultation, problems with, 336
Auscultatory findings, 120–122
Autoregulatory resistance, 22–23

Balke protocol, 142, 143f–144f
Bassler hypothesis, 369
Bayes' theorem, 272–273, 272f, 273f
  critique of, 279
Beta-blockers, 325, 325f, 363, 494
  mechanisms, 494–496
Bezett's formula, 223
Bicarbonate, 31, 31f
Bicycle ergonomic workloads, oxygen requirements of, 139, 140t
Bicycle stress, 434
Bicycle tests, 138–139
  supine *vs.* upright, 139
Blood flow, coronary, 22, 23f, 24, 25f
Blood flow regulation, physiology of, 49–51
Blood pressure. *See also* Pressure pulse product
  recovery, 346–347, 349f
Blood pressure measurement
  automated, 339
  simultaneous, on opposite arms, 338, 338f
Blood pressure recording
  correctable sources of error, 336–338
  problems with auscultation, 336
  reliability, 335
Blood pressure response (during exercise), 339, 349
  with age, 340, 341f
  and body surface area, 386, 387f
  cardiomyopathies and, 347
  hypertensive, 340–342. *See under* Hypertension
    in CAD patients, 342, 343f
  hypotensive, 344–346
    early in exercise, 344
    late in exercise, 344, 345f
  with ischemia, 344–346
  medications and, 347–348
  normal, 339–340
  in patients with resting hypertension, 340–341, 408, 410f
Body surface area (BSA), 384, 386, 387f–388f
Body surface maps (BSMs), ECG
  and exercise, 526–527
Body weight, and oxygen consumption, 139, 140t
Bradycardia, sustained relative, 114
Bradycardia-chronotropic incompetence, 294, 294f
Bruce protocol, 141–142, 142f–144f, 146
Bruce stages, 145t
Bundle branch blocks. *See also* Left bundle branch block; Right bundle branch block
  digital computer simulation of, 515
  rate-related, 260
Bypass graft surgery, coronary artery
  diagnostic value of angina, 182
  postoperative exercise performance, 182–183, 183f
  pre- and postoperative ST-segment depression, 182
  prediction of ischemia and postoperative testing, 181–182, 181t
  prediction of postoperative results, 180–181
  serial postoperative exercise testing, 183–184
Bypass patients, evaluation of, 179–180

CA lead, 105
Calcium, coronary, 525, 526f, 528, 529f
Calcium blockers, 496–497
Carbohydrates, 31–32
Carbon dioxide (CO_2), 321f. *See also* Partial pressure of carbon dioxide
Carbon dioxide production (VO_2), 385, 386f. *See also* Oxygen uptake (VO_2)
Carbon monoxide, 487
Cardiac catheterization, 284t, 345

Cardiac failure, chronic
aerobic activity and severity of, 320t
Cardiac ischemia. *See* Ischemia
Cardiomyopathy(ies), 329, 347, 499
hypertrophic, 408–409, 410f
Cardiopulmonary resuscitation (CPR)
drugs for, 92t
CASS study—1982, 289
Catecholamines, 16, 498–499
CB lead, 105, 105f
CC_5, 105, 109–110, 235f
Cedars Emory Quantitative Analysis program (CEQUAL), 444, 447
Chest pain. *See also* Anginal pain; Pain
evaluation of patients with, 78–79
and normal coronary arteries, 327, 333
clinical syndromes, 328–331
prevalence, 327–328
prognosis, 332–333
therapy, 332
treadmill findings, 331–332
Chlorthalidone, 502
Chronotropic incompetence (sick sinus syndrome), 113, 114f, 242–243, 293–294, 293f, 294f
Circadian influence, 153
Circumflex disease, 450f–451f
Clonidine, 503
Clothing, 158
CM_5, 105, 106, 108–110, 261
Coarctation of thoracic aorta, 394–396, 394f–396f
Cold, 35
Collateral formation, coronary
stimulus to, 46
exercise, 46–47
Collaterals, intracoronary, 45–46
Compressive resistance, 23
Computer simulation of human ECG, digital, 515–516
optimal ECG lead locations, 516
Computer technology, 513–514. *See also specific topics*
digital processing, noise reduction, and measurement accuracy, 518–519, 518f
Computerized measurements in exercise systems, advantages of, 519
Conditioning, age and, 21–22, 147, 148t
Conduction disturbances, 254–257, 257f–259f, 260–264, 261f, 263f–264f, 266
accelerated conduction. *See* Wolff-Parkinson-White (WPW) syndrome
Congenital heart disease, pediatric. *See under* Pediatric exercise testing
Congenital heart failure, and valvular dysfunction, 82–83
Congenital long QT syndrome (LQTS), 257, 259f
Congestive heart failure patients
contraindications to exercise testing, 88
exercise testing in, 319, 323f
evaluation, 81
exercise duration, 324
instrumentation, 324
and prediction of events, 324–325
VO_2max, 322
heart rate, 324, 325f
Contingency table, 273, 275t
Contractility, 14, 15f, 16, 494. *See also under* Ischemia
Cooper Clinic study—2000, 289, 290f, 291. *See also* Ischemic ST segments
Cornell (exercise) protocol, 145
Coronary arteries
collaterals, 45–47
and ischemia, 44–48
pressure relationships of left ventricle and, 53, 54f–55f
vasomotion, 44–45, 45f
Coronary artery disease (CAD), 113–115, 117, 118, 120, 136, 195, 262, 279, 359. *See also specific topics*
diagnosis, 419
MPI, 464, 464t
exercise and prevention of, 370–371
Hollenberg exercise score and, 520, 522
hypertensive response and, 340
mortality predicted by two-vessel, 304f
population groups and, 279–280
prevalence, 277f, 279–280, 279t, 354
prognosis, 421
QRS and, 219
severity, 79
estimating, 175
significant occlusive CAD in asymptomatic subjects, 525–526, 526f
and upsloping ST segments, 192, 195f
Coronary artery narrowing, 282, 282f
Coronary blood flow, 22, 23f, 24, 25f
Coronary collateral formation
stimulus to, 46
Coronary resistance, 22–24
Coronary size related to workload, 47–48
Correct classification rate, 275
CS_5, 105, 106
Cuts, misaligned, 445

Deaths, 196f. *See also* Mortality
  case histories of patients who died, 92–93, 94f–95f, 96, 97f–98f
  sudden, during exercise, 368–369
Defibrillator, 91
Delta heart rate, 294, 296
Diabetes, 484–485
Diastolic blood pressure, 409, 410f. *See also* Left-ventricular end-diastolic pressure
Diazepam, 501–502
Diffusion (respiration), 37
Digital processing, 518–519, 518f. *See also* Analog-to-digital (A-D) conversion; Computer simulation of human ECG
Digitalis, 228, 488–490
Digoxin, 489
Dipyridamole, 52f, 429, 434–436, 464t, 494. *See also* Stunning, post-persantine
Diuretics, 502–503
Dobutamine, 131, 431, 432, 436–437
Drugs, 131
  and blood pressure response, 347–348
  in emergency kit, 91, 92t
  metabolic abnormalities and, 481, 506. *See also specific abnormalities; specific drugs*
  psychotropic, 499–502
  reported to alter exercise-induced ST-segment changes, 486t
Duke Score, 302
Duke study—1978, 288

Ebstein's anomaly, 401–402
Echo imaging, indications for, 129
Echocardiography, stress, 127–129, 132
  accuracy, 131, 131t
  images, 129, 130f
    evaluation of, 130
  methodology, 129
  vs. nuclear studies, 132
  in prognosis, 132
Ejection fraction (EF), 414, 415, 418, 419, 421
Electrocardiogram (ECG) database, comprehensive normal and exercise, 527
Electrocardiograms (ECGs), 137, 163–164, 190. *See also* Computer technology; *specific topics*
  digital computer simulation of normal, 515–516
  in history of stress testing, 1
  of patients who died, 92–93, 94f–95f, 96, 97f–98f
Electrocardiographic (ECG) changes, 190. *See also specific patterns*
  conventional
    distribution of ST depression, 203–204, 204f
    horizontal *vs.* downsloping ST segments, 195–198, 197f
    intraobserver agreement, 202–203
    magnitude of ST depression, 201–202
    normal exercise ECG ST and J point, 190–191, 192f
    ST depression in recovery only, 198, 199f
    ST integral and slope, 198–200, 200f
    time course of ST depression, 200–201, 201t, 202f
    upsloping ST segments, 192, 194–195, 194f
  unconventional, 207–214, 208f, 210f–215f
Electrocardiographic (ECG) complex, normal, 191f
Electrocardiographic specifications, 104
Electrode positions and attachments, 158, 159
Ellastad protocol, 142–144f, 147
Emotional stress test, 153
Encainide, 491
Endorphins, 65–66
Endothelin, 330
Environmental factors, 370
Esophageal dysfunction, 330–331
Estrogens, 313–314, 485
Exercise
  amount needed, 370–371
  quantity and quality to maintain fitness, 370
Exercise capacity
  and prediction of events, 324–325
  in sedentary and active men, 145, 146f
Exercise duration, 297–298, 324
Exercise intensity, 147, 148t, 149–151, 149f
Exercise stress test report, M.H.I., 166–167
Exercise test
  equipment and supplies necessary to test safely, 90–92
  in sports, type of, 371
  termination
  indications for, 89–90, 383t
  when to terminate, 88–89
Exercise testing. *See also* Stress testing
  indications for, 77–83
    assessing severity of disease and prognosis, 79

chest pain, 78–79
evaluation of functional capacity, 81–82, 82f
evaluation of therapy, 79
screening for latent coronary disease, 79–80, 80f
sports medicine, 83
stimulus to motivate change in lifestyle, 83
parameters to be measured in, 103–104, 123. *See also specific parameters*
reliability, 6–7
risks reported in literature, 96, 99
Exercise training. *See* Training

2-F-18 fluoro-2-deoxyglucose (F-18 FDG), metabolic imaging with, 428, 467, 469, 470, 470f
Fallot's tetralogy, 398–399, 400f–402f, 401
False-positive and false-negative tests, 275, 284–285. *See also* Sensitivity of (stress) tests; Specificity of (stress) tests
Fascicular block, 256–257, 257f–258f
Fatty acid oxidation inhibitors, partial, 505
Fatty acids, 32. *See also* Free fatty acids (FFAs)
Flecainide, 491
Flow reserve, 341
Follow-up, extended, 176
Fontan procedure, 402–403, 403f
Free fatty acids (FFAs). *See also* Fatty acids
and ischemic myocardium, 67, 505
Froelicher Score, 302–303

Gastroesophageal reflux (GER), 331
Gated cardiac blood pool, 418, 420f–421f
diagnosis, 419, 421
diastolic function, 419
interpretation of results, 419
risk stratification and prognosis, 421
systolic function, 418–419
Gating, verifying correct, 446
Gender. *See* Sex differences
Glucose metabolism, 31–32
Guanethidine, 503–504

Handrail support, 160
Hearing, threshold of, 336, 337f
Heart
efficiency, 24
substrate use in the, 31–32
Heart murmur. *See* Aortic murmur
Heart rate recovery, 296
Heart rate response to exercise, 112–115, 114f, 115f
Heart-rate-targeted testing, 138
Heart rate(s) (HR), 16–18, 18f, 24, 25f, 294, 295f. *See also* ST/HR; ST/HR slope
beta-blockers and, 495
in congestive heart failure patients, 324, 325f
delta, 115, 116f
HR recovery ST loop, 212–213, 213f
intrinsic, 497–498
submaximal target, and test termination, 89–90
with training, 19–20, 20f
Heart sounds
first and second, 120–121
third, 121
fourth, 121
Heart volume. *See* Stroke volume
Heart Watch—1978, 288
Heat, 34–35, 34f
Hemodynamic responses, 173–174
His' bundle, 264
Hollenberg treadmill exercise score, 520, 522
"Hump sign," 231
Hyperpnea, exercise, 36
Hypertension. *See also under* Blood pressure response
after coarctectomy, 394–395, 394f–396f
antihypertensive drugs, 502–505
blood pressure response in patients with resting, 340–341, 408, 410f
early detection of labile, 81
severe, 87–88
systolic, 396f, 397
Hyperthyroidism, 483
Hypertrophied myocardium, 341–342
Hypertrophies, digital computer simulation of, 515
Hyperventilation, 207f, 482–483, 483f
and orthostatic changes, 229–231, 232f
Hypokalemia, 228
Hypotension. *See under* Blood pressure response
Hypothyroidism, 484
Hypoxia, 31, 61
ischemia and, 33–34

Inferior leads, ST-segment depression only in, 228
Inferior wall ischemia, 452f–453f
Internal contractile element work, 26

Intramyocardial perfusion, 48–49, 49f. *See also* Myocardial perfusion imaging
  and ischemia, 48–53, 50f
  physiology of blood flow regulation, 49–51
  transmural flow distribution, 51–52
  vasodilator reserve, 52–53, 52f
Intramyocardial tension, 26–27
Ischemia, 31, 43, 71–72. *See also* Myocardial ischemia; *specific topics*
  blood pressure response with, 60, 344–346
  contractility, wall motion, and, 60–62, 61f
  coronary arteries and, 44–48
  digital computer simulation of, 515
  direction of ST vector and, 70–71, 70f
  EKG criteria for, 303
  future strategies for improving quantitation of, 526–529
  inferior wall, 452f–453f
  intramyocardial perfusion and, 48–53, 50f
  isometric and isotonic exercise and, 152, 153
  lateral wall, 450f–451f
  left ventricle and, 53, 55–57, 62–64
  localization by ECG patterns, 233
  metabolic and mechanical events associated with, 58, 59f
  oxygen supply *vs.* demand and, 43–44
  pain and, 64–66, 359–360
  posture and pressure fillings and, 57–58, 58f
  screening of asymptomatic subjects for, 523–525
    improvement in, 528–529
  stroke work and, 64
  subendocardial, 198, 242
  time intervals and, 53, 55–56, 56f
  transmural, 233, 515–516
  trigger mechanisms for, 48
Ischemic cascade, 128, 128f
Ischemic dilation, transient, 456f–457f, 460f–461f
Ischemic disease, chronic, 464–465
Ischemic myocardium. *See* Myocardium, ischemic
Ischemic ST segments. *See also* ST-segment depression
  and mortality, 288, 289f, 304f
Ischemic syndromes, acute, 465
Isometric and isotonic exercise, 152, 153
Isometric test, 151–152
  combined with isotonic exercise, 152–153
Isoproterenol, 499

J junction, 197f
J point, 190–191, 192f, 194, 194f, 195, 387, 389f, 390f
James protocol, 383t, 384f, 388f

Kawasaki disease, 406–407
Kligfield index, 209
Korotkoff sounds, 336–339

L-Arginine, 505
Lactate, and ischemic myocardium, 67
Lactate metabolism, 31, 32
Lateral wall ischemia, 450f–451f
Lawsuits, 99
Lead strength (ST/R), 207–208, 208f
Lead systems, 105
  bipolar leads, 105–107, 105f–107f
  conventional 12 leads, 107
  mixed-lead systems, 109–110
  precordial maps, 108–109, 109f
  XYZ orthogonal leads, 108
Leads
  localization with right precordial, 234
  optimally distorted, 106
Left anterior descending (LAD), localization of proximal or distal, 234
Left anterior descending (LAD) disease/narrowing, 219, 221, 226, 233
Left anterior descending (LAD) ischemia, 447, 448f–449f
Left anterior division block, 256, 257f–258f
Left anterior hemiblock, 256, 257f
Left anterior oblique (LAO) view, 438, 439f, 443
Left bundle branch block (LBBB), 214, 216–217, 253, 254, 260, 262–264, 263f, 455
Left main equivalent, suspected, 87
Left posterior hemiblock, 256–257
Left ventricle, pressure relationships of coronary arteries and, 53, 54f–55f
Left-ventricular dynamics in women, 314
Left-ventricular end-diastolic pressure (LVEDP), 58, 62, 62f, 64, 65f, 261, 261f, 263, 263f, 329, 520
  ST depression and, 211, 211f
Left-ventricular hypertrophy (LVH), 201, 341–342, 375
  and myocardial function during exercise, 341–342
Left-ventricular (LV) length (L), 415
Left-ventricular outflow tract obstruction, 392

Left-ventricular stroke volume (SV), 62–64
Left-ventricular (LV) volume (V), 415, 421f
Lidocaine, 490
Lifestyle change, motivating, 83
Limited challenge, 280
Lithium, 500–501
Long QT syndrome (LQTS), congenital, 224, 257, 259f

Master's test, 90, 137, 286
Maximum heart rate (MHR), 149–151
  age and, 150, 151t
    conditioning and, 147, 148t
    fitness and, 149–150, 149f
Maximum stress testing, 150
Medication. *See* Drugs
Memorial Heart Institute Exercise Stress Test Report, 166–167
Memorial Heart Institute (M.H.I.) database, 357, 359
Memorial Heart Institute protocol, 157–165, 167
  examination and explanation, 160
  exercise, 160, 161
  questionnaire and informed consent, 157–158
  timing, 157
Memorial Medical Center follow-up study—1975, 286–288
Metabolic acidosis, 482
Metabolic equivalents (METS), 141, 145, 146f, 147t, 173
Methyldopa, 503
Metoprolol, 436
Mitral murmur, 121, 122f
Monitoring, 161–163
Morise Score, 302–303
Mortality, predictors of, 150, 287–288, 291f, 303, 304f. *See also* Deaths
  age, 298–299, 300f
  ischemic ST segments, 288, 289f, 304f
MUGA (multiple gated acquisition), 418
Multivariate analysis, 301–302
Muscle mass, effect of, 16
Myocardial efficiency, 24
Myocardial infarction (MI), 113, 196, 287, 288, 291f
  acute, 466
  and angina, 328
  digital computer simulation of, 515
  future strategies for improving quantitation of, 526–529
  vs. ischemia, diagnosis of, 447, 449
  predictive value of previous, 299–300, 301f
  silent, 353
  size. *See also* QRS
    validation studies of regional transmural ischemia and, 515–516
  in sports, 369
  stress testing after, 169, 176
    abnormal stress test responses, 172–174
    advantages and benefits, 169–170
    estimating the extent of CAD, 175
    protocols, 151, 152f, 171
    reliability of abnormalities, 174–175
    safety and patient selection, 170–171
Myocardial ischemia. *See also* Myocardium, ischemic
  P-wave changes and hemodynamic changes with, 519–520
  silent, 353, 364–365
    analysis of M.H.I. database, 357, 359
    angina equivalent, 361
    clinical strategy, 360–361
    detection, 356–357, 357f
      markers, 358t, 359, 359t
    implications, 360
    mechanisms and pathophysiology, 354–355
    medical treatment, 363–364
    pain perception, 355–356
    prevalence, 353–354
    prognosis, 359–360
    ST depression and normal coronary arteries, 354
    ST depression with prior negative test, 363
    surgical treatment, 364
  threshold of, 136
Myocardial perfusion imaging (MPI), 414, 421–422. *See also* Intramyocardial perfusion
  diagnosis, 462–465, 464t
    results, 464
  "hibernating" myocardium, 467
    metabolic imaging for defining, 467, 468f–471f, 469, 470, 471f
  perfusion defects, causes of reversible, 459, 462
  perfusion-metabolic mismatch, tracer combinations for defining, 469–471, 471f
  prognosis, 466
  risk stratification, post acute MI, 466
  tracers, 422–425
  unstable angina, 465–466
Myocardial perfusion scintigraphy, causes of defects on, 462, 463t

Myocardial scarring, 294, 295f
Myocardium, 180
  echocardiography to identify viable, 132
  hypertrophied, 341–342
  ischemic. *See also* Myocardial ischemia
    biochemical changes in, 66–68
    free fatty acids and, 67, 505

Naughton Protocol, 322, 323t
Nicotine, 487–488
Nitrates, 437, 492–493
  long-acting, 493
Nitric oxide (NO), 50
Nitroglycerin, 65f, 467, 468f–469f, 493
Nucleotides, 32
N.Y. Heart Classification III and IV, 320t, 323

Observer bias, 337–338
Orthostatic changes, hyperventilation and, 229–231, 232f
Oxygen. *See also* Arteriovenous oxygen
  partial pressure of, 23
Oxygen consumption, 115–117, 142, 144f
  body weight and, 139, 140t
  and duration of exercise, 323f
  duration of work and, 117, 117f
  estimation of, 145–147, 147t
    VO_2 estimate *vs.* direct measurement, 147t
  treadmill stage and, 117, 118f
Oxygen demand
  myocardial, 24
  vs. oxygen supply, 27, 27f
    and ischemia, 43–44
Oxygen transport, 321–322
Oxygen uptake, maximum (VO_2max), 17, 18f, 26f, 28–29, 399, 400f, 407, 408f
  caveats in the use of, 321–322
  in congestive heart failure patients, 322, 324, 325
  mean values for, 28, 29t
  measurement in normal patients, 319–320
Oxygen uptake (VO_2), 17–18, 386f
  and work during submaximal exercise in children, 384, 385f

p FOX inhibitors (partial fatty acid oxidation inhibitors), 505
P wave changes, 227–228, 519–520
P waves, 110
Pain. *See also* Chest pain
  anginal *vs.* nonanginal, 272–273, 274f, 282–283, 312, 313f. *See also* Anginal pain
  ischemia and, 64–66, 359–360
Pain perception in silent myocardial ischemia, 355–356
Palpitation, 122
Paroxysmal atrial tachycardia (PAT), 246–247
Partial pressure of carbon dioxide (Pco_2), 23, 29, 30f, 36, 482, 483f
Partial pressure of oxygen (PO_2), 23
Pediatric exercise testing, 381–382, 409–410
  arrhythmia with normal heart, 403–404, 404f
  complete congenital heart block, 404–405, 405f, 406f
  congenital heart disease and, 389–390, 392, 394–399, 401–403
  congenital long QT syndrome, 406
  equipment, 382
  exercise protocols, 382–383, 383t
  hypertension, 407–408
  hypertrophic cardiomyopathy, 408–409, 410f
  Kawasaki disease, 406–407
  measured responses during exercise testing, 383–388, 384f–391f
  reasons for clinical, 382
  sickle cell anemia, 407, 408f
Percutaneous transluminal coronary angioplasty (PTCA), 169, 170
Perfusion. *See* Intramyocardial perfusion; Myocardial perfusion imaging
Pericardial constraint, 62f
Pericardial hypothesis, 62
Pericarditis, 63f
Persantine. *See* Dipyridamole
pH, 29, 31, 31f, 32, 482–483, 483f
Pharmacological stress, 131
Phenothiazines, 501
Phosphorylase, 32
Population groups, 279–280
Positron emission tomography (PET), 428
Postexercise period, management during, 91
Posture, 57–58, 58f
PQ interval/segment, 255
  short, 231, 243, 255
  sloping, 228, 230
PQ junction, 229
Precordial leads. *See* Lead systems
Predictive value of tests, 276, 276t–277t
Premature ventricular contractions (PVCs), 88, 163, 248–250, 250f, 374
  "ominous," 249
  during recovery, 251, 252f
  ST segments in exercise-induced, 251–252
Pressure pulse product, 111–112, 112f, 113f

Prevalence of disease, 277–278
and exercise-induced ST depression, 278, 278f
and predictive value of tests, 276, 276t–277t, 277f
Prinzmetal's angina, 204–205, 328–329
Propranolol, 497–498, 498f
Prostoglandins, and ischemic myocardium, 67–68
Psychotropic drugs, 499–502
Pulmonary artery pressures, left ventricle and, 56–57, 57f
Pulmonary valvular stenosis, 397–398, 397f, 398f
Pulse. *See* Heart rate
Pulsus alternans, 122
Pyruvate metabolism, 31

Q wave and QT intervals, 220–221, 221f
congenital long QT syndrome, 224, 257, 259f
prolonged QT, 222–224, 223f
QT dispersion, 221–222
Q waves, 231f
septal, 221, 222, 375
QRS changes, 215–216, 219
changes in QRS axis, 219
changes in S waves, 220
R-wave amplitude, 216–218, 217f. *See also* R-wave amplitude
QRS duration, 491
increased, 219
QRS score, Athens, 219, 220f
QRS (vector), 68, 70, 70f, 515–520
QT interval(s). *See also* Q wave and QT intervals
corrected (QT_c), 222, 223, 223f, 259f
prolonged, 257, 258f. *See also* Long QT syndrome
Quinidine, 490
QX/QT ratio, 220–221, 221f

R-wave amplitude, 214f, 216–218, 217f, 252
R-wave responses to exercise, 216, 216f
R wave(s), 110, 207, 210f, 211, 244, 244f. *See also* QRS
increased, with atrial extrasystoles, 218
ST elevation in leads with, 205f
Radionuclide angiography (RNA), 414–415
diagnosis, 415–416, 416f–417f
indications, 418
prognosis, 416, 418
Radionuclide techniques, 176, 414. *See also* Gated cardiac blood pool; Myocardial perfusion imaging
adrenergic agonists, 431
anatomic correlation, 443–444
image acquisition, 437–438
planar imaging, 438–439, 439f
image interpretation
ancillary findings in ischemia, 448f–450f, 449, 452, 452f–454f, 456f–461f
causes of "reversible deficits" other than ischemia, 455, 459, 462
infarct *vs.* ischemia, 447, 449
preliminary observations, 444–446
quantitation, 449, 454
quantitative polar map displays, 446–447
reverse redistribution, 455
protocols, 431–432, 432f–433f, 434–437
SPECT, 414, 423, 427, 428, 439–440, 440f–442f, 442–444, 448f–454f, 463
stress, 429
vasodilators, 429–430
Ramp protocol, 145
Rate-related bundle branch blocks, 260
Reassurance, 161
Record preparation, 164–165
Recovery period, 163–164
Rehabilitation, cardiac, 367
exercise testing in, 367, 377
confirmation of improvement or detection of progression, 378–379
discharge exercise test after coronary event, 378
exercise prescription, 378
exercise testing prior to outpatient rehabilitation, 378
Relaxation, abnormal, 61
Repolarization, 283–284
early, 206–207, 207f, 372
Respiration, 35–37
rate *vs.* depth, 36–37
Respiratory data during stress testing, 118. *See also* Oxygen uptake
Respiratory gas exchange ratio (R), 118–120
Revascularization, postoperative, 182–183
unsuccessful, 183, 183f
Rhythm disturbances, 368. *See also* Arrhythmias
Right bundle branch block (RBBB), 260–262, 261f, 455
Risk ratio, 287t

S waves, changes in, 220
Safety, exercise test
equipment and supplies necessary to, 90–92

Safety factors and precautions, 86, 100, 170–171
Sensitivity of (stress) tests, 273–277, 275t–277t, 279, 280, 281t, 287t
Septal defect, atrial, 401
Septal hypertrophy, asymmetrical, 88
Septal Q waves, 221, 222, 375
Sestamibi (MIBI), Tc99m, 425, 426t, 431–432, 432f–433f, 464t, 465–467, 468f–469f
Sex differences, 19, 309, 316. *See also* Women
  in findings according to symptoms, 312, 313f
  in prevalence of CAD, 309–310, 310f, 311f
  in stress test results, 279t, 280
Sheffield ST-segment integral, 520, 521f
Sick sinus syndrome. *See* Chronotropic incompetence
Sickle cell anemia, 407, 408f
Single photon emission computed tomography (SPECT), 414, 423, 427, 428, 439–440, 440f–442f, 442–444, 463
Sinus arrhythmia, 396f
Sinus tachycardia, 325f
6-minute-walk test, 322–323
Skin preparation for electrodes, 158, 159
Sodium bicarbonate, 31, 31f
Sotolol, 496
Specificity of (stress) tests, 273, 275–277, 275t–277t, 279, 280, 281t, 287t
Sports. *See also* Athletes
  effects of exercise training on ST depression and exercise capacity, 376–377
  exercise testing in, 377
    alerting patient and physician to occult dysfunction, 376
    evaluating drug regimens, 377
    following progress in known disease, 376
  risks of coronary events in
    infarction, 369
    rhythm disturbances, 368
    sudden death, 368–369
Sports medicine, 83
ST changes
  false positive, 190, 228–231, 230f–232f, 233–234, 235f
    false-positive tracings due to computer averaging, 229
  sensitivity and specificity of, 310–312
ST heart rate index (Kligfield index), 209. *See also* ΔST/ΔHR index
ST-heart rate slope, 208
ΔST/ΔHR index, 523, 524f. *See also* ST heart rate index
ST/HR slope, 110–111, 315, 522–523
ST hysteresis (HR recovery ST loop), 212–213, 213f
ST integral and slope, 198–200, 200f
ST/R, 207–208
ST-segment depression. *See also* Electrocardiographic (ECG) changes; Ischemic ST segments; *specific topics*
  asymptomatic, 361, 362f
  computer measurements used to evaluate, 520, 521f
  convex, 231
  and coronary events, 288, 290f, 291, 291f
  and coronary heart disease survival, 289, 290f
  decreased R + ST depression, 218
  digitalis-induced, 488–489
  downsloping in V3 and V4, 198
  exercise-induced, 374–375
    duration, 375
  fictitious/false positive, 190–191
  in inferior leads only, 228
  intermittent, 209, 210f, 211
  with long diastolic filling, 211–212, 212f
  magnitude, 291f, 292
  mechanism of, 68, 69f
  and mortality, 291f, 304f
  with nodal premature contractions, 214, 215f
  in post-MI testing, 172
  posture, filling pressures, and, 57–58, 58f
  resting, increased with exercise, 201
  rounded, 213–214, 214f
  septal Q waves and, 221, 222, 222f
  severe, 89
    at rest, 88
  slowly upsloping, 195
  ST evolving toward normal with exercise, 209
  time of onset, 291–292, 291f
  time of recovery from, 292–293
ST-segment depression curves, and CAD, 278, 278f
ST-segment elevation, 174
  in AVR, 233
  ischemia and, 71, 233
  in leads with Q waves, 206, 206f
  in leads without Q waves, 204–205, 205f
  at rest, 206–207, 207f, 376. *See also* Repolarization, early
  and test termination, 90
  in V1, 233

ST segments. *See also* Electrocardiographic (ECG) changes; *specific topics*
segment variability, 231, 233
Starling's curves, 15f
Starling's law, 14
Stenosis, 45f, 121, 204, 525. *See also* Aortic stenosis; Valvular stenosis
idiopathic hypertrophic subaortic, 88
STJ, 519
Stress, types/modes of, 131
Stress echocardiography. *See* Echocardiography
Stress testing, 429. *See also* Exercise testing; *specific topics*
capacity to predict coronary events, 80, 80f
contraindications, 84, 100
absolute, 86–87
relative, 87–88
history, 1–6
predictive implications, 271–272, 287t, 298–299, 298f, 299f, 303–304. *See also specific topics*
estimating disease prevalence, 277–278, 277f, 278f
of exercise test scores, 301–303
false-negative tests and, 284–285
false-positive tests and, 283–284, 284t
limited challenge and, 280
long-term follow-up studies, 285–291, 287f, 287t, 289f, 290f
manipulation of data to produce scores, 303
population groups and, 279–280, 279t
of previous MI, 299–300, 301f
sensitivity and specificity, 273–277, 275t–277t, 279, 280, 281t
preparation for test, 136–137
requirements, 135–136
Stress testing protocol(s), 135, 136, 154. *See also specific topics*
comparison of various, 142, 143f–144f, 145
Stress tests
continuous, 138–139, 140t, 141–142
intermittent, 137–138
single-load, 137
Stroke volume (SV), 11–12
defined, 11
preload and, 12–14, 12f, 13f
and training, 14, 15f
Stroke work, and ischemia, 64
Stunning
myocardial, 49
post-persantine, 460f–461f
Supine *vs.* upright bicycle tests, 139
Supraventricular extrasystoles, 244
Surgery, bypass. *See* Bypass graft surgery
Sympathetic tone, increased, 229
Syndrome X (microvascular angina), 314–315, 329–332. *See also* Chest pain, and normal coronary arteries
Systole(s), 23, 54f. *See also* Atrial extrasystoles
Systolic and diastolic time intervals, 27–28, 53, 55–56, 56f
ratio of systolic to diastolic time interval (SPTI/DPTI), 56
Systolic blood pressure (SBP), 344, 345f, 347, 348f, 394, 408, 409f–410f
normal and abnormal, 346, 346f
peak, 343f
Systolic hypertension, 396f, 397

T waves, 375, 387, 389f
alterations
deep T wave inversions, 225
normalization of inverted T waves, 224–225, 225f
peaked T waves, 225, 226f
tall T waves, 225–227, 226f
pseudonormalization, 224
in V2, peaked, 233
Ta wave (wave of polarization), 190, 191, 193f
Tachycardia. *See also* Ventricular tachycardia
paroxysmal atrial, 246–247
sinus, 325f
Teboroxime, Tc99m, 425, 426t
Technetium 99m (^{99m}Tc), 414
Technetium 99m (^{99m}Tc) labeled agents/tracers, 415, 424–425, 428
biologic properties, 425, 426t
imaging equipment, 425, 427–428
indications for, 427–428
Temperature, 34–35
Tension time index, 25, 26f
Tetralogy of Fallot, 398–399, 400f–402f, 401
Tetrofosmin, Tc99m, 425, 426t, 432f–433f, 464t
Thallium (Tl), 431, 470, 471f
Thallium 201 (Tl-201), 422, 426t, 432f–433f, 440, 442, 462, 464, 464t, 467, 488
Thallium 203, 422–424
Thiazides, 502
Thoracic pump, abdominal, 13
Thyroid abnormalities, 483–484
Tidal volume, ventilation and, 118, 119f

Tocainide, 490
Total working capacity (TWC), 391f, 392, 394, 408, 409f
Training
  and diastolic and systolic volume, 12, 12f
  and ST depression and exercise capacity, 376–377
Training methods
  duration, 21
  frequency, 20
  intensity, 20–21
  mode, 21
Transmural flow distribution, 51–52
Transmural ischemia, 233, 515–516
Treadmill echocardiography, 129. *See also* Echocardiography, stress
  methodology, 129
Treadmill exercise score, Hollenberg, 520, 522
Treadmill protocol. *See* Naughton Protocol
Treadmill stage, and oxygen consumption, 117, 118f
Treadmill stress, 434
Treadmill test, 141, 141f, 331–332
Tricyclic antidepressants, 499–500

U waves, 234, 235f
Ultrafast, ECG-gated, x-ray computerized tomography (ultrafast-CT), 525, 526f, 528, 529f

VA study, 291
Valium. *See* Diazepam
Valvular stenosis. *See also* Aortic stenosis; Stenosis
  pulmonary, 397–398, 397f, 398f
Vasodilator reserve, 52–53, 52f
Vasodilators, 429–430, 504
Vasomotion, 44–45, 45f
Vasoregulatory asthenia, 229
Ventricular arrhythmias. *See under* Arrhythmias
Ventricular contractions. *See* Premature ventricular contractions
Ventricular dysplasia, arrhythrogenic right, 254
Ventricular ectopy, 173
  in CAD patients, 249–252, 250f, 252f
Ventricular ectopy, reproducibility of, 254
Ventricular fibrillation (VF), 253
Ventricular tachycardia (VT), 252, 402f
  defined, 252
  exercise-induced sustained, 253
  exercise testing to evaluate spontaneous, 253
  idiopathic right ventricular outflow tachycardia, 254
  nonsustained, 252, 253
Vessels left ungrafted (VLU), number of, 181t
Viscous resistance, 22

Walk test, 6-minute, 322–323
Walk-through phenomenon, 120
Wall motion, 446
  contractility, ischemia and, 60–62, 61f
Wall thickening, segmental, 446
Weight, and oxygen consumption, 139, 140t
Wolff-Parkinson-White (WPW) syndrome, 260, 265–266, 265f–266f, 455
Women. *See also* Sex differences
  ST changes in
    mechanisms, 313–315
    sensitivity and specificity of, 310–312
  strategy to separate true- from false-positive, 315
  stress testing in, 309, 316
Work up bias, 303
Working capacity. *See* Total working capacity
Workload, heart rate and, 19, 20f

XYZ orthogonal leads, 108

CPSIA information can be obtained at www.ICGtesting.com
Printed in the USA
BVOW11*1639200714

359671BV00002B/7/P

9 780195 159288